ETHNIC CONSIDERATIONS
IN
FACIAL AESTHETIC SURGERY

ETHNIC CONSIDERATIONS IN FACIAL AESTHETIC SURGERY

Editor

W. Earle Matory, Jr., M.D., F.A.C.S.
A New You Plastic Surgery Medical Group
Irvine, California

Illustrator
Kim Hogatt

Lippincott - Raven
PUBLISHERS
Philadelphia • New York

Acquisitions Editor: Danette Knopp
Manufacturing Manager: Dennis Teston
Production Manager: Maxine Langweil
Production Editor: Loretta Cummings
Cover Designer: Karen Quigley
Indexer: Deana Reese Fowler
Compositor: Maryland Composition
Printer: Toppan Offset

Printed in the Singapore

9 8 7 6 5 4 3 2 1

Library of Congress Cataloging-in-Publication Data

Ethnic considerations in facial aesthetic surgery / editor, W. Earle Matory, Jr. ; illustrator, Kim Hogatt.
p. cm.
Includes bibliographical references and index.
ISBN 0-7817-0292-5
1. Face—Surgery. 2. Surgery, Plastic. 3. Race. I. Matory, W. Earle (William Earle), 1950– .
[DNLM: 1. Face—surgery. 2. Surgery, Plastic—methods. 3. Ethnic Groups. WE 705 E84 1997]
RD119.5.F33E87 1997
617.5′20592—dc21
DNLM/DLC
for Library of Congress

97-22014
CIP

To my wife, Yvonne,
and our two wonderful sons, Earle III and Adam,
for all their support and love

And to my caring parents, Deborah and Bill,
for the many tangible and intangible gifts
they have shared with me through the years

Contents

Contributing Authors xi

Foreword xv
Blair O. Rogers

Preface xix
W. Earle Matory, Jr.

Section I: General Considerations

1 **Patient Selection for Aesthetic Surgery in the Non-Caucasian: Practical Guidelines** 3
Mark Gorney

2 **Psychological Considerations** 11
Maisha Hamilton-Bennett and W. Earle Matory, Jr.

3 **Addressing the Needs of the Hostile Patient and Preventing the Unhappy Patient** 21
W. Earle Matory, Jr.

4 **Medicolegal Considerations** 27
W. Earle Matory, Jr.

5 **Anthropologic and Physiologic Considerations** 31
Blair O. Rogers

Section II: Definitions of Beauty

6 Parameters of Caucasian Attractiveness 39
Hale Tolleth

7 Definitions of Beauty in the Ethnic Patient 61
W. Earle Matory, Jr.

8 The Definition of Beauty in the Northern European 85
Rod J. Rohrich and Jeffrey M. Kenkel

Section III: Skin Care for People of Color

9 Skin Care—Editor's Commentary 99
W. Earle Matory, Jr.

10 Skin Care for Patients of Color 121
Kathryn K. Leverette and Yolanda L. Moore

11 Skin Care for People of Color 139
Rebat M. Halder and Sharon E. Bridgeman-Shah

Section IV: The Aging Patient

12 Aging in People of Color 151
W. Earle Matory, Jr.

Section V: Abnormal Scarring

13 Abnormal Scarring—Editor's Commentary 173
W. Earle Matory, Jr.

14 Disorders of Excessive Scarring 179
Raphael C. Lee, Mary Capelli-Schellpfeffer, and Elton X. Tinsley

Section VI: The African American Patient

15 The African American Patient—Editor's Commentary .. 195
W. Earle Matory, Jr.

16 Ethnic Considerations in the African American Patient .. 197
Fred J. Stucker

17 Rhinoplasty in the African American Patient 213
W. Earle Matory, Jr.

Section VII: The Asian Patient

18 The Asian Patient—Editor's Commentary 247
W. Earle Matory, Jr.

19 **The Asian Patient** 253
Leonard Gray, Edmond A. Zingaro, and Edward Falces

20 **Facial Surgery in the Asian Patient** 263
John A. McCurdy, Jr.

21 **The Filipino and Polynesian Patients** 285
Marco Rizzo

Section VIII: The Hispanic Patient

22 **The Hispanic Patient—Editor's Commentary** 303
W. Earle Matory, Jr.

23 **Facial Surgery in the Hispano-American Patient** 307
Oscar M. Ramírez

Section IX: The Mediterranean Patient

24 **The Mediterranean Patient—Editor's Commentary** 323
W. Earle Matory, Jr.

25 **The Mediterranean Nose** 327
Lorelle N. Michelson, George C. Peck, Jr., and George C. Peck

Section X: The Middle Eastern Patient

26 **The Middle Eastern Patient—Editor's Commentary** 339
W. Earle Matory, Jr.

27 **Facial Surgery in the Middle-Eastern Patient** 343
Bahman Teimourian and Saeed Marefat

28 **The Middle Eastern Nose** 363
Bahman Guyuron

Section XI: The Northern European Patient

29 **The Northern European Patient—Editor's Commentary** 373
W. Earle Matory, Jr.

30 **Rhinoplasty in the Northern European Patient** 379
Brian P. Maloney and E. Gaylon McCollough

Subject Index 399

Contributing Authors

Sharon E. Bridgeman-Shah, M.D.
Chief Resident, Department of Dermatology, Howard University College of Medicine, 2041 Georgia Avenue, NW, Washington, D.C. 20060

Mary Capelli-Schellpfeffer, M.D., M.P.A.
Assistant Professor, Clinical Surgery, Occupational Medicine, Electrical Trauma Research Program; Director, Hyperbaric Oxygen Unit, The University of Chicago, Section of Plastic and Reconstructive Surgery, 5841 South Maryland, MC 6035, Chicago, Illinois 60637

Edward Falces, M.D.
1150 Bush Street, Suite 4-B, San Francisco, California 94109

Mark Gorney, M.D.
1150 Bush Street, Suite 4-B, San Francisco, California 94109

Leonard Gray
1150 Bush Street, Suite 4-B, San Francisco, California 94109

Bahman Guyuron, M.D., F.A.C.S.
Clinical Professor of Surgery, Case Western Reserve University, 29017 Cedar Road, Lyndhurst, Ohio 44124

Rebat M. Halder, M.D.
Professor and Chairman, Department of Dermatology, Howard University College of Medicine, 2041 Georgia Avenue, NW, Washington, D.C. 20060

Maisha Hamilton-Bennett, Ph.D.
Clinical Consultant, Chemical Dependency, Advocate Trinity and Bethany Hospitals, 2320 East 93 Street, Chicago, Illinois 60617

Jeffrey M. Kenkel, M.D.
Assistant Professor, Department of Plastic Surgery, The University of Texas Southwestern Medical Center at Dallas, 5323 Harry Hines Boulevard, Dallas, Texas 75235-9132

Raphael C. Lee, M.D., Sc.D., F.A.C.S.
Professor of Surgery; Organismal Biology and Anatomy, Departments of Surgery and Organismal Biology and Anatomy, University of Chicago Hospitals, 5820 South Ellis Avenue, Chicago, Illinois 60637

Kathryn K. Leverette, C.M.E.S.
National Certified Medical Esthetics Specialist, The Solutions Center, 530 East Eighth Street, Suite 103, Oakland, California 94606

Brian P. Maloney, M.D., F.A.C.S.
4553 North Shallowford Road, Suite 60-C, Atlanta, Georgia 30338

Saeed Marefat, M.D.
Plastic Surgeon, 3289 Woodburn Road, Suite 330, Annandale, Virginia 22003-6800

W. Earle Matory, Jr., M.D., F.A.C.S.
Director, A New You Plastic Surgery Medical Group, 250 East Yale Loop, Suite A, Irvine, California 92604

E. Gaylon McCollough, M.D.
1600 South 20th Street, Birmingham, Alabama 35205-4916

John A. McCurdy, Jr., M.D.
Assistant Clinical Professor, Department of Surgery, University of Hawaii, John A. Burns School of Medicine, 1188 Bishop Street, Suite 2402, Honolulu, Hawaii 96813

Lorelle N. Michelson, M.D., F.A.C.S.
Clinical Assistant Professor, Department of Surgery, University of Medicine and Dentistry of New Jersey, New Jersey Medical School, Newark, New Jersey 07103

Yolanda L. Moore, M.P.S.
c/o Kathryn Leverette, P.M.E., The Solutions Center, 530 East Eighth Street, Suite 103, Oakland, California 94606

George C. Peck, M.D.
The Peck Center, 1200 Route 46, Clifton, New Jersey 07013

George C. Peck, Jr., M.D.
Associate Attending, Department of Plastic and Reconstructive Surgery, St. Barnabas Hospital, Old Short Hills Road, Livingston, New Jersey 07013

Oscar M. Ramírez, M.D., F.A.C.S.
Clinical Assistant Professor, Johns Hopkins University, Department of Plastic Surgery, University of Maryland, School of Medicine, 1212 York Road, Suite B101, Baltimore, Maryland 21093

Marco Rizzo
Suite 401, 1329 Lusitana Street, Honolulu, Hawaii 96813

Blair O. Rogers, M.D., F.A.C.S.
Professor of Clinical Surgery, Department of Plastic and Reconstructive Surgery, University Hospital, New York University Medical Center; Manhattan Eye, Ear, and Throat Hospital, 550 First Avenue, New York, New York 10016

Rod J. Rohrich, M.D., F.A.C.S.
Professor and Chairman, Department of Plastic Surgery, The University of Texas Southwestern Medical Center at Dallas, 5323 Harry Hines Boulevard, Dallas, Texas 75235-9132

Fred J. Stucker, M.D., F.A.C.S.
Professor of Medicine, Department of Otolaryngology/Head and Neck Surgery, Louisiana State University Medical Center, P.O. Box 33932, 1501 Kings Highway, Shreveport, Louisiana 71130-3932

Bahman Teimourian, M.D.
Clinical Professor, Department of Plastic Surgery, Georgetown University School of Medicine, 3800 Reservoir Road, NW, Washington, D.C. 20007

Elton X. Tinsley, M.D.
5841 South Maryland, MC 6035, Chicago, Illinois 60637

Hale Tolleth, M.D.
Suite 14, 2425 East Street, Concord, California 94520

Edmond A. Zingaro, M.D.
1150 Bush Street, Suite 4-B, San Francisco, California 94109

Foreword

> The bewildered comment of any 5th century Athenian upon our society . . . would surely be "Yes, I can see all the works of the great civilizations; but why can't I meet any civilized persons? I only encounter specialists, artists who know nothing of science, scientists who know nothing of art, philosophers who have no interest in God, priests who are unconcerned with politics, politicians who only know other politicians."
>
> —*W. H. Auden*

The broad scope of this fascinating book deals with strategies to address the cultural and anatomic considerations in aesthetic surgery in the faces of African American, Asian, Hispanic, Middle-Eastern, Filipino-Polynesian, and Northern European people.

The great Anglo-American poet, W. H. Auden, when commenting on modern specialization, compared the creative, all-encompassing curiosity of ancient Greek artists, scientists, and writers to the present age of categorized specialists. As plastic surgeons, are we to be criticized as mere surgical specialists, who only know surgical technique *per se* of Caucasians and know nothing of anthropology, anatomy, and comparative morphology of African Americans, Hispanics, and Asians? Let us hope not!

Despite the increasing number of precise anthropologic techniques that have been described in plastic surgery literature within the last two decades, there is a distinct lack of sophistication in the anatomic and morphologic information relevant to the patient of color. If we as plastic surgeons are concerned with the aesthetics of facial proportions, it would seem that more anatomic information about various ethnic groups would give us a firmer base from which to develop, interpret, analyze, and speculate upon the variations that depart from the so-called "norm." Plastic surgeons should be in the forefront of efforts to gather and compile clinically useful data on ethnic facial differences.

HISTORICAL PERSPECTIVE

When tracing the interest of the plastic surgery community in performing aesthetic plastic surgery in the Black patient, we find that interest in publishing relevant articles began in the 1960s. Perhaps it is not just coincidental that it was in the 1960s that civil rights laws were passed by the United States Congress that permitted Blacks in the United States to finally achieve a recognition of their rights on all levels in the United States society. This would include the right and interest to seek a plastic surgeon in order to make changes in facial anatomy.

In looking through the plastic surgery literature, we can trace articles that reflect the increasing interest in cosmetic surgery in the African American patient. Publications of note include O'Connor in 1967, Millard in 1967, Rees in 1969, Falces et al. in 1970, Snyder in 1971, Rogers in 1974, Bernstein in 1975, Ship in 1975, de Avelar in 1976, Stucker in 1976, Meyer and Kesselring in 1977, Sheen in 1978, and Millard in 1980.

PERSONAL PERSPECTIVES

Compared to the experiences of other surgeons, those of us who entered the practice in the mid-1950s already had some patients who were of Asian background, especially those originating from mainland China, Taiwan, Japan, and the Philippines. Soon after I entered private practice in 1956, I received many Chinese patients from New York City and the surrounding counties who had originally been patients of one of the plastic surgeons who trained me but who unfortunately passed away about the time I entered the practice. His thoughtful private secretary, who knew of my interest in China during World War II, thought the Chinese patients might be more comfortable under my care. I performed my first rhytidectomy on a Chinese patient in the mid-1950s. I was worried that she might develop periauricular and postauricular keloids. Fortunately, this did not occur in this woman, who has been my very close friend ever since. She accompanied me to visit Professor Ruyao Song when I made my first trip to China in 1980, after President Nixon had opened the Chinese diplomatic channels in the late 1970s. She was my interpreter for all of the meetings I had with Chinese plastic surgeons in Canton, Shanghai, and Peking. It was from this meeting that, as Editor of *Clinics in Plastic Surgery,* I invited Dr. Ruyao Song to become the guest editor of a special issue on the up-to-date standards of Chinese plastic surgery entitled "One-Stage Reconstructions."

My interest in operating on the African American patient arose early in my practice, when I came into contact with many Black nurses and surgical scrub technicians who assisted me and were part of a very congenial team at Manhattan Eye, Ear, and Throat Hospital. When I started in practice in 1956, I had already studied for two years during the senior part of my resident training in plastic surgery with Dr. Lyndon A. Peer at the St. Barnabas Hospital in Newark, New Jersey.

During that residency program, approximately 30% to 35% of our patients were African Americans. Many patients who came to us in those early years presented with congenital abnormalities and automobile and other accident injuries. Very few, if any, sought aesthetic procedures. Consequently, it was fascinating for me to have as my associates in the Manhattan Eye, Ear, and Throat Hospital's operating room Black friends and members of the surgical team who constantly expressed a curiosity about cosmetic surgery possibilities for themselves or for family members. It was during those years that many plastic surgeons believed that to perform a standard blepharoplasty on a Black patient would result in hypertrophic scarring and even the dreaded possibility of keloid formation. We did not know of or understand the "neutral triangle" that exists from the lateral-most extensions of both lateral canthi across the nasal bridge extending down to the base of the lateral-most extension of the nostrils, which permits a surgeon to perform various aesthetic plastic surgery operations without abnormal scarring.

I performed my first blepharoplasty on my chief scrub nurse, who was my constant companion in the operating room. He was a good-looking, tall, Black North Carolinian, who was approaching his 60s. He asked me if I would correct his severe blepharochalasis. When I told him that I was not sure whether he might form hypertrophic or keloid scars, since there was nothing in the literature to otherwise correct this impression, he volunteered to free me of any responsibility if these scars occurred. Therefore, taking the bit between my teeth, I performed the operation. It was totally successful, with no vestiges of hypertrophic scarring either in the eyelids themselves or in the lateral canthal regions. Following this experience, I felt more confident that I could selectively perform aesthetic blepharoplasties in

Black patients, given careful selection and avoidance of surgery on patients with existing abnormal scarring. During the decade following the Civil Rights Act passage in Congress, we saw a more rapid increase in the number of African Americans presenting for blepharoplasty.

In the late 1960s, I performed a facelift on a "volunteer" Black female patient who was afraid of losing her job because of facial aging. It was perhaps fortuitous that while she had a fairly dark complexion, she also had freckles of her cheeks, nose, and forehead, most likely traceable to her Scottish grandmother. I felt, perhaps unwisely, that given her Northern European heritage, she might be less predisposed to the development of hypertrophic or keloid scarring. This proved to be the case. Her operation was completely successful, without any untoward healing.

I became much bolder when a very dark-skinned Black school teacher from Harlem approached me because of her aging face. She was afraid that her features would reveal to the New York City school system that she was much older than she had told them at the time she was hired. She wished to continue teaching underprivileged children in Harlem for as long as she could physically "stand on her own two feet," as she put it. At the time she came to me she was 75 years old and extremely vigorous, thoroughly delightful, and extroverted. We discussed the potential risks of surgery. The surgery was totally successful, and she retained her job. She retained her dynamism in her approach to life, leaving a lasting impression upon me. Each year that has passed following this operation, I have received three to four postcard greetings from her, from different parts of every continent, as she has been cruising around the world spreading her exuberance. Just this past Christmas, I received my usual Christmas card from her wishing me many hearty Christmas benefits. She reminded me that she was still as in love with life as she had been when I first operated on her more than 20 years ago.

For my first chin-neck lift in an African American, I was fortunate to operate on someone I had known for many years. An old friend, who was a very famous nightclub entertainer and singer requested a correction of his "inherited" double chin. The neck lift was complication-free. From this experience, I surmised that aesthetic surgery is possible and permissible in most Black patients, if they do not show preoperative signs of hypertrophic scarring or keloid formation. One must pay particular attention to the smallpox vaccination site, which commonly hypertrophies in the ethnic patient. One should also pay special attention to something that has been cited in Japanese literature: avoidance of rotating and suturing the facial and neck flaps with any undue tension. The development of the SMAS technique, which reduces the factor of skin tension, has, in my experience, further reduced the likelihood of postrhytidectomy abnormal scarring.

W. Earle Matory, Jr., the extremely perceptive editor of this volume, emphasizes that the American Society of Plastic and Reconstructive Surgeons has noted that 19.6% of cosmetic surgery patients are in the African American, Hispanic, and Asian ethnic subgroups. He points out that by the mid-21st century over 50% of the United States population will be of Asian, African American, or Hispanic descent. Plastic surgeons need to understand the varied surgical needs of ethnic populations.

Earle Matory's interest in plastic surgery in patients of color goes back a dozen years to one of his earliest presentations at a medical meeting, on the subject of "Fifteen Year Experience With Non-Caucasian Rhinoplasty," presented to the National Medical Association, meeting in San Francisco, California in August 1982. A subsequent presentation with the same title received commendation in the Plastic Surgery Resident's Competition at the meeting of the California Society of Plastic Surgeons at Scottsdale, Arizona in April 1983. From 1983 to 1986, each year saw a number of presentations of his experience with plastic surgery in this population. In 1986, he and Edward Falces of San Francisco published their fascinating and informative essay, "Non-Caucasian Rhinoplasty: A 16-Year Experience," in the *Journal of Plastic and Reconstructive Surgery.* The importance of this work is confirmed by its nomination for the Robert Barrett Brown Award, given by the American Association of Plastic Surgeons.

In every year since 1986, Dr. Matory has given presentations at national medical meetings, especially in the United States and abroad, on the surgery, aesthetics, and aging of various aspects of the ethnic face. In 1991 he was the author of an informative chapter in the book, *Male Aesthetic Surgery,* edited by Eugene Courtiss, the title of which is "Cosmetic Surgery in the Black Male." In 1993, he contributed "Aesthetic Surgery in the African-American Face" to a volume edited by M. Cohen.

Now that these personal surgical experiences in Black patients have been recalled in the previous paragraphs, I believe it is now appropriate for me to sit back and enjoy the following chapters by Earle Matory and his renowned faculty of authors, who have so willingly shared their outstanding expertise in plastic, reconstructive, and aesthetic surgery!

Blair O. Rogers, M.D.

BIBLIOGRAPHY

Auden WH. The Greeks and us. In: *Forwards and Afterwards.* New York: Random House; 1973:3.

de Avelar JM. Personal contribution for the surgical treatment of Negroid noses. *Aesthet Plast Surg;* 1976:1;81.

Bernstein L. Rhinoplasty for the Negroid nose. *Otolaryngol Clin North Am;* 1975:3;783.

Falces E, Wesser O, and Gorney M. Cosmetic surgery of the non-Caucasian nose. *Plast Reconstr Surg;* 1970:45;317.

Matory WE Jr and Falces F. Non-Caucasian rhinoplasty: a 16-year experience. *Plast Reconstr Surg;* 1986:77;239.

Matory WE Jr. Aesthetic surgery in the African-American face. In: M. Cohen, editor. *Mastery of Surgery: Plastic and Reconstructive Surgery.* Boston, Massachusetts: Little, Brown and Co.; 1993.

Matory WE Jr. Cosmetic surgery in the black male. In: Eugene Courtiss, editor. *Male Aesthetic Surgery.* St. Louis, Missouri: C. V. Mosby, Co.; 1991:170–184.

Matory WE Jr. Rhinoplasty and adjunctive procedures in the African-American. In: Robert Russell, editor. *Surgery Educational Foundation Instructional Courses.* St. Louis, Missouri: C. V. Mosby, Co.; 1990:72–85.

Meyer R and Kesselring UK. Sculpturing and reconstructive procedures in aesthetic and functional rhinoplasty. *Clin Plast Surg;* 1977:4;15.

Millard DR. Alar margin sculpturing. *Plast Reconstr Surg;* 1967:40;337.

Millard DR. The alar cinch in the flat, flaring nose. *Plast Reconstr Surg;* 1980:65;669.

O'Connor GB, McGregor MW, Shapiro L, and Tolleth H. The bulbous nose. *Plast Reconstr Surg;* 1967:39;273.

Rees TD. Nasal plastic surgery in the Negro. *Plast Reconstr Surg;* 1969:43;13.

Rogers BO. The role of physical anthropology in plastic surgery today. *Clin Plast Surg;* 1974:1;439.

Sheen JH. *Aesthetic Rhinoplasty.* St. Louis, Missouri: Mosby; 1978.

Ship A. Alar base resection for wide ala. *Br J Plast Surg;* 1975:28;77.

Snyder GB. Rhinoplasty in the Negro. *Plast Reconstr Surg;* 1971:47;572.

Song RY. One stage reconstructions. *Clin Plast Surg;* 1982:9;Issue 1.

Stucker FJ. Non-Caucasian rhinoplasty. *Trans Am Acad Ophthalmol Otolaryngol;* 1976:82;417.

Preface

Why write a book on ethnic considerations in aesthetic surgery? The perception of beauty held by most U.S. citizens is based on Northern European ideals. The cosmetic surgeon's training is a reflection of this perspective.

According to the 1990 census, approximately 30% to 35% of the United States population is not Caucasian. The American Society of Plastic and Reconstructive Surgeons notes that 19.6% of cosmetic surgery patients are currently represented by these subgroups. Each ethnic group has subcategories that further compound the complexities of identifying and surgically creating attractive features. Within the racial designation of Asian or Oriental, one finds widely variant features, e.g., in Northern versus Southern China, in Thailand or Vietnam versus the South Pacific, and the Native American in comparison to the East Indian. The same applies to the Hispanic patient, who may have Castillian features or conversely may mirror characteristics of the Central or Southern African people.

The population of non-European groups within the United States is increasing 2 to 18 times as fast as the Caucasian population. Anticipated percentage increases in the next ten years are as follows: Caucasian, 6%; Asian, 107%; Hispanic, 53%; Native American, 38%; and the African American, 13%. The U.S. Census Bureau projects that the current non-European population of 25% will increase to 33% by the year 2000. By the year 2056, over 50% of the U.S. population is expected to be of non-European descent. This text has been written to facilitate the education of today's plastic surgeon in preparation for these dramatic changes in our cosmetic surgery clientele.

The plastic surgeon faces significant challenges in trying to address the cultural and surgical presentations of such varied ethnic populations. Our distinguished cadre of contributing authors have combined their experiences and expertise to identify the ideal characteristics of beauty within each major ethnic category. Many of the techniques described are similar to those used in the Caucasian patient. More often than not, these masterful surgeons have developed unique methodologies that provide consistently excellent results. The diversity of these methods is best illustrated by the input of two or more authors sharing their favored techniques. We have also incorporated several disciplines that are pertinent to the ethnic patient undergoing aesthetic surgery, including psychologic, medicolegal, anthropologic, scarring, and skin care considerations. Distinctive parameters and definitions of beauty have also been outlined in very practical detail. This text reviews appropriate surgical strategies as well as pitfalls that one may encounter when addressing the needs of the ethnic patient.

SECTION I

General Considerations

Ethnic Considerations in Facial Aesthetic Surgery, edited by W. Earle Matory, Jr.
Lippincott–Raven Publishers, Philadelphia © 1998.

1

Patient Selection for Aesthetic Surgery in the Non-Caucasian: Practical Guidelines

Mark Gorney

There is no excellent beauty that hath not some strangeness in the proportion.
— Sir Francis Bacon

In the United States the growing popularity of aesthetic plastic surgery among both men and women of all ethnic groups has, unfortunately, created a carnival-like atmosphere of which advertising by dubiously qualified practitioners is only one aspect. In this climate it becomes imperative to establish clear criteria for patient selection; without these, there will be an inevitable parallel increase in patient dissatisfaction and litigation.

In the 1990s we have seen a major increase in requests for aesthetic surgery in individuals of color. In a culture as appearance conscious as ours, not only show business personalities perceive the effects of aging as an impediment to career advancement. Additionally, aesthetic improvement is seen by many non-Caucasian individuals as a method of better adaptation to the standards of appearance promulgated by our media.

IDENTIFYING THE IDEAL CANDIDATE

Who, then, is the "ideal" candidate for aesthetic surgery? There is no such thing; however, the surgeon should certainly seek those personality factors that will enhance the phys-

M. Gorney: San Francisco, California 94109

ical improvements desired. There are, in most cases, clear indications of who will do well and enjoy the results. A person who is obviously intelligent and preferably educated and who listens (rather than merely hearing) and clearly understands the pros and cons is a good candidate. Individuals who have a clearly discernible physical problem about which they have an appropriate but not neurotic concern are good candidates. People whose jobs require them to look attractive or who must compete with younger individuals are reasonable candidates.

By the same token, however, one should be aware that such people may have major ego structure flaws that require constant admiration as psychic nourishment. These individuals are also highly critical and prone to dissatisfaction with their appearance. The problem, in this instance, may not be physical but a psychological one. Instead of being improved by elective surgery, the problem may be acutely aggravated.

Someone with a sense of humor is always a better candidate than a dour, anxious individual. Plastic surgery patients are in a category by themselves and should be evaluated with the utmost care. Generally speaking, men make more difficult patients than women. They do not tolerate pain as well and are generally fussier. They also cannot usually hide their scars as casually under make-up or clever hairdos.

It is a fundamental mistake to assume that the non-Caucasian individual is looking to become more "westernized" for greater acceptability in our society. Most often those individuals are looking to improve their body image purely within the idealized concept of their own particular ethnic group. The wide and low Negroid nose can be made less so without looking ridiculously out of place on the face on which it sits. The heavy Asiatic "single eyelid" can be corrected without making it look like a parody of a "Western" eyelid. The delicate body frame of a young Korean woman looks foolish with large and heavily augmented breasts that are totally out of context with her heredity. What is usually requested is improvement, not conversion.

CONTRAINDICATIONS TO AESTHETIC SURGERY

There are basically two major categories for rejection of any patient seeking aesthetic surgery. One is anatomical unsuitability; the other is emotional inadequacy. Of these, emotional inadequacy is by far the more important. It is reviewed here on a purely pragmatic basis. The inexperienced surgeon must learn early to differentiate between healthy and unhealthy reasons for seeking to change essentially normal anatomy. It becomes absolutely critical to develop a sixth sense regarding motivation because a substantial number of poor results are based on emotional dissatisfaction rather than technical failure.

In all ethnic groups, there is a variable stigma attached to individuals seeking aesthetic improvement. In some non-Caucasian ethnic groups, it may add a significant element of guilt to a preexisting distorted body image. Jacobson and others (1) neatly liken the body image to a gyroscope. When it is functioning well, we do not notice it. It does not decide the course or steer the ship. In a storm, however, the ship becomes difficult to steer if the gyroscope is not functioning.

Obviously, every patient seeking plastic surgery cannot be referred for psychiatric evaluation, nor is it necessary. Patients seeking aesthetic surgery believe that they are trying to do something positive about their problems. It is the plastic surgeon's responsibility to determine whether the "problem" is actually in, say, the nose or in the mind. If they are asked to see a psychiatrist, they might consider themselves failures. In all likelihood they will walk out and never come back to you. Seldom do patients have sufficient self-awareness to realize that their problems lie more in their minds than in the physical parts they wish corrected. Our insightful Editor, one of my former plastic surgery residents, suggests a strategy that he sometimes finds useful. Dr. Matory feels that the emotionally distraught or the neurotic patient senses a need for emotional support. Suggesting that a psychiatrist may be able to lend this support during the patient's peri-operative course may open the door to pre-surgical diagnostic and therapeutic psychiatric input. Those that successfully receive psychiatric approval for surgery may lend themselves to surgical treatment.

CRITERIA TO ASSESS THE GRAY ZONE OF EMOTIONAL INADEQUACY

There are no objective criteria in this gray zone. The criteria are not only subjective but also totally different for patient and physician. The patient has an idea of what s/he wants; the surgeon knows, more or less, what can be done. The problem is for the two to communicate as accurately as possible beforehand. It is much easier to arrive at a prior mutual understanding than to look back retrospectively with regret. In the eyes of the law, however, responsibility of selecting the patient rests squarely on the surgeon's shoulders.

For example, there are significant differences in the psychodynamics of the male versus the female rhinoplasty candidate. Jacobson and others have pointed out that both sexes have positive psychological expectations and a conscious wish for attractiveness; women, however, more frequently wish to change themselves to feel more attractive. Men seem more interested in changing others' attitudes toward them. The male patient, according to Jacobson and others, more often than the female patient, shows the following characteristics:

1. A family or cultural background conflicting with his present life. This is a particularly important red flag.
2. Ambivalance or discomfort with sexuality and sexual preferences.
3. A self-deprecating attitude and feelings of inadequacy.
4. Familial conflict and either conscious or subconscious shame related to ethnic background. Failure to screen this category of patients almost invariably leads to trouble when the patient returns to his friends and family and encounters a chorus of sneering disapproval. This is a clear prelude to spasms of guilt, dissatisfaction, and a visit to the attorney's office.

The characteristics of the individual least likely to be satisfied with his post-operative result, regardless of ethnic background, can be formed into the useful acronym SIMON:

Single
Immature
Male
Overexpectant
Narcissistic

There are often identifiable common traits in certain types of aesthetic surgery candidates. For example, patients with outstanding or "lop" ears often demonstrate a hostile, aggressive "chip on the shoulder" attitude. Most often, they have inherited their deformity from a parent who also suffered ridicule in childhood. Cleft lip/palate patients often have reclusive, involutional personality patterns. Patients seeking rhinoplasty, on the other hand, may show a guilt-tinged, second-generation rejection of their ethnic background masked by excuses, such as not photographing well. Sometimes it is not so much a desire to abandon the ethnic group as it is to be viewed as individuals. Infrequently, one may encounter individuals who want to rid themselves of specific physical attributes associated with their particular ethnic group.

Motivation, rather than specific psychodynamics, should be the plastic surgeon's overriding concern. Is there a pragmatic desire to improve appearance, or is there pathological projection of subconscious problems onto a physical fault? Contrast these two commonly heard statements: "I don't like my nose; it's too big for my face and I don't photograph well." "I've always been terribly self-conscious about my nose. My father's family all have noses like this. I HATE IT!" Many patients can say anything convincingly; however, the second statement should trip a red flag and invite further inquiries into the patient's real motivation.

Strength of motivation is important and has a startlingly close relationship with patient satisfaction. A strongly motivated patient will have less pain, a better post-operative course, and a significantly higher index of satisfaction, regardless of the result.

PATIENT SELECTION AND LIABILITY POTENTIAL

Despite all of this, it is possible to establish some nearly objective criteria for patient selection and liability potential (Fig. 1). Such criteria are discussed herein in order of descending importance.

Objective Deformity Versus Patient Concern

Two extremes of patient selection are as follows:

1. The patient who has a major deformity but demonstrates minimal concern (Fig. 1, lower right-hand corner).
2. The patient who has a minor deformity that causes extreme concern (Fig. 1, upper left-hand corner).

The latter represents the poorest candidate. One seldom sees the patient depicted in the lower right-hand corner, but the majority of patients seeking aesthetic surgery fall somewhere on a diagonal band between the contralateral corners. The decision to accept or reject a patient for surgery must be the surgeon's ultimate responsibility. I have found it very useful to note, after the initial visit, on a "tic–tac–toe" type of diagram, my coded impression of where the patient fits. Thus, when a patient, whom I dimly recall, expresses interest in proceeding with the surgery, a glance at the chart with the X in the appropriate square serves as a reminder.

Great Expectations

Experience invariably teaches the plastic surgeon to avoid patients who expect surgery to change their whole life. Consider the likely outcome in operating on someone who has a large, wide, fat nose and significant hang-ups. With great probability, the result is likely to be someone with a thinner, more delicate nose and exaggerated post-operative hang-ups. Certainly, a reasonable degree of positive change is expected and usually occurs; however, aesthetic surgery, regardless of excellence, is dubious therapy for severe personality disturbances.

The Demanding Patient

The individual who brings pictures from magazines, drawings, and exact specifications should be suspect, as a general rule. Such a person has little insight into the realities of reconstructive surgery and, by definition, forces the surgeon to attempt to fulfill expectations

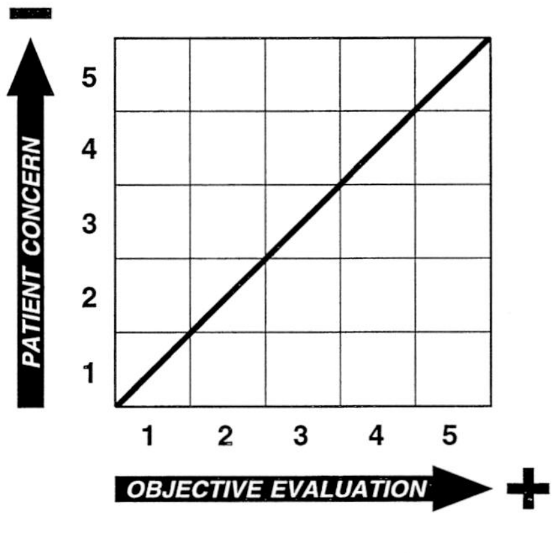

Figure 1. A graphic plot of the patient's objective deformity as judged by the surgeon versus the patient's degree of concern about the deformity.

that cannot be realized. More than likely, this type of patient is very explicit, very fussy, and very demanding about tiny imperfections and will not understand the fact that you are working with human tissue, not clay.

The Indecisive Patient

We have already discussed the relationship between motivation and result. To the question, "Doctor, do you think I ought to have this done?" an appropriate response may be, "This is a decision that I cannot make for you. I will neither encourage nor discourage this operation. I can only tell you what I think we can accomplish. If you have thought about it carefully and feel strongly that you would like to have it done, you will probably be satisfied with the results. If you have any doubts at all, you might want to think about it further." It is very difficult to dissuade a jury or an arbitration panel when one of the patient's principal complaints is that s/he was "talked into" the surgery.

The Immature Patient

For reasons other than growth and development, one should carefully evaluate the degree of maturity in the young candidate. There is, of course, no linear relationship between maturity and age. Immature individuals often have excessively romantic and unrealistic expectations regarding the effect of the plastic surgery. When confronted with a mirror postoperatively, they sometimes exhibit disconcerting shock reactions and alarming behavior. If they have been talked into the surgery by a relative or friend, this only compounds the problem. The adolescent boy seeking rhinoplasty may be the most likely patient to express post-operative dissatisfaction.

The Secretive Patient

Some applicants make a fetish of absolute secrecy about their surgery. Besides the fact that such arrangements are difficult to guarantee, exaggerated concern regarding this aspect of the operation strongly suggests a significant degree of guilt about what they are contemplating.

Familial Disapproval

I prefer that the immediate family members be in agreement with the proposed operation and may refuse to do it if they are not. Too often failure to communicate or an unsatisfactory result produces an automatic "See, I told you so!" reaction. This only intensifies the patient's feelings of guilt, dissatisfaction, and associated emotional stresses. In certain groups aesthetic surgery may be viewed as a rejection of one's ethnic background, and, successful or not, such surgery commonly causes a host of problems with the patient and with the family and peers.

Failure to Establish Rapport

An experienced aesthetic surgeon can usually determine within minutes of entering the examining room whether the individual sitting in the chair will become a patient. Within moments of the opening conversation, there are often discernible "bad vibes." One of the most significant mistakes in plastic surgery is to take on as a patient someone whom one truly dislikes. A clash of personalities cancels out all other factors, regardless of the "challenge" of the case.

The "Surgiholic"

Beware of the patient who has had multiple or repeated aesthetic procedures. Such a patient obviously has a severe and probably incorrigibly distorted body image. Aside from the technical difficulties involved, you will suffer comparison with the other surgeons.

AN OUNCE OF PREVENTION

There should be a frank discussion of fees and costs either by the surgeon or by someone in the surgeon's office. Experience has shown that payment in full and in advance for cosmetic surgery tends to diminish subsequent unhappiness with the final results. However, pre-payment obviously does not eliminate post-operative dissatisfaction.

1. One of the most valuable and least expensive investments you can make is a chalkboard in every examining room. All illustrations and diagrams should be on the chalkboard and not on the permanent record. Unless you can duplicate exactly what you have drawn, a permanent record may come back to haunt you. This is particularly so in the case of imaging devices.
2. In counseling the patient, avoid the use of complex medical terminology. Use simple, understandable language and tailor your explanations to your impression of patient's capacity to understand. Do not make any promises, stated or implied. Do not patronize your patient but do encourage questions; an informed patient is a good patient.
3. It is an ironclad rule in our office never to accept patients at the first visit. I ask them to go home, think about what I have told them, and return (at no fee). I ask them to write down any questions, and at the second visit, I go over the highlights of our original conversation and cover, once again, the most significant complications that might occur. When I am convinced that patients are well and truly motivated and understand clearly what I have told them, then, and only then, do I allow them to book the surgery.
4. At surgery, it is axiomatic that all patients under local anesthesia be adequately sedated. No permit should be signed after sedation is administered, since it may be held to be invalid. All members of the surgical team should understand clearly that the patient, under the influence of narcotics, can misinterpret the most innocent words or jokes and that these can come back to haunt them. Under no circumstances should there be arguments of any kind, even in jest. There should be no swearing for any reason. Assistants and observers should be warned to save expressing any doubts for later. There is no such word as "Oops!" in the operating room, whether the surgeon drops a hemostat or severs an artery. It helps to talk to the patient and be highly visible at the beginning and end of the procedure. It is extremely therapeutic to have music in the operating room if the surgery is being performed while the patient is under local anesthesia. It not only diffuses the unfamiliar and terrifying atmosphere, but also tends to cover up the sounds of the operating room, which of themselves are extremely anxiety producing.
5. The surgeon should always report to the family members immediately after the operation. If they are not present, a telephone call may be the least expensive investment any surgeon can make. A visit on the evening prior to the operation is immensely reassuring to the patient and builds rapport. If patients are admitted to a hospital, the surgeon should be the last person the patients see before going under the anesthetic and the first face that they focus on in the recovery room. Discharge instructions should be clear, specific, and in writing. The operating surgeon's availability during the first few days is essential. If the surgeon signs out, it should be to someone equally competent, and the patient should be notified of this ahead of time.
6. When dressings come off, there will be innumerable questions, all of which require simple, reassuring answers. There will be fewer questions and the patient will be less anxious if many of these questions have been addressed pre-operatively.

RECOMMENDED READING

Jacobson WE, et al. Psychiatric evaluation of male patients seeking cosmetic surgery. *Reconstr Surg* 1960;26:356.

MacGregor FC, Shaffner B. Screening patients for nasal plastic operations. *Psychosom Med* 1950;12:277.

Meyer E, et al. Motivational patterns in patients seeking elective plastic surgery (women who seek rhinoplasty). *Psychosom Med* 1960;22:193.

Palmer A, Blanton S. Mental factors in relation to reconstructive surgery of nose and ears. *Arch Otolaryngol* 1952;56:148.

Stern K, Fournier G, LaRiviera A. Psychiatric aspect of cosmetic surgery of the nose. *Can Med Assoc J* 1957;76:469.

Ethnic Considerations in Facial Aesthetic Surgery, edited by W. Earle Matory, Jr.
Lippincott–Raven Publishers, Philadelphia © 1998.

2

Psychological Considerations

Maisha Hamilton-Bennett
and W. Earle Matory, Jr.

Beauty is truth, truth beauty
—that's all ye know on earth,
and all ye need to know
— John Keats

Reverence for beauty is a fundamental cultural norm throughout the world. Valuing beauty is so intrinsic that it organizes and influences national attitudes, beliefs, feelings, and behaviors. Although the United States is a "salad bowl" of races, ethnicities, and cultural groups, it is the European–American depiction of beauty that dominates varied cultural perspectives.

How does this prevailing veneration for Western standards of beauty impact women, men, and children of color? Depending on hereditary considerations and the degree of racial admixture, the pigmented races manifest features ranging from African to Asian to Occidental.

Drs. Rod Rohrich, Halle Tolleth, and W. Earle Matory, Jr., in their chapters elsewhere in this text, have defined certain concepts of beauty and provided in-depth historical, artistic, physiologic, and anatomic discourses on physical features that we humans use to innately define attractiveness. This seventh sense seems to be influenced by several factors, which are components of the individual personality growth and development (1):

1. Genetics: Subconscious perspectives of self are defined, at least in part, by inherited traits. Formation of self-perspective is at least partially defined before leaving the womb.

M. H. Bennett: Hamilton Wholistic Healthcare, Ltd., Chicago, Illinois 60601-7401
W. E. Matory, Jr.: A New You Plastic Surgery Medical Group, Irvine, California 92714

2. Family: Interpersonal nurturing from family members during early development is also significant in personality development and aesthetic perspective.
3. Environment: Societal influences as promoted by peers, teachers, media, etc., contribute further to perceived self-value, self-esteem, and self-acceptance. Members of society are drawn toward a tendency to conform.

There are common components among the latter two factors that counter self-acceptance. For example, there may be familial or societal influences that do so by denigrating the ethnic characteristics of an individual or that promote the physical characteristics of the dominant culture. "Your nose is too broad and too flat!" "The tip of your nose should be more pointed and your lips thinner!" The steady bombardment by media of Northern European faces with aquiline features indirectly, but powerfully, imparts perceived self-value, self-esteem, and self-acceptance. Additionally, social and peer acceptance may be compromised.

Conversely, the former two contributions, genetics and family, may bolster self-acceptance and self-preservation, thus contributing to common statements that may contradict leanings toward cosmetic surgery. "You were born that way, and you should stay that way!" "God made you as you are and you should not change!" Personal worth is largely translated in early life by the care and nurturing of the family unit. It is defined by individual character, spirit, and motivation, not by external physical features. The individual of color who is a good candidate for surgery emotes self-confidence but seeks to change specific features of concern.

The majority of individuals of color, as is true for the Caucasian, seek facial surgery for aesthetic improvement. Perhaps one has a facial flaw that can be surgically eliminated or significantly reduced. Ethnically identifying features are valued; therefore, changes are not sought to diminish ethnic identity. Facial surgery might, in fact, be sought to enhance an ethnic standard of beauty, for example, enlarging the lips in an African American. Or perhaps the individual is pursuing a career that demands cosmetic changes such as a permanent eyeliner to facilitate make-up application or cheek implants to change facial shape. Facial surgery used to improve career opportunities and successes is more consistently deemed justifiable by family and peers. Physical change for cosmesis has long been an innate part of human culture dating back over 2,000 years. In the South Pacific, Central Africa, and Asia, the presence and cultural significance of scarification, lip or ear expansion, and permanent tattooing have been well documented.

Individuals of color are no less influenced than the rest of the nation by a socially established, strong, positive correlation between youthful appearance and beauty. In the perpetual pursuit of youth, women and men of all colors are motivated to undergo facial aesthetic surgery.

All who live in America are affected by Euro–American standards of beauty, depending on three interacting variables:

1. The degree to which the individual values Euro–American standards of beauty.
2. The extent to which his/her own physical features conform to these standards, particularly those that are most salient to that individual's definition of beauty.
3. The worth ascribed both internally by self and externally by others to his/her traits, talents, and achievements.

This chapter outlines the following concepts that may be helpful in the surgeon's assessment of surgical appropriateness in individuals of color: dynamics of self-criticism; defining psychological stability; assessing psychological suitability; and when surgery should be avoided.

DYNAMICS OF SELF-CRITICISM

Healthy self-esteem derives from the right balance of internal and external recognition for one's significant achievements, talents, and personal qualities. Self-hatred, on the other hand, is a phenomenon stemming from negative comparisons of oneself with others.

Arenas for self-versus-other comparisons include four dimensions of life: the mental, the emotional, the spiritual, and the physical/material. In comparison, the individual perceives himself/herself to be significantly lacking. Self-hatred is a syndrome that typically includes the self-perception of one or more major defect, shortcoming, or despised feature.

Primary sources of self-hatred among individuals of color are related to perceived physical/material defects and shortcomings, as opposed to those in the mental, emotional, or spiritual dimensions. All ethnicities in America considered, women have typically been more concerned about achieving physical beauty, while men have been more focused on achieving economic success. However, among African Americans, Asians, and Hispanics, both men and women appear to be equally concerned about achieving both physical beauty and economic successes.

The tendency to ascribe nearly equal value to achieving physical and material successes can be traced to socioeconomic development worldwide. For example, the cultural and fiscal development of the Philippines and Korea, spurred by U.S. military input, strongly influences goal orientation. With regard to beauty and finances, the great divergence for many individuals of color from American norms commonly leads to self-denigration as a result of the pervasive and constant exposure to the American standard of beauty, strong societal reverence for financial success, and the tremendous barriers encountered by individuals of color in trying to achieve these norms. As we see growing changes in migration patterns and population trends in the U.S.A., the importance of physical and material successes transcends all ethnic groups.

While the male Caucasian has many avenues available for achieving economic success, individuals of color, in general, are far more limited. Technology and circumstance, in many instances, have allowed the Northern European woman to attain the American standard of physical beauty and financial success. Any similar goals perceived by the individual of color constitute a far greater and more complex challenge. Some physical features cannot, practically, be changed, even with recent scientific advances. For example, while skin tone and shades of lightness and darkness can be altered, the reality of skin color emanating from the presence of melanin is forever present in the colored races. For those individuals seeking ethnic change, unalterable features, which do not fit the American standard of beauty, may constitute major barriers.

American culture promotes the high value of physical Euro–American beauty and material successes through televised and printed media. Most individuals of color have a high degree of self-esteem and reject the emulation of Euro–American standards of beauty. Individuals of color suffering from glamorization of Euro–American standards or from self-hatred pursue those standards in an attempt to be more like the majority culture.

For African American, Hispanic, and Asian women, the physical features that seem most important to defining beauty are skin color, hair texture and length, nose width, lip thickness, eye color, and size of hips and buttocks. For African American, Hispanic, and Asian men, similar features are important: skin color, hair texture, nose width, lip thickness, eye color, but also including a key significance attached to genital endowment.

Relentless pursuit of cosmetic changes to be physically more similar to the dominant ethnic group is consistent with strong emulation and may represent self-hatred. Self-hatred can also occur when one perceives defects or shortcomings in the mental/intellectual or in the emotional/interpersonal dimensions. Notions of intellectual inferiority, especially during the school years, when the foundations of self-concept and self-esteem are established, can contribute to self-criticism or self-hatred. Feelings of interpersonal powerlessness can produce similar conceptions. Chronically being perceived as the recipient of social injustices, coupled with the incapacity to overcome these injustices, commonly leads to anger that may be vented toward the doctor.

Large numbers of a group may negatively compare themselves with the group in power: for example, widespread use of lightening creams in Japan and in Nigeria or the common use of platform shoes in Vietnam. These types of feelings may foster disdain for one's own group as a whole. When members of the majority group are perceived to achieve successes based on physical attributes, material possessions, career successes, power to control outcomes, and intellectual strengths, then it is not surprising that members of the minority would seek to escape feelings of inferiority by imitating the successful majority group.

Most patients of color who seek cosmetic surgery are searching for physical refinement within the physical parameters of attractiveness within their own ethnic group. A few individuals of color seek facial surgery due to these feelings of inferiority and/or self-hatred. Individuals may opt to change as many features as necessary to duplicate Euro–American beauty or to escape their ethnic characteristics. They may start with the most despised feature and change others as other significant factors allow, e.g., economics, effectiveness of the procedure, and tendency not to form keloids. It would not be unusual for such individuals to engage in a syndrome of behaviors including the regular use of skin lighteners, election of a hair weave, extensions, or a wig, choice of wearing light brown or green contact lenses, and, if affordable, seeking surgery on a characteristic ethnic feature like the nose. This person may avoid marrying anyone darker than himself/herself "for the sake of the children" and might use a clothespin, their thumb and forefinger, or some other device to pinch the children's noses so that they grow narrow and pointed rather than broad and flat.

DEFINING PSYCHOLOGICAL STABILITY

Basis of Psychological Stability: Wholism

A thorough patient assessment is essential to identify patients appropriate for cosmetic surgery and to rule out potentially problematic patients (2–4). Psychological stability, a crucial requisite to any operative candidate, is based on the concept of wholeness, defined as well-being in four dimensions of life: physical/material, mental, emotional, and spiritual. Psychological disease occurs when there is a lack of wholeness, incompleteness, lack of harmony with the energy of the universe, and lack of balance internally. Psychological stability and well-being occur when balance and harmony are restored and maintained (Fig. 1).

Mental Dimension

Definition

The mental dimension includes acquiring knowledge, information, and problem-solving techniques, producing ideas, creating thoughts, and forming opinions.

Goal

The goal is to seek the truth. The basic skills are thinking, analysis, judgment, and creativity.

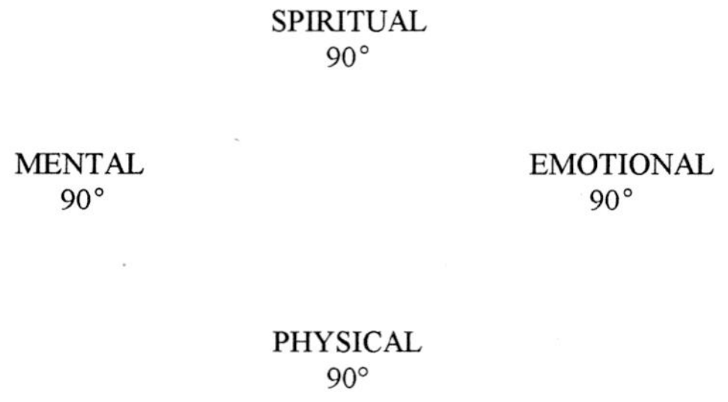

Figure 1.

Spiritual Dimension

Definition

The spiritual dimension concerns the relationship between individuals and God, a Higher Power, or the Universe; understanding the purpose of one's life on earth.

Goal

The goal is to help the individual clarify purpose and values and the choices that exemplify them.

Belief in a Higher Power provides an external source of support. The individual is no longer totally reliant on self and can share responsibility with another force. Enhancement of the spiritual dimension contributes to the clarification of conceptions and beliefs referable to education, family life, physical appearance, money, work ethics, relationships, violent behaviors, religion, sports, career, and the like.

Emotional Dimension

Definition

The emotional dimension concerns the acknowledgment and expression of a full range of feelings, identification of internal sources of excitement, the giving and receiving of love, and the formation and maintenance of strong, healthy, honest, mutually loving relationships.

Goal

Development of the emotional dimension seeks to enhance self-esteem, love of self, and to promote interpersonal harmony, love of others.

What one possesses is an artificial index of self-worth. Emotional growth helps individuals to make the shift from "I'm OK because I have money or some material possession" or "I'm OK because I have light skin and a narrow nose" to "I'm OK because I give my talent back to life" or "I'm OK because my inherited features are beautiful."

Physical/Material Dimension

Definition

The physical/material dimension concerns the achievement of physical healthiness, wellness, and fitness through nutrition, exercise, physical activities, and sports and the achievement of material comfort through the acquisition of objects, goods, and money.

Goal

The best route to material/financial success is through an individual identifying his/her God-given talents and developing them. For some, physical traits or perceived physical flaws may require cosmetic surgery.

ASSESSING PSYCHOLOGICAL SUITABILITY

Diagnosable mental illnesses impair cognitive and/or emotional and/or behavioral processes, thus compromising decision making, particularly with regard to cosmetic surgery. The psychologically impaired may be unable to fully appreciate the objectives, processes, or outcome of cosmetic surgery. A gross overall assessment of psychological stability can be performed by the psychotherapist and sometimes by the surgeon by evaluating impairments in orientation, memory, judgment, rational thinking, and reality testing indicative of psychopathology and/or cognitive disorders.

Mental Disorder

The presence of any psychological disorder that meets criteria established in the *Diagnostic and Statistical Manual of Mental Disorders* (5), as outlined in this section, should prompt the surgeon to exercise caution before initiating any aesthetic procedure. Each category of mental disorder is characterized by a syndrome of signs, symptoms, and features that may negatively impact the patient's ability to make an informed decision regarding cosmetic surgery. Organic mental disorders feature a psychological or behavioral abnormality associated with transient or permanent dysfunction of the brain. Substance use disorders are characterized by undesirable behavioral changes associated with frequent use of substances that affect the central nervous system. The essential features of schizophrenic disorders include the presence of certain psychotic features during the active phase of the illness, characteristic symptoms involving multiple psychological processes, delusions, hallucinations, or certain disturbances in the form of thought during some phase of the illness.

Affective disorders are characterized by "a disturbance of mood, accompanied by a full or partial manic or depressive syndrome, that is not due to any other physical or mental disorder." In anxiety disorders, "anxiety is either the predominant disturbance or anxiety is experienced if the individual attempts to master the symptoms." Somatoform disorders are characterized by the presence of "physical symptoms suggesting physical disorder for which there are no demonstrable organic findings or known physiological mechanisms and for which there is positive evidence, or a strong presumption that the symptoms are linked to psychological factors or conflicts." The essential feature of dissociative disorders is "a sudden, temporary alteration in the normally integrative functions of consciousness, identity, or motor behaviors." Factitious disorders are characterized by "physical or psychological symptoms that are produced by the individual and are under voluntary control."

Personality Disorders

The presence of another category of psychological aberrancy, personality disorders, may not automatically rule out a candidate for cosmetic surgery. However, the presence of a personality disorder should certainly prompt the surgeon to require a fuller evaluation of the patient before entertaining surgery. In personality disorders, "personality traits, enduring patterns of perceiving, relating to, and thinking about the environment and oneself, are inflexible and maladaptive, and cause either significant impairment in social or occupational functioning or subjective distress." Patients with any mental disorder diagnosis may seek cosmetic surgery for the wrong reasons. They may be disappointed with the results when their lives do not change and as a result may initiate some legal action against the surgeon.

Diagnostic Instruments

The following instruments constitute techniques used for pre-operative psychological assessment for the appropriateness of cosmetic surgery.

Hamilton Assessment of Life Balance

This instrument assesses psychological stability in the four dimensions of life. In the mental arena, it explores the extent of the patient's knowledge and information about the surgical procedure: process, outcome, prognosis, side effects, and the like. It also assesses the patient's thoughts and opinions about both the magnitude of the perceived problem and the ramifications of the intended surgery, and the self-image of the individual and other members of her/his ethnic group.

In the physical/material arena, this instrument allows exploration of non-surgical options to achieve the desired outcome. The patient assesses whether the aesthetic result can be achieved by using makeup contouring or other camouflage techniques like clothing/accessories. The patient's psychiatric history and expectations regarding surgical changes are evaluated to determine clarity and decisiveness of thought.

In the emotional arena, the Hamilton test explores the patient's current feelings and the emotional expectations of surgery. It explores the healthiness of existing interpersonal relationships as well as feelings about standards of beauty to which the individual, peers, and family members ascribe.

In the spiritual arena, this instrument explores the patient's values, life purpose, and goals. The compatibility of surgery with personal values and life purpose can be established in an effort to determine the advisability of surgery.

Hamilton Assessment of Self-Esteem

This instrument measures the following factors:

- Overall happiness and satisfaction with life
- General successes in life
- Marital status and level of satisfaction
- Parental status, satisfaction, and performance
- Employment status, satisfaction with job performance
- Career path, satisfaction with progress
- Internal or external locus of control
- Personal effectiveness and impact on others in the community and society
- Individual's adherence to the individual's standards of beauty

Hamilton Standards of Beauty Questionnaire

The individual is asked to describe his/her own features, as well as the characteristics that are deemed ideal, to family members, to members of the same ethnic group and relative to men and women in the majority culture. The patient is asked to describe his/her spousal relationship and perceived attractiveness to the spouse and dating history and attractiveness to individuals of the same and other ethnicities.

The patient rates his/her own features and those features listed below, using the following scale as well as the nature of the contemplated change:

- Like very much, like somewhat, neutral, dislike somewhat, dislike a lot
- Would change if money were not an object
- Will definitely change as soon as able

The patient is asked to rate the following features according to relative importance of each to attractiveness:

- Skin color (very dark, dark, medium, light, very light)
- Natural hair texture (straight, wavy, coarse, kinky)
- Hair length (long, medium, short)
- Nose width (wide, medium, narrow)

- Lip thickness (thick, medium, thin)
- Natural eye color (dark brown, light brown, green, blue, gray)
- Hips and buttocks (high and round, round, medium, flat)

WHEN SURGERY SHOULD BE AVOIDED

Patients who have a diagnosable mental illness or who are seeking unrealistic, culturally questionable, or ethnic changes are not good candidates for facial aesthetic surgery. An assessment battery, including the mental status exam, a comprehensive diagnostic interview, the Hamilton Assessment of Life Balance, the Hamilton Assessment of Self-Esteem, and the Hamilton Standard of Beauty Questionnaire, attempts to define the appropriateness of surgical intervention or lack thereof. Screening concepts are key to making this decision.

Screening

The first step in patient screening is the interview by the surgeon. If the surgeon believes that the surgery requested is a feasible way to meet the patient's objectives but is unsure of psychological stability, one may recommend psychotherapeutic input for a comprehensive assessment. This intervention will provide a written report of significant findings and recommendations. The surgeon should discuss this report with the patient, exploring at length the significant findings and the recommendations.

Inviting one or more significant other to participate in the discussion with the surgeon and in the assessment process with the psychologist will provide additional information about the patient's psychological stability, motives, and expectations. Significant others may share relevant details about the realism and about cultural and ethnic implications of the cosmetic changes sought. One may also gain insight into the perceptions of family and friends.

The surgeon should give honest feedback to patients seeking ethnic changes. When surgery is not felt to be appropriate, the patient should be advised that surgery is not the most effective or practical way to achieve the perceived goals, to boost self-esteem, or to satisfy other psychological needs. Patients seeking culturally questionable or ethnic conversion may benefit from the input of a mental health professional.

The Persistent Patient

A patient may insist on ethnic changes despite recommendations and counseling to the contrary. Allow the patient sufficient time to consider all the presented information, perspectives, and alternatives. If the patient does not have a mental disorder and is legally competent to make such decisions, then the surgeon may opt to perform surgery. Ensure that appropriate consents are signed. Family members, peers, and office staff should serve as witnesses to confirm an informed and understood consent.

Families and friends are important participants in the peri-operative sequence. Family and friends who agree with a patient's decision to undergo surgery can serve as sources of support to the patient and as allies to the surgeon. Significant others who are anxious about the patient's decision will benefit from discussions with the surgeon and staff. Those who do not support the decision will reap the greatest benefit from a meeting with the surgeon.

Predicting the Unhappy Patient

It is possible to both predict and prevent unhappy patients.

At age 23, Sharon was a single woman of Korean descent, who had dated infrequently and, in fact, had never had a boyfriend. She worked in a clerical support position where she performed what she perceived as fairly meaningless duties reasonably well, received reasonably good performance evaluations, and was rewarded by a modest salary. Sharon, however, was generally unhappy with her job, her social life, and her self-perceptions, as suggested by her shabby dressing tendencies.

Shortly after enrolling in psychotherapy, Sharon sought cosmetic surgery to alter her depressed nasal dorsum and her broad, flared tip. Sharon was convinced that these features were responsible for her social inadequacies and her lack of advancement at work.

Without the benefit of a comprehensive psychological assessment, Sharon underwent osteoplastic rhinoplasty. The surgeon reported an excellent outcome. Sharon was so pleased with the results that she abruptly discontinued psychotherapy, stating that now her life was perfect, so therapy was no longer needed.

Six months later, Sharon called her therapist, angry and crying. She was seeking the name and address of the surgeon so that she could litigate, claiming, between sobs, that despite the surgery, her life had not improved.

This unfortunate sequence could have been avoided. An astute surgeon or psychological assessment would have red-flagged Sharon as a poor surgical candidate based on both her affective disorder and her unrealistic expectations of improving her lot in life. The psychological assessment instruments would have better defined the extent of her low self-esteem, her lack of life balance, and perhaps her distorted perceptions of beauty.

WAYS TO AVOID PSYCHOLOGICAL UNREST

Key to a successful outcome for the patient and surgeon is a strong positive relationship between the patient and the surgeon. Doctor/patient relationships are built on honest, genuine, caring communications. The surgeon must relay details about the surgical procedure and, equally important, feelings of caring and concern for the patient. Talk in a fashion that the patient can understand. The surgeon should listen respectfully to the patient's thoughts and feelings and respond empathically. From this type of dialogue can grow a relationship that is warm and respectful and one that may shield the surgeon against litigation.

Hand-written notes by the patient as well as the surgeon that define the surgical objectives may reduce the risks of litigation. Such a document should be written in clear terms defining what surgery can accomplish and what it cannot. If the surgeon is undertaking the procedure with reservation, it may be appropriate to document these reservations in writing.

Another way to enhance the chances of patient unhappiness is to operate under undesirable circumstances, e.g., a patient who does not pass surgical or psychological screening, one with whom the surgeon finds it impossible to develop a positive rapport, or one who sees the surgeon for the first time and wants surgery the next day. Exceptions to the latter are few.

DEALING WITH THE UNHAPPY PATIENT

Effective counseling of the unhappy post-surgery patient can diminish the likelihood of litigation. The surgeon must listen closely to establish the basis of the patient's dissatisfaction. If the concerns seem unfounded, then the surgeon must find a way to reassure the patient. If there are merits, the surgeon should communicate empathy for the patient's well-being as well as a sincere commitment to identify options that will address the concerns.

CONCLUSION

Standards of beauty should not be purely Euro–American. Adherence to such standards serves only to reinforce low self-esteem based on a feeling that one can be attractive only if one conforms to the Euro–American norm.

Ideally, facial cosmetic surgery should achieve optimal aesthetics that are satisfactory for the individual and that are compatible with the characteristics of attractiveness appropriate for the individual ethnic background.

REFERENCES

1. Cassem NH. *Massachusetts General Hospital handbook of general hospital psychiatry*. 3rd ed. St. Louis: Mosby Year Book, 1991.
2. Herskowitz J, Rosman NP. *Pediatrics, neurology, and psychiatry—common ground, behavioral, cognitive, affective, and physical disorders in childhood and adolescence*. New York: Macmillan, 1982.
3. Halleck SL. *Law in the practice of psychiatry: a handbook for clinicians*. New York: Plenum Medical, 1980.
4. Kaplan HI, Sadock BJ. *Comprehensive textbook of psychiatry V*. 5th ed. Baltimore: Williams & Wilkins, 1989.
5. American Psychiatric Association. *Diagnostic and statistical manual of mental disorders*. 4th rev. ed. Washington, D.C.: American Psychiatric Association, 1994.

Ethnic Considerations in Facial Aesthetic Surgery, edited by W. Earle Matory, Jr.
Lippincott–Raven Publishers, Philadelphia © 1998.

3

Addressing the Needs of the Hostile Patient and Preventing the Unhappy Patient

W. Earle Matory, Jr.

Refusal to operate in many instances is less an act of cowardice than of wisdom.
— Robert Goldwyn

The importance of understanding your patient's needs, personality, and his/her goals cannot be overstated. Of greatest significance in the ethnic patient is a natural, improved appearance. One should avoid the operated look at all costs. Ideally, one should remain within the parameters of the ethnic background, particularly if this is translated as a key desire of the patient. It is equally important to remain within the parameters of the patient's gender. An exaggerated dorsal height or cephalic tip rotation in an individual with otherwise strongly Asian or African American features may create significant disharmony. Feminization of the male nose may lead to disastrous consequences for the patient as well as for the surgeon. Several recommendations are discussed herein.

Encourage patients to bring photographs of features they like as well as ones that they do not like. Liked or disliked photographs of family members will best identify surgical outcomes that can realistically be achieved. Video imaging may also clarify realistic versus unrealistic goals.

W. E. Matory, Jr.: A New You Plastic Surgery Medical Group, Irvine, California 92714

KNOW YOUR PATIENT

This can be aided by asking the following key questions:

1. What features would the patient like to change? Insist on a priority list.
2. What is the patient's motivation? Is it for career-related goals versus vanity? Or is it at the request of a friend or spouse?
3. How long have the features been a concern? How do these features practically affect daily activities?
4. Why is the patient presenting now? Has there been a major psychological change, like divorce or a broken relationship?
5. What do peers or family members think about this physical change? Are they supportive, contrary, or unaware? Beware of patients that have shared their plans with no one. They may be attempting to suppress family traits or may be denying family or peer resistance. The latter may come forth post-operatively to haunt the patients and to make the surgeon's life miserable.
6. Are the patient's goals and perspectives realistic? Try as best you can to translate realistic goals to the patient by drawings or video imaging.
7. Has there been a recent tragic or stressful event such as job lay-off, divorce, spousal dispute, or death in the family? Each of these events may contribute to an unhappy outcome, regardless of the post-operative result.
8. Has there been prior psychiatric treatment? If so, be aware that the treatment described by the patient may not be factual or complete. The alcoholic or the smoker may note substance abuse but may minimize the quantity or severity. Other psychiatric illnesses are likely to have similar presentations. Obtain written clearance from the attending psychiatrist or psychologist.

CHARACTERIZE THE PATIENT'S PERSONALITY AND THE SURGEON'S ABILITY TO INTERACT WITH THE PATIENT

Intelligence should be assessed, particularly the patient's ability to understand details, risks, and options of surgery. Perceived goals should also be assessed using photographs, drawings, and/or video imaging. It can be helpful to ask the patient what popular or visible media talents have features that they like versus those that they do not. They will identify individuals who have undergone an ethnic transformation or they will say contrarily that they do not want to undergo such a transformation.

DETERMINE PERSONALITY

The fastidious dresser with refined jewelry or meticulously matched garb may be particularly demanding post-operatively. Conversely, the individual of low economic station may be anticipating a surgical outcome that will elevate his/her position in life. In most instances surgical input is appropriate. One should be aware that the impoverished patient undergoing surgery is more likely to litigate. One should be especially cautious with unkempt or unhygienic presentations.

Keep the surgical plan simple, using proven techniques with the least degree of visible signs of surgery.

Psychological liability should be assessed by reviewing the patient's interactions with all staff members. Demanding or infantile characteristics may be more apparent to other staff than it may be to the surgeon.

EVALUATE SPOUSAL/FAMILY/PEER SUPPORT

Be sure to inquire about the degree of support that has been attained from family members and peers. Encourage office visits that include a spouse, family member, or friend. The better the pre-operative understanding of the patient and an additional party, the clearer the understanding of the peri-operative concerns or post-operative untoward outcomes. Lack of familial or peer support for the ethnic patient undergoing cosmetic surgery is far more common than it is not. Religious mores may dictate that "God made you that way and you should stay that way!" Family members often perceive plastic surgery of the face as an effort to erase a family trait.

The fact that aesthetic surgeons take healthy patients, make them sick, endanger their lives, and take their money for performing a procedure that is often perceived as ethnicity transforming may well induce perjorative feedback and cajoling from family members or ethnic peers. Litigation may follow the suboptimal outcome in the ethnic patient when incited or persuaded by peer and family input.

ENCOURAGE MULTIPLE PRE-OPERATIVE OFFICE VISITS

Get to know your patient well and vice versa. The more you interact, the better you will be able to address patient needs. With a more detailed sense of perceived goals, you will be better able to avoid undesired surgical outcomes. This may also prepare the surgeon's ability to deal with unforeseen circumstances.

RED FLAGS

The following list of potentially problematic characteristics should alert the surgeon to impending peri-operative difficulties.

Unrealistic Expectations

The individual who has broad cheek bones or thick or dark nasal and facial skin and presents with perceived goals demonstrated by photographs of Farrah Fawcett or Cheryl Tieg is a very unlikely candidate for a satisfactory surgical outcome in spite of notable improvements.

Non-Compliance

It is often necessary to be graphic in your description of the importance of following post-surgical instructions. Patients who ignore time restraints, office appointment schedules, or advised physical restrictions may compromise surgical outcome. In spite of patient non-compliance, the surgeon is perceived as the origin of any peri-operative complications.

The Indecisive or Vague Patient

"Doctor, what do you think is wrong with me? I would welcome your opinion." This presentation is always problematic. This patient's self-esteem is probably low, and his/her feelings of inferiority may be heightened by mentioning characteristics that the patient was heretofore unaware of. If a patient cannot identify where you should operate, do not oblige.

The Perfectionist

This individual is seldom satisfied with anything. No matter how positive the surgical outcome, the patient will never be pleased.

The Individual with Minimal Deformity

Heightened anxiety about a relatively minor deformity should raise suspicions that there may be underlying psychopathology. Upon surgical correction of the inconspicuous deformity, the true problem is rarely resolved.

The Shopper

These patients are often seeking a better surgeon, a better price, or a doctor that is more sympathetic to their concerns. More often than not, these individuals are seeking a surgeon who will guarantee an outcome.

The "Surgiholic"

The physician should recognize this individual as being psychologically unhealthy. Repeated submission to surgical procedures represents sparks of masochism, which may indicate psychotherapeutic intervention.

The Secretive Patient

The individual who tells no one that s/he is undergoing surgery, including a spouse or family member, should raise concerns. In addition, patients may hide portions of their medical history, including psychiatric or somatic pathologies. Tell-tale signs include denial that the patient has had prior cosmetic surgery when physical stigmata are readily apparent. Unwillingness to undress for proper examination and refusal to be photographed are common presentations. One should avoid operating on an individual who is unwilling to share pertinent information.

The Rude or Pushy Patient

This patient is most often recognized by your office staff. This individual may present a particularly positive image with the surgeon but is particularly troublesome for the support staff. Rarely does surgery ever change this general demeanor. Conversely, an operative procedure is more likely to exacerbate the innate malevolence.

The Unkempt Patient

An unshaven, unwashed, or untidy appearance may indicate acute depression or some other psychopathology. While this state of mind and appearance may be temporary, these external signals imply an inappropriate time for surgery.

An Individual Who Writes an Excessively Long Letter to Arrange the Initial Consultation

This personality trait is often deceiving. The letter will often include high praises for you, the new surgeon, along with an extremely detailed account of his/her dissatisfaction with the outcome of the prior surgeon. While it is true that some individuals communicate best in writing, this presentation may reflect difficulty with communication or perseverance tendencies.

The Special Patient

Special demands, refusal to take photographs, tardiness for office visits, and relaying social or work obligations as explanations for missing appointments characterize this patient.

This inability to follow standard office routine may represent the patient's inability to give up control. This trait may become more problematic after surgery.

The Patient Whom the Surgeon Dislikes

Incompatible characteristics may lead the surgeon to be uncomfortable with the patient or family members. Once the surgeon operates, this is the surgeon's patient for life. It is best to refer such a patient to another surgeon.

The Indigent Patient

Medicaid patients are presenting more frequently for facial aesthetic surgery. While it is everyone's right to undergo cosmetic surgery, one must discern whether the motivation for this procedure is appropriate based on other obligations or priorities in life, like children or jobs. Individuals of lower economic station are more likely to sue.

The Unfocused Patient/The Poor Listener

You are talking about risks and the patient interrupts you to ask how soon she can wear a bathing suit. Lack of retention, misinterpretation, or gross maljudgments are common in this type of patient.

In summary, while these exclusions from your patient pool may seem exhaustive, this list is presented to identify potentially problematic patients. Common sense and clinical judgment should guide clinical decision making.

GENDER

Irrespective of the ethnic group, females tend to be more understanding and tolerant. Conversely, males are more demanding, spend less time listening, and are more likely to fuss about little things.

Many surgeons concur with the impression that men are the most challenging of cosmetic patients. Pain tolerance is less and impatience is greater than in the female counterpart. Men are frequently out of touch with their emotions, often denying feelings of inadequacy. There is a general fear of intimacy or dependency, along with the denial of pain. Uncontrolled pain or unalleviated anxieties are exhibited in other ways, which tend to be less direct and more difficult to deal with. Pre-operative paranoias and social maladjustments often heighten or magnify post-operatively. Pre-operative sexual inadequacies may translate into subtle or flagrantly aberrant social interactions and hostilities. These problem situations are often in association with aesthetically acceptable results.

The Ethnic Male

The Hispanic, Asian, or African American man, by my perspective, is the greatest psychological challenge to the plastic surgeon. Every trait known in the Caucasian man, including anxiety, maladjustment, impatience, feelings of inadequacy, fear of intimacy/dependency, pain denial, or paranoia, may be magnified in the ethnic man. These individuals often perceive the plastic surgeon as a representative of the Establishment. If all goes well peri-operatively, there may be an outpouring of support, often associated with gift giving and referral of other patients. Conversely, if the outcome is less than satisfactory, all of the social ills for hundreds of years may be consciously or subconsciously thrust upon the surgeon. The surgeon may become the enemy and every interaction between you/your staff and the patient becomes inflammatory or even hostile.

Be cautious with the ethnic man. Pay attention to these premonitory characteristics to guide patient selection.

HOW TO SURVIVE A HOSTILE RAGE

Anticipate the rare but substantially disruptive and hostile patient: No matter how exceptional your bedside manner or your surgical skills, you may encounter the angry or violent patient. It may be advantageous to keep the patient affiliated with your practice.

Pre-operatively identify the potential need and stronger likelihood of secondary surgery in the ethnic patient. Ensure that the patient understands your office policies regarding the associated secondary surgical fees, including facility, anesthesiology, and surgical fees. Confirm the patient's understanding in writing.

Encourage frequent follow-up visits. The working patient and the male patient are least likely to keep follow-up appointments. Encourage follow-up through your staff or, if necessary, call your patient directly. Evening or weekend appointments may occasionally be necessary to ensure patient contact.

Have a list of known mediators and select the mediator most appropriate for this particular patient, based on your knowledge of the patient and of the mediator:

1. Patient care coordinator. This individual should be trained to acquaint the patient with the surgeon and the practice. Patient screening is probably the most pivotal role for the patient care coordinator. Pre-operative rapport that is established is usually adequate to keep the patient in contact with your practice until you can achieve a satisfactory outcome.
2. A friendly second opinion. Known non-competitive associates who are patient and understanding may be able to provide supportive perspectives that will allow continued input from your practice to the patient.
3. A former patient. Some patients may benefit by interacting with a former patient who has had similar surgery, with or without an adverse outcome, that can help the patient to adjust to his/her present post-surgical status and the subsequent revisions that may be necessary.
4. An aesthetician. Work with an aesthetician/make-up artist who is qualified to address the needs of the recovering patient with ethnic background. Aesthetic skin covers may allow daily functioning during the recovery phase, thus optimizing patient adjustment. An aesthetician that is uncomfortable with ethnic skin may further aggravate the problem.

Common sense, clinical judgment, and peri-operative support mechanisms will diminish the frequency and optimize the support of the dissatisfied patient.

RECOMMENDED READING

Edgerton MT, Langman MW. Psychiatric considerations. In: Courtiss EH, ed. *Male aesthetic surgery*. St. Louis: Mosby, 1991.

Goldwyn R. Patient selection. In: Courtiss EH, ed. *Male aesthetic surgery*. St. Louis: Mosby, 1991:12–17.

Matory WE Jr. Cosmetic surgery in the black male. In: Courtiss EH, ed. *Male aesthetic surgery*. St. Louis: Mosby, 1991:170–184.

Matory WE Jr. Personal notes, 1995.

Ethnic Considerations in Facial Aesthetic Surgery, edited by W. Earle Matory, Jr.
Lippincott–Raven Publishers, Philadelphia © 1998.

4

Medicolegal Considerations

W. Earle Matory, Jr.

Facts are to the mind the same thing as food to the body. On the due digestion of facts depends the strength and wisdom of the one, just as vigor and health depend on the other. The wisest in counsel, the ablest in debate, and the most agreeable in the commerce of life, is that man who has assimilated to his understanding the greatest number of facts.
— Burke

To the ethnic patient cosmetic surgery is stepping beyond the edge. While make-up application is generally accepted except within religious circles, cosmetic surgery may be perceived as taboo by many members of most ethnic subcultures. Any surgical procedure may therefore cause considerable stress both internally and externally.

It is crucial that the surgeon create a relationship based on understanding and mutual respect. Understand that ethnic patients represent the minority in a cosmetic surgery practice. This patient population is particularly sensitive because of family and peer pressure. These individuals are usually uncomfortable in the plastic surgeon's office. It is easy to understand why the ethnic patient may not be at ease when exposed to European faces among the lay media, the office personnel, and the office literature.

Many patients of color are working individuals who find it difficult to get off work during regular hours. Time is therefore very important. Given an extra wait in your recovery room, inherent feelings of uneasiness may be magnified. These factors make the ethnic patient particularly vulnerable to medicolegal suggestion or directive, especially when motivated by peers and family.

WHAT MOTIVATES THE MEDICOLEGAL CLAIM

Claims usually develop when there is a lack of communication between the surgeon's office and the patient. Listen to your patients and their needs. Make the expectations of the

W. E. Matory, Jr.: A New You Plastic Surgery Medical Group, Irvine, California 92714

surgical procedure clearly understood by both you and the patient and family members/peers. Doctors are perceived as being busy. You, as a member of the Establishment, may also be perceived as someone who may be antagonistic to the patient's goals. Encourage patient follow-up utilizing the techniques described in Chapter 3.

Most patients presenting to an attorney raise the same question: Why did I end up with the result that I now experience? Frequently, the patient will state that the surgeon did not explain how the patient got the suboptimal outcome. If the surgeon did talk to the patient after surgery, the complaint is that the surgeon did not explain details of the surgery before the operation. One can sometimes allay these feelings by encouraging multiple pre-operative discussions with the patient, attended by a friend or spouse and with the confirmation of an office staff member.

Over-inflated patient expectations often contribute to litigation. Try your best to limit the patient's expectations by explaining what can as well as what cannot be done. Video imaging in the ethnic patient may be particularly helpful in this regard. Some suggest that you have the patient write out his/her expectations. You may follow with a letter detailing what your expectations are, thus eliminating any later questions about whether you actually performed the service that you said you would perform.

EMOTIONS THAT CONTRIBUTE TO LITIGATION

Four common emotional reactions have been cited in the precipitation of medicolegal actions: disappointment, anger, surprise, and financial stress. To prevent or alleviate these patient responses, one must understand their etiology.

Inattention or indifference to patient feelings and failure to appreciate a patient's time and importance are key factors that contribute to anger. Loss of control that accompanies any surgical procedure tends to precipitate anxiety that may progress to anger. Recovery time that may have been outlined to the patient pre-operatively is often unconsciously denied, thus propagating dissatisfaction and frustration. Routine post-operative office visits may be perceived as an invasion of the patient's daily schedule, and any delay in recovery further exacerbates this situation. While most patients of color carry a high degree of respect for the medical profession, peri-operatively the surgeon may be projected as an extension of other unrelated social ills.

The patient of color may interpret or misinterpret the overtures of the surgeon and his/her staff. Ethnic resentments may surface. There may be a lack of appreciation for appointments that are designed to support the patient and conversely may be perceived as a waste of time.

Surprise

An unanticipated outcome may be perceived as mismanagement. Patients of color may be overpowered by the Establishment presence, which may diminish listening capacity.

Disappointment

Disappointment is usually a reflection of not meeting anticipated goals. If the surgical goals include cultural assimilation, no matter how positive the surgical outcome, disappointment may result.

Dramatic improvements that may be accomplished with one procedure in the Caucasian more often than not require multiple procedures in the patient of color. If the patient does not understand, dissatisfaction may result.

Financial Stress

Many individuals of color may be expending their cash reserves or borrowing to have cosmetic surgery. Finance plans that are readily available place patients in an awkward position, particularly if they are unhappy with their surgical outcome. Should secondary surgery be necessary to enhance appearance or to address complications, inability to afford such a procedure may precipitate litigation.

HOW TO MINIMIZE FACTORS THAT MAY PRECIPITATE LITIGATION

Informed Consent

It is the surgeon's obligation to clearly define surgical options, peri-operative details, and the most commonly noted along with the most serious complications. On the other hand, the patient's listening capacity may be impaired by education level, anxiety about surgery, or language barriers. Cultural differences between the patient and the surgeon may also compromise communication.

The consent must clearly identify the potential need for secondary surgery and the patient's responsibility for hospital-, anesthesiology-, and surgeon-related expenses. The concept is particularly important for the patient with limited financial resources. Multiple preoperative office visits assist the translation of this information. Encourage discussions with a spouse or friend. Use visual adjuncts to translate information, including drawings, slide presentations, videotapes, video imaging, or pre- and post-operative photographs. Train office personnel to assist in the translation of the pertinent information to the patient and friend/spouse.

Being Prepared to Address the Unhappy Patient

No matter how exceptional your bedside manner or surgical skills, you may encounter an angry or violent patient. As best possible, you should anticipate the rare but substantially disruptive and hostile patient. Keep the patient affiliated with your practice as long as possible. It is hoped this will cement your relationship with the patient and allow additional opportunities to satisfy patient needs.

Ensure that the patient understands the strong or likely potential need for secondary surgery pre-operatively. Make sure that s/he understands your office's financial policies with regard to secondary surgery so that s/he may plan this in the budget and thus avoid surprises.

Frequent pre-operative and post-operative follow-up visits are key to optimize patient understanding and post-operative reassurance. The working patient and the male patient are least likely to keep follow-up appointments. Direct your staff to communicate the importance of a follow-up. It may be necessary for you to call your patients directly or to have evening or weekend appointments to expedite patient care.

Have a list of individuals who may serve to mediate. Select the mediator most appropriate for the particular patient, based on your knowledge of the patient's personality, logic, and his/her concerns:

1. Patient care coordinator. This individual should be trained to spend more time with each patient than the surgeon does. In so doing, preoperative rapport is usually optimized, allowing the patient to stay connected to your practice.
2. A friendly second opinion. Known non-competitive surgeons who are patient and understanding may be able to provide supportive perspectives that will allow continued input from your practice to the patient.
3. A former patient. Some patients may benefit by interacting with a former patient who has had similar surgery, with or without an adverse outcome, and who can help the patient to adjust to his/her present post-surgical status and any revisionary surgery that may be necessary.
4. An aesthetician. Work with an aesthetician/make-up artist who is facile with ethnic skin. Aesthetic make-up may allow daily functioning during the recovery phase, thus lessening patient dissatisfaction. An aesthetician that is uncomfortable with ethnic skin may further aggravate the problem.

RECOMMENDED READING

Cole NM. Limiting risk of medical liability—a surgeon's view. In: Courtiss EH, ed. *Male aesthetic surgery*. St. Louis: Mosby, 1991:18–23.

Edgerton MT. The plastic surgeon's obligation to the emotionally disturbed patient. *Plast Reconstr Surg* 1975;55:83.

Edgerton MT, Langman MW. Psychiatric considerations. In: Courtiss EH, ed. *Male aesthetic surgery*. St. Louis: Mosby, 1991.

Goldwyn R. Patient selection. The importance of being cautious. In: Courtiss EH, ed. *Male aesthetic surgery*. St. Louis: Mosby, 1991:12–17.

Gorney M. Patient selection: an ounce of prevention. In: Courtiss EH, ed. *Male aesthetic surgery*. St. Louis: Mosby, 1991.

Horan DW. Limiting risk of medical liability—a lawyer's view. In: Courtiss EH, ed. *Male aesthetic surgery*. St. Louis: Mosby, 1991:18–23.

Ethnic Considerations in Facial Aesthetic Surgery, edited by W. Earle Matory, Jr.
Lippincott–Raven Publishers, Philadelphia © 1998.

5

Anthropologic and Physiologic Considerations

Blair O. Rogers

Then describe the man fully grown and the woman, and their measurements, and the nature of their complexions, colour, and physiognomy.
— Leonardo da Vinci, *Dell Anatomia*, Fogli B, Vol. I, Chap. III

Anthropologic and physiologic differences in various ethnic groups have long been a fascination of mine. Analysis of these differences enables identification of subgroups that exhibit a higher risk for certain deformities and diseases. Let me share some interesting facts.

In general, Blacks uniformly have the smallest ears of the three major groups: Blacks, Caucasians, and Asians. Most Blacks and Melanesians have a small, rounded concha with a deficient lobule. Interestingly, the majority of Lapps belong to this type; their lobules are usually completely attached. In general Asiatics of the yellow and brown races have the largest ears, and Blacks generally have the smallest ears. The external ear in the White races is commonly intermediate in size between those of the Asiatics and those of the Blacks. Dinaric and Armenoid anthropologically White ethnic groups generally have long ears, almost rectangular in shape, with large fleshy lobules.

Pre-auricular cysts and sinuses occur 5–10 times more frequently in Blacks and Asians than in Caucasians. Pre-auricular appendages are somewhat more common than pits, sinuses, or fistulae, occurring in ~1.5% of the White population. In a routine physical examination of 3,660 White American schoolchildren, Selkirk found 34 cases of pre-auricular cysts or fistulae or an incidence of ~1 in 100 or 1% of the population and an incidence of 5.2% in 346 Black children studied. Females apparently outnumbered males four to one in their susceptibility to the inheritance of congenital auricular fistulae in both Caucasians and Blacks. Aird reports that these pit or sinus defects occur as frequently as in 5–10% of the population in parts of Asia and Africa, thus representing a 5- to 10-fold increase among

B. O. Rogers: Manhattan Eye, Ear, and Throat Hospital, New York, New York 10021

Asians and Africans as compared with White Europeans. Ride observed a 10–14% incidence of pre-auricular pits in the Asiatic population groups of Hong Kong.

There is a much greater incidence of protruding ears in the Celtic groups, which include the Irish, Scottish, some English, and Breton peoples, than in any other group in the White population. Deafness or a hearing impairment may be more likely than previously assumed in any child with protruding ears.

Cryptotia is approximately nine times more prevalent in the Japanese than in Blacks or Caucasians. Studies of New York City longshoremen have shown that hearing acuity among Blacks is superior to that of Caucasians in the higher auditory frequencies. Otosclerosis is very rare among Asians and Blacks; it occurs seven times more frequently among Caucasians than in Blacks in the United States.

Irrespective of age, normal vision is more prevalent in people of color. Myopia is chiefly a disorder of White populations, and its incidence is exceedingly low in African Blacks, American Indians, and Polynesians.

Isolated cleft lip occurs much less frequently in Blacks. Cleft uvula incidence is much lower in the American Black than in the White populations, but cleft uvula in the White is also only one-tenth as common as in the Navajo and other Native American groups.

The shape of the nose varies among populations throughout the world. In general, for example, the nasal bones are relatively large and prominent in Western Europeans, less so in Eastern Europeans such as the Slavs, and much less prominent, smaller, and flatter in people of color. Vertical, oblique, and horizontally directed nostrils are characteristic features of the three basic nasal types: leptorrhine (narrow nose), mesorrhine (medium nose), and platyrrhine (broad nose). Narrow or leptorrhine nostrils are more commonly found in the Northern European and Mediterranean populations, obliquely directed or mesorrhine nostrils are chiefly characteristic of Asians, and flat, platyrrhine nostrils are most frequently seen in Blacks.

The Black African nose often has a low, broad, slightly depressed nasal root; the bridge is usually concave or straight, of a low or medium height, and of great breadth. The tip is commonly thick and bulbous and the nostrils very thick and flaring, with the long axes directed transversely. The whole nose is generally short and very broad at the tip and in the alar margins.

The Asian nose in profile, in contrast to the Black or Caucasian nose, is strongly concave. It has a nasal root and bridge usually much lower than the Black's. Often the Asian nose shows practically no elevation of the root. The root is not as broad and the bridge is often much narrower than that of the Black. The moderately wide nostrils and tip are frequently short and often snubbed in many Asians. The tip is usually not bulbous, and the alar margins are much thinner and less flaring than those of the Black.

The physical differences in the nasal types are perhaps greater in the Caucasoid nose than in people of color. Europeans show a marked diversity of nasal shapes and these have challenged many a physical anthropologist who attempts to develop any clear-cut reference index. In general, however, certain truisms concerning nasal types in Europe and in European–Americans have stood the test of time as emphasized by an extensive description of these differences in an article by Rogers published in 1974.

In Blacks and in Native Americans, septal deviation is seldom seen. Kubota believed that in Japan septal deviation was more frequent in patients with long and narrow faces and narrow nasal shapes. Comparative anatomic studies of the nose have been made in Caucasians, Native Americans, and Blacks. In Blacks, the pyriform crest varies considerably as it descends and curves medially. In some individuals it tends to blend into the alveolar ridge, thus bringing the pyriform aperture floor closer to the level of the nasal floor. In others, it tends to blend into the anterior maxillary spine. Rarely is there a tendency for it to help in forming the superior maxillary spine as it frequently does in Caucasians. Williams found that on the average the width between the pyriform aperture was 4 mm greater in Blacks than in Caucasians. Bridger believes that inspiratory curves in Black nostrils are deeper and more complete. Thus, some authors suggest that the expanded nostrils of the Black might physiologically help to provide a great physical endurance. On the basis of these findings, Williams concluded that Black nostrils in a White person are not conducive to good breathing, while Caucasian-type nostrils and pyramids do not allow good breathing in people of color.

Variations in the attachment of the inferior turbinate to the lateral nasal wall as it relates to the nasal floor and the relationship of the floor of the pyriform aperture to the floor of the vestibule further indicate that the function of these distinctly different Caucasian and Black types of noses "was meant to be different." A Black with a Caucasoid type of nasal pyramid with a high clinical index often complains of definite disturbances in breathing. Similarly, a Caucasian with an external nose and vestibule and a clinical nasal index similar to that of a Black often has disturbances in breathing. It has therefore been suggested that from a reconstructive surgical standpoint, the problem for the surgeon is to alter the shape and size of the nasal cavity and the vestibule so that these structures will function physiologically more in keeping with the patient's ethnic characteristics.

The overall width of any nose, to the eye of the viewer, is primarily determined by the width of the nasal tip and the width of the nasal bones. Whenever one major ethnic group marries another in which there is a wide diversity in ethnic types, one type of nose will often be inherited as dominant. Thus, Davenport and others have demonstrated that in Black–Caucasian mixtures, the offspring are more likely to inherit the broader Black nose rather than the narrower Caucasoid nose. In 1928 Dunn found that the broad nose dominated the narrow nose in its prevalence among offspring of ethnic Hawaiians and Caucasians.

In populations in whom a major ethnic cross-breeding occurs, such as in Blacks and Native Americans, the higher convex nasal bridge of the Native American is dominant in the sibling inheritance pattern over the flatter concave nasal bridge of the Black. In addition, in European–Eskimo admixtures, the higher European nasal bridge is dominant over the flatter, wider, Eskimo nasal bridge.

In terms of certain congenital deformities, studies of scaphocephaly, one of the deformities found in Crouzon's disease, for example, show there is a marked difference in the scaphocephalic head form of Blacks compared with Caucasians and Asians, thus suggesting different patterns of skull growth in these three major ethnic groups. Polydactylism, for an example, occurs nine times more frequently in Black than in Caucasian newborns. Inguinal hernias seem to be five times more prevalent in Black than in Caucasian newborns, and umbilical hernias are nine times more common in Black newborns. Basal cell carcinomas predominate chiefly in light-skin groups, especially among the Irish, Scottish, and Scandinavian ethnic groups, since their skin cancers are most commonly actinic, whereas in the other major groups, the Black and the Asian, the predominant skin cancers are squamous cell carcinomas that frequently arise in regions of thermal and chemical irritation and/or ulceration. In Blacks, melanomas are found almost exclusively on the most weakly pigmented areas, the palms and especially the soles of the feet. From the standpoint of cosmesis and aesthetics, the following statement by the Committee on Cosmetics of the American Medical Association is of ethnic interest: "Because of the fact that Negro skin has natural protection in its high melanin content, elderly Negroes often appear deceptively young." Keloids, of course, are chiefly a problem in Blacks and to a lesser extent in some Asians.

A number of hematologic diseases are restricted primarily to members of certain ethnic groups: sickle cell anemia in Blacks, thalassemia in persons of Mediterranean origin, and pernicious anemia in Caucasians. Specific hematologic differences between the major ethnic groups and between lesser sub-divisions of these ethnic groups have been increasingly reported in the literature within the last 4 decades. Healthy African Americans, without tropical diseases, liver disease, malnutrition, or parasitic infestations, have significantly elevated levels of all immunoglobulins as contrasted with comparable White Americans. Significantly higher serum cholesterol levels exist in the White ethnic groups of Western Europe as compared with the lower levels in Asians.

In a review of 30,398 consecutive live births recorded at hospitals in Brooklyn, NY, U.S.A., from 1952 to 1955, anomalies of the central nervous system were shown to be four times more common in Caucasian than in Black infants. Spina bifida, meningocele, and hydrocephaly often occurred together. Congenital malformations occur more frequently in White ethnic groups than in Blacks in a ratio of 2 : 1.

The reader interested in a much more detailed enumeration and listing of ethnic disease and deformity patterns is referred to Richard's comprehensive text, *Le Facteur Racial dans la Pathologie*. These many anatomic and physiologic considerations make us privy to the many clinical applications that are described elsewhere in this text.

The literature defines most facial differences among ethnic groups, based upon anthropologic, anthropometric, or photographic studies of young adults. The faces of elderly persons, regardless of their ethnic group, are less reliable as anthropologic parameters, because of the pathologic and anatomic ramifications of aging. Chief among these are the loss of skin elasticity and muscular and skeletal atrophy. Among those features characteristic of the aging face that make anthropometry unreliable are the sagging or changing of soft tissue points of measurement. Ear lobules tend in most older people to elongate and droop due to the loss of elasticity. This is especially true of many Eastern Mediterranean peoples such as Syrians, Lebanese, Greeks, and Turks, whose lobules tend to become longer with age. The soft tissues of the nasal tip frequently drop with advanced age, much more noticeable in these latter mentioned groups. Absorption of buccal fat pads in the cheeks, sagging and drooping of the eyelids and their adjacent canthal landmarks, and destructive changes in dentition tend to make any facial measurements based upon any or all of these features extremely variable and therefore unreliable. The consistency achieved by Farkas in the use of anthropologic measurements in young adults, by contrast to older adults, was demonstrated in the work of Churchill et al. in which different anthropomorphic facial and body increments in 15 different race/age/national origin–specific groups were studied.

RECOMMENDED READING

Aird I. *A companion to surgical studies*. Edinburgh: Livingstone, 1949:360.
Alhady SMA, Kandian S. Keloids in various races. *Plast Reconstr Surg* 1969;44:564.
Altemus LA. The incidence of cleft lip and palate among American Negroes. *Cleft Palate J* 1966;3:357.
Altmann F. Malformations of the auricle and the external auditory meatus: a critical review. *Arch Otolaryngol* 1951;54:115.
Altmann F, Glasgold A, MacDuff JP. The incidence of otosclerosis as related to race and sex. *Ann Otol* 1967;76:377.
Becker PE, ed. *Humangenetik*. Stuttgart: Georg Thieme Verlag, 1964.
Berg JW. Some intercountry and intergroup differences in histological types of cancer. *J Chronic Dis* 1970;23:325.
Bridger GP. Physiology of the nasal valve. *Arch Otolaryngol* 1970;92:543.
Churchill E, Robinow D, Erskine P. Factor analyses of anthropometric data for fifteen race-age-national origins specific groups. Presented at the IXth International Congress of Anthropological and Ethnological Sciences, Chicago, Aug. 28 to Sept. 8, 1973.
Cottle MH. From lectures given during a course: Introduction to fundamentals of reconstructive surgery of nasal septum and external nasal pyramid. Illinois Masonic Hospital, Chicago, Oct. 3–10, 1953.
Cottle MH. The structure and function of the nasal vestibule. *Arch Otolaryngol* 1955;62:173.
Davenport CB. Post-nasal development of the human outer nose. *Proc Am Philos Soc* 1939;80:175.
Davenport CB, Steggerda M. *Race crossing in Jamaica*. Washington, D.C.: Carnegie Institute, 1929.
Farkas LG. The position of anthropology from the view-point of plastic surgery. *Anthropologie* 1968;6:3.
Farkas LG, WK. Morphology of adult after repair of isolated cleft palate in childhood. *Cleft Palate J* 1972;9:132.
Fomon S, et al. Physiological principles in rhinoplasty. *Arch Otolaryngol* 1951;53:256.
Frazier TM. A note on race-specific congenital malformation rater. *Gynecology* 1960;80:184.
Gates RR. Études sur le croisement des races. III. Nouvelles observations concernant les oreilles, en particulier les lobes. *J Hum Genet* 1954;3:95.
Holm S. Les état deis refvvion oculaine les palenegrides au Gabon, Afrique Equatoriale Francaise. *Acta Ophthalmol [Suppl]* 1937;13:1.
Ivy RH. Congenital deformities recorded on birth certificates in Pennsylvania, 1961–1965: with special reference to racial influence on incidence. *Plast Reconstr Surg* 1968;41:50.
Jost G, Meresse B, Torossian F. Étude des la jonction entre les cartilages latéraux du nez. *Ann Chir Plast* 1973;18:175.
Karayalcin G, Rosner F, Sawitsky A. Quantitative serum immunoglobulins in healthy Negroes. *NY State J Med* 1973;751.
Karsai LK, Bergman M, Young BC. Hearing in ethnically different longshoremen. *Arch Otolaryngol* 1972;96:449.
Lewis MG. Malignant melanoma in Uganda. *Br J Cancer* 1967;21:483.
Morel-Fatio D, Pales L. Considérations ethnographiques sur l'étiologie des chéloides. *Ann Chir Plast* 1956;1:11.
Oluwasanmi JO. Keloids in the African. *Clin Plast Surg* 1974;1:179.
Richard JJ. *Le facteur racial dans la pathologie*. Paris: Gauthier-Villars, 1963.
Richardson ER. Cleft uvula: incidence in Negroes. *Cleft Palate J* 1970;7:669.

Ride L. Discussion. Trans 11th Assembly of International Federation of Eugenic Organizations. *Arch Int Klaus Stiftg* 1935;10:42.
Rogers BO. The role of physical anthropology in plastic surgery today. *Clin Plast Surg* 1974;1:439.
Schwarz M, Becker PE. Anomalien, Missbildungen und Krankheiten der Ohren, der Nase und des Halses. In: Becker PE, ed. *Humangenetik*. Stuttgart: Georg Thieme Verlag, 1964.
Selkirk TK. Fistula auris congenita. *Amer J Dis Child* 1935;49:431.
Sesgin MZ, Stark RB. The incidence of congenital defects. *Plast Reconstr Surg* 1961;27:261.
Shapiro RN, et al. The incidence of congenital anomalies discovered in the neonatal period. *Am J Surg* 1958;96:396.
van der Linden W, Nakayama F. Gallstone disease in Sweden versus Japan: clinical and etiologic aspects. *Am J Surg* 1973;125:267.
Verlee DL. Ophthalmic survey in the Solomon Islands. *Am J Ophthalmol* 1968;66:304.
Williams RI. The nasal index: anthropological and clinical. *Ann Otol Rhinol Laryngol* 1956;65:171.
Williams RI. Physiology of the nose in reconstructive surgery. *Rocky Mountain Med J* 1954;51:352.
Ziegelmayer G. Aussere Nase. In: Becker PE, ed. *Humangenetik*. Stuttgart: Georg Thieme Verlag, 1964:56–81.

SECTION II

Definitions of Beauty

Ethnic Considerations in Facial Aesthetic Surgery, edited by W. Earle Matory, Jr.
Lippincott–Raven Publishers, Philadelphia © 1998.

6

Parameters of Caucasian Attractiveness

Hale Tolleth

The face is the soul of the body.
— Wittgenstein

Santayana declared, "Beauty as we feel it is something indescribable: What it is or what it means can never be said" (1). Pope said, "It is not a lip or eye we beauty call but all the joint force and full result of all" (2). The concept of beauty conjures in us a mental picture of the very special, whereas attractive is more a part of ordinary experience. We attempt to define, describe, and analyze it because, as Taschek said, "No other object in the visual world has so much salience for us, so much power over us, as the human face" (3).

Aside from the aesthetic sensation produced by the contemplation of the beautiful, there are practical necessities to determine the parameters of human attractiveness. Mere intuition and opinion are not enough. Shakespeare anticipated this when he wrote, "Beauty is bought by the judgment of the eye and not altered by the base sale of chapmen's [peddler's] tongues" (4). Determining the essence and nature of this quality has occupied us individually and collectively at least from the time of the Egyptians 4,000 years ago (5–15). Unfortunately, the artistic rules that we believe must have aided Thutmose in creating the Nefertiti bust have been lost and must be intuited from the work itself (16). Similarly, the "classical canons" of the Greeks that have survived through the work of Renaissance scholars are so few and trivial as to be of little use. We impute from the sculpture of the Greeks what they believed to be ideal, though even that may be a questionable enterprise since many of the widely admired Greek sculpture pieces are Roman copies (17–18).

The development of Greek art and sculpture beginning almost a millennium before the Common Era has had an enormous influence on Western ideals of human beauty (19). The sculpture of the 6th and 7th centuries B.C.E., although of great aesthetic interest, appear

H. Tolleth: Concord, California 94520

stiff, angular, and geometric. However, by the 4th century sculptors had developed a fluidity and harmony of such appeal that Phidias was said to give a "new conception of the divine" in his work (18). To explain the remarkable development of exquisite sculpture of the human form, it has been suggested that models were used and the sculptor modified and corrected, working until the piece was "ideal"—which may express a too facile and simplistic explanation of the process of creation and development of an art over an extended period of time. The gradual evolution of what constituted ideal shape, proportion, and the aesthetically pleasing appears more likely to have developed from experience, constant practice, and trial and error. Unlike the Romans who produced realistic or idealized portraits, the Greek sculptor was expected to produce a god-like ideal.

For the most part we, trained or untrained, are able, without apparent effort or analysis, to perceive the most attractive (20–21). Surprisingly, within a culture there is considerable agreement as to who are the beautiful, but it is of greater interest that perception of beauty may cross time, cultural, or ethnic lines contrary to commonly held opinion (22–25).

To avoid the inadequacies created by unqualified opinion, dubious presumption, uncertain observation, or unsupported intuition, the research into the nature of attractiveness has focused on measuration and recording, creating means and averages of certain limited groups, seeking in general the "normal" and the limits of normal (26–28). Often the subjects have been evaluated by some sort of judging panel with the characteristics of the studied group varying widely in terms of age, ethnicity, celebrity, or attractiveness (29–33). The characteristics of the chosen then are evaluated. There is an implicit assumption that the average would be attractive; however, it has been shown that the attractive may very well differ substantially from this (34–36). Although we persist in these efforts, virtually any sculptor or portraitist will point out that virtually imperceptible changes in line, curve, angle, texture, or color may seriously alter the perception of beauty.

If surgeons and orthodontists have focused their attention on attractive subjects, hoping that a formula might be adduced, the psychologists and sociologists have, especially in the recent past, looked at the viewer of the subject as an important part of the issue, confirming Hume's observation in the 1700s that "beauty in things exists in the mind which contemplates them" (37), or the commonly repeated cliché from Hungerford who said in 1843 that "beauty is in the eye of the beholder" (38).

The question as to why attractiveness is so valued is beyond our scope; however, it deserves comment. For example, the psychologists Dion and Berscheid entitled an article, "What Is Beautiful Is Good," and many others have opined that those who are attractive have multiple advantages that the less attractive do not (39–41). Research into this aspect of human appearance seem to have been delayed since it was speculated that the researchers were uncomfortable were they to find that beautiful is better. It would be discomfiting if it were found that dates were made and mates chosen on the basis of appearance rather than the presumably sounder criteria of honesty, intelligence, humor, skills, etc. Be that as it may, it has been found that attractive women are perceived as more intelligent, better potential wives, more charming, etc. Attractive children are treated differently, rated as more intelligent, receive more attention, and get better grades than the less so. Attractive men get better jobs and are economically more successful (45). Apparently this situation crosses cultural and time lines and has been true historically as well, recalling that Helen had a face that was "able to launch a thousand ships." It has been further posited that in an evolutionary sense attractiveness may create survival advantage, and capacity to perceive attractiveness is not very different from other kinds of discriminative judgment clearly previously demonstrated in many animal species (46–48).

Keeping in mind that "our ability to make almost any kind of judgment or calculation far exceeds our capacity to understand how we make them," can we determine general or specific characteristics of attractiveness (49)? Symonds states that there are only two absolute criteria for attractiveness, age (youthfulness) and good health, implying that signs of aging or evidence of disease or deformity are serious detriments to the perception of beauty (50). Relative criteria are the appearance of high status or dominance, which may explain some of the rather odd human pairings observed and peculiar twists of fashion. Fashion, or its imitation, is apparently an attempt to emulate those perceived to have status or power and will therefore enhance the person who imitates. The use, then, of the beautiful or powerful to sell products is clearly a sound business judgment.

Specific anatomical characteristics have been determined to be attractive and include a full head of hair, smooth complexion, large eyes, small nose, full lips, slightly protrusive lower face, high cheekbones, and so forth (51–53). Features of negative value include significant disproportion, asymmetry, excessive size, abnormal shape, convexity of the profile, retrusion of the chin, laxity of the skin associated with aging, thinness of lips, large nose, absent, irregular, or discolored teeth, excessive show of the gums, and so forth. Here one might introduce the concept of "too," which the lay person uses to describe any inadequacy of feature, such as too big, too little, too thin, too fat, etc. The limits of "too" for the individual patient may seem ill defined but are arguably no less adequate than reliance on arbitrary averages or opinion.

If "too" is a parameter for the ordinary person and millimeters the tool of the researcher, "god-like" was the measure of perfection for the Greeks in sculpture and it fit well their concept of the perfect mind and body in a well ordered universe. The unifying basis between life, art, the gods, and universe was believed to be mathematics. Perfection, harmony, and balance could surely be revealed by the study of numbers and theorems of Pythagoras. According to the Pythagoreans, "Everything is arranged according to the numbers" (54). The concept had such appeal that the secrets revealed by the study of mathematics as a source of perfection became a central part of the ritual and teaching of secret societies of architects, masons, and medieval guilds of the Middle Ages. One of the remarkable events in mathematics was the concept of "pi," the ratio of the circumference to the diameter of the circle. It seemed almost mysterious in its implication and powerful in its wide application in mathematics and geometry. Similarly, the concept of the golden mean or "phi" produced profound influence on aesthetics since it supplied a rational basis for analysis and supported the philosophy of a well ordered universe.

THE GOLDEN PROPORTION

Phi, so-called after Phidias, the Greek sculptor, was mathematically most clearly defined in the 1200s by Leonardo of Pisa called Filius Bonacci, or Fibonacci, an Arab-trained mathematician of exceeding skill who had brought the concept of zero into use in the Mediterranean world of trade (55–56). In solving what appeared to be a trivial problem regarding the number of rabbits that would be obtained starting with a pair and reproducing regularly, the solution indicated a sequence of numbers: 1, 1, 2, 3, 5, 8, 13, etc. The sequence can be carried to infinity adding any two adjacent numbers to produce the next in the sequence. Each number of any pair is in the same ratio to any other pair, that is, 5 is to 8 as 8 is to 13 and so forth. The ratio of these numbers is 1.618 and is known as phi. It has been called the golden number; its reciprocal 1/1.1618 is 0.618 and is said to be the single number in mathematics whose reciprocal is 1 less than the primary number. A line *ABC* in which *AB*/*AC* is equal to *BC*/*AB* is called a golden section. A rectangle with sides of the ratio is called a golden rectangle; similarly, an isosceles triangle is called golden if the sides are 1.618 and the base 1 (Fig. 1). A spiral equivalent to the spiral of the chambered nautilus, a pentagram, and other figures can be created using phi, further confirming some kind of "universality" and special quality of the number.

Although aesthetic satisfaction may be enjoyed by the mathematically inclined, more consequentially this peculiar proportion occurs repeatedly in nature: petals in a sunflower, leaf arrangement on a stem, relationship in length between a phalanx and its metacarpal, even distances between certain points on the human face; the examples are almost innumerable (57–60). In Greek architecture the golden proportion is said to have been used in the design of the Parthenon. To mention a trivial example, it may be no accident that filing cards are 3×5 or 5×8 in., representing examples of the golden rectangle. There appears to be no obvious good reason why the golden mean, triangle, rectangle, and so forth would be preferred over any other proportion; however, Guggenheim has stated that there are general biologic needs that influence aesthetic judgment: clarity and simplicity for orientation,

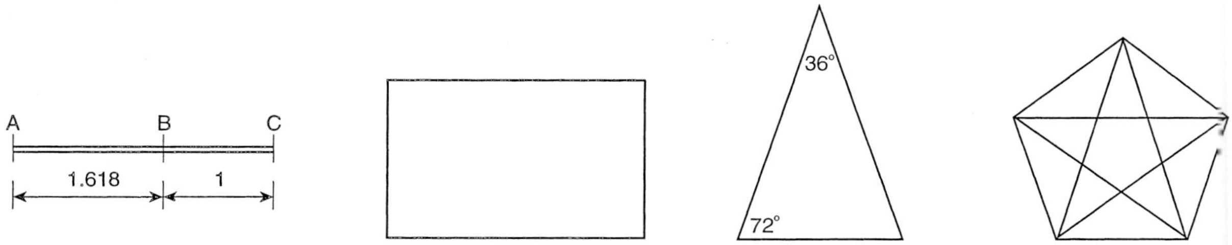

Figure 1. The golden line where *AB* is to *AC* as *BC* is to *AB*. The golden rectangle represents unbreakable unity (see text). The golden triangle has a base of 1 and sides of 1.618, and finally the pentagram has five equal sides formed of five golden triangles. Each of the lines forming the star has golden relationships between segments.

balance and unity for tranquility and good function, and variety and tension for stimulation (1, 12). The golden rectangle represents "unbreakable unity and lively tension" (49). If one were to consider the aesthetic merits of the golden section of the line previously mentioned, there has, in fact, been work done to show that it is not necessarily preferred over other segmented lines, although the golden rectangle has been shown to be clearly preferred. In the human face, the golden proportion has been thoroughly discussed by Ricketts and others (58–60), and Marquardt has created a pentagram-based overlay that can be used in analysis of aesthetic relationship problems of the face (Figs. 2 and 3) (61).

APPRAISAL

An observer appraises appearance first "by the eye," taking in the overall shape, size, color, texture, animation, expression, posture, and so forth, being able in a brief time to assess the whole and even the degree of attractiveness. It has been observed "that the typical product of the mature artist is so intricate that only intuitive perception is capable or orga-

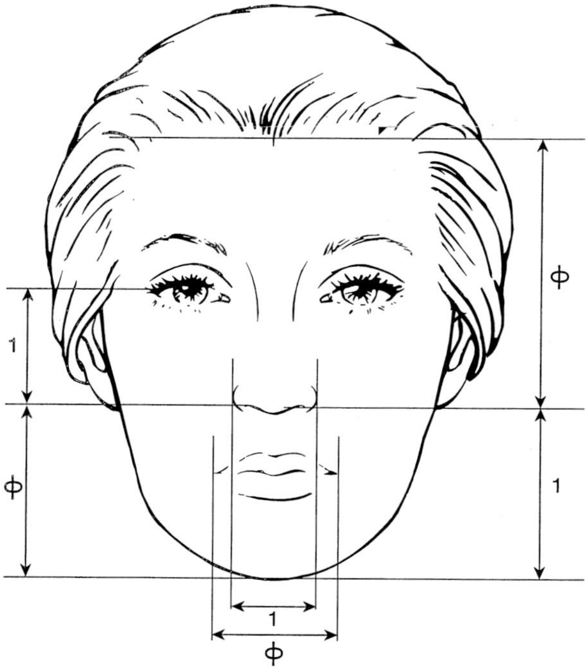

Figure 2. Examples of golden relationships of the face. (Modified from Ricketts RM. Divine proportion in facial esthetics. *Clin Plast Surg* 1982; 9:401.)

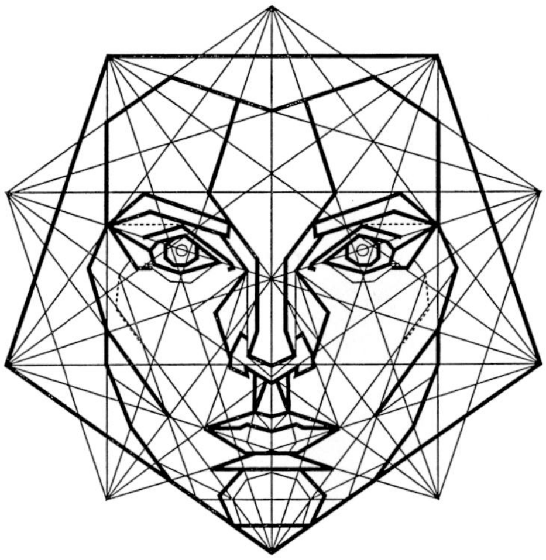

Figure 3. The computer diagram designed as a plastic overlay developed by Marquardt for aesthetic analysis of the face.

nizing and unifying the multiplicity of forces that make up the whole" (12). It is important to note that the face is not a static object but a particularly dynamic one. Focusing exclusively on the static face as in pictures, photographs, x-rays, painting, or sculpture is to seriously impair the adequacy of one's understanding of the distinctive status of the human face as an object of aesthetic judgment.

Subjective judgment does not meet easily identifiable criteria; however, the necessity to alter or modify human physiognomy requires an evaluative system. For example, one could describe hair as rich, thick, brown, short, curly—creating a sufficiently accurate word picture for the hairdresser. As a practical matter, little would be gained by counting hairs, measuring diameter of hair shafts, determining light reflectance, and so forth. Clearly, useful analysis is one that fits the task, suggesting that observation and intuitive capacity may be acceptable tools. Symmetry can be both estimated or measured depending on the need. Certain parameters such as volumes, masses, curves, and shapes can be measured, but the effort and tools required are often so cumbersome that estimation will be preferred. Similarly, texture and other characteristics can be more meaningfully described with well chosen language.

If an orderly scheme is chosen, one might evaluate first the whole proceeding from the general to the specific or the larger to the smaller. First, the general shape and volume of the cranium in relationship to the face on at least three views are noted (Fig. 4) (62–63). The rel-

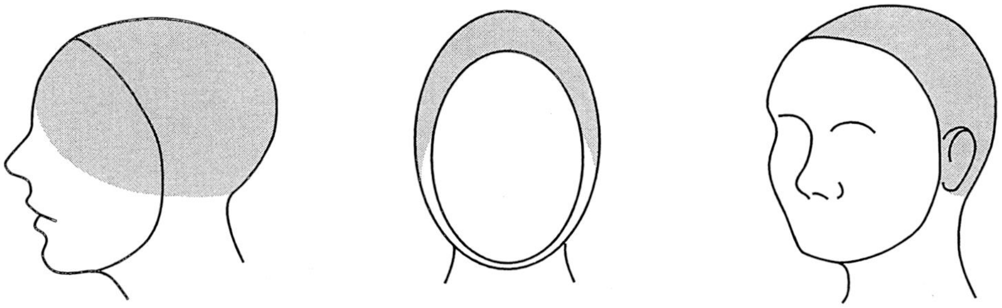

Figure 4. The volume and shape of the cranium, though often obscured by hair, are of significance in appraising the whole. No single view adequately defines its appearance.

ative length and breadth of the head and the shape of the face are determined (Fig. 5). The volume estimation of the mid and lower face using the scheme of Barnett and Whitaker is useful (Fig. 6) (64). The curves of the face from the front and profile views are described (Fig. 7) and then the convexity or concavity of the face and facial inclination (Figs. 8 and 9). Legan and Burstone have described a specific measurement of facial convexity (Fig. 10) (65).

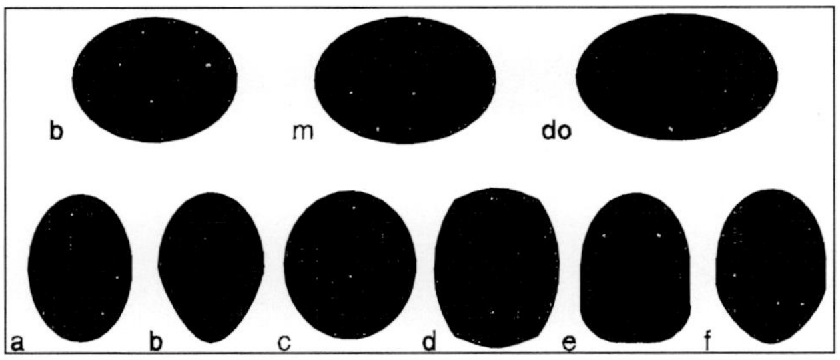

Figure 5. *B-M-DO* indicate the anthropological description of cranial length from the top view: brachycephalic *(B)*, meso- or normocephalic *(M)*, and dolichocephalic *(DO)*. Facial shape is almost infinite, but a simple system includes oval **(A)**, heart **(B)**, round **(C)**, square **(D)**, compound round head and square jaw **(E)**, and compound round head and oval jaw **(F)**.

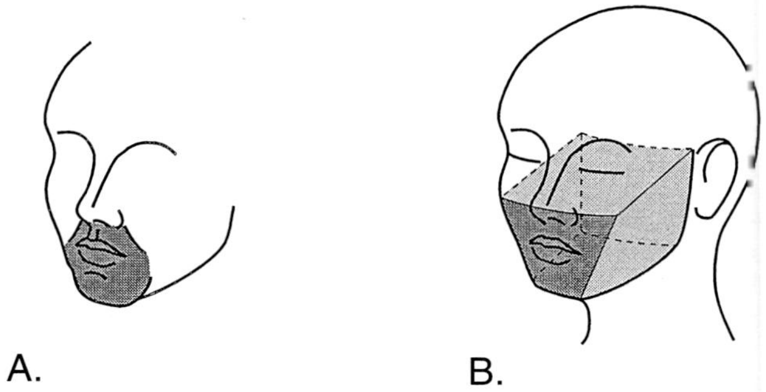

Figure 6. A: The sculptor's "mouth barrel," virtually the primary focus of attention in the human face. **B:** The volume of the lower face delineated by Barnett and Whittaker is useful in appraising the volumetric form and relationship.

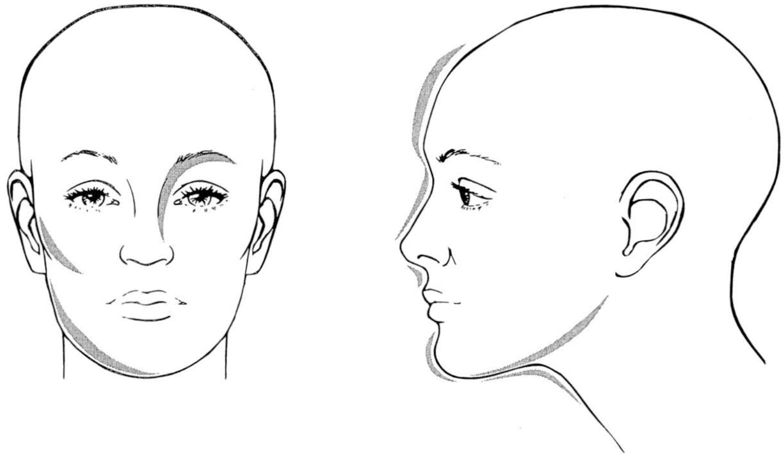

Figure 7. The "curvilinear consideration" where consonant curves contribute to harmony. Angularity in any of these in the female face may diminish attractiveness. (Modified from Peck.)

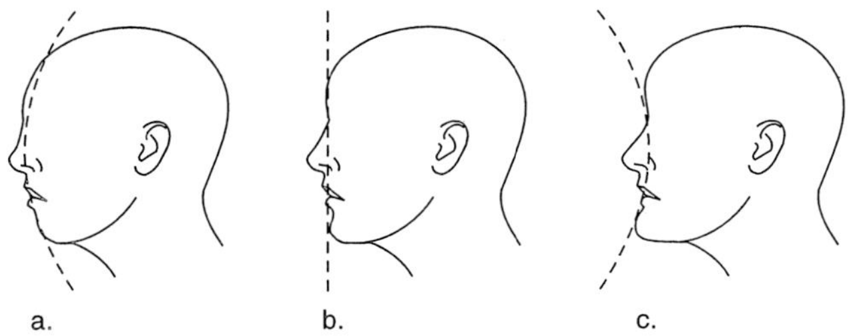

Figure 8. A–C: Another appraisal method describes the appearance of convexity or concavity of the profile.

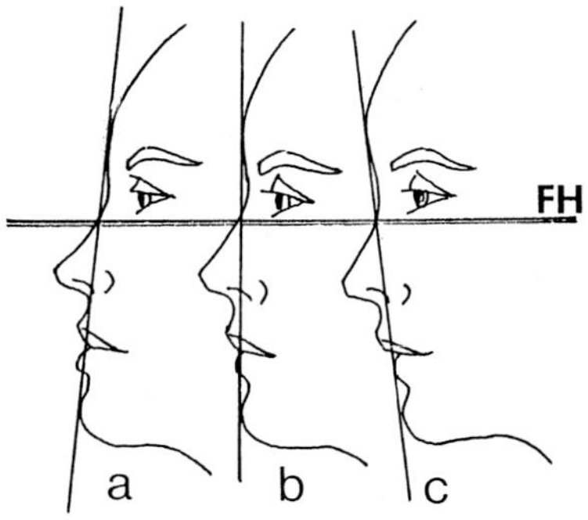

Figure 9. Facial inclination relative to the Frankfort horizontal. Each profile is essentially equivalent, indicating the potential reduction of attractiveness as the face is altered from the vertical.

PROPORTIONS

With no more than the eye and a ruler, rapid appraisal of a face will produce considerable information and inform the examiner as to the source of some problems and the rough degree of variance from acceptable norm. Proportional evaluation is simply recalled and diagrammed with ease either by dividing the face in halves or thirds (Figs. 11 and 12). Horizontal and vertical guidelines are illustrated by the grid in Fig. 13, indicating that the ovoid face can be described with a grid that is five eye widths wide and eight eye widths long. The eyes sit on a line equidistant from vertex to chin. With that as a primary reference line, the position of the eyebrow is drawn, which allows a line to be drawn upon which the nose sits equidistant between brow and chin. Equidistant from the base of the nose and the chin

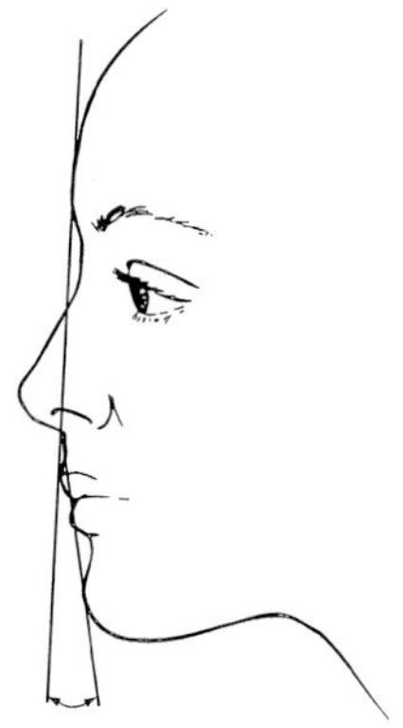

Figure 10. Angle of facial convexity using glabella, subnasion, and pogonion points. Legan indicates normal is 12° (range 8–16°).

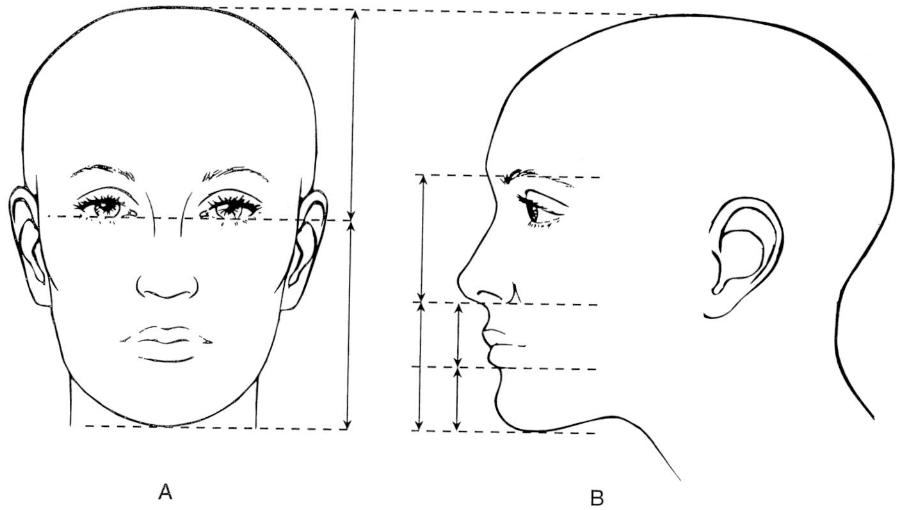

Figure 11. The classical and simplest of the proportion systems. **A:** The eyes sit on line halfway between the top of the head and the chin. **B:** The brow to base of columella distance is equal to the base of columella to chin distance and the line upon which the lower lip sits divides equally the distance from the base of the columella to the chin.

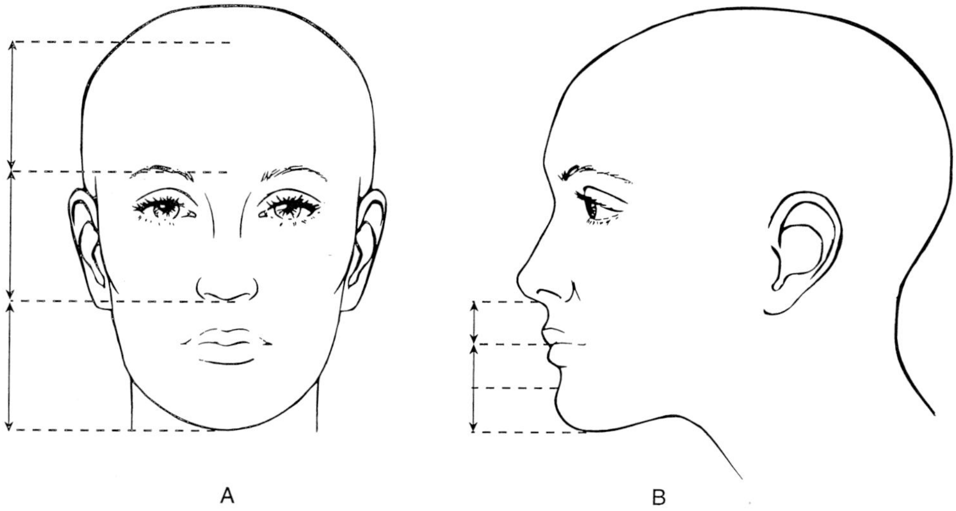

Figure 12. Another classical system of proportion that divides the face into thirds. **A:** Chin to nose, nose to brow, and brow to trichion. **B:** Similarly the lower third can be divided into thirds: Base of nose to lip embrasure is one-third and embrasure to chin is two-thirds.

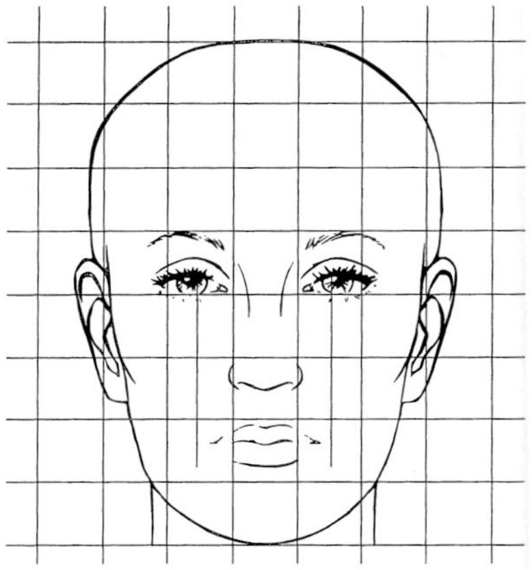

Figure 13. A classical grid showing that the face as five eye widths wide and eight eye widths vertically; the eyes are one eye width apart and the mouth is two eye widths, or about in line with the medial pupil margin. The top of the ear is at the eyebrow level and the ear lobules at or below the nasal alae.

is a line upon which the vermilion lips sit. This is an exceedingly simple system, although the system of thirds may be used as shown in Fig. 12. This divides the face from trichion to chin as equal thirds and the distance from base of columella to chin into thirds also. The top of the ear is roughly on a level with the eyebrow; the ear sits approximately one ear length back from the lateral brow. The medial canthi are one eye width apart and the nose at the region of the alae is very slightly wider than that. The corners of the mouth are on a vertical dropped from the medial pupil. Refinement of the proportion systems has been done by percentages and also by careful measurement. In a specific problem, reference to the extensive tables from the careful work of Farkas provides extensive linear and angular measurements. Many of the measurements used in the various diagrams presented here represent modification or rounding off of his figures, which were made on a relatively limited group of 6- to 18-year-old boys and girls apparently randomly chosen.

CEPHALOMETRICS

Since the early 1930s when Broadbent developed an analysis system of the lateral x-ray of the head, cephalometrics have become a primary tool for the orthodontist (66). Schendel

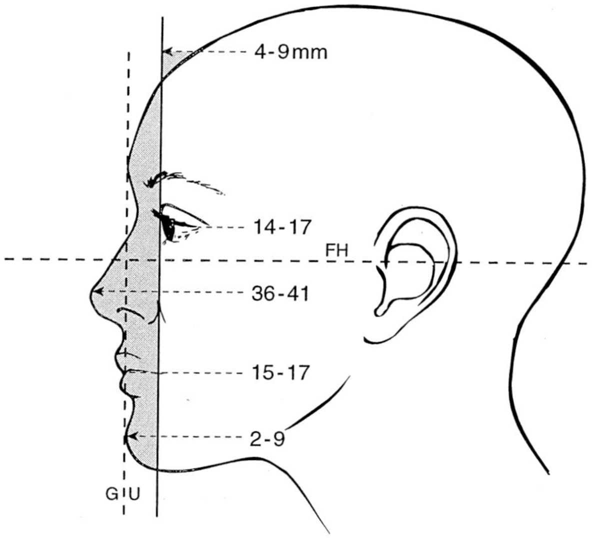

Figure 14. Vertical facial plane at right angles to the Frankfort horizontal at the position of the cornea. GU labels the vertical facial plane as described by Gonzalez-Ulloa. (Modified from Farkas LG. *Anthropometry of the head and face in medicine*. New York: Elsevier North Holland, 1981.)

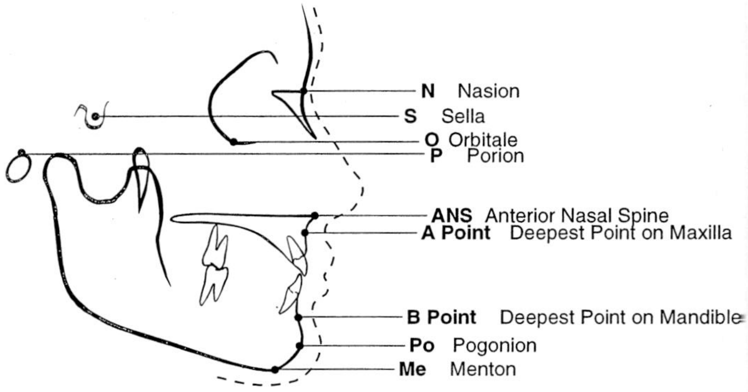

Figure 15. Scheme for labeling profile points on the lateral cephalogram.

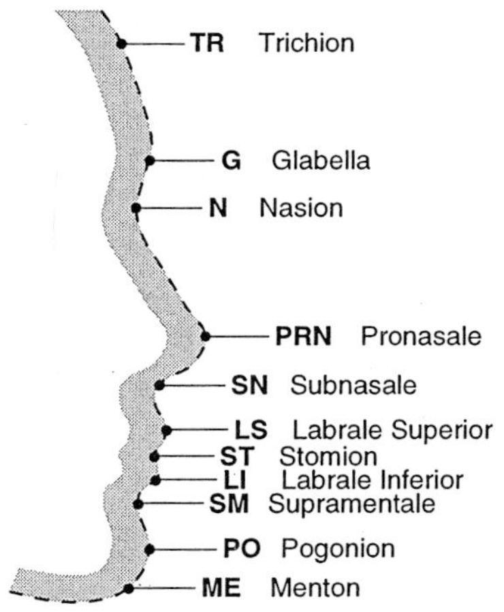

Figure 16. The scheme used for labeling soft tissue points on the lateral cephalogram.

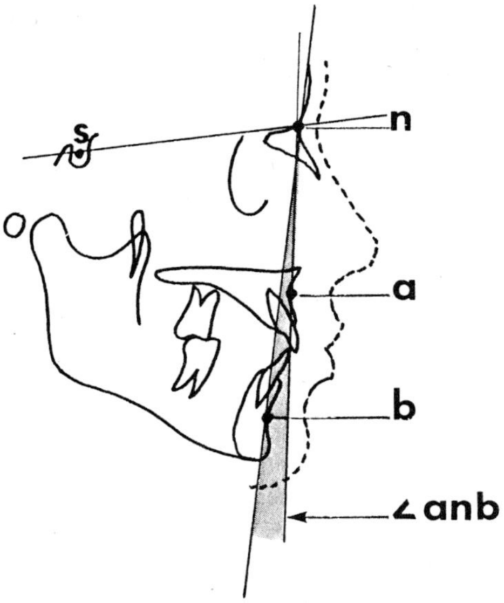

Figure 17. Angles *Sna* and *Snb* or angle *anb* describe the relative positions of maxilla and mandible. *Sna* is 82°, *Snb* 80°, and *anb* 2°.

notes that "what began as a relatively simple dental analysis has become a more complex skeletal analysis enhanced by soft tissue standards" (67). The sophistication has increased greatly and average measurements and standards of normality are relatively secure. Diagnosis, planning, and determination of treatment results are facilitated. Inevitably, multiple systems have been put forward, each with putative advantage and no method preferred or used by all (68–72). One must be clear that serious primary disadvantages are built in: Profile represents only a single view of a complex three-dimensional structure, and there may be as little as 60% correlation with clinical diagnosis (67). Although two-dimensional evaluation is simple, the human face is least commonly observed from the lateral vantage point, and there is an uncertain relationship with aesthetics or estimate of attractiveness. Both conceptual and technical handicaps have been described (74). Though cephalometric analysis is simple, rapid, standardized, and widely used, the information obtained is essentially skeletal and dental and reference points are relatively arbitrary and have limited application to aesthetics.

A primary reference line in cephalometrics is the Frankfort horizontal, a line traced from the superior border of the auditory canal to the infraorbital rim on the lateral head film; in the living subject, the line is traced from the upper attachment of the tragus to the palpable infraorbital rim (Fig. 14). With standardization the Frankfort horizontal is commonly ad-

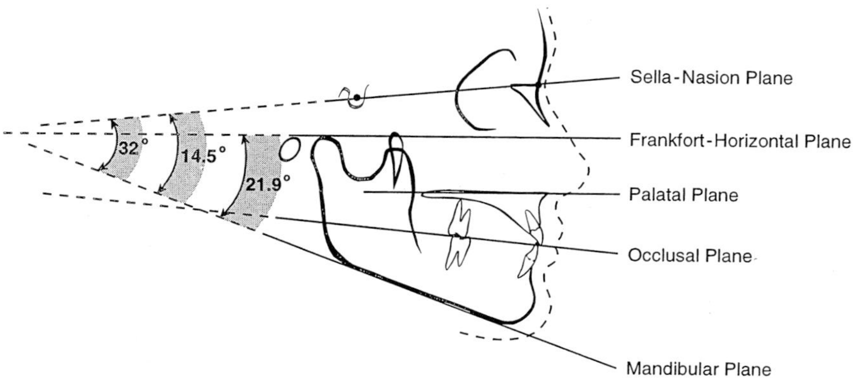

Figure 18. Angular measurements made on the lateral cephalogram to indicate relative vertical position. The palatal plane is usually within 2–3° of the Frankfort horizontal. The mandibular plane angle when increased or steep describes the "long" lower face.

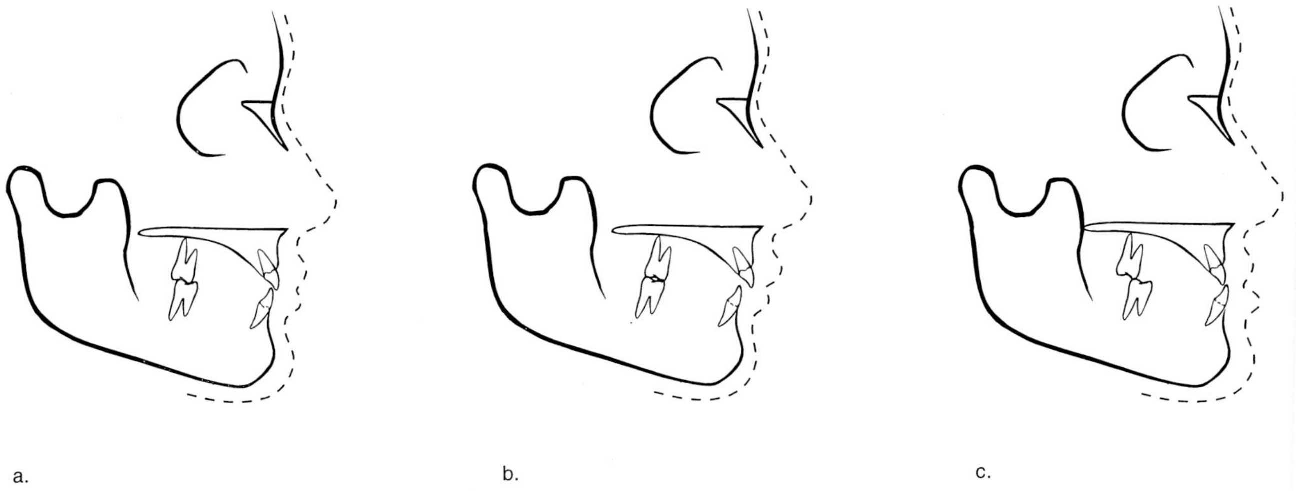

Figure 19. Edward Angle classified malocclusion (or occlusion) as Class I, II, or III based on the relative position of maxillary and mandibular first molars. **A:** Class I (normal relationship); **B:** Class II (retrognathic); **C:** Class III (prognathic).

justed to be parallel to the floor, although that may not represent the usual head posture. A vertical line intersecting the Frankfort plane at right angles at the glabella or the cornea has been used as a reference to describe the anteroposterior position of the facial features, its convexity or concavity, and relative position of nose, lips, and chin (15, 27, 28).

Reference points are marked on the lateral cephalogram as shown in Fig. 15. Similarly, soft tissue points can be marked as in Fig. 16. Note that the terms and abbreviations may vary from author to author, although the points are essentially the same. The plane from sella to nasion is also a primary reference plane. A line drawn from nasion point *A* in the anterior maxilla or to point *B* in the mandible allows the creation of angle *ANB* and describes the relative anteroposterior position of the maxilla and mandible in reference to each other (Fig. 17).

A series of planes have been used to describe the relative proportion and position of the mid and lower face, including the *S-N* plane, Frankfort horizontal, the palatal plane, the occlusal plane, and the mandibular plane as shown in Fig. 18.

It may be necessary in a given case to determine the position of the teeth, soft tissue, and skeleton since the correction of a problem may require alteration of any or all of the three elements (76). Further, the movement or change of a single element will inevitably and often uncertainly affect the other two. Edward Angle, the father of orthodontics, declared that dental occlusion (or malocclusion) should be described as Class I orthognathic, where the maxillary and mandibular first molars occluded as in Fig. 19. In Class II, or retrognathic, the maxillary molar appears to precede the mandibular, and in Class III, or prognathic, the mandibular molar appears to excessively precede the maxillary molar (77). Profiles would then appear to be straight in Class I, midface protrusive in Class II, and lower jaw protrusive in Class III. Further refinements are commonly used and a given patient may be described as either dental class or skeletal class.

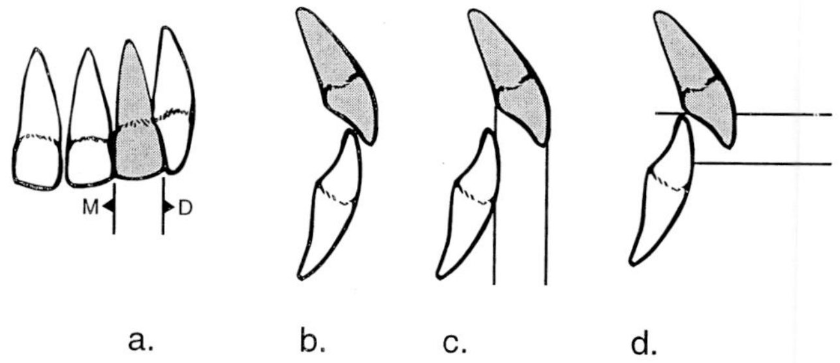

Figure 20. **A:** The mesial *(M)* aspect of the tooth, a lateral incisor, is closest to the midline and distal *(D)* is posterior. **B:** In normal occlusal relationship the upper incisor does not overlap the lower incisor by more than a third of the visible lower incisor. **C:** Overjet in which the upper incisor precedes the lower. **D:** Overbite where the upper incisor overlaps the lower incisor.

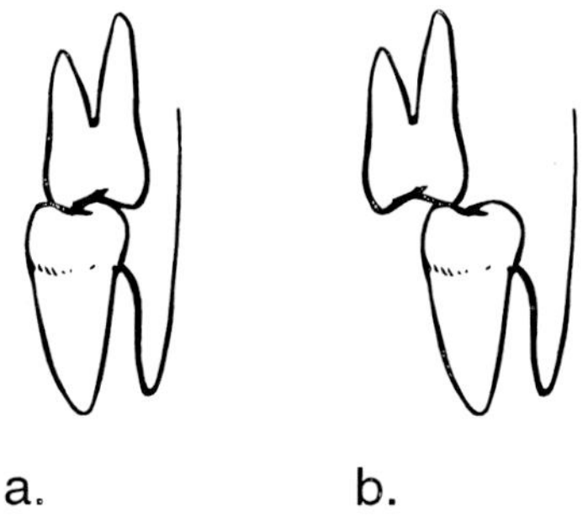

Figure 21. A: Normal molar relationship. **B:** Posterior cross-bite occurs when the lingual cusp of the maxillary molar is lingual to the mandibular molar.

A few relationships in regard to the teeth may be useful for the non-dentist, including overbite, in which the incisors overlap, and overjet, in which the upper incisors precede the lower (Fig. 20). Open bite is present when the anterior teeth do not occlude when the posterior teeth are in contact or vice versa.

In describing cross-bite the dental descriptive terms of mesial, distal, lingual, labial, and buccal must be used. The mesial surface of the tooth is closest to the midline, and the distal posterior (Fig. 20). Labial or buccal surfaces are on contact with the lip or cheek, and the lingual with the tongue (Fig. 21). Anterior cross-bite, then, occurs when the upper teeth are lingual to the lower and posterior cross-bite when the molars are excessively lingual or buccal.

Angle and subsequently others repeated the idea that normal or good occlusion was related to good harmony of the face; however, in recent years it has been shown that improvement in occlusion may result in poor aesthetics and adequate occlusion may have little relationship to attractiveness. However, anteriorly positioned incisors (buck teeth), "excessive show" of the gingiva, lack of a relaxed lip seal, overclosure, open bite, malposed teeth, poor relationship between tooth sizes, discoloration, or restorations result in a significantly diminished appearance. The plastic surgeon may substantially improve patient satisfaction with appropriate referrals to the dentist, orthodontist, or prosthodontist. It is noteworthy that the lips are supported by the teeth and attractive lips are not excessively protrusive; however, they are full since flattening or thin lips suggests the changes of age. Lombardi, Ricketts, and others have described a "golden" relationship between tooth size, but agreement in this regard is not uniform.

PREFERRED FEATURES

Critics in the various fields of aesthetic endeavor have employed a lexicon of terms that have been applied to human facial attractiveness but are abstract and virtually immeasurable: harmonious, proportional, rhythmic, symmetrical, dynamically symmetrical, balanced, elegant, luminous, unified, complex, interesting, regular, and so forth. Researchers in an attempt to quantify objectively have for the most part relied on numerical scales or used terms that are fairly straightforward, but consistency is lacking and comparison between studies difficult.

Returning to basics, the straight profile, particularly in the male, is considered more attractive than the convex, although in females this is less important. The fuller, slightly protrusive lower face pattern is preferred, with the attractive being slightly more prognathic than the average—again, particularly in males. Attractive eyes are associated with full cheekbones, which, when less full or with a small maxilla, may make the eyes appear exophthalmic. The flatter cheekbone and retruded or flat midface due to a small maxilla are considerably less desirable. In profile the more nearly the cheek line parallels the nose the more attractive. It has been said that flat cheeks "do the most harm" to the female face; protrusive lips and large noses are less harmful, retrusive chin is the least damaging. Low (more acute) angle of the mandible has more appeal than a high angle (more obtuse) in the male. A natural gentle hollow of the cheek along the line of occlusion is preferred to its absence (62–78).

Although asymmetry is disadvantageous, only facial asymmetry >3% is clinically discerned and the apprehension of symmetry is determined by context. Relative visual importance of features was determined by Cross, who reported that lay judges said that eyes are the most important 34% of the time, mouths and smile 31%, hair 10%, skin color 10%, nose shape 5%, and face as a whole 15% (22). Berry reported that the order of importance is mouth, eyes, hair, and nose (79). Cross also believed that ability to detect beauty differs widely depending on age, sex, or race, although other researchers have indicated the opposite.

Cunningham described what was perceived as important for attractiveness in men: expressive features, large eyes, mature features with large chin, and prominent cheekbones. Further, the appearance of sexual maturity, dominance, height, social status, grooming, high status clothing, sociability, and approachability were all judged as of importance. Berry agreed for the most part that the male might have components of a baby face with some child-like features, that is, large, round eyes and elevated eyebrows, but believed a small chin more attractive. Romm suggested that females preferred "a rugged" look tempered with softness (80). McKelvie in his research found subjects equated widely separated eyes and short noses as youthful and pleasant, long noses as male, passive, and unpleasant. Big mouths were perceived as male, active, and strong, whereas narrow mouths were passive or weak. Hinckleman in the *History of Ancient Art* described the Greek ideal as having a low forehead, eyebrows of "grace" that grew together, blond hair, smooth, round chin without a dimple, lower lip fuller than the upper, and a nose that was straight or slightly concave in profile. Finally, Romm described the features which Phryne, the mistress of Praxiteles (375–330 B.C.E.), the sculptor had: regular and symmetric features, high cheekbones, mouth with perfect cupid's bow, lower lip fuller than upper, nose in a straight line from its root, and a chin on a vertical plane of the face (81).

FACIAL AREAS

Forehead

The forehead is an area of the face almost devoid of interest except when too great in expanse, without appropriate hairline or distorted by a fault: wrinkles, creases, flatness, protrusion, excessive bossing, absence of eyebrows, etc. Commonly, the inexperienced artist will diminish its vertical height as though it were unimportant; women will frequently cover it with hair. It is bounded superiorly by "trichion" or central hairline point, which is not apparent on the skull, laterally by the temporal line marking the origin of the temporalis muscle, and inferiorly by the brows or supraorbital rim. It has been described as protruding, flat, or sloping, but more accurately it is curvilinear in all dimensions with minimal flatness in the central portion and bossing just above the superorbital rim in the male (Fig. 22). One need only to examine the cut calvarium or the curvilinearity of a hat band to confirm this. It was noted on a limited number of calvaria that the arcs of the forehead had radii of 160–185 mm and were analogous to the curves of an egg without significant flattening. Similarly, on profile the arcs of the forehead parallel the origin of the temporalis muscle (Fig. 23).

Eyes

The eyes are one eye width apart, a classical canon borne out by careful measurement. Canthi appear to be on a horizontal line; however, the lateral canthus is slightly higher and more posterior than the medial. Rarely, except in pathologic states, are the lateral canthi lower. Visible sclera is approximately three times as wide as high and the areas of the sclera should be visually equal on either side of the iris. The upper lid crosses the iris neither above its margin nor touching the pupil. The lower lid margin is found at the level of the

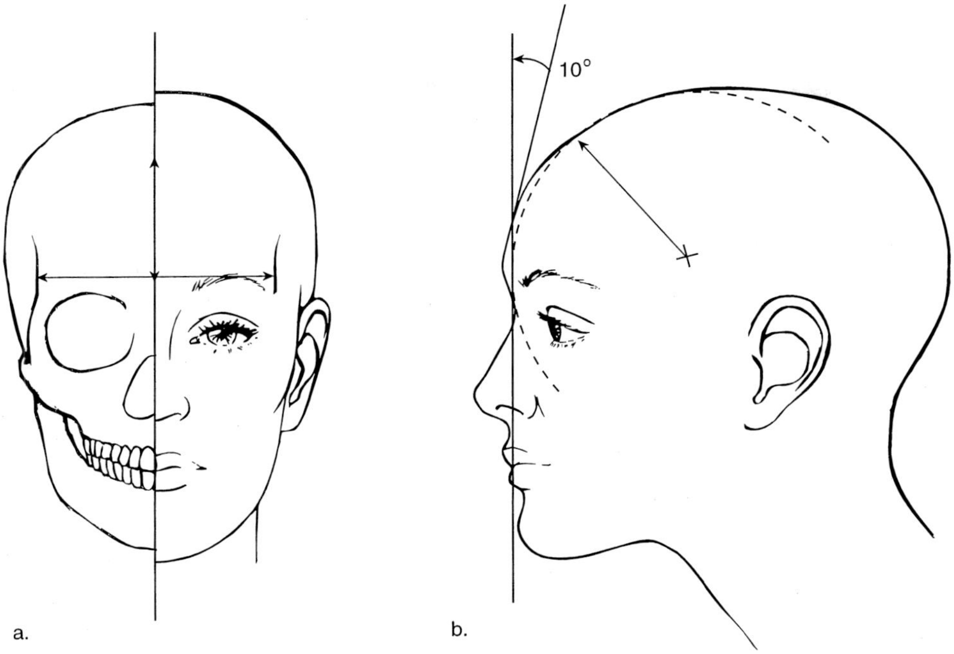

Figure 22. A: Height of brow, glabella to trichion, is one-third of face height, as measured by Farkas ~115 mm in the male and 109 mm in the female. Width at supraorbital level is ~118 mm in males and 114 mm in females. **B:** The "slope" of the forehead is ~10°. The curve of the forehead is a regular arc very slightly flattened in the lower midportion.

iris or slightly below. More than a millimeter or two below would give the appearance of "excessive scleral show." The primary lid fold is 7–12 mm above the lid margin, although it may be indistinct with deep orbits, aging, or in non-Caucasian eyes (Fig. 24).

Lid margin curves are slightly asymmetric with very slight medial elevation on the upper and very slight depression on the lower, as shown in Fig. 25. Upper lid margin curvature is greater than that of the lower. The most anterior portion of the cornea is posterior to the supraorbital and infraorbital rim.

Average eye width in males is 31.2 mm and in females 30.7. The aperture or vertical distance between lid margins is 10.4 in males and 11.1 in females, confirming the view that women appear to have larger eyes than men.

Eyebrows vary immensely in size, shape, position, and luxuriousness of hair growth. Male eyebrows are flatter, more luxuriant, and closer to the lid margin than females, lying directly over the bony orbit or slightly below. In females the eyebrow is arched, with the

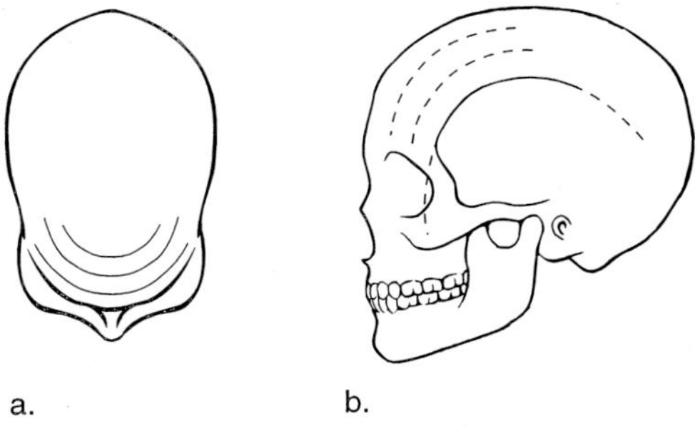

Figure 23. A: Forehead curve appears to be a series of regular parallel arcs. **B:** From lateral view the curve of the forehead again is a regular arc parallel with supratemporal line.

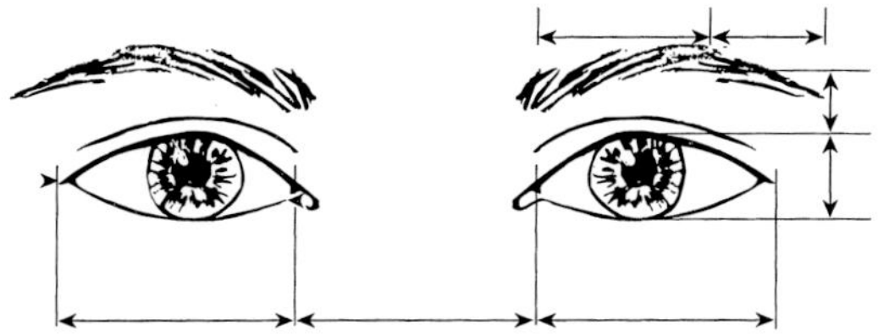

Figure 24. The eyes are essentially one eye width apart, with the highest point of the eyebrow at the junction of the medial two-thirds and the lateral one-third. The distance between lids is 10–11 mm, and the distance between upper lid margin and lowest part of the eyebrow is 11–13 mm in the male and 12–15 mm in the female.

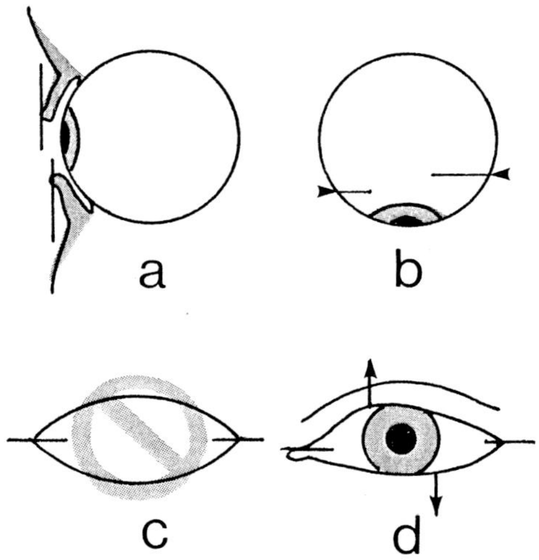

Figure 25. **A:** The upper lid precedes the lower. **B:** The lateral canthus is posterior to the medial canthus. **C:** Contrary to the poet's view, the eye is not almond shaped. **D:** The margin of the upper lid has a greater curvature than the lower, and there is very slight elevation of the medial upper lid and a very slight depression of the lateral lower lid as shown. The lateral canthus is superior to the medial.

highest point at the junction of the medial two-thirds and the outer third and lies just above the bony rim. The pattern of eyebrow hair is variable but has virtually been ignored both by cosmetologists and plastic surgeons. Medially, it is oblique or almost vertical and becomes more horizontal lateralward. The upper and lower portions of the lateral third of eyebrow hair travel in opposite directions. The brows may almost meet, but ideally they begin on a vertical line with the medial canthus. Laterally they extend beyond the lateral canthus by a variable distance. Size, shape, and position are often altered in females by perceived cosmetic necessity and often require trimming as they commonly begin to luxuriate in the late middle age, particularly in men.

Eyelashes, longer and thicker on the upper lid, begin more medially than on the lower. From an aesthetic view they should be curved and sufficiently dark to frame and accentuate the eye, increasing interest. When eyelashes are sparse, pale, or straight, the lids may have an unattractive, glabrous appearance.

Nose

As the most protrusive and prominent feature of the face, the nose has a remarkable range of sizes, shapes, facets, planes, angles, highlights, and shadows. Mere measurement is inadequate to describe its complexity or the harmony of its parts and relationships to the adjacent features and face as a whole. The nasal surgeon must be able to determine aesthetic value of a given nose and perceive whether there is imbalance of shape, line, weight, or tonality of its surface. The barrenness of mere angle and linear measurements on a flat piece of paper or film is demonstrated as we compare them to the living three-dimensional nose. In Fig. 26 important highlights and shadows are indicated. In Fig. 27 the general dimensions and averages are noted. In Fig. 28 the nose from the inferior view is illustrated, although there is wide variation between races.

In the Caucasian nose, unlike many Greek sculptures, there is a depression and definite

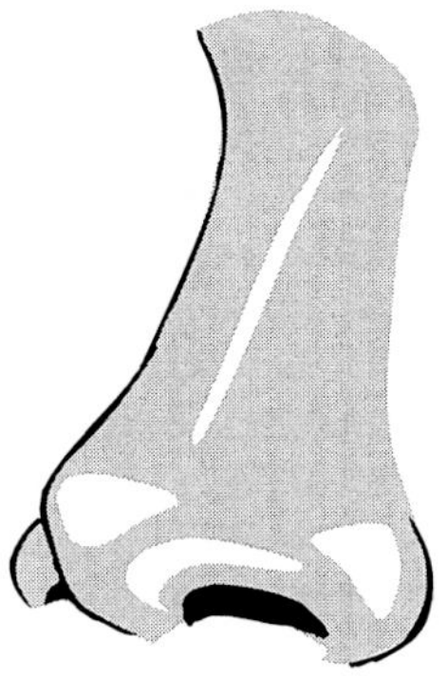

Figure 26. A diagrammatic representation of the important highlights and the shadow that overlies the soft tissue triangle, giving advantageous definition to the nasal tip.

angle between glabella and radix proceeding inferiorly to a relatively straight or slightly concave line distinguished at the tip by a slight "break." The axis, of course, is vertical and the nose symmetrical from side to side with alae that are smooth in contour and not excessively thick or fleshy. The nostrils are symmetric and the alar margins are described as smoothly curved without arching. The columella from the inferior view is not tubular but shaped like an inverted funnel due to the flare of the medial crura at the base of the columella (Fig. 28). On the profile view the columella shows ~4 mm; the hidden or excessively hanging columella is perceived as a cosmetic defect. A round, boxy, or large tip is less desirable than a sculpted tip, which demonstrates a highlight or several and a distinctive shadow formed by the "soft triangle" as in Fig. 26. The nasolabial angle has a wide variation and is, of course, in part dependent upon the position and appearance of the lip; it is aesthetically advantageous if it exceeds 90° but does not exceed 105 or 110°. It is noted the nostrils are symmetrical and should not ordinarily exceed 10–12 mm in length.

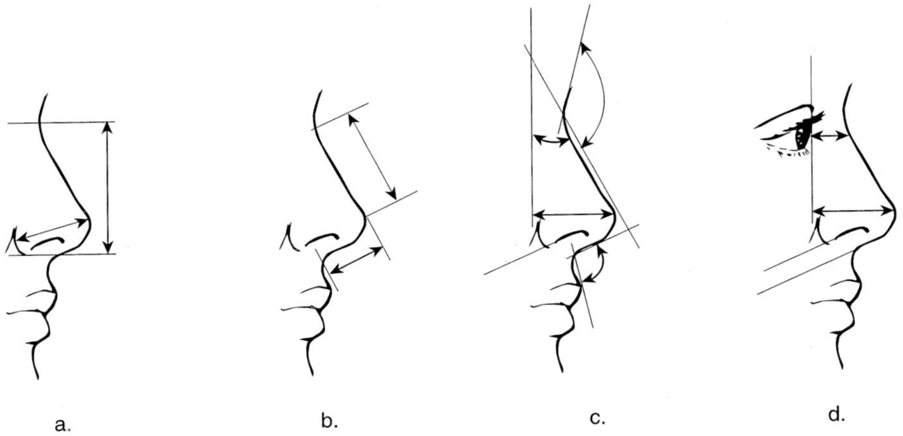

Figure 27. A: The nose from nasion to columella is ~53 mm in the male and ~49 mm in the female. From alar crease to tip is 35 mm in the male and 31 mm in the female. **B:** The length of nose from nasion to tip is ~49 mm in the male and ~45 mm in the female. From columellar base to tip is 21 mm in the male and 19 mm in the female. **C:** Nasofrontal angle, highly variable, measures 120–135°. The angle of the nasal bridge measured from vertical to Frankfurt horizontal varies from 30 to 40°. The nasolabial angle is aesthetically most pleasing between 95 and 105°. **D:** Columellar "show" varies from 2 to 5 mm. The bridge is ~14–17 mm anterior to the cornea and the tip of the nose and ~36–41 mm from the vertical facial plane.

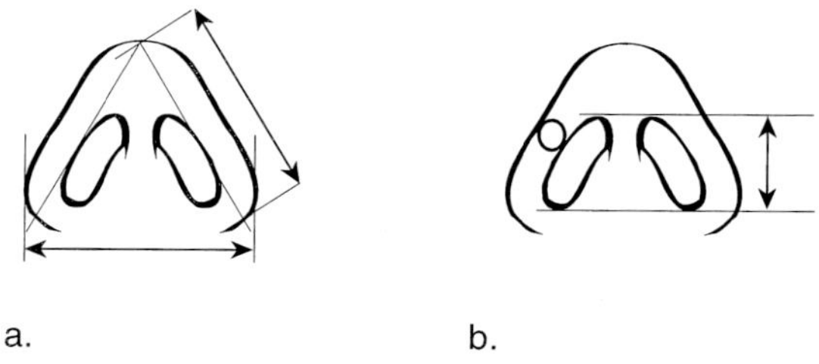

Figure 28. The "equilateral triangle" of the aesthetic nose. **A:** The sides are ~35 mm in the male and ~31 mm in the female. **B:** The alar thickness is ~5 mm in the female and ~6 mm in the male. The length of the columella is ~11 mm. Note that the columella resembles an inverted funnel rather than a column.

Mouth

Current fashion suggests that the lips should be very full, and the apparent thinning of the lip with the loss of the white line, flattening, and turning in is viewed negatively as a part of the aging process. The artist and sculptor view the complex of cutaneous upper and lower lip, vermilion, and chin as the "mouth barrel" and consider it to be of primary importance in expressing emotion, contrary to the commonly held belief that the eyes "are the windows of the soul." According to Faigin, the eyes confirm, by movement of the forehead, eyebrows, and tissue about the eyes, the validity of what the mouth and lower face are expressing.

Classic proportions indicate that the upper lip is slightly thinner and wider and precedes the lower lip (Figs. 29 and 30). The mouth barrel vertically is about one-third of the face and the distance from base of the columella to the mouth fissure is approximately one-third of the distance between base of columella and chin. Vermilion lips sit on a line halfway between the nose and chin.

The ideal width of the mouth fissure can be determined by dropping a vertical line from the medial pupil (Fig. 13). Rounding off the figures from Farkas, the mean width in males is ~53 mm (range 45–60 mm) and 50 mm in females (range 43–56 mm) (Figs. 29 and 30).

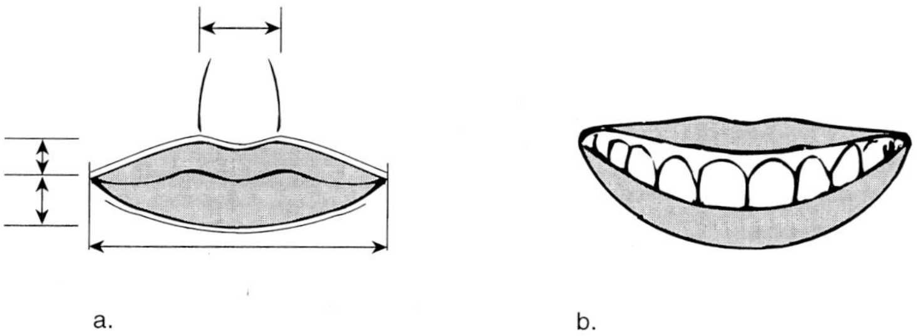

Figure 29. A: The width of the philtrum is 10–11 mm at the junction with the vermilion. The upper lip vertical height is 8.5–9 mm, and the lower lip 9.5–10 mm. The lips are ~57–62 mm in width, a few millimeters less than the distance between the center of the pupils. No differences between the white line on upper and lower lip. **B:** No more than 2 mm of gingiva should show, or a gummy smile is seen. Apparent regular decrease in the size of the teeth from anterior to posterior is most aesthetic. Relative size of the teeth for the most attractive smile is a matter of controversy (see text).

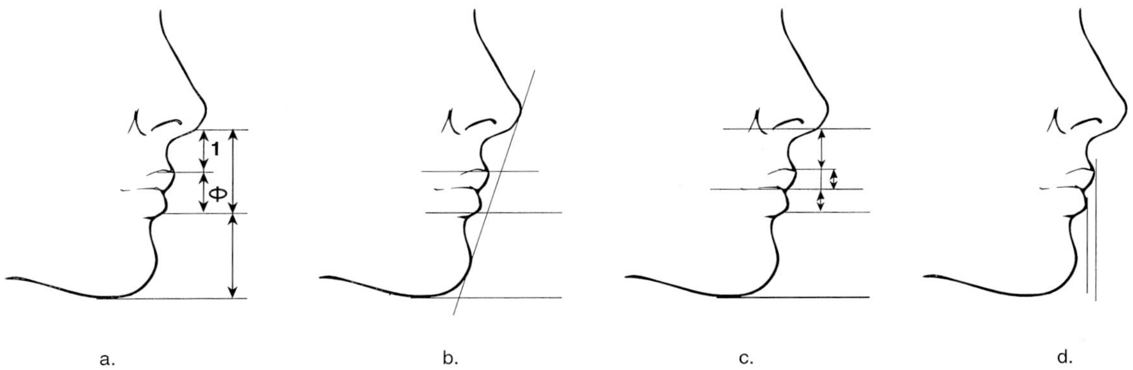

Figure 30. A: Classically the distance between columellar base to the lower lip line and lower lip to chin is one to one. It is pointed out that a golden relationship between cutaneous upper lip and upper–lower lip vermilion may exist. **B:** Oblique E-line of Ricketts: The upper lip should be 4 mm behind this and the lower lip 2 mm. **C:** According to Farkas, the cutaneous upper lip measures 1.9 mm in the male and 9.9 mm in the female, the upper lip vermilion 8.9 mm in the male and 8.4 mm in the female, and the lower lip vermilion 10.9 mm in the male and 9.7 mm in the female. **D:** The upper lip precedes the lower in an ideal relationship.

Upper lip length in males is 15 mm (range 10–20 mm) and 12.5 mm (range 7–18 mm) in females. The vermilion of the upper lip averages 9 mm in males and 8.5 mm in females. The vermilion of the lower lip is 10.4 mm in males and 9.7 mm in females. The upper lip precedes the lower lip as shown in Fig. 30D. Ricketts, using the "E line," describes the upper lip as 4 mm posterior to that line and the lower lip 2 mm posterior (Fig. 30B).

The Cupid's bow contour of the upper lip line in youth is defined by the white line extending the width of the lip; it fades to non-existence laterally on the lower lip. The philtrum is variably prominent and contributes to attractiveness of the lip as two columns extend from the base of the columella slightly diverging on either side of a philtral dimple. It too diminishes with age (Fig. 31).

The aesthetics of the lips and mouth in repose are no more important than the appearance of the mobile lips with various expressions. Particularly, as the lips widen into a smile or grin, the gums and teeth are revealed. Extensive information about the size, shape, relationships, and color of the teeth is available in the dental literature, since these factors are of particular importance in prosthetics. The possible golden relationship between adjacent teeth has been explored by Ricketts, Lombardi, Preston, and others. The gingiva exposed in a smile or grin is aesthetically disadvantageous when it exceeds 2–3 mm and may be indicative of a long midface (Fig. 29B). The lips in repose should appear to close without effort.

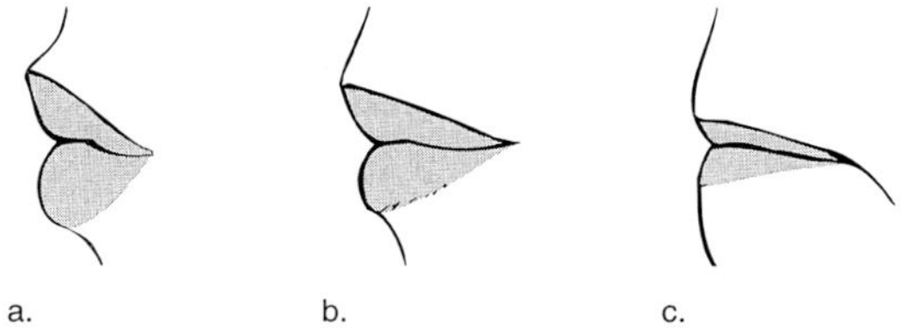

Figure 31. A: Infant's lip with marked fullness of vermilion and sharp definition and prominent white line. **B:** The adult lip maintains some fullness, but this and the white line diminish with age. **C:** The aged lip, thin and convex with an imperceptible white line.

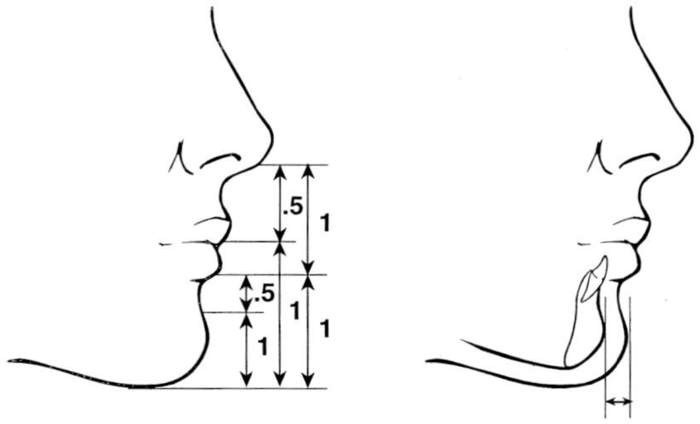

a. b.

Figure 32. A: Proportion schemes to aid in determining chin and lip dimensions and proportions. Lower lip vermilion divides equally the distance between the base of the columella and the chin; base of columella to commissure is one-half distance from crease to chin. **B:** Thickness of chin soft tissue is highly variable measuring from 10 to 14 mm.

Chin

The chin is the lower part of the mouth barrel defined superiorly by the mental crease separating the gentle slightly concave curve of the cutaneous lower lip from the convex chin (Fig. 32). There may be a slight vertical central depression, crease, or dimple that may be viewed as attractive, although the Greeks considered it a defect. Laterally the chin flows smoothly into the line of the mandible laterally and inferiorly until with aging the submental crease may define it excessively, giving a knob-like appearance. The telling view of the chin is from the inferior position, with the ideal being a symmetrical parabola. Vertical creasing of the chin occurs with excessive contraction of the mentalis in the attempt to maintain a lip seal in certain malocclusions and retrusion of the chin or mandible.

Volume, shape, and protrusion of the chin are often contrasted with those characteristics of the nose, with a change in one affecting the impression of the other. The protrusion and

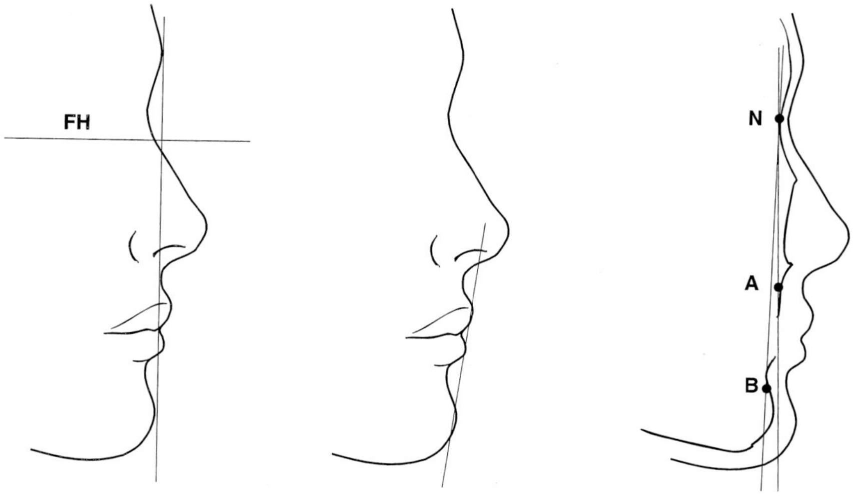

a. b. c.

Figure 33. A: Gonzales-Ulloa proposed that maximum chin protrusion point should be on a vertical line dropped from Frankfort horizontal at the glabella. **B:** Riedel's method indicates that the point of maximum chin protrusion is on a line drawn from the upper and lower lips. **C:** Angle *ANB* (see Fig. 17) indicates the position of the mandible and by inference the chin.

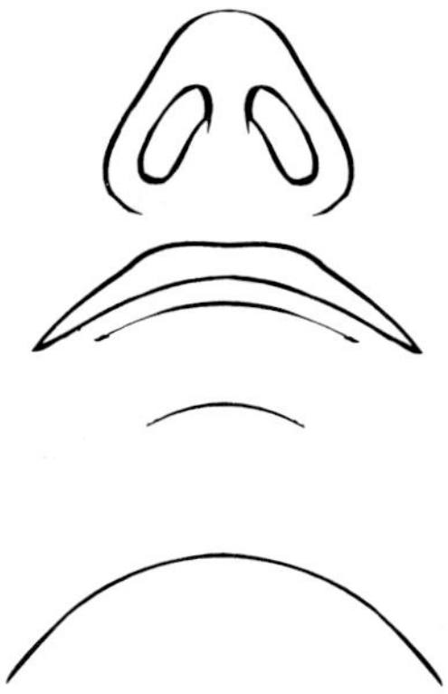

Figure 34. The inferior view reveals the parabolic curve of the mandible and the consonant curves of the lips and chin.

length are dependent on underlying maxillary and mandibular position and the highly variable thickness of the soft tissue. Repositioning of the chin by moving the mandible or osteoplastic genioplasty with a bony chin is somewhat problematic insofar as soft tissue change, since there may not be a one-to-one response. Vertical dimension change may result in an increase or obliteration of the mental crease, creating serious aesthetic disadvantage. Chin implants and soft tissue reduction may both be followed by subtle aesthetic contour problems. The need for and degree of correction of protrusion or retrusion can be determined by reference to the vertical facial plane (Fig. 33), the plane of facial convexity (Fig. 8), measurement from the vertical corneal plane (Fig. 14), and evaluation of *ANB* angle on the cephalogram. Again, attention should be paid to the inferior view where the consonant curves of the upper lip, vermilion, and chin should be noted and preserved (Fig. 34).

The soft tissue chin varies in thickness from 10 to 14 mm. Anterior position movement of mandible may result in a one-to-one change. Soft tissue in advancement genioplasty may only be 80% and chin setback may result in only a 25% change.

Cheek

It has been noted that the greatest harm to the female face is an inadequate prominence of the cheek. Two characteristics are primary: the highlight of the prominence and the cheek shadow. From the profile view it has been noted that the cheek is more attractive the more closely the line parallels the dorsum of the nose. The cheek prominence is distinguished as a highlight almost ovoid in shape related most easily to the orbit. If the Frank-

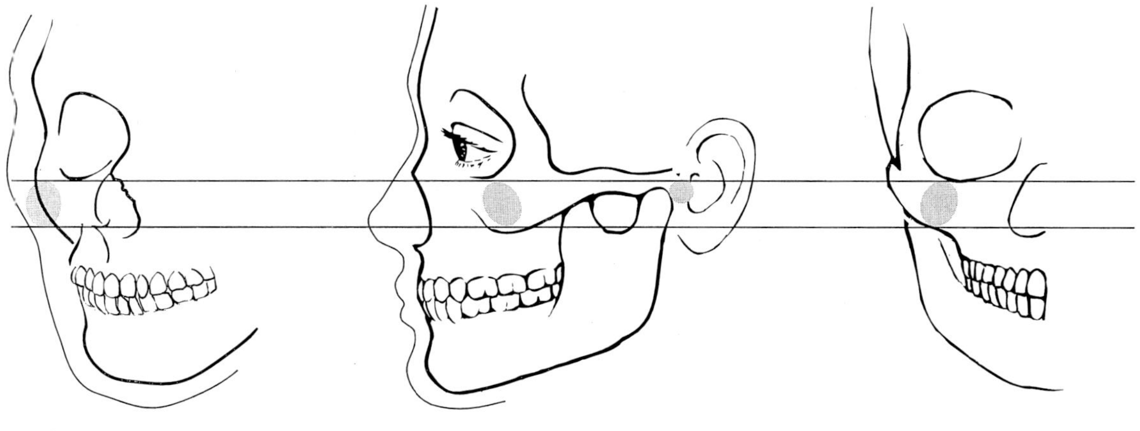

Figure 35. The oval prominence of zygomatic highlight may be related to the inferior lateral "corner" of the orbital rim on both skull and face.

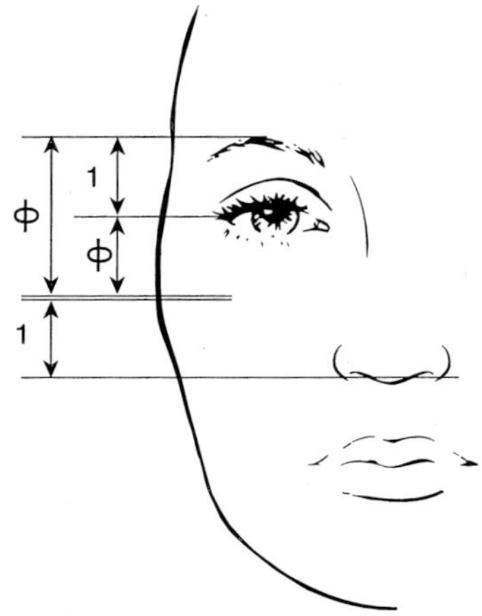

Figure 36. Determining the area of maximum prominence of the cheek using Ricketts' method; phi is the golden number, 1.618. The shadowed area beneath the zygomatic prominence indicates the shadow of the ideal cheeks; it curves upward corresponding at first to the occlusal plane obliquely toward the tragus.

fort horizontal is determined, the high point of the cheek will be ~1 cm below that line and 1 cm posterior to the lateral orbital rim (Fig. 35). Ricketts has located the high point of the zygoma using the golden mean, as in Fig. 36. The hollow of the cheek corresponds roughly to the occlusal plane or above a line drawn between the ear lobule and the ala. Manipulation of this shadow by removal of cheek fat or adding cheek implants requires sophisticated judgment since excessive hollowness is a serious disadvantage.

SUMMARY AND CONCLUSIONS

Beauty or attractiveness is defined with difficulty both subjectively and objectively, although there has been no lack of opinion. Though the difficulties are great, there is a pressing need for guidelines because of our increasing technical capacity to alter human facial form. Both the viewer and the subject have been the objects of considerable and progressively more sophisticated research by psychologists, orthodontists, surgeons, and others. The oft-repeated clichés—Beauty is in the eye of the beholder, Media determine what is attractive, and Beauty differs from culture to culture—are widely but not universally accepted. However, if they contain a grain of truth, they contribute little to the illumination of the problem. Use of measurement systems, proportions, the golden proportion, cephalometry, x-rays, photography, and mapping methods will be helpful in solving certain problems, allowing the surgeon to regularize or bring features within the bounds of normal. One anticipates, however, that exquisite harmony of form, texture, color, and proportion and, for that matter, beauty and attractiveness are sufficiently evanescent and subjective to remain within the province of the poet and artist.

REFERENCES

1. Santayana, G. *The Sense of Beauty*. 1896.
2. Pope, A. *An Essay on Criticism*, Part I. 1711.
3. Taschek WK. Faces, masks and the grotesque: on objectivity in aesthetic judgement. In: McNamara JA, ed. *Esthetics and the treatment of facial form, vol 28*. Ann Arbor: University of Michigan, 1992:41–64.
4. Shakespeare, W. *Love's Labor Lost, Act II, Scene I*. 1594–1595.
5. Cox NH. Facial harmony. *Am J Orthod* 1971;60:175.
6. Foltyn JL. Dead beauty: some thoughts in preservation, memorialization and destruction of beauty in death. Presented at the London School of Economics, April 1993.

7. Meerdink JE, Garbin CP, Leger DW. Cross-gender perceptions of facial attributes and their relation to attractiveness: do we see them differently than they see us. *Percept Psychophys* 1990;48:227.
8. Melli C, Giorgini S. Aesthetics in psychosomatic dermatology. *Clin Dermatol* 1984;2:180.
9. Phillips C, Tulloch C, Dann C. Rating of facial attractiveness. *Commun Dent Oral Epidemiol* 1992;20:214.
10. Loverpel EH. On facial balance and harmony. *Angle Orthod* 1937;7:81.
11. Lew KKK, Soh G, Loh E. Ranking of facial profiles among Asians. *J Esth Dent* 1992;4:128.
12. Arnheim R. The face and the mind behind it. In: McNamara JA, ed. *Esthetics and the treatment of facial form, vol 18*. Ann Arbor: Center for Human Growth and Development, University of Michigan, 1993.
13. Powell NJ, Humphreys B. *Proportions of the aesthetic face*. New York: Thieme-Stratton, 1984.
14. Powell SJ, Rayson RK. The profile in facial esthetics. *Br J Orthod* 3:207.
15. Valentine CW. *The experimental psychology of beauty*. Berkeley: University of California Press, 1962.
16. Gombrich EH. *The story of art*. Englewood Cliffs: Prentice Hall, 1978.
17. Sweeny J, Curry T, Tzedakis Y. *The human figure in early Greek art*. Athens: Greek Ministry of Culture, Washington: National Gallery of Art, 1987.
18. Ehrenzweig A. *The hidden order of art*. Berkeley: University of California Press, 1967.
19. Carpenter R. *The esthetic basis of Greek art*. Bloomington: Indiana University Press, 1959.
20. Samuels CA, Ewy R. Aesthetic perception of faces during infancy. *Br J Dev Psychol* 1985;3:221.
21. Sternglanz S, Gray JL, Murakami M. Adult preferences in infantile facial features. *Anim Behav* 1977;25:108.
22. Cross JF, Cross J. Age, sex, race and the perception of facial beauty. *Dev Psychol* 1971;5:433.
23. Iliffe AH. A study of preferences in feminine beauty. *Br J Psychol* 1960;51:267.
24. Martin JG. Racial ethnocentrism and judgement of beauty. *J Soc Psychol* 1964;63:59.
25. Wagatsuma E, Kleinke CL. Rating of facial beauty by Asian-American and California females. *J Soc Psychol* 1979;109:299.
26. Farkas LG. *Anthropometry of the head and face in medicine*. New York: Elsevier North Holland, 1981.
27. Farkas LG, Hreczko TA, Kolar JC, Munro IR. Vertical and horizontal proportions of the face in young, adult North American Caucasians: revision of neoclassical canons. *Plast Reconstr Surg* 1985;75:328.
28. Farkas LG, Sohm P, Kolar JC, Katic MJ, Munro IR. Inclinations of the facial profile: art versus reality. *Plast Reconstr Surg* 1985;75:509.
29. Milord JT. Aesthetic aspects of faces: a (somewhat) phenomenological analysis using multidimensional scaling methods. *J Pers Soc Psychol* 1978;36:205.
30. Moyers RE. Evolution of concepts of the face. In: McNamara JA, ed. *Esthetics and the treatment of facial form, vol 28*. Ann Arbor: Center for Human Growth and Development, University of Michigan, 1993:27–40.
31. McNamara JA, Brust EW, Rioco ML. Soft tissue evaluation of individuals with an ideal occlusion and a well-balanced face. In: McNamara JA, ed. *Esthetics and the treatment of facial form, vol 28*. Ann Arbor: University of Michigan, 1992:115–146.
33. Arndt EM, Travis F, Lefebvre A, Niec A, Munro IR. Beauty and the eye of the beholder: social consequence and personal adjustments for facial patients. *Br J Plast Surg* 1986;39:81.
34. Arnett GW, Bergman RT. Facial keys of orthodontic diagnosis and treatment, part II. *Am J Orthod Dentofac Orthop* 1993;103:395.
35. Peck S, Peck L. Concept of facial esthetics. *Angle Orthod* 1970;40:284.
36. Czarnecki ST, Nanda RS, Currier GF. Perceptions of a balanced facial profile. *Am J Orthod Dentofac Orthop* 1993;104:180.
37. Hume, D. *Essays: Of Tragedy*. 1741–1742.
37. Motoyoshi M, Namura S, Arai HY. A three-dimensional measuring system for the human face using three-dimensional photography. *Am J Orthod Dentofac Orthopaed* 1992;101:431.
38. Hungerford, M. *Molly Bawn*. 1878.
40. Bersheid E. An overview of the psychological effects of physical attractiveness. In: Lucker GW, Ribbens KA, McNamara JA, eds. *Psychological aspects of facial form—monograph 11*. Ann Arbor: Center for Human Growth and Development, University of Michigan, 1980:1–24.
41. Berscheid E, Gangestad S. The social psychological implications of facial physical attractiveness. *Clin Plast Surg* 1982;9:289.
42. Bhatia AF. Facial profile esthetics and acceptance. *Ind J Dent Res* 1989;2:45.
43. Dion KK, Berscheid E, Walster E. What is beautiful is good. *J Pers Soc Psychol* 1972;24:285.
44. Kligman AM, Graham JA. The psychology of appearance in the elderly. *Dermatol Clin* 1986;4:501.
45. Marshall J. Looks count, study on earning power. *San Francisco Chronicle*, November 2, 1993.
46. Klopfer PH. Sensory physiology and esthetics. *Am Sci* 1970;58:399.
47. Sutherland NS. Shape discrimination by animals. *Exp Psychol Soc* 1962.
48. Zolman JF. Stimulus preferences and form discrimination in young chicks. *Psychol Rec* 1969;19:407.
49. Arnheim R. *Art and visual perception*. Berkeley: University of California Press, 1974.
50. Symons D. *The evolution of human sexuality*. New York: Oxford University Press, 1979.
51. Cunningham MR, Barbee AP, Pike CL. What do women want? Facialmetric assessment of multiple motives in perception of male physical attractiveness. *J Pers Soc Psychol* 1990;59:61.
52. McKelvie SJ. Effects of feature variations on attributes for schematic faces. *Psychol Rep* 1993;73:275.
53. Perrett D, May K, Yoshikawa S. Facial shape and judgements of female attractiveness. *Nature* 1994;368:239.
54. Ghyka M. *Geometry of art and life*. New York: Dover, 1977.
55. Huntly HE. *The divine proportion: a study in mathematical beauty*. New York: Dover, 1970.
56. Gardner M. Mathematical games—the multiple fascinations of the Fibonacci sequence. *Sci Am* 1969;220:116.
57. Mitchison AV. Phyllotaxis and the Fibonacci series. *Science* 1977;196:270.
58. Levin, EI. Dental esthetics and the golden proportion. *J Prosthet Dent* 1978;40:244.
59. Ricketts RM. Divine proportion in facial esthetics. *Clin of Plast Surg* 1982;9:401.
60. Preston JD. The golden proportion revisited. *J Esthet Dent* 1993;5:247.
61. Marquardt SR. *Pentagram analysis human face*. Symposium, California Society of Plast Surgeons, Monterey, CA, 1992.
62. Tolleth H. Concepts for the plastic surgeon from art and sculpture. *Clin Plast Surg* 1987;14:585.
63. Tolleth H. Facial contours and proportions from an artist's point of view. In: Ousterhout DK, ed. *Aesthetic contouring of the craniofacial skeleton*. Boston: Little, Brown, 1991:59–70.

64. Barnett A, Whitaker L. Facial form analysis of the lower and middle face. *Plast Reconstr Surg* 1986;78:158.
66. Broadbent BH Sr, Broadbent BH Jr, Golden WH. *Bolton standards of dentofacial developmental growth.* St. Louis: Mosby, 1975.
67. Schendel SA. Surgical corrections of dentofacial deformities. In: Bell WH, ed. *Modern practice in orthognathic and reconstructive surgery*. Philadelphia: Saunders, 1992.
68. Burstone CJ, James RB, Legan H, Murphy GA, Norton CA. Cephalometrics for orthognathic surgery. *J Oral Surg* 1978;36:269.
68. Legan HL, Burstone CJ. Soft tissue cephalometric analysis for orthognathic Surg. *J Oral Surg* 1980;38:744.
69. Delaire J, Schendel SA, Tulasne JF. An architectural and structural craniofacial analysis: a new lateral cephalometric analysis. *Oral Surg* 1981;52:226.
70. Sassouni V. A classification of skeletal facial types. *Am J Orthod* 1969;55:104.
71. Sassouni V. *The face in five dimensions*. Morgantown: School of Dentistry Publications, West Virginia University, 1962.
72. Steiner CC. Cephalometrics for you and me. *Am J Orthod* 1953;39:729.
73. Moyers RE, Brookstein FL. The inappropriateness of conventional orthodontics. *Am J Orthod* 1979;75:599.
74. Obwegeser HL, Marentette LJ. Profile planning based on alterations in positions of the bases of the facial thirds. *J Oral Maxillofac Surg* 1986;44:302.
75. Gonzales-Ulloa M. A quantitative method for the appreciation of the morphology of the face. *Plast Reconstr Surg* 1964;34:241.
75. Lombardi RE. The principles of visual perception and their clinical application to the denture esthetics. *J Prosthet Dent* 1973;29:358.
77. Angle, E. H. *The Treatment of Malocclusion of the Teeth*. 7th ed. Philadelphia: S. S. White Co., 1907.
77. Cunningham MR. Measuring the physical in physical attractiveness: quasi-experiments on the sociobiology of female facial beauty. *J Pers Soc Psychol* 1986;30:925.
78. Lu KH. Harmonic analysis of the human face. *Biometrics* 1965;21:491.
79. Berry DS, McArthur LZ. Perceiving character in faces: the impact of age-related craniofacial changes on social perception. *Psychol Bull* 1986;100:3.
80. Romm S. Art, love and facial reality. *Clin Plast Surg* 1987;14:579.
81. Romm S. *The changing face of beauty*. St. Louis: Mosby Year Book, 1992.
82. Faigin G. *The artist's complete guide to facial expression*. New York: Watson-Guptill, 1990.

Ethnic Considerations in Facial Aesthetic Surgery, edited by W. Earle Matory, Jr.
Lippincott–Raven Publishers, Philadelphia © 1998.

7

Definitions of Beauty in the Ethnic Patient

W. Earle Matory, Jr.

Ask a toad what is beauty . . . ; he will answer that it is a female with two great round eyes coming out of her little head, a large flat mouth, a yellow belly and a brown back.
— Voltaire

The vast array of physical features and proportions that are present in the patient of color represents a tremendous challenge to the plastic surgeon.

Distinctive anatomic and physiologic concepts pertinent to each major ethnic group will be reviewed. Concepts of attractiveness are influenced by a number of factors including ethnic and family characteristics, social disposition, and media personalities. The faces of the 1970s and 1980s like Jaclyn Smith, Christie Brinkley, and Cybill Shepherd have been "spotted" by ethnic models with Caucasoid features like Louise Vyent (Fig. 1). The 1990s, however, have displayed a vast array of colorful hues and facial characteristics, including those of Beverly Johnson, Iman, Whitney Houston, Florence Griffith-Joyner, and Oprah Winfrey (Fig. 2). Hispanic and Asian representation is growing as exemplified by the strikingly attractive features of Barbara Carrerra and Connie Chung. In reviewing these distinctive faces, it is clear that any analysis of attractiveness is a study in ethnic and individual diversity.

At the University of Massachusetts, we performed an analysis of facial characteristics in people of color (Fig. 3). Three independent examiners were utilized to identify 400 attractive male and female models representing different ethnic groups. Groups that were evaluated included African American, Hispanic, Asian, Middle Eastern, and Caucasian. Anthropometric measurements and angles, 26 in number, were obtained in male and female models (Fig. 4). Aesthetic parameters of the face were assessed, including Frankfort horizontal, neoclassical canon of facial proportion, golden aesthetic proportions, and facial shapes (Table 1).

W. E. Matory, Jr.: A New You Plastic Surgery Medical Group, Irvine, California 92714

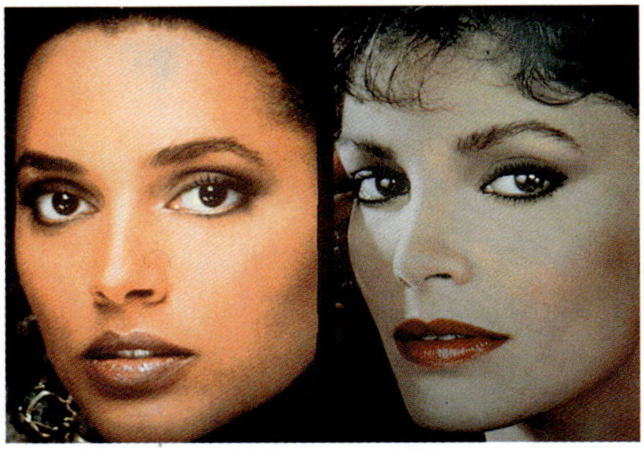

Figure 1. Media models of the 1970s and 1980s were occasionally of color, but more often than not associated with Caucasian-like features.

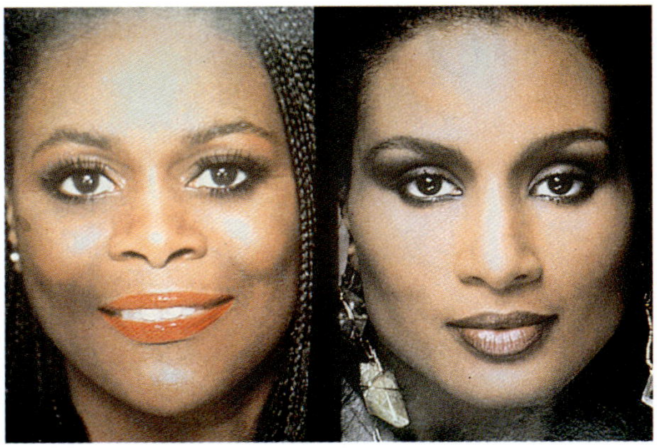

Figure 2. The late 1980s and 1990s have yielded a significant increase in the number and variety of representations from various ethnic groups as well as varied facial characteristics.

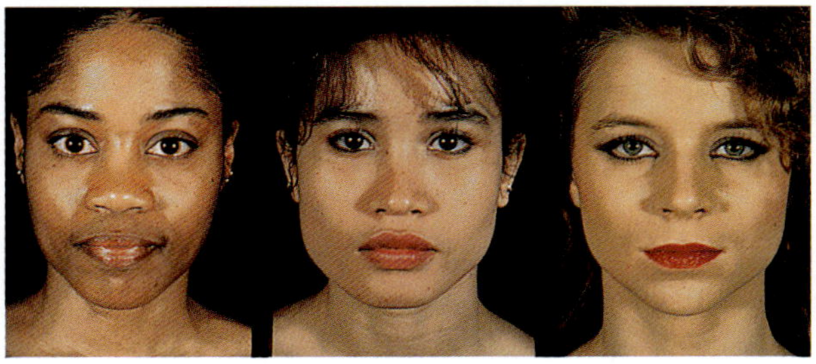

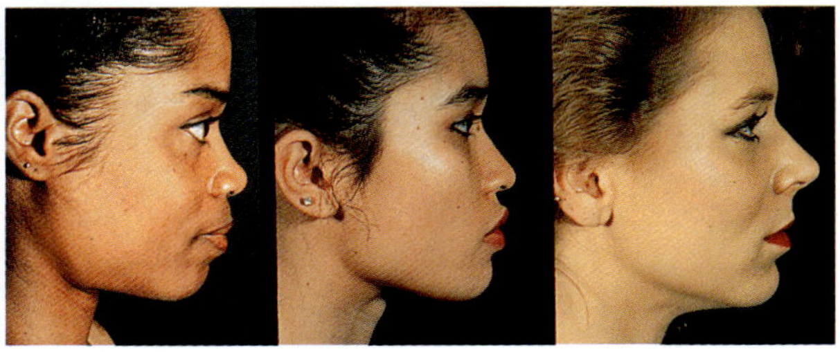

Figure 3. There are many differences as well as similarities that can be noted in comparison views of attractive African American, Asian, and Caucasian models. Note that the Frankfort horizontal is observed in the Caucasian model, but to lesser extents in the other facies. Nasal length is shorter in the more pigmented races with wide variations in the columella–labial angle. Each demonstrates an oval face with prominent cheekbones. Full lips are aesthetically compatible with widened nasal width and intercanthal width.

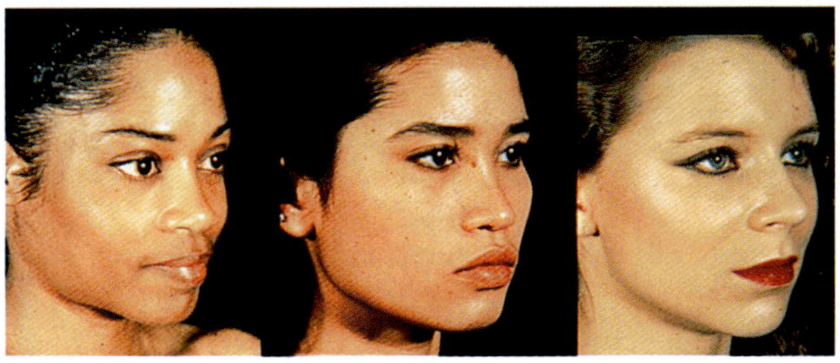

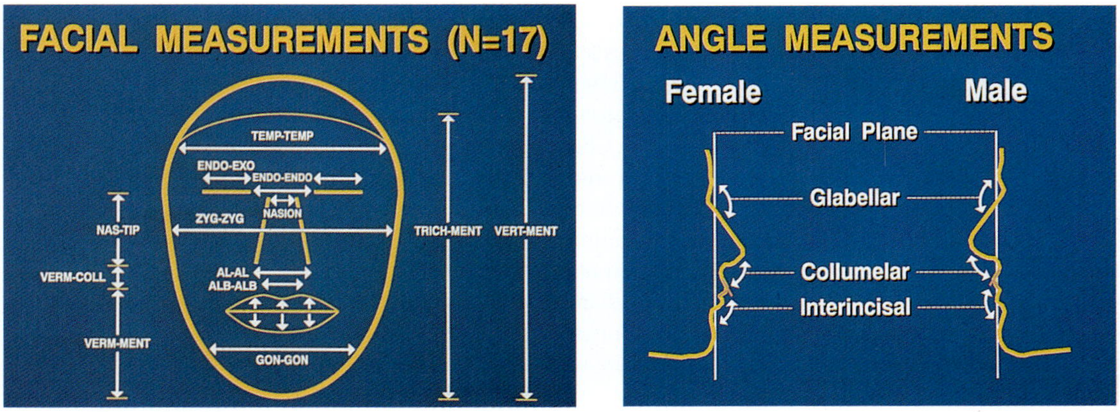

Figure 4. Facial balance and harmony were assessed by calculating a number of facial and angle measurements in each respective ethnic group.

Table 1. *Angle measurements (females)*

	African American			Caucasian
	Narrow	Moderate	Wide	
Frankfort horizontal	+	+	+	+
Glabellar	151 ± 2	144 ± 2	142 ± 2	142 ± 2
Columellar	94 ± 3	95 ± 3	106 ± 2	104 ± 5
Incisal	32 ± 3	31 ± 2	30 ± 2	26 ± 4

Comparative angle measurements ( ) are noted for the narrow, moderate, and wide African American face in comparison to the Caucasian face. Incisal angles tended to be more acute in the wide African American versus the columella angle, which appeared to be more obtuse.

ETHNIC BACKGROUND

Of note, the ethnic background of aesthetic models was quite varied. Caucasian models (Fig. 5) tended to have an admixture that included French, German, Norwegian, Baltic, Slavic, and/or English (Table 2). The African American (Fig. 6), on the other hand, was most commonly mixed with American Indian and Eastern European or Hispanic (Table 3). East Indian, Samoan, Eskimo, and Asian heritages were less common. Anthropometric measurements discerned three categories of facial characteristics in each ethnic group, including narrow, moderate, and wide. We found that nasal and facial dimensions fell into these respective categories, within each of the different ethnic subgroups (Table 4). A similar description was used to describe features in the African American by McNeil (Table 5).

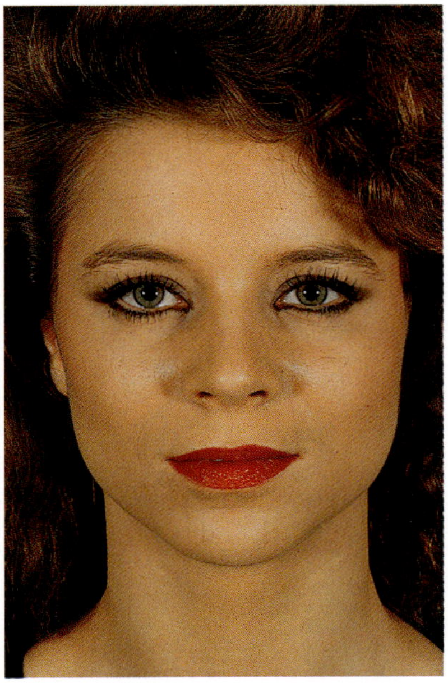

Figure 5. Caucasian models in the study tended to have a diverse heritage.

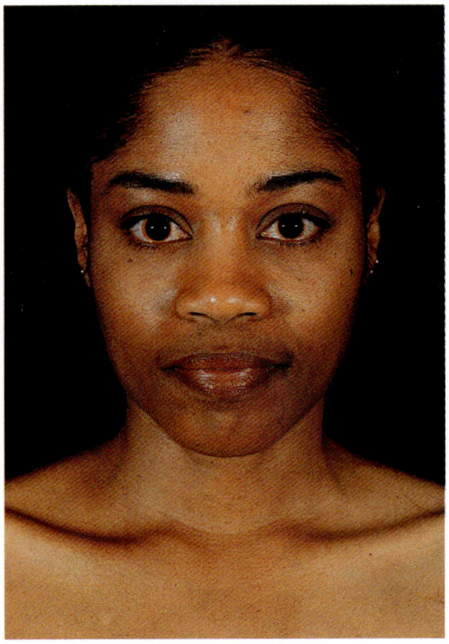

Figure 6. Racial admixture was very common among the African American and to a lesser extent the Hispanic patient. Caucasian populations were mixed to a limited degree, particularly relevant to other Asian groups within the same region.

Table 2. *Aesthetic considerations: Caucasian*

	Female	Male
French	10	9
German	8	10
Norwegian	6	5
Baltic	4	5
Slovak	2	1
Total	30	30

The diverse heritage of Caucasian models in the study.

Table 3. *Aesthetic considerations: African American*

	Female	Male
Eastern European	8	0
American Indian	10	1
Hispanic	8	5
East Indian	2	5
Samoan	1	1
Eskimo	1	0
Asian	1	1
Total	31	13

Racial admixture among ethnic groups in the study.
[a] Dominant ethnic background.

Table 4. *Analysis of attractive female and male models*

	Wide	Moderate	Narrow
African American	20	20	20
Hispanic	20	20	20
Asian	20	20	20
Polynesian	20	20	20
Middle Eastern	20	20	20
Caucasian	20	20	20

Our analysis spaned several ethnic groups and both sexes. Within each category we noted subcategories of wide, moderate, and narrow faces.

Table 5. *African American face*

Negroid
Caucasoid
Miscegenated ideal composite

Our findings were consistent with similar conclusions described by McNeil in his description of the African American face. He perceived that there were individuals of African American background with Caucasoid and those with Negroid facies and there was a category of individuals with mixed features.

Table 6. *Aesthetic parameters of the face*

Frankfort horizontal
Neoclassical canons of facial proportion
Golden aesthetic proportions
Facial shapes

The key focus of our work in the evaluation of various ethnic groups was based on four aesthetic parameters of facial attractiveness.

Table 7. *Aesthetic considerations in the African American: results (%)*

	Narrow		Moderate		Wide	
	Male	Female	Male	Female	Male	Female
Frankfort horizontal	82.6	98.3	73.5	64.0	32.6	33.2

In the African American, the Frankfort horizontal was commonly noted in the narrow and moderate faces, but to a lesser extent in the wide face.

PARAMETERS OF ATTRACTIVENESS

Historically described components of attractiveness include the Frankfort horizontal, neoclassical canons of facial proportion, golden aesthetic proportions, and facial shapes (Table 6).

Frankfort Horizontal

The Frankfort horizontal, defined as a plane perpendicular to a line drawn between the intraorbital rim and the tragus, has been interpreted as an ideal facial plane. For attractive female models in these study, the Frankfort horizontal was felt to be a common characteristic in those with narrow and moderate features (Fig. 7; Table 7), but less so in individuals with wide facial features (Fig. 8). The same patterns were consistent in the male.

Neoclassical Canons of Facial Proportion

Neoclassical canons of facial proportion as originally described by scholars and artists of the Renaissance based on classical Greek canons (Farkas) were felt to be inconsistent in each of the ethnic categories. The concept of being able to divide the face into three equal parts or the cranium and face into four equal parts was noted in <8.4% and <3.2% of individuals in the study, respectively. Subnasion-to-stomion distance varied considerably

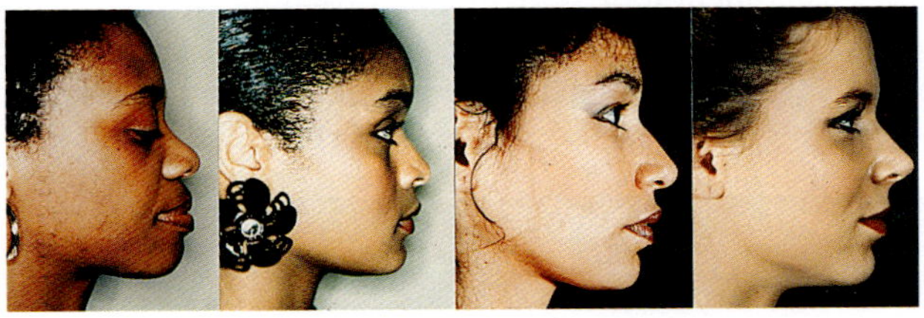

Figure 7. The Frankfort horizontal line is noted to lesser degrees as one appraises lateral views of the attractive Caucasian, Hispanic, and African American models.

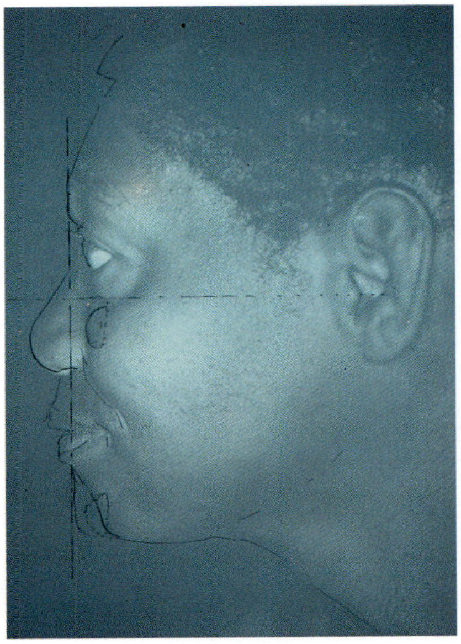

Figure 8. The Frankfort horizontal is defined as a line perpendicular to a line drawn from the tragus to the infraorbital rim. It theoretically establishes the ideal facial plane. With use of this criterion, malar and chin augmentation may optimize facial planes in this patient.

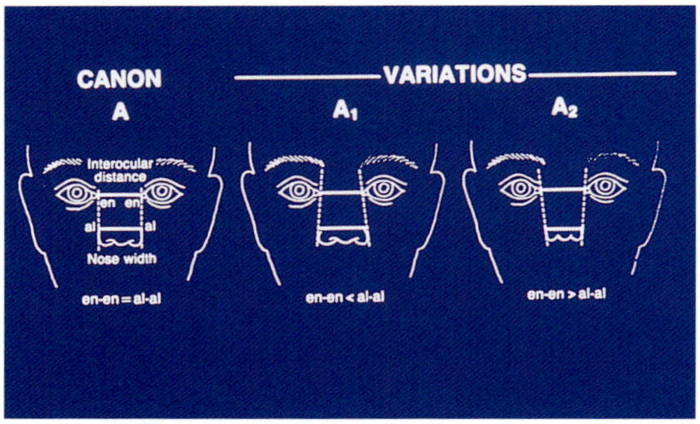

Figure 9. Farkas also noted inconsistencies of neoclassical canons of facial proportion including three section, four section, morbid nose, interocular distance, and nasal oval canons.

among individuals of each ethnic group. Enopth-enopth was almost uniformly smaller than the enopth-exopth distance in contrast to the equal enopth-enopth (en-en) to enopth-exopth (en-ex) distance (Fig. 9).

Golden Aesthetic Proportions

A dramatic consistency was noted in the applicability of golden aesthetic proportions to the ethnic face. The phidias, 1:1.618 as measured by the Ricketts caliper (Fig. 10) (Rocky Mountain Orthodontics), correlated extremely well with a number of facial relationships, for example, vert-ment to zyg-zyg, trich-ment to temp-temp, and trich-ment to gon-gon. These ratios define ideal length and width relationships of the face, i.e., facial shape (Table 8). The most common attractive facies (Table 9) in females were oval, diamond, and square

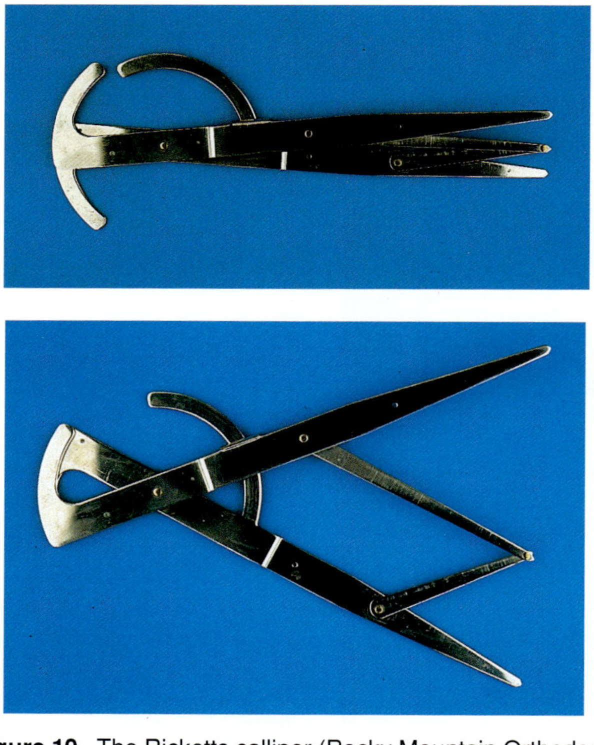

Figure 10. The Ricketts calliper (Rocky Mountain Orthodontics) is a useful instrument in defining ideal facial proportions.

Table 8. *Horizontal–vertical relationships (females, n = 60)*

	African American				
	Narrow	Moderate	Wide	Caucasian	Facial shape
Vert-ment vs. phi × zyg-zyg					
Equal to	+ 8/10	+ 9/10	+ 9/10	+ 26/30	Oval
Less than	– 0/10	– 0	– 1/10	– 4/30	Diamond
Greater than	– 2/10	– 1/10	– 0/10	– 0/30	Square
Trich-ment vs. phi × temp-temp					
Equal to	+ 6/10	+ 8/10	+ 9/10	+ 24/30	Oval
Less than	– 0/10	– 0/10	– 1/10	– 4/30	Diamond
Greater than	+ 4/10	– 2/10	– 6/10	– 2/30	Heart/rectangle
Trich-ment vs. phi × gon-gon					
Equal to	+ 5/10	+ 6/10	+ 6/10	+ 16/30	Oval
Less than	– 1/10	– 2/10	– 2/10	± 9/30	Diamond
Greater than	+ 4/10	– 2/10	– 2/10	± 5/30	Round/rectangle

Note the consistency of these phi values.

Table 9. *Aesthetic considerations in the African American: results (%)*

	Narrow		Moderate		Wide	
Facial shape	Male	Female	Male	Female	Male	Female
Oval	38	74	33	78	23	72
Heart	51	18	42	10	36	13
Rectangular	10	2	12	4	25	5
Other	2	6	13	8	16	10

The oval-shaped face is more common in the female versus the heart-shaped face in the male.

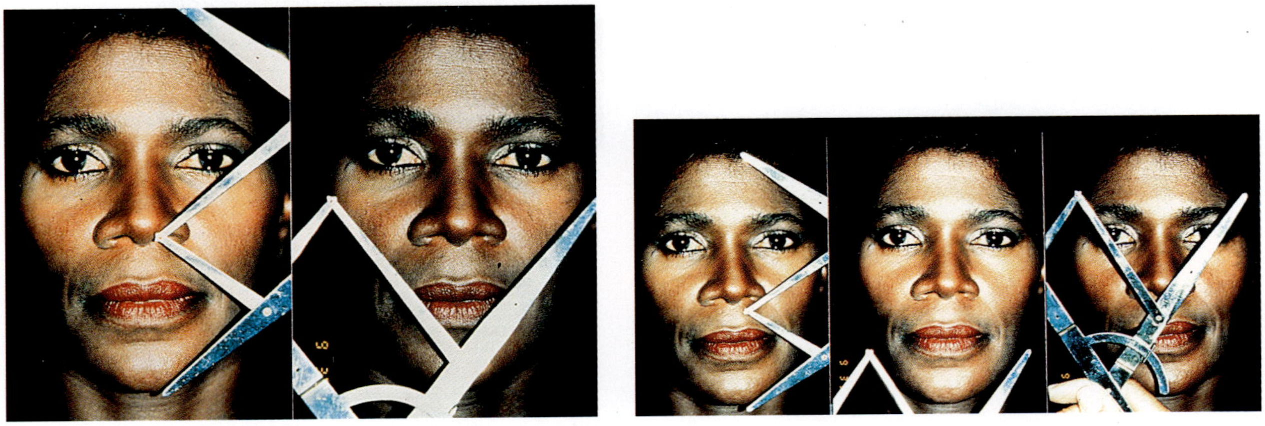

Figure 11. Vertex–menton maintains a ratio of 1 : 618 with the zygoma to zygoma width in the attractive model. The trichion–menton maintains a phi relationship with the temp-temp and also with the gon-gon. These relationships define an oval face. These were common findings noted in the overwhelming majority of attractive models.

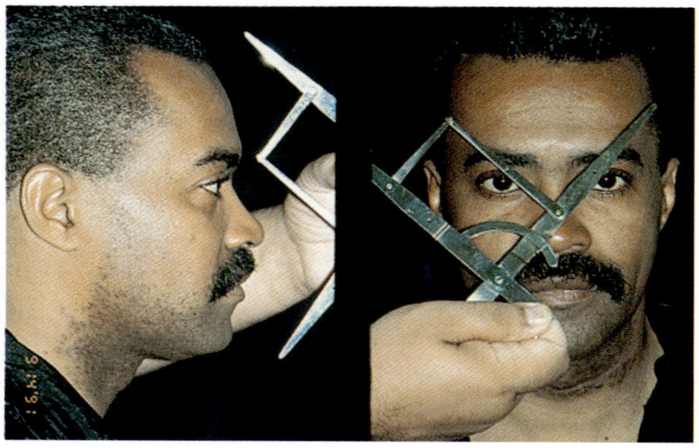

Figure 12. In the male, the vertex–menton maintains a phi relationship with the temp-temp as well as with the zyg-zyg. This overall relationship defines a heart-shaped face, commonly noted in the male.

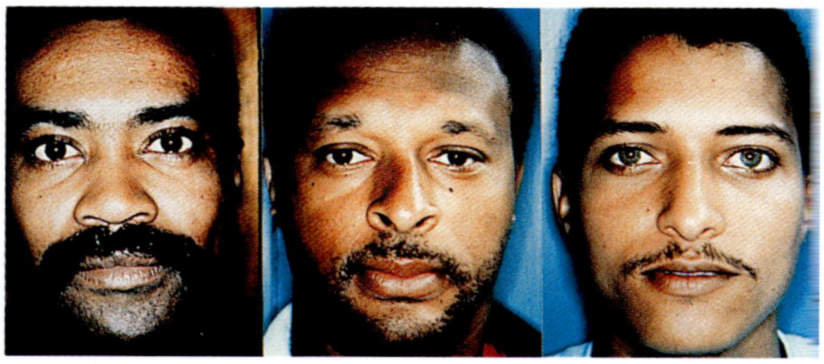

Figure 13. The heart-shaped face was most consistent in the attractive male. However, some oval shapes were noted.

(Fig. 11), with a broader temp-temp distance noted in most males, in which the more common shape was heart (Fig. 12). Oval shapes in the male were occasionally noted and occasionally discerned as feminizing (Fig. 13).

The phi relationship was also consistent with nose, nose/eye/lip, and nose/lip/chin relationships. A complementary basal view is observed when the subnasalis to tip-defining point has a 1:1.618 ratio with the al-al distance (Fig. 14). An equilateral triangle is more commonly seen in the attractive Caucasian female (Fig. 15). Alar flaring is more commonly apparent in the male and female with wide features. Canons of beauty as described by Broadbent and Matthews, which suggest that the attractive nose lies between vertical lines drawn through the inner canthus, were not consistently noted (Fig. 16). When features of narrow, moderate, and wide male and female facies were assessed, only a few Caucasian

A 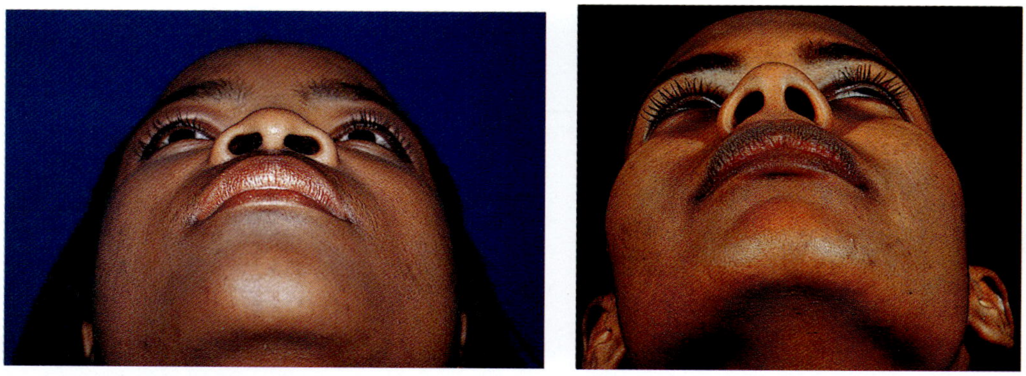 B

C 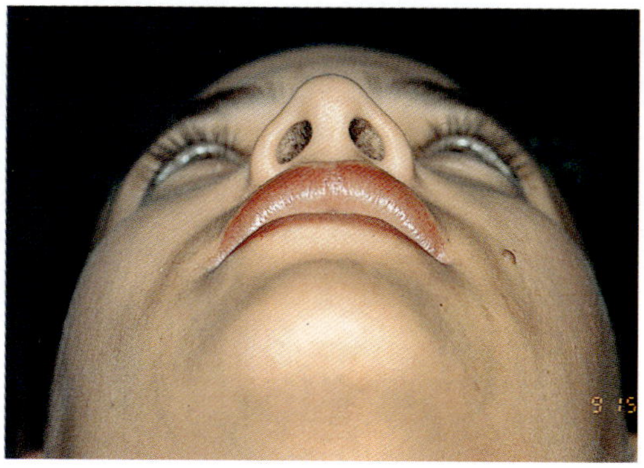

Figure 14. Alar bases are noted in the attractive African American female, wide **(A)**; moderate **(B)**; and narrow **(C)**. The interalar distance to tip height is ~1 in the narrow face versus 1:1.618 in the attractive wide face.

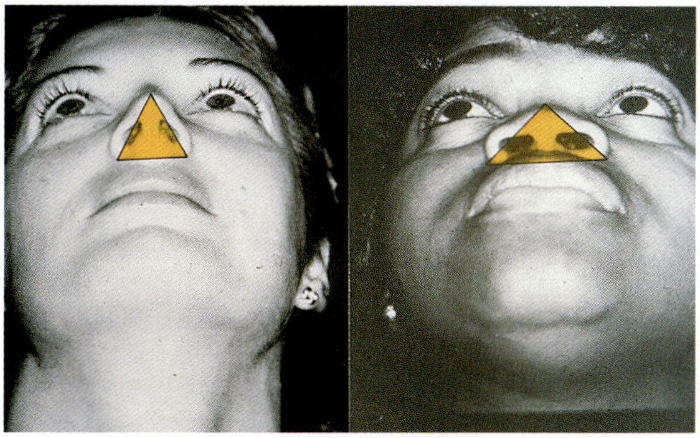

Figure 15. This figure allows comparison of the attractive Caucasian with narrow features versus the African American with wide features. In both patients the interalar distance exceeds the en-en.

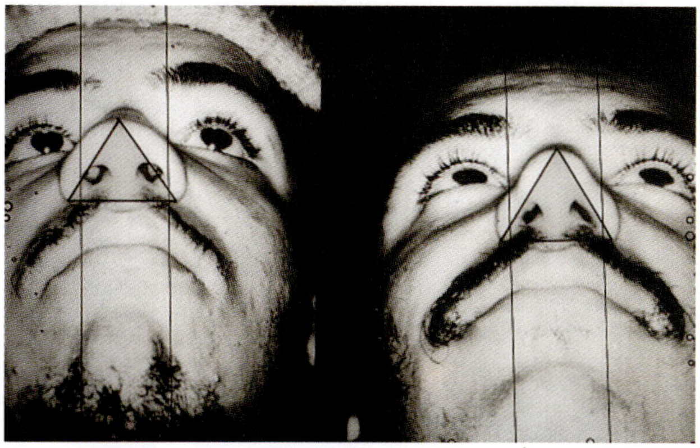

Figure 16. The canons of beauty as described by Broadbent and Matthews, suggesting that the attractive nose between vertical lines drawn through the intercanthus was not consistently noted in our attractive models or in postoperative patients. (With permission *Plast Reconstr Surg*, 77:239, 1986.)

models with narrow features were found to have alar width to be within the intercanthal lines (Fig. 17). For the attractive male and female models in each group, the distance between alar attachment to the cheek was found to be phi with the en-en distance and equal to en-en (Fig. 18).

In the lateral view, effort was made to assess nasal length relative to other facial proportions. In the African American female (Table 10), the nasion was uniformly no higher than the palpebral fissure (Fig. 19). In Asian and Hispanic models, the nasion was located at a level between the palpebral fissure and the supratarsal fold, in contrast to the Caucasian model in which the nasion was very consistently at or near the supratarsal fold (Fig. 20). In the Caucasian male, the nasion was almost uniformly at the level of the supratarsal fold, even in the presence of a dorsal hump deformity (Fig. 21). In Hispanic, Asian, and African American males, nasions were located between the palpebral fissure and the supratarsal fold, with the wide African American male nasion being located at the midpalpebral fissure (Table 11). The nasion to tip-defining point was found to have a phi relationship with the inferior brow subnasally, the distance from the lower lid margin to the oral commissure. For the male, nasal length has a phi relationship with the distance between the inferior brow and the upper lip vermilion border and in the young patient from the upper lid margin to the commissure (Fig. 22).

The glabellar, columellar, and incisal angles that were observed are seen in Table 12. Individuals with narrow features had measurements very similar to the Caucasian measurements, while those with wider features had more obtuse glabellar and incisal angles. The incisal angles are consistent with the open bite deformities commonly seen in the African

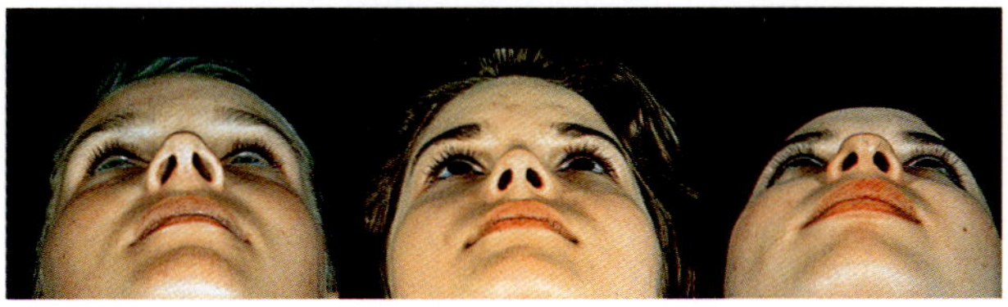

Figure 17. When features of narrow, moderate, and wide male and female facies were assessed, only a few Caucasian models with narrow features were found to have alar width to be within the intercanthal lines. For the attractive male and female models in each ethnic group, the distance between alar attachment to the cheek was found to have a phi relationship with the en-en distance.

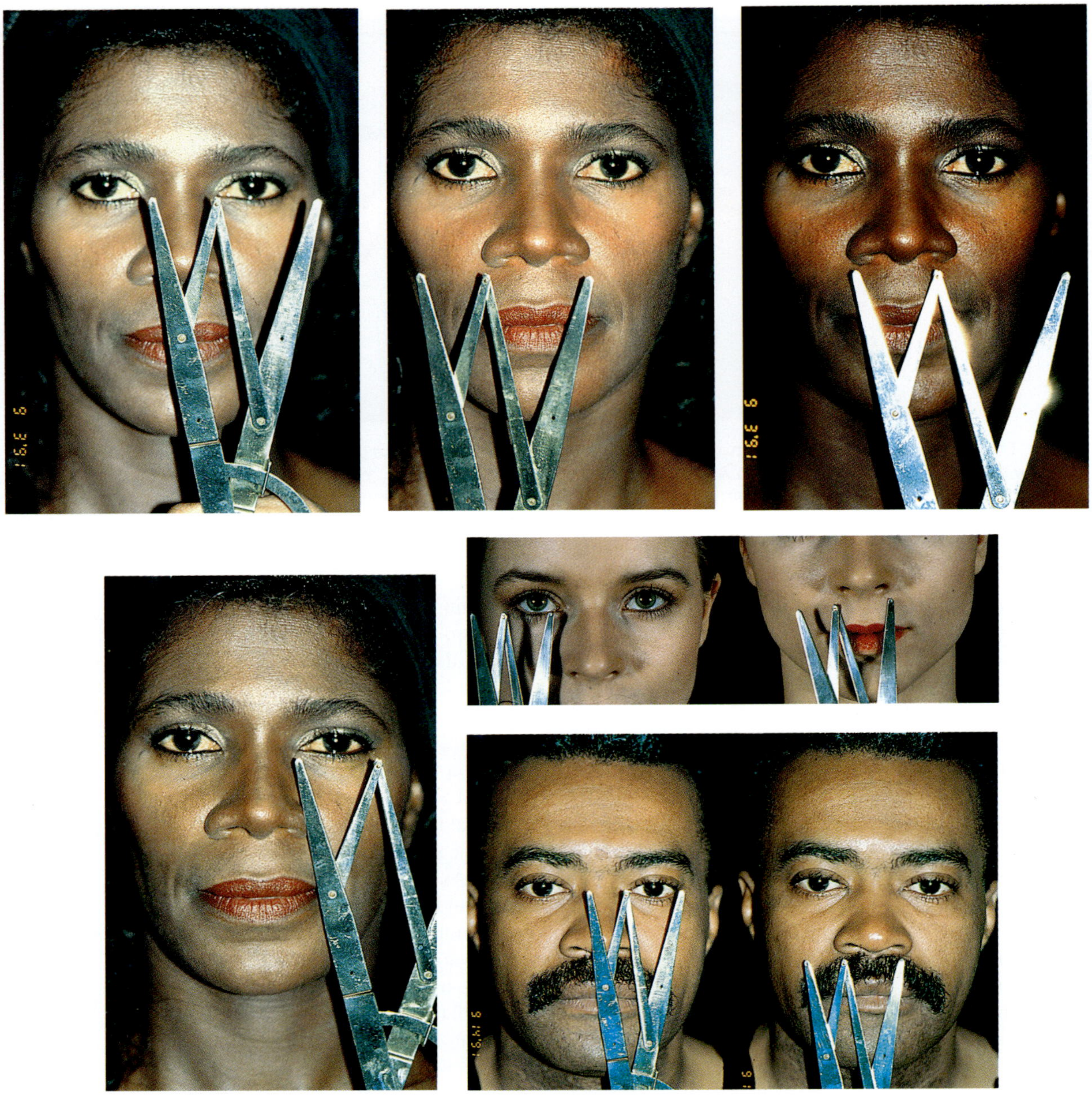

Figure 18. The interalar distance, in the vast majority of attractive models, was equal to the canthal width, not the en-en distance.

Table 10. *Location of the nasion (females, n = 60)*

Nasion	African American			Caucasian
	Narrow	Moderate	Wide	
Palpebral fissure (PF)	+ 10/10	± 4/10	– 1/10	± 0/30
Between PF and STF	– 0/10	± 4/10	± 7/10	– 4/30
Supratarsal fold (STF)	– 0/10	– 2/10	– 2/10	+ 26/30

In the Caucasian female, the nasion is added just below the supratarsal fold. In the Hispanic Castilian and in the Middle Eastern female, the nasion may extend above the supratarsal fold. In the Asian, African American, and wide Hispanic face, the nasion sits at the mid to low palpebral fold.

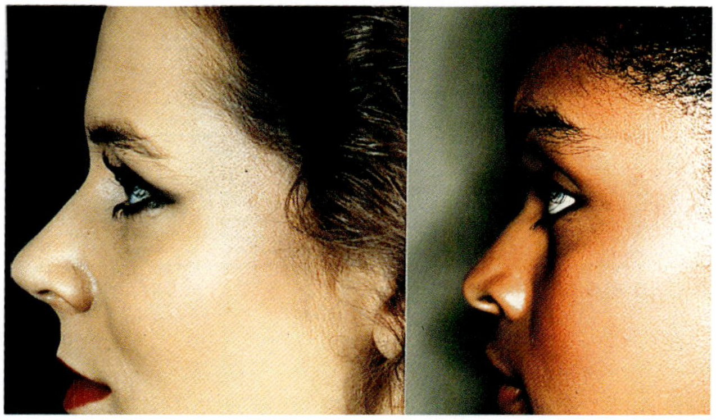

Figure 19. Comparison of nasion position in the moderate Caucasian and moderate African American.

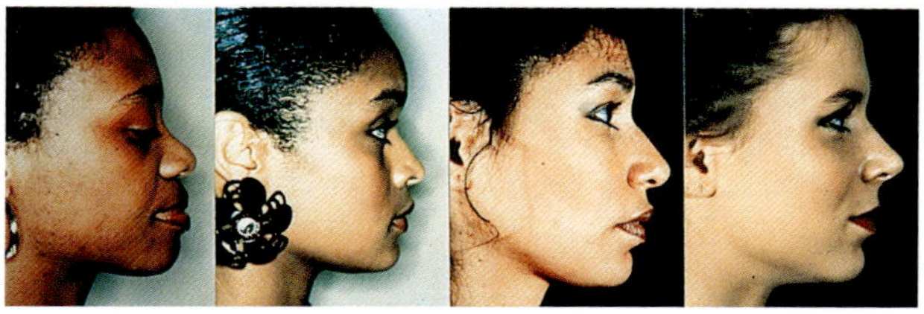

Figure 20. In the lateral view of the Caucasian, Hispanic, and moderate and wide African American, one notes a decreasing nasion height (from right to left).

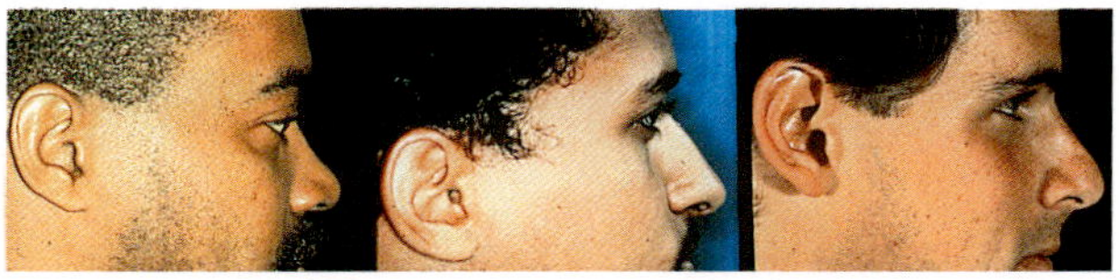

Figure 21. The nasion in the Caucasian male is within 1–2 mm of the supratarsal fold in contrast to the wide African American with the nasion sitting between the supratarsal fold and the palpebral fissure.

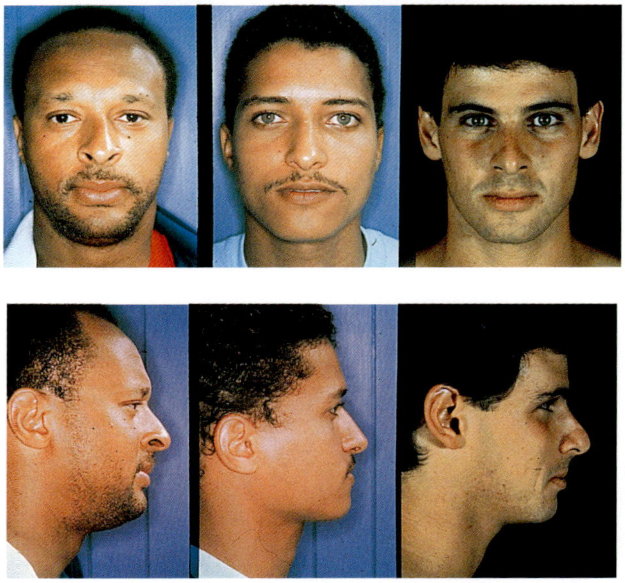

Figure 22. In the attractive male model, nasal length has a phi relationship with the distance between the inferior brow and the upper lip vermilion border (and in the young patient from the upper lid margin to the commissure).

Table 11. *Location of the nasion (male, n = 60)*

	African American			
Nasion	Narrow	Moderate	Wide	Caucasian
Palpebral fissure (PF)	+ 10/10	± 3/10	− 0/10	− 1/30
Between PF and STF	− 0/10	± 6/10	+ 7/10	− 4/30
Supratarsal fold (STF)	− 0/10	− 1/10	− 3/10	+ 25/30

The position of the nasion as noted in the attractive male models.

Table 12. *Angle measurements (females)*

	African American			
	Narrow	Moderate	Wide	Caucasian
Frankfort horizontal	+	+	+	+
Glabellar	151 ± 2	144 ± 2	142 ± 2	142 ± 2
Columellar	94 ± 3	95 ± 3	106 ± 2	104 ± 5
Incisal	32 ± 3	31 ± 2	30 ± 2	26 ± 4

The angles ( ) that were observed are presented here.

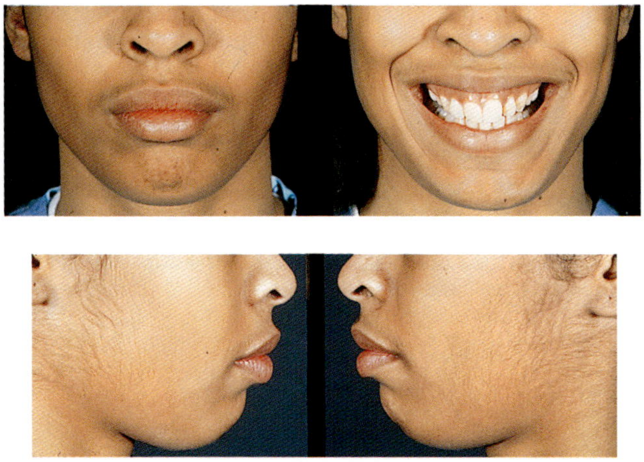

Figure 23. Open bite deformities are common in the African American and Asian, primarily due to obtuse incisal angles. This phenomenon is frequently associated with microgenia and malar hypoplasia.

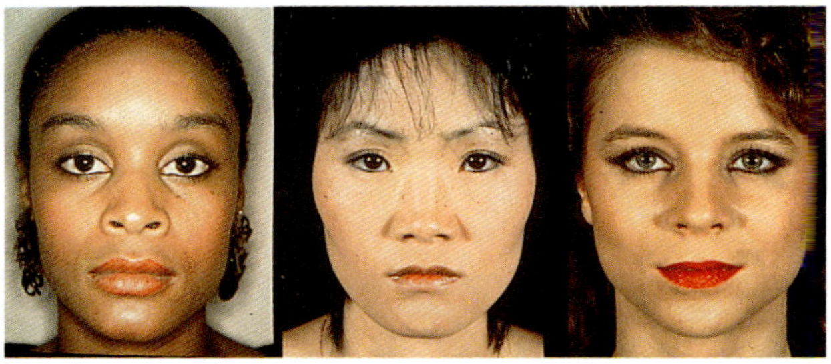

Figure 25. Asian features in the narrow and moderate faces demonstrate obtusely oriented middle crura.

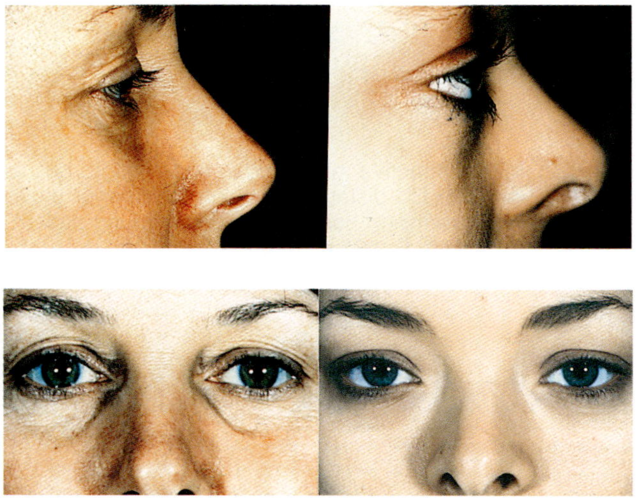

Figure 24. The middle crura, frequently seen in the Caucasian and measuring 6–10 mm, is rare in all but the narrow African American and Hispanic faces. When observed in the patient of color, the middle crura is typically short and obtusely oriented.

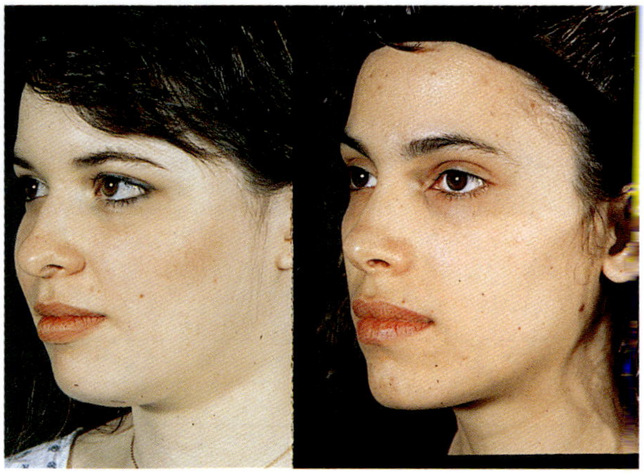

Figure 26. Hispanic features in the narrow and moderate facies demonstrate middle crura comparable with those of the Caucasian.

American and in the Asian (Fig. 23). Malar hypoplasia and microgenia are commonly associated. The columellar angles are often sharper in the African American female consistent with the shorter columella.

Middle crura were frequently observed in the Caucasian, measuring from 4 to 10 mm (Fig. 24). Middle crura were particularly short or non-existent in the African American and were more obtuse in the Asian (Fig. 25). Hispanic features in the narrow and moderate facies demonstrate middle crura measuring 3–4 mm in length comparable with that of the Caucasian (Fig. 26).

THE NOSE

Nasal attractiveness is determined by facial proportion. Analysis of ethnic features in the attractive nose is best outlined by four nasal templates that can be used in each of the respective ethnic noses. Features outlined in the African American template (Fig. 27A) may be utilized in the wide African American, the wide Asian, and the wide Hispanic nose. These faces are often accompanied by thick skin about the tip as well as a wide nasal base and pyramid. The moderate African American, Asian, and Hispanic and the wide Caucasian noses may have features similar to the Asian nasal template (Fig. 27B). The African American with American Indian heritage, the Northern Asian, and the Middle Eastern nose characteristically have dorsal humps or a high nasion that may extend onto the glabella (Fig. 27C). The Caucasian with narrow features, as well as narrow facies of any ethnic group, may have features similar to that in the Caucasian template (Fig. 27D).

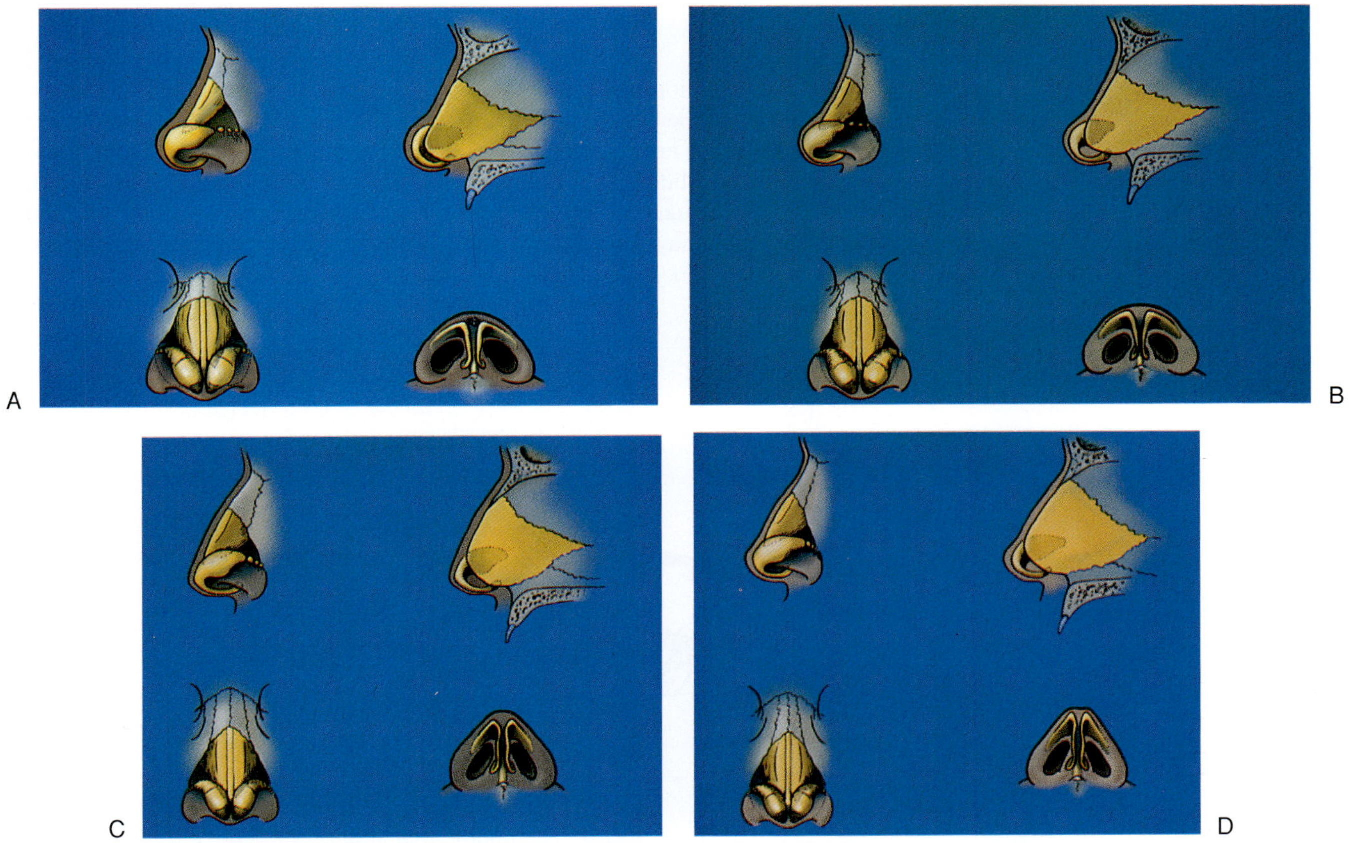

Figure 27. Rhinoplasty templates for the different ethnic groups. **A**: African American; **B**: Asian/Hispanic; **C**: Castillian Hispanic; and **D**: Northern European.

THE EYES

Upper Eyelids

The following discourse will outline clinically significant anatomic variations that thus may benefit from an armamentarium of approaches to address the clinical need.

Upper Lid Supratarsal Fold

Presence or absence of the supratarsal fold influences the perceived size and width of the eye. Figure 28 depicts the left eye with and without a supratarsal fold. In the presence of a fold, the human eye perceives an increased width of the palpebral fissure. Asians born with the crease seem to have larger eyes and may be culturally perceived as more alert and friendly than those without a fold. In addition, the application of make-up in the presence of a supratarsal fold is far simpler than that achieved in the absence of the crease. Surgeons' frequent requests for eyelid surgery from Asian patients are prompted by a desire to have a bright-eyed, open look in contrast to the hooded eye that to some translates as a lack of openness.

When the supratarsal fold is present, a variety of presentations may be noted (Fig. 29). According to Chen, the lid may exist without a crease; with a parallel crease, a non-continued or segmented fold, a partial or incomplete crease, or multiple creases; nasally tapered in contrast to the crease that insets into the upper lid margin; and with a parallel crease in contrast to the semi-lunar crease as seen in the Caucasian. The cadaveric dissections of Doxanas and Anderson have discerned that the fundamental difference lies in the point of fusion of the orbital septum onto the levator aponeurosis.

Caucasians

The anterior and posterior orbital septum fuses just cephalad to the inset of the levator aponeurosis and to the superior tarsal border located 8–10 mm above the lid margin (Fig. 30). Terminal fibers of the levator aponeurosis insert into the subdermal surface of the pretarsal and preseptal upper lid skin. As the levator contracts to elevate the upper lid, a crease forms just above the supratarsal border. The skin overlying the crease forms a fold. As aging progresses, hooding may develop as a result of redundant pre-aponeurotic fat pad descending through a weakened outer skin envelope (dermatochalasis).

Asians

In the absence of a supratarsal crease, a low-point effusion of the posterior and anterior septum results in a fatty prominence extending close to the superior lid margin (Fig. 31). The pre-aponeurotic fat pad is also descendant, with both pads contributing to a fuller

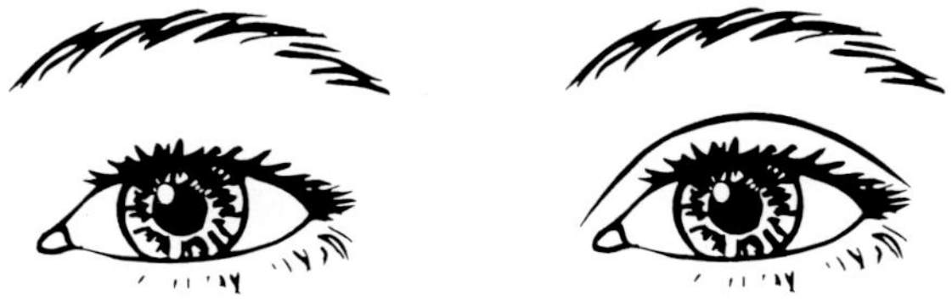

a. b.

Figure 28. A and B: The supratarsal crease when present gives the impression of a larger palpebral fissure.

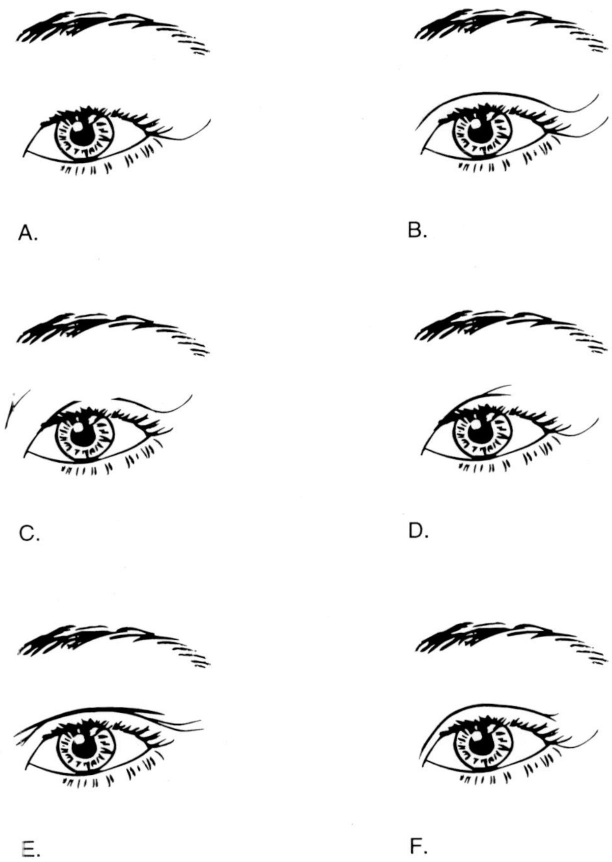

Figure 29. A host of presentations can be noted in the Asian eyelid as described by Chen. **A:** Absent supratarsal fold; **B:** a full supratarsal fold with a parallel crease; **C:** non-continuous or segmented supratarsal fold; **D:** an incomplete crease; **E:** multiple creases; **F:** nasally tapered crease with or without lateral flare.

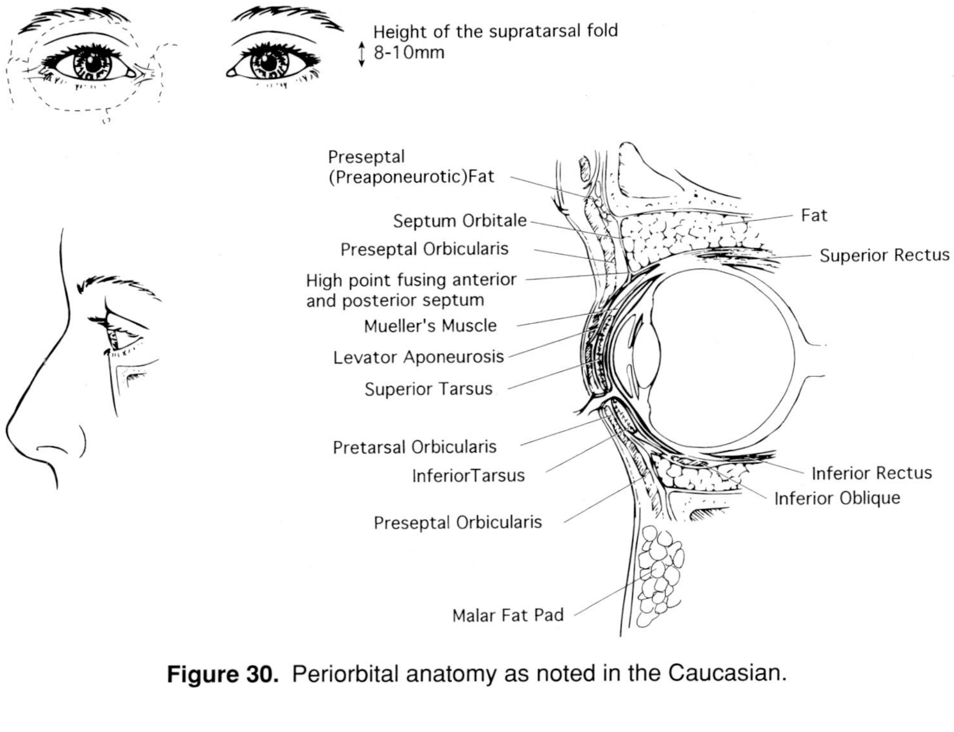

Figure 30. Periorbital anatomy as noted in the Caucasian.

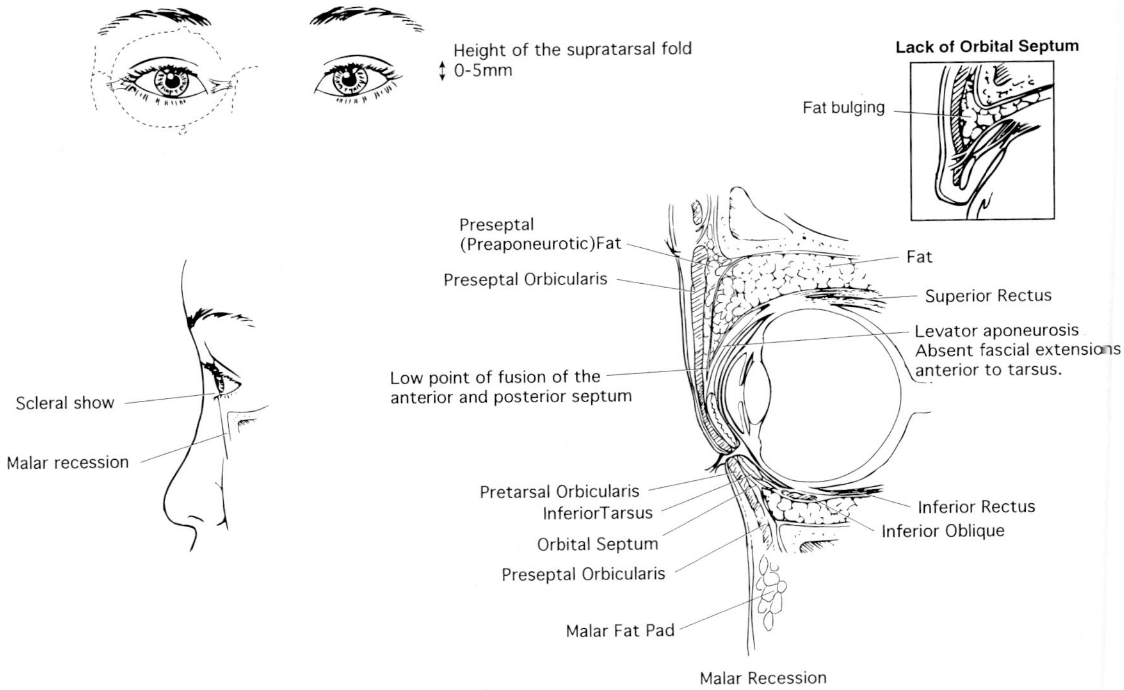

Figure 31. Periorbital anatomy as noted in the Asian.

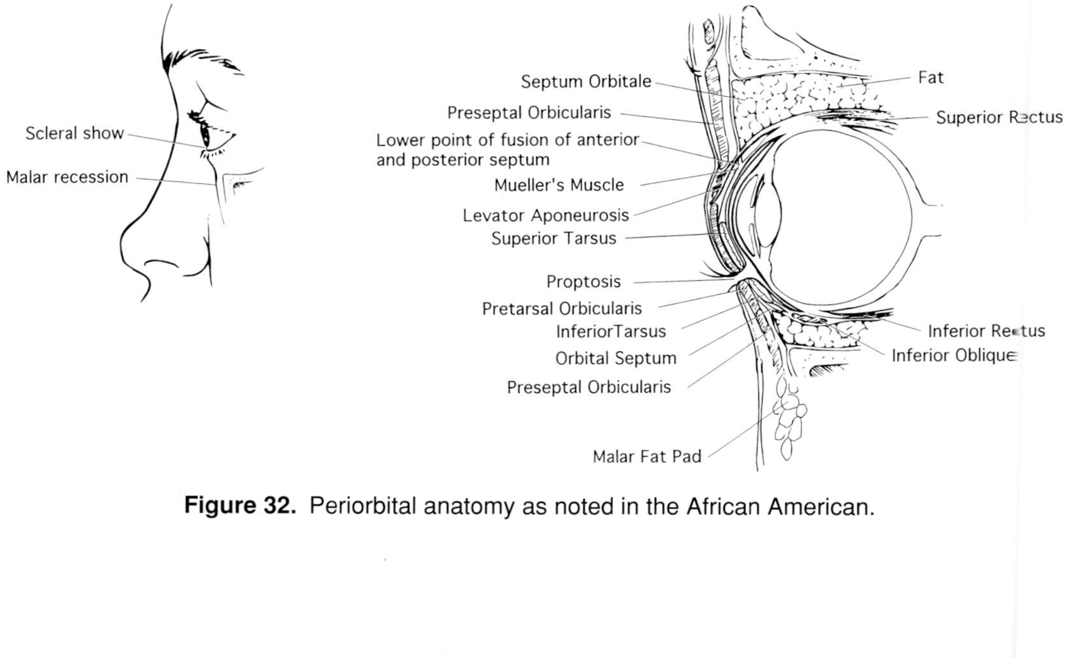

Figure 32. Periorbital anatomy as noted in the African American.

appearance of the eyelid. The presence of these fatty layers, along with the absence of levator extensions to the subdermal plane. In the elderly patient, skin laxity progresses, making upper lid fullness greater.

African Americans

The tarsus is shorter, ~5–8 mm in height (Fig. 32). The supratarsal fold resulting from insertions of the levator aponeurosis typically sits at ~6–8 mm. The relatively lower position of the fusion of the anterior and posterior septum commonly contributes to upper lid fullness that is commonly exacerbated by aging and dermatochalasis.

Epicanthal Folds

Webbing just anterior to the medial canthus occurs much more commonly in children in each ethnic group than in adults. The origin of the epicanthus is highest at an earlier age

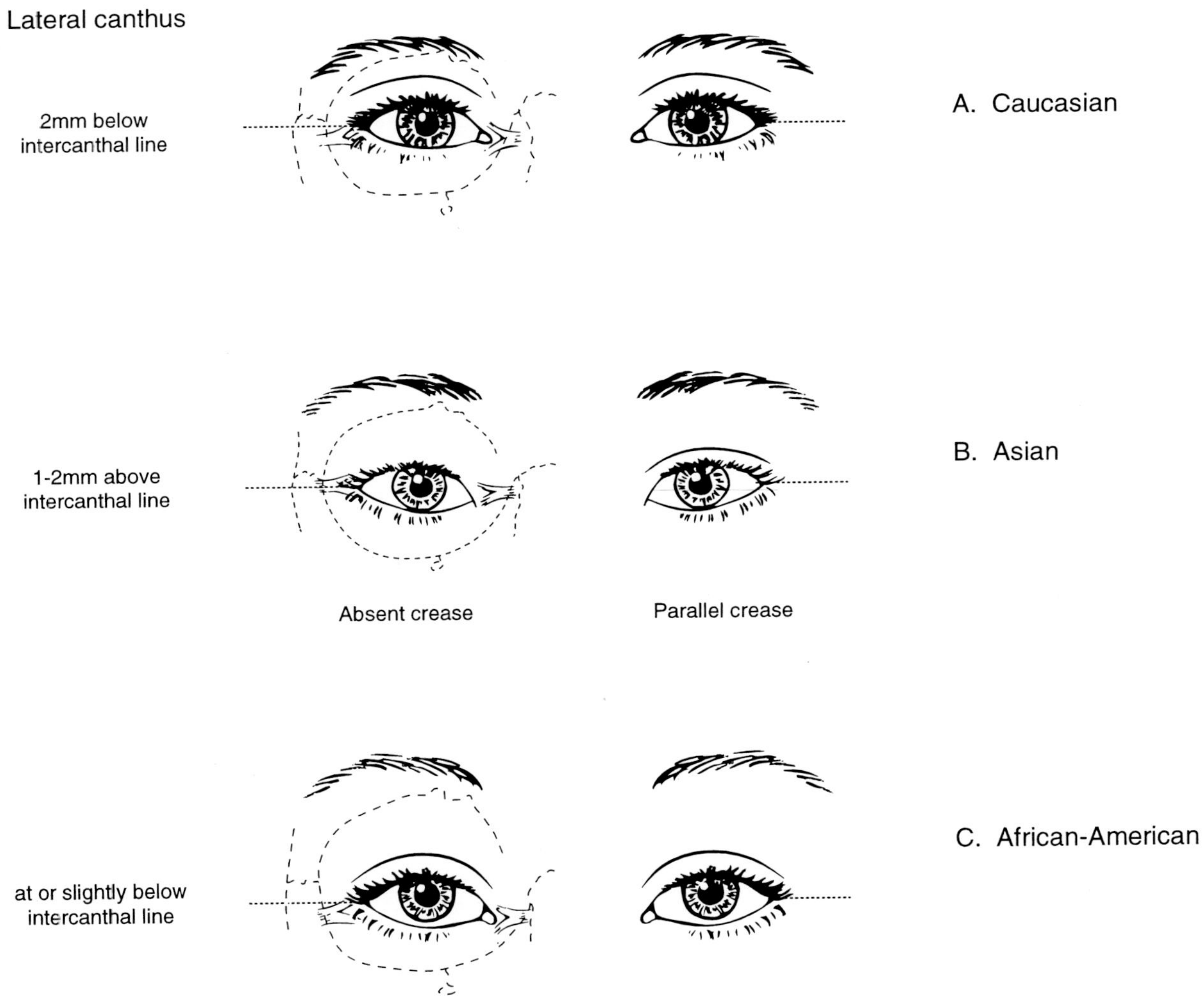

Figure 33. Comparative anatomy of the eyelids. Note the higher lateral canthal position relative to the medial canthus in the Asian versus the other two ethnic groups. The nen-ex distance is much less in the Asian lid, particularly in the presence of epicanthal folds. The vertical width of the palpebral fissure is greatest in the African American and is frequently associated with 1–3 mm of scleral show.

and descends as one becomes an adult. Epicanthus supraciliaris may begin as high as the brow and extend inferiorly to the lacrimal sac. Epicanthus palpebralis rises above the tarsus and may extend to the infraorbital rim. As one matures, there is a tendency toward epicanthus tarsalia with a fold arising from the upper lid crease and extending to the medial canthus. Epicanthus tarsalia is the type of webbing seen most commonly in the Asian. As the nasal bridge becomes more defined, the epicanthus diminishes. The lateral canthus in the Caucasian is ~5° higher than that of the medial canthus in contrast to 8° in the African American and 10° in the Asian (Fig. 33).

In the Asian, the intracanthal width is usually much wider than the en-ex distance. The palpebral fissure in most Asians is typically several millimeters shy of the vertical fifths as defined by neoclassical facial proportions (Fig. 34).

Lower Eyelids

Prominence of the lateral malar bone in the Caucasian, along with well positioned malar fat, yields prominent cheekbone (Fig. 29). Anterior malar hypoplasia in the Asian and the

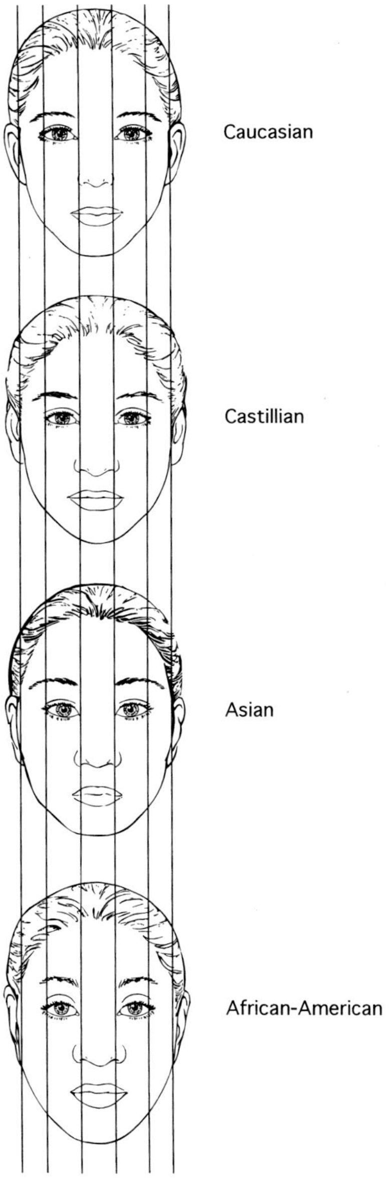

Figure 34. Theoretically the face can be divided into equal fifths with lines landing on anatomic features such as the inner and outer canthus as defined by neoclassical canons. However, this canon does not apply in most attractive faces irrespective of ethnic background.

African American (Figs. 30, 31) contributes to proptosis along with a lower position of the lid margin and resultant scleral show. Scleral show and malar fat pad descent progress with aging, particularly in the Asian and African American populations.

FACIAL RELATIONSHIPS

The importance of phi relationships in the face has been noted earlier in this chapter. In Fig. 35 we can see several anatomic differences among the ethnic groups. The trichion is commonly higher in the Hispanic, Asian, and African American. The glabella angle is often more obtuse in the pigmented races. The supratarsal fold tends to be at a lower position in a number of ethnic groups. The relative differences between the columella angle and tip-defining points are noted in viewing the line through the Caucasian tip-defining point. The position of the nasal spine is fairly consistent in faces of similar size. Chin resection is commonly noted in the Asian and African American.

RISK FACTORS FOR THE PATIENT OF COLOR

The origin of many individuals of color from the Mediterranean and the African and Asian continents (Fig. 35) exposes the plastic surgeon to a number of disease entities from

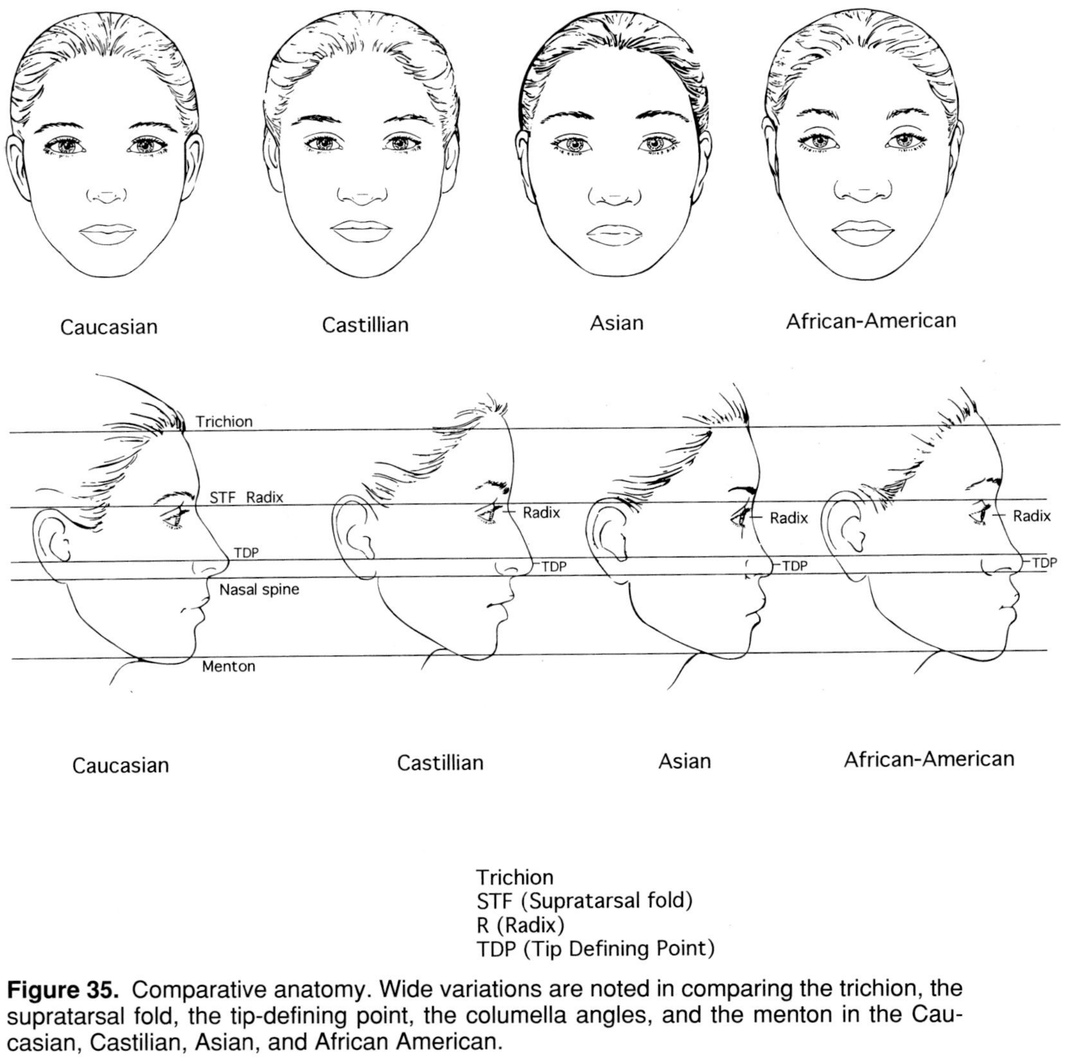

Figure 35. Comparative anatomy. Wide variations are noted in comparing the trichion, the supratarsal fold, the tip-defining point, the columella angles, and the menton in the Caucasian, Castilian, Asian, and African American.

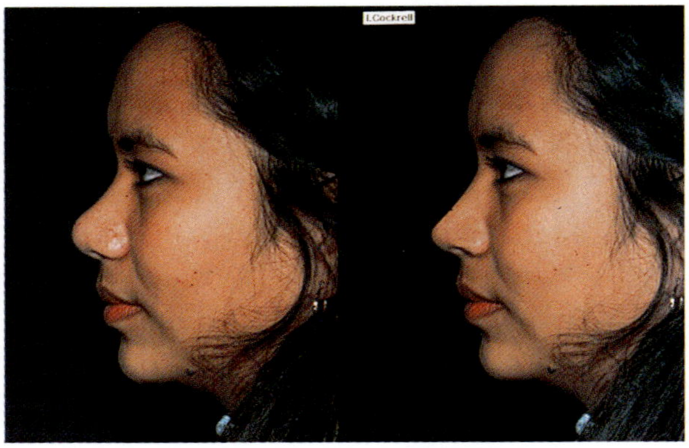

Figure 36. This 30-year-old Filipino woman presented for nasal surgery. The surgeon's assessment suggested the need for dorsal augmentation and lateral infracture without any adjustments in the tip or alar base. Anticipated surgical goal was outlined. In spite of the patient's impressions that she needed tip enhancement, an alar wedge resection is advised by another surgeon, she was very satisfied with the imaging and the subsequent surgical outcome as outlined.

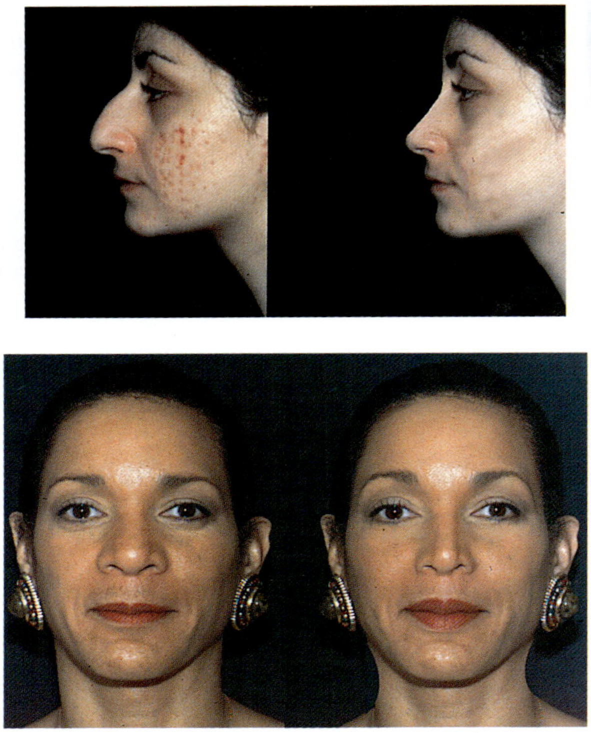

Figure 38. This 24-year-old Syrian woman *(top)* and 48-year-old African American woman *(bottom)* presented with a thick dorsum and tip. Osteocartilaginous reduction would lead to blunting of the bridge and tip. Imaging was used to illustrate the benefits of the slight dorsal augmentation and onlay tip graft to better define the nasal lobule.

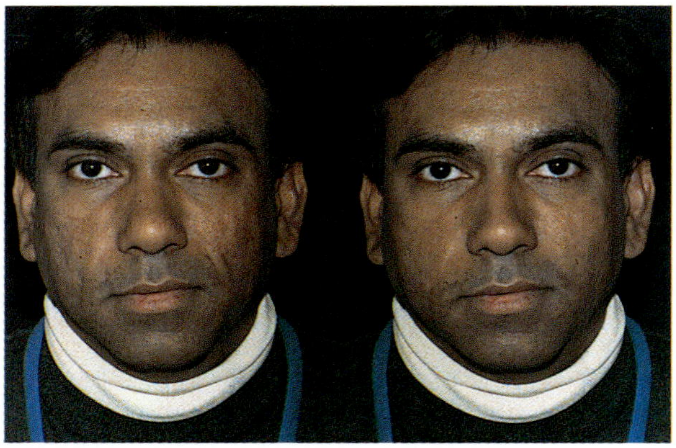

Figure 37. The excessive dorsal bony and cartilaginous elements of the East Indian nose are best addressed with minimal hump resection and 1- to 3-mm reduction in tip length. The tip should be adjusted first and dorsal planing follows. The East Indian and Middle Eastern noses often have an enlarged skin envelope that does not follow the reduced osteocartilaginous volume. The tip can be foreshortened, but excess skin is best accommodated using tip cartilage grafts to increase anterior projection and tip height. Dorsal bridge adjustment follows the desired tip position. In both the male and the female, the dorsal height may match the tip aesthetically in contrast to the desired supertip depression in the Caucasian female.

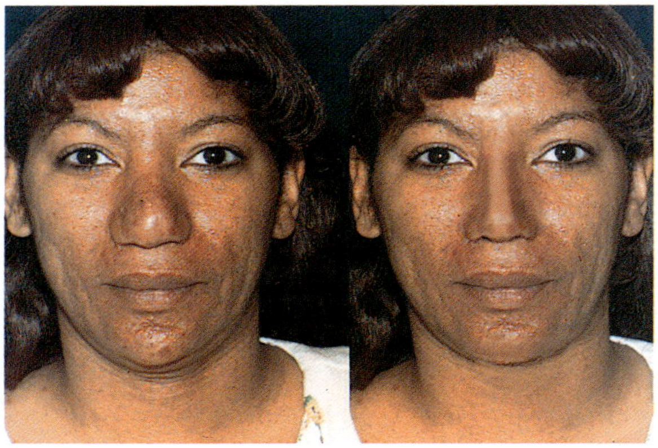

Figure 39. This is the desired outcome opted for by a patient with an excessively thick and glabrous tip skin. Given this goal, the only way to achieve this degree of reduction was with a direct dorsal midline skin resection that was selected by the patient.

each respective area. Some of the most common but subtly striking of these include several hemoglobinopathies that have teleologically been protective against falciparum malaria. Thalassemia major and minor are frequently seen in Middle Eastern populations. Fetal hemoglobin replaces the more typical hemoglobin A, resulting in susceptibility to red cell malformation and microcytosis. Thalassemia major patients are usually sickly and die by the age of 30. Thalassemia trait (minor) trait, on the other hand, may allow long-term survival with minimal symptoms. Severe anoxia, however, may precipitate vaso-occlusive phenomena like papillary necrosis of the kidney. Mild anemias are frequent.

Sickle cell disease is far more common with sickle cell trait noted in as many as 10% of African American patients. Anoxia, acidosis, dehydration, stress, and infections may precipitate acute painful hemolytic crises in those with sickle cell disease. Acute aplastic crises may occur in association with parvo virus infection or folate deficiency.

Glucose-6-phosphate dehydrogenase deficiency occurs in 10% of the African American population. The glucose-6-phosphate dehydrogenate deficiency compromises the ability of the red cell to produce NADPH. Thus, the red cell is not protected against oxidizing drugs like primaquine, proveisate, phenacetin, aspirin, chloramphenicol, vitamin K, sulfonamides, suiphones, and naphthalene (moth balls). In this condition, also referred to as fauvism, the acute hemolysis that occurs is self-limiting but may present as a diagnostic dilemma.

Pre-operative histories, in Middle Eastern, Asian, and African patients, should query familial or personal histories consistent with hemolytic or hypoxic crises. Food and medications that pre-operative hemolytic anemias should be awarded. Awareness of the frequency of these pathologies and a high degree of suspicion will ensure a safe peri-operative course. Food and medications that precipitate hemolytic crises should be avoided.

IMPROVING AESTHETIC ACUMEN FOR PATIENTS OF COLOR

Rhinoplasty is perhaps the greatest challenge for the cosmetic surgeon. Tracing paper is an excellent way to prepare for surgery and to outline various surgical options. Sketching allows input from the patient as well as relates to his/her aesthetic goals.

A more natural outcome is achieved with the least amount of surgery possible. Determining how much surgery will be necessary to achieve a satisfactory outcome is very difficult unless one utilizes video imaging as shown in Figs. 36–45. The importance of achieving an improved but natural appearance in the patient of color cannot be overstated.

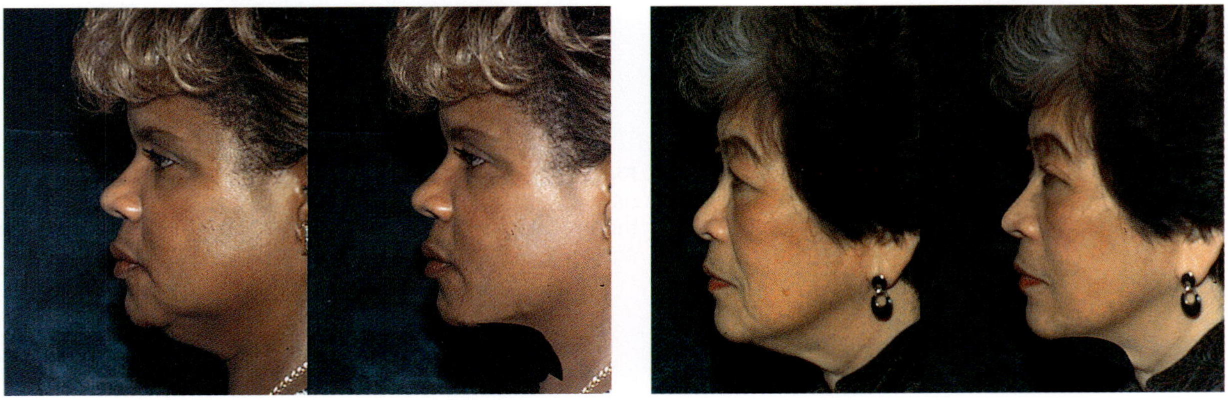

Figure 40. Dark shadows under the eyes softened by resuspending the malar fat pad, lateral lid skin resection, and neck lift.

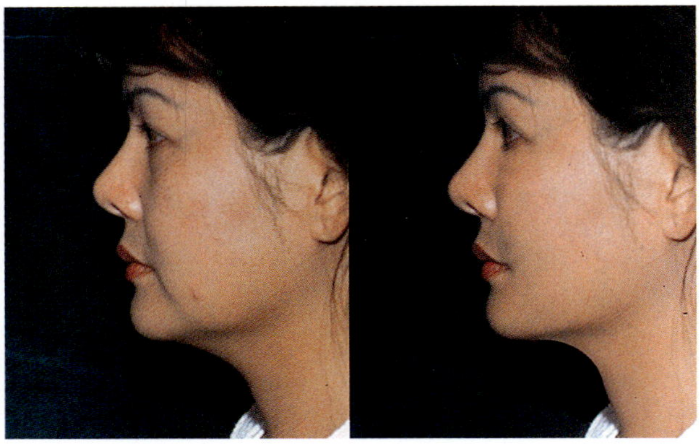

Figure 41. This patient presented, complaining of early jowl formation. Intraoral incisions were used to perform zygomatic major and levator anguli plication.

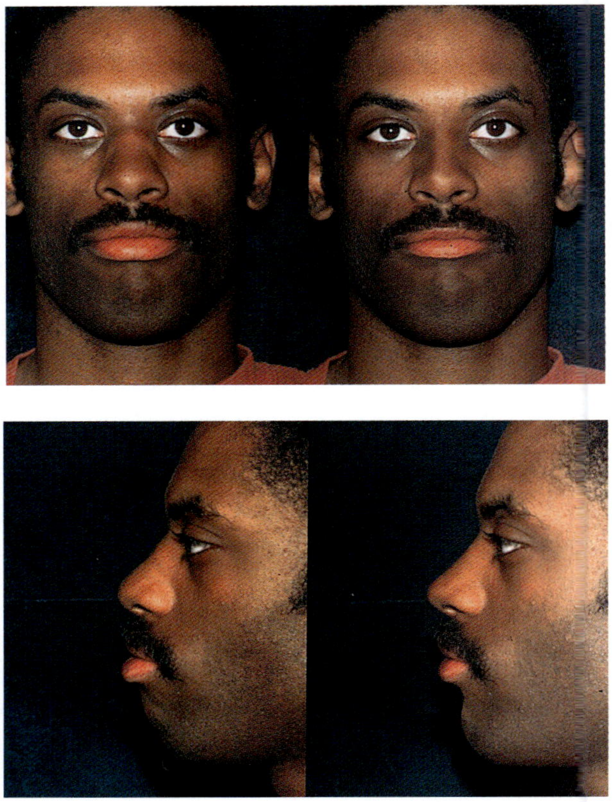

Figure 43. Determining the amount of desired lip reduction is very difficult to achieve. In this patient dorsal rasping and augmentation with lateral infracture along with a mucosal reduction would yield this outcome.

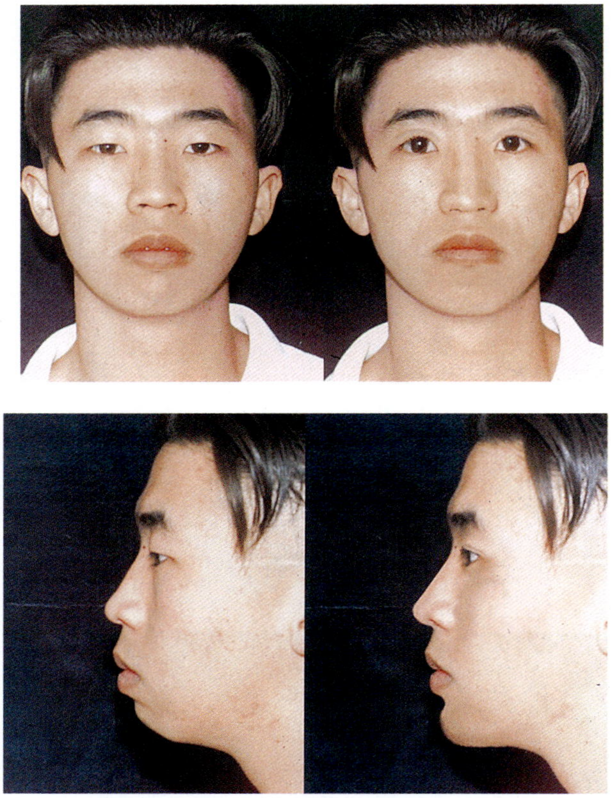

Figure 42. Chin augmentation with a Mental oval-shaped implant, suction-assisted lipectomy, along with dorsal augmentation and onlay tip grafting.

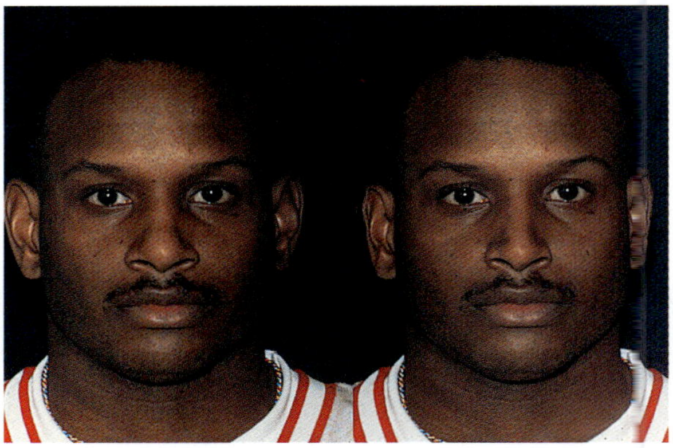

Figure 44. The anxieties and lifelong stresses of the individual with protuberant ears can be realistically alleviated through otoplasty. Depicting anticipated results optimizes the surgeon's ability to translate the anticipated goals.

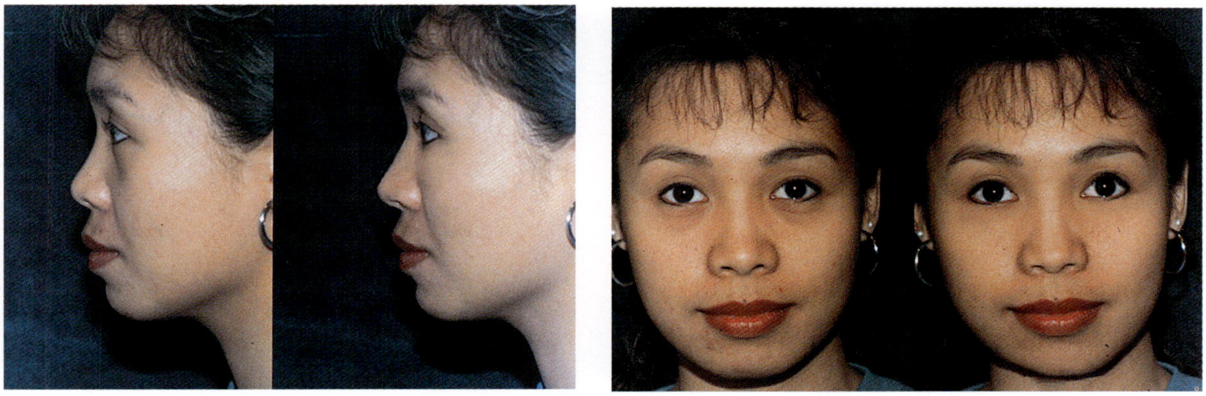

Figure 45. Video imaging is particularly helpful in outlining surgical goals in the Asian nose. Patients commonly request improvements in the dorsum and tip. How subtle or how dramatic a change is requested is difficult to discern. Expectations are clarified, making patient satisfaction easier to achieve.

RECOMMENDED READING

Chin WPD. Upper blepharoplasty in the Asian patient. In: Putterman AM, ed. *Cosmetic oculoplastic surgery*. 2nd ed. Philadelphia: Saunders, 1993.

Chin WPD. A comparison of Caucasian and Asian blepharoplasty. *Ophthalmol Pract* 1991;9:216–222.

Doxanas MT, Anderson RL. Oriental eyelids: anatomic studies. *Arch Ophthalmol* 1984;102:1232–1235.

Farkas LG. *Anthropometry of the head and face in medicine*. New York: Elsevier North Holland, 1981.

Farkas LG, Sohm P, Kolar JC, et al. Inclinations of the facial profile: art vs. reality. *Plast Reconstr Surg* 1985;75:509.

Farkas LG, Hreczko TA, Kolar JC, Monroe IR. Vertical and horizontal proportions of the face in young adult North American Caucasians: revision of neoclassical canons. *Plast Reconstr Surg* 1985;75:328.

Gonzales-Ulloa M. Quantitative method for the appreciation of the morphology of the face. *Plast Reconstr Surg* 1964;34:241.

Huntley HE. *The divine proportion: a study in mathematical beauty*. New York: Dover, 1970.

Johnson CC. Epicanthus. *Am J Ophthalmol* 1986;66:939–946.

Lew K, Loh E. Ranking of facial profiles among Asians. *J Aesthet Dent* 1992;4:128.

Loverpel EH. *On facial balance and harmony*. Engle Orthodontics and Dann, C. *Rating of facial attractiveness*. Community Dental and Oral Epidemiology, 1992;20:214.

Matory WE Jr, Falces E. Non-Caucasian rhinoplasty: a sixteen year experience. *Plast Reconstr Surg*. 1986;77:239.

Millard DR Jr. The Oriental eyelid and its surgical revision. *Am J Ophthalmol* 1964;57:646–649.

Preston JD. The golden proportion revisited. *J Aesthet Dent* 1993;5:247.

Ricketts RM. Divine proportion in facial aesthetics. *Clin Plast Surg* 1982;9:401.

Romm S. *The changing face of beauty*. St. Louis: Mosby YearBook, 1992.

Steiner CC. Cephalometrics for you and me. *Am J Orthod* 1953;39:729.

Tolleth H. Concepts for the plastic surgeon from art and sculpture. *Clin Plast Surg* 1987;14:585.

Tolleth H. Facial contours and proportions from an artist's point of view. In: Ousterhout DK, ed. *Aesthetic contouring of the craniofacial skeleton*. Boston: Little, Brown, 1991:59–70.

Ethnic Considerations in Facial Aesthetic Surgery, edited by W. Earle Matory, Jr.
Lippincott–Raven Publishers, Philadelphia © 1998.

8

The Definition of Beauty in the Northern European

Rod J. Rohrich and Jeffrey M. Kenkel

Beauty is truly in the eye of the beholder.
— Hungerford

The face, more than any other part of the body, defines our individuality. Each face is distinguished from another by the size and shape of distinct features and specifically by the relationship of these features to each other. The presence of physical beauty does much more than distinguish one from another—it positively influences all aspects of our daily lives. What constitutes beauty is, to a great extent, influenced by ethnic and cultural patterns (1).

Plato recognized the importance of physical beauty and felt its secret lay in the harmonious proportion of facial features. He related the face to the number 3 (the number by which all things were determined). He divided the face into three segments: from hairline to eyes, eyes to upper lip, and from upper lip to chin. He found the ideal face to be two-thirds as wide as it was high. It was felt that the nose needed to be straight or fall in a slightly depressed line from its root to the forehead (23).

As plastic surgeons concerned with facial and nasal aesthetics, we recognize the importance of facial proportions as well as the influence ethnicity has on nasal deformities. Farkas's work on the anthropometrics and morphometrics of the nose with respect to ethnicity is significant. He found significant racial disparity specifically among columellar width, nasal tip projection, and angulation of the nares (Fig. 1; Table 1). Type II was found to be most common in Caucasians (52.8%), type III in Asians (52.8%), and type VI (50%) was the most frequently found angle of the nares in Blacks (14).

R. J. Rohrich and J. M. Kenkel: Department of Plastic Surgery, University of Texas Southwestern Medical Center, Dallas, Texas 75235-9132

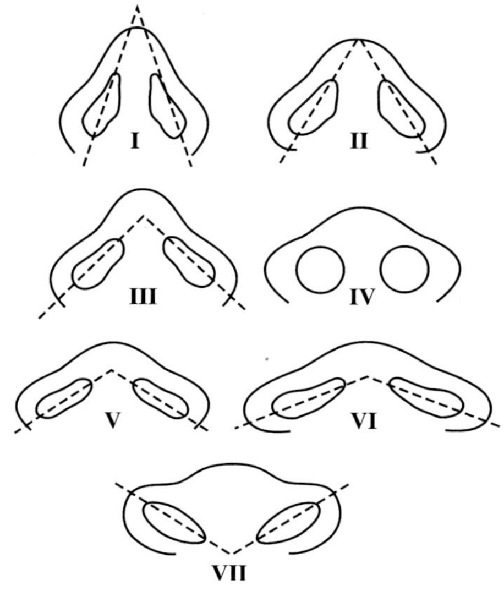

Figure 1. Nostril types with inclination. (Reprinted from Farkas LG, Hreczko TA, Deutsch CA. Objective assessment of standard nostril types—a morphologic study. *Ann Plast Surg* 1983;11:381, with permission.)

AESTHETIC FACIAL PROPORTIONS

Aesthetically pleasing faces have certain proportions and relationships in common. In evaluating a patient for rhinoplasty, one must recognize and analyze facial proportions to determine the aesthetic goal. Facial relationships commonly found in attractive Caucasian women and men will be described. Variations for the Middle Eastern, African American, Asian, and Hispanic will be noted.

The face is divided by horizontal lines into thirds adjacent to the menton, alar base, supraorbital notch (brow), and hairline (Fig. 2). The upper line varies with hairstyle and patient age and is least important in nasal/facial diagnoses. The lower face (distance between alar base and menton) is further subdivided into an upper third and a lower two-thirds by a transverse line bisecting the oral commissures. A transverse line through the labial mental groove divides the distance from stomion to menton in a one-to-two ratio (5,6) (Fig. 3). Fa-

Table 1. *Inclination of the medial longitudinal axis of symmetrical nostrils in the study group*

Type of nostril	Racial origin	No. of subjects	Percent of type	Inclination ()
I	Caucasian	53	100.0	70–90
II	Caucasian	66	85.7	55–69
	Asian	10	13.0	
	Black	1	1.3	
III	Caucasian	6	15.4	40–54
	Asian	28	71.8	
	Black	5	12.8	
IV	Asian	3	60.0	0
	Black	2	40.0	
V	Asian	10	90.9	25–39
	Black	1	9.1	
VI	Asian	2	11.1	10–24
	Black	16	88.9	
VII	Black	5	100.0	−50

Reprinted with permission from Farkas LG, Hreczko TA, Deutsch CA. Objective assessment of standard nostril types—a morphometric study. *Ann Plast Surg* 1987;14:599.

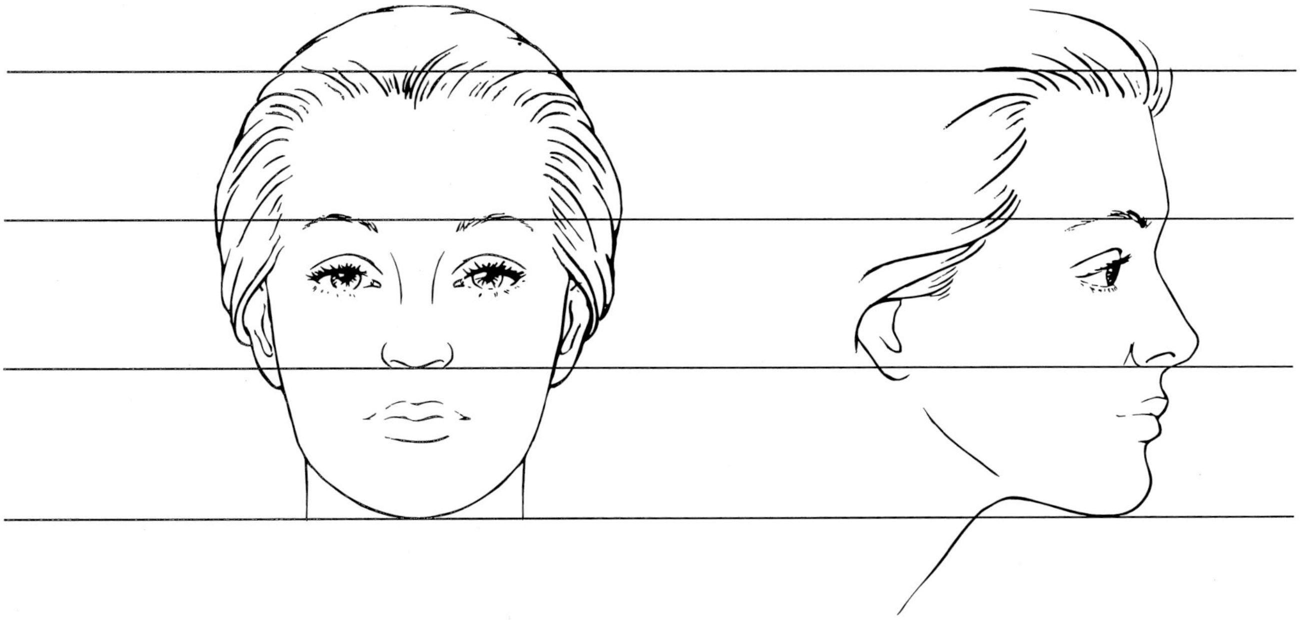

Figure 2. Division of face by horizontal lines.

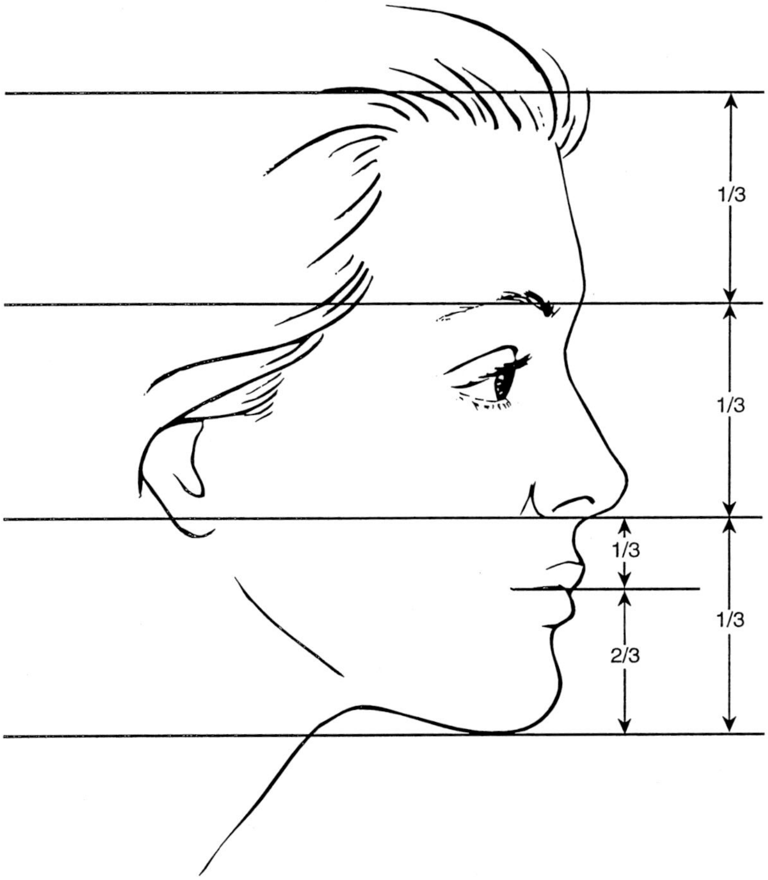

Figure 3. Stomion-to-menton ratio.

cial proportions are slightly different depending on ethnicity. For example, in African Americans, the lower face has a greater vertical dimension than the midface, which in turn has a greater vertical dimension than the upper face. Bimaxillary protrusion is common, and a Le Forte I setback maxillary osteotomy and/or mandibular surgery may improve the Black facial profile and should be discussed with the patient (6,7,8). Maxillary retraction is also quite common in the African American, Hispanic, and Asian. Northern Asians have a long midface and nose as well as bimaxillary protrusion. Each may benefit from orthognathic manipulation.

One must use caution when augmenting nasal dorsal projection in Asians as this often creates an undesirable illusion of an even longer nose (7).

Byrd has further refined facial analysis such that ideal facial dimensions are specific for a given face and not a generic mean of features pooled from a number of attractive faces. He calculates ideal nasal length with respect to facial proportions of either the lower face or the midface [middle facial height should be equal to or slightly less (3 mm) than the lower facial height]. Ideal nasal length equals the distance from stomion to menton or is equal to 0.67 × midfacial height. Ideal nasal tip projection equals 0.67 × ideal nasal length (*RT*) (Fig. 4). A natural horizontal facial plane is determined by drawing a line perpendicular to a plumb line superimposed over the head with the eyes in straightforward gaze (Fig. 5) (9).

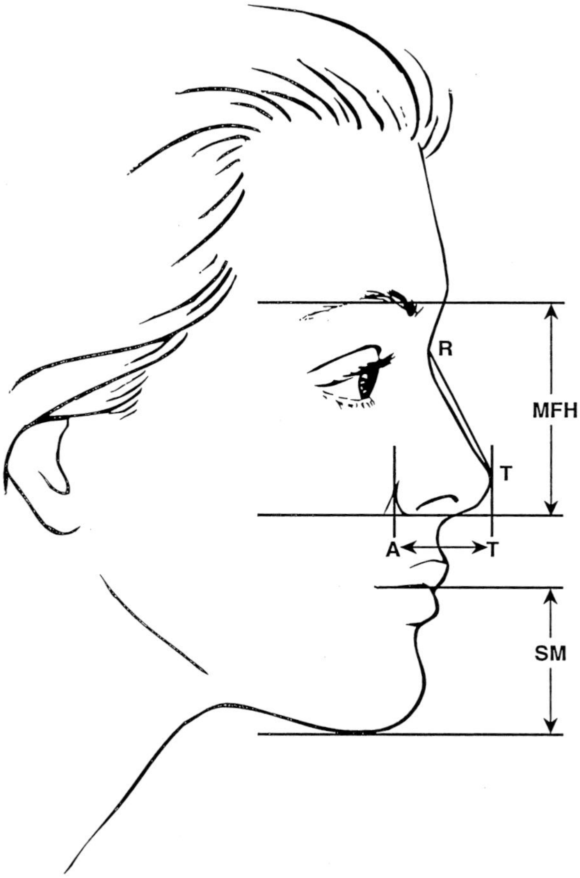

Figure 4. Byrd's facial analysis.

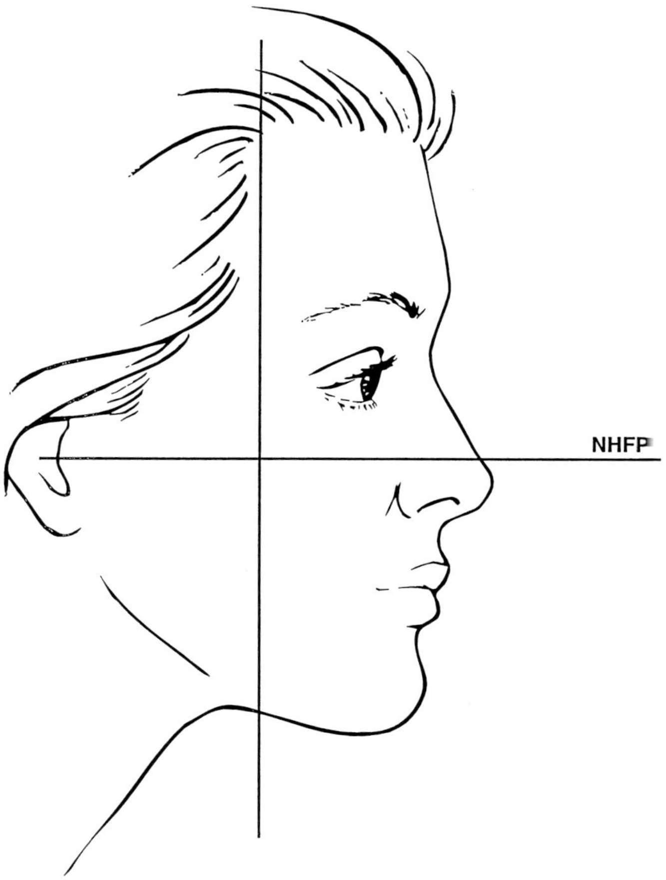

Figure 5. Natural horizontal facial plane.

AESTHETIC NASAL PROPORTIONS

The presence or absence of nasal deviation is a key contribution to nasal aesthetics. A line is drawn from the midglabella to the menton. This line should bisect the nasal bridge, upper lip, and Cupid bow. In patients with normal occlusion, the midline is the vertical line between the two central incisors (Fig. 6) (5,6).

The nasal dorsum is outlined by two slightly curved, divergent lines beginning at the medial supraciliary ridges and extending to the tip-defining points. The width of the bony base is noted and should be 75% of the normal alar base (Fig. 7). Alar base width should equal the intercanthal distance or the intercanthal width of one eye (Fig. 8).

If the alar base width is wider than the intercanthal distance, then one must determine if this is secondary to increased interalar width or alar flaring. The normal degree of alar flaring in the Caucasian female is 2 mm outside of the alar base. If the degree of alar flaring is excessive (>2 mm), then alar base resection should be considered. Nostril sill resection may be indicated if the interalar width is felt to be too broad (Fig. 9) (5,6,10,11,12). Each alar rim is assessed for symmetry and should have a slight outward flare in the inferior lateral direction (Fig. 10). The tip-defining points are characterized by two equilateral triangles from the supratip area to the apex of the domes, to the columella–lobule angle (Fig. 11). A tip modification may be required if any of the points are not anatomically correct (5,6,13,14). In contrast, the nose in many African Americans and Hispanics is wide based with prominent alar flare and/or increased interalar width (Fig. 12) (8). Common findings in the Asian nose are depicted in Fig. 13 (7).

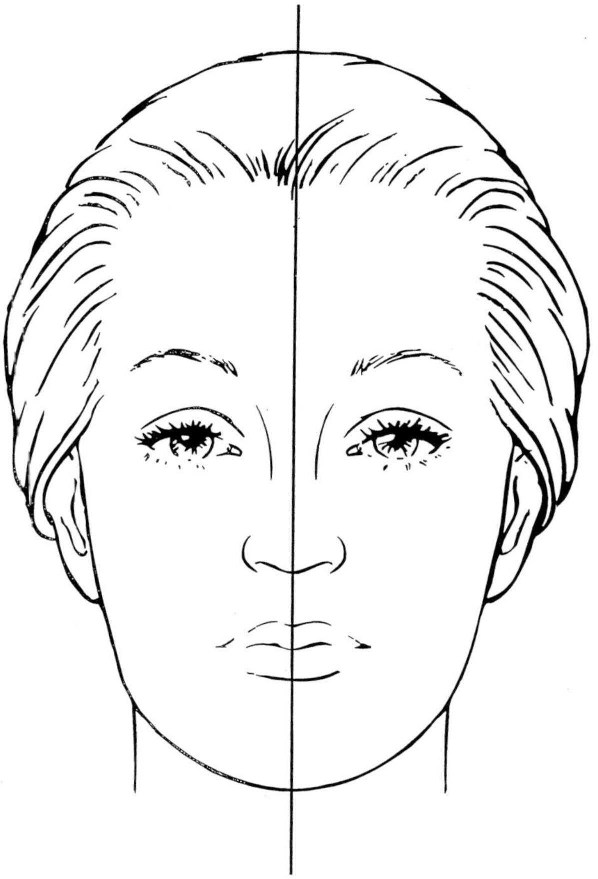

Figure 6. Bisection of face.

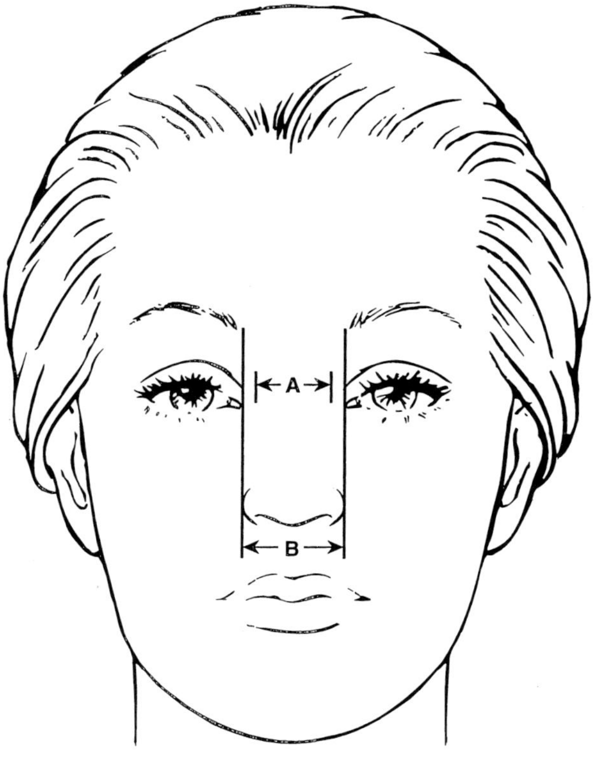

A = .75B

Figure 7. Relationship of bony base to alar base.

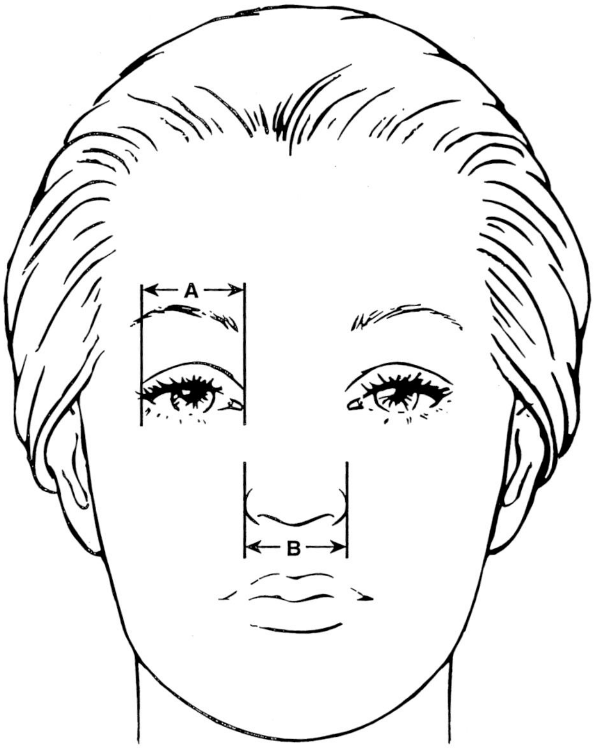

A = B

Figure 8. Relationship of alar base to intercanthal base.

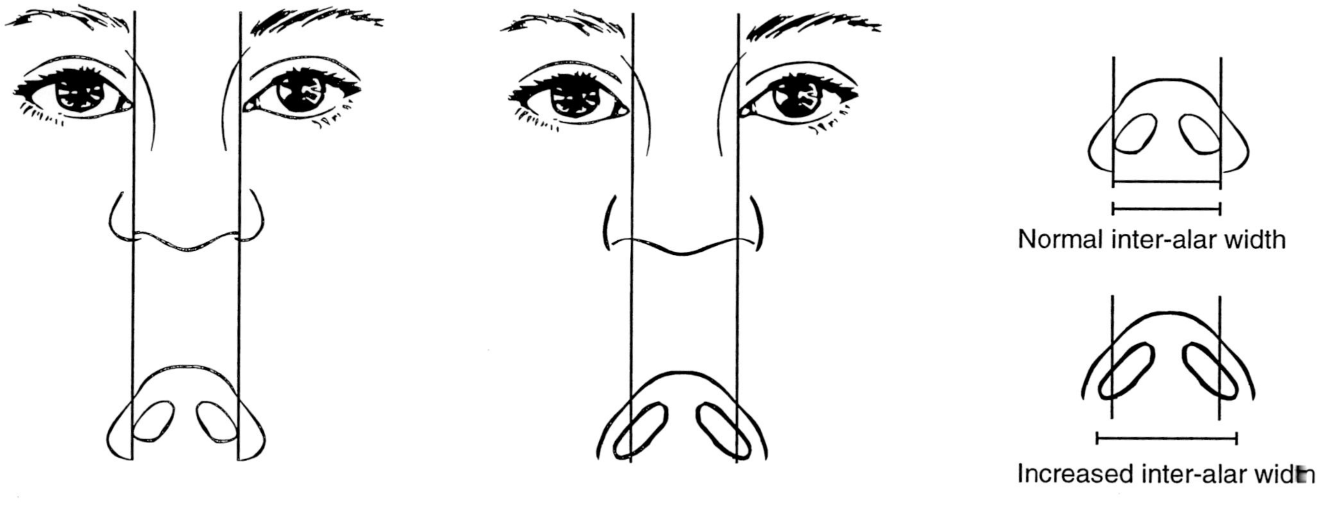

Alar flaring,
normal inter-alar width

Increased inter-alar width

Figure 9. Alar flaring versus interalar width.

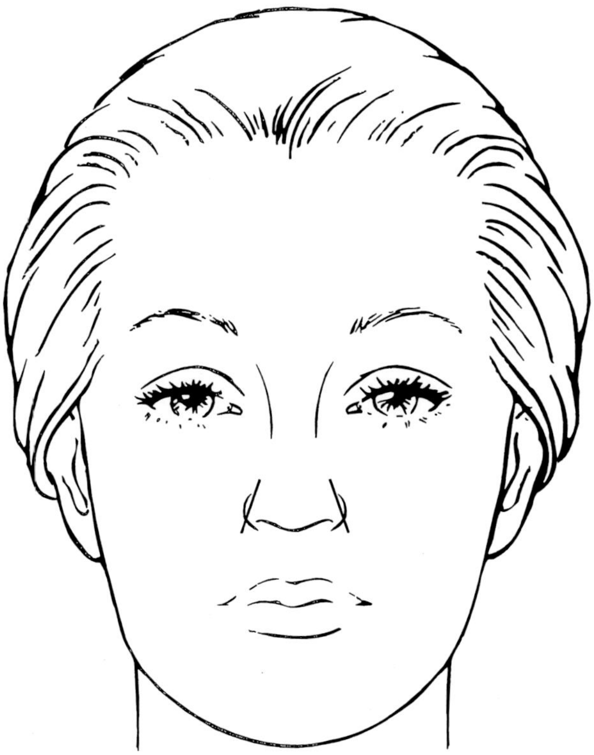

Figure 10. Alar flare.

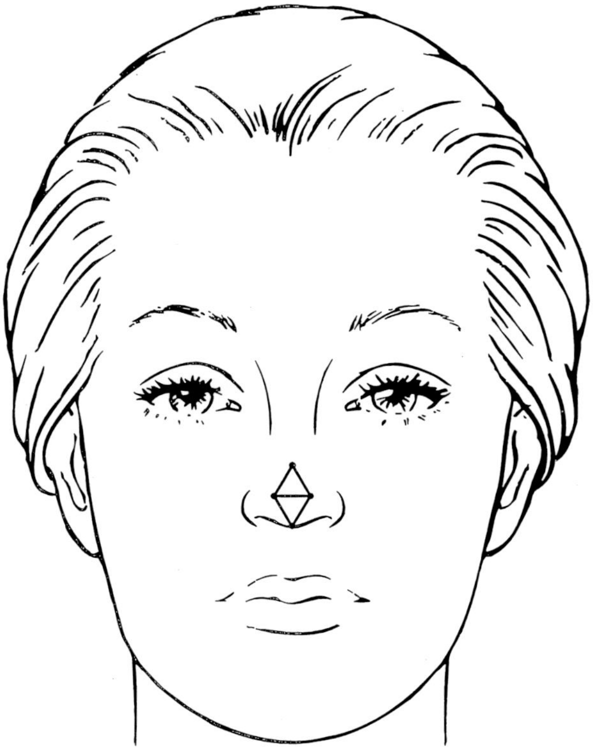

Figure 11. Tip-defining points.

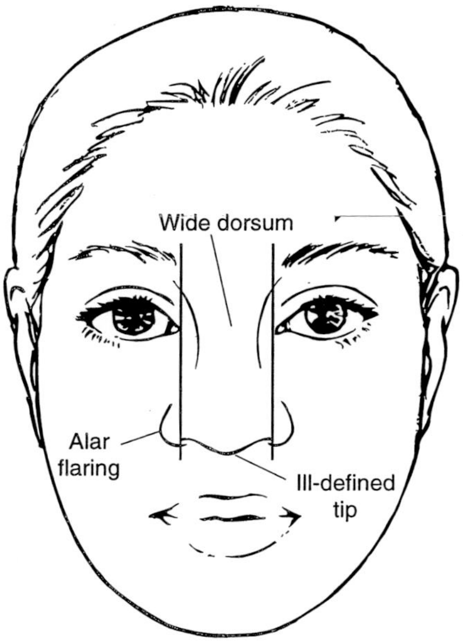

Figure 12. Typical nasal aesthetics in the African American.

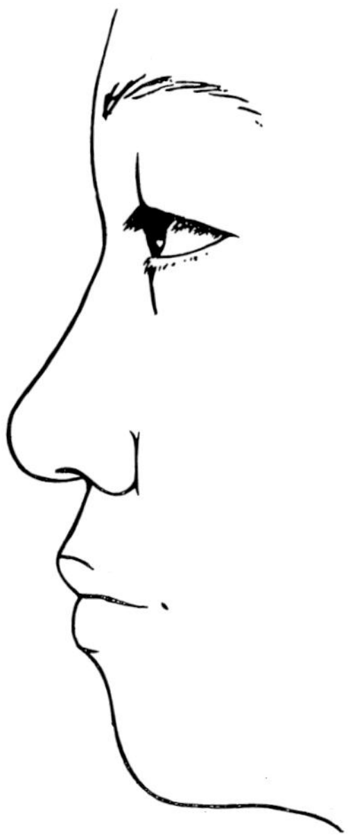

Figure 13. Many Asians have thickened ala, wide alar base, acute columellar–labial angle, and poor tip projection. (Adapted from Flowers RJ. Rhinoplasty in Oriental patients: repair of the East Asian nose. In: Daniel RK, ed. *Rhinoplasty aesthetic plastic surgery*. 2nd ed. Boston: Little, Brown, 1993.)

When the columella is inspected, on frontal view, the outline of the alar rims and columella should resemble a seagull in gentle flight (Fig. 14). If this curvature is too pronounced, the hanging columella may require reduction. A straightened gull wing implies a retracted columella, which often requires augmentation. The basal view of the columella and the outline of the nasal base forms an equilateral triangle with a lobule-to-nostril ratio of one to two (Fig. 15). The nostrils have a slight teardrop shape, with the long axis from base to apex in a slightly medial direction (5,6). African Americans often have a shortened columella with ovoid nostrils (11). Small, transversely oriented nostrils are often seen in the Asian (7).

When examining a patient in profile, one must assess the position and depth of the nasofrontal angle. This angle begins at the infrabrow area and forms a gentle, concave curve that connects the brow to the dorsum. The deepest portion of the nasofrontal angle should lie between the upper eyelash and the supratarsal fold with the eyes in natural horizontal gaze (Fig. 16). Unfortunately, an adequate guideline for accurately assessing the depth of the nasofrontal angle has not been defined, although the distance from the cornea to the nasal/facial angle has been suggested by Byrd (9).

The nasal dorsum in women lies ~2 mm behind a line drawn from the radix of the nasofrontal angle to the tip-defining points (Fig. 17). The dorsum is slightly higher in men. In Blacks, Asians, and Hispanics, the nasal dorsum is often depressed, often requiring augmentation. In those of Middle Eastern or Castillian background, a dorsal osteocartilaginous hump may be accompanied by globellar prominence (8).

Nasal tip projection is evaluated. With normal upper lip projection, a line is drawn from alar–cheek junction to the tip of the nose (Fig. 18). A vertical line is drawn adjacent to the most projecting part of the upper lip. Tip projection is considered normal if 50–60% of the tip lies anterior to the vertical line. If the tip is >60%, it overprojects and may require reduction. If <50%, tip projection is inadequate and often benefits from augmentation (5,13). With utilization of Byrd's analysis, tip projection is equal to 0.67 × RT (ideal nasal length) (9). Nasal tip projection in Blacks is usually somewhat less and can be estimated by 0.5 × nasal length (Fig. 19). Less tip projection is common in Asians, Hispanics, and African

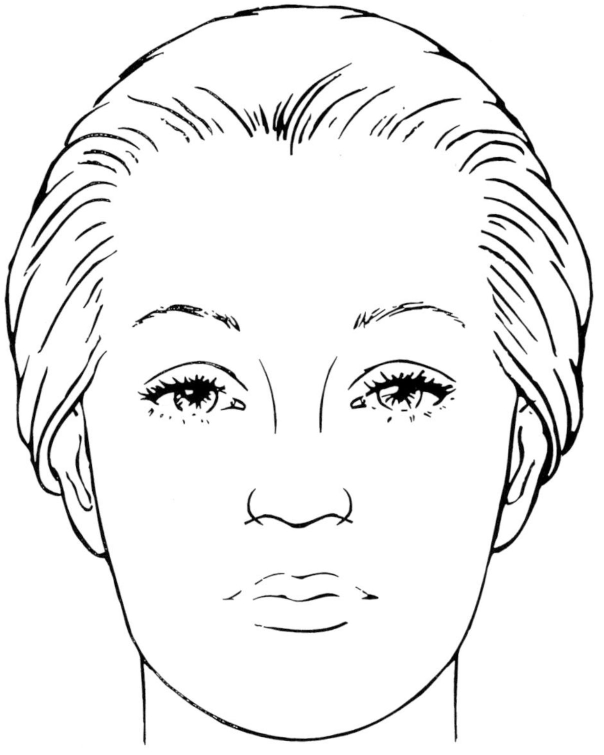

Figure 14. Outline of alar rims and columella.

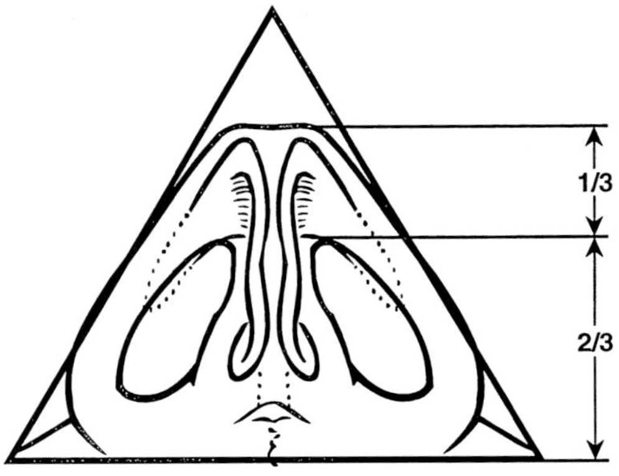

Figure 15. Basal view of lobule/nostril complex.

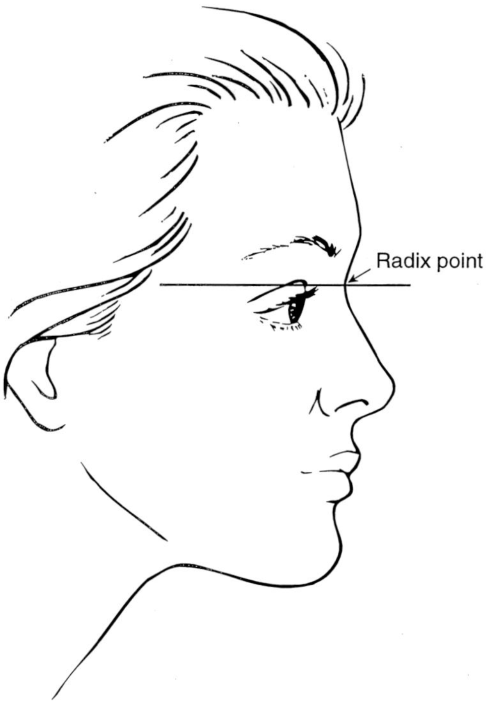

Figure 16. Deep portion of nasolabial angle.

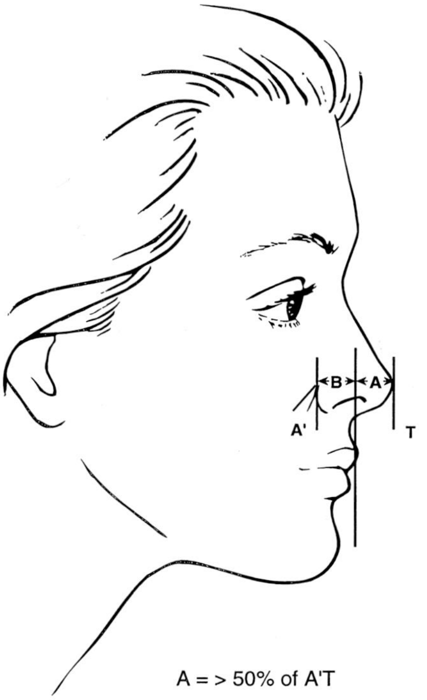

Figure 18. Nasal tip projection.

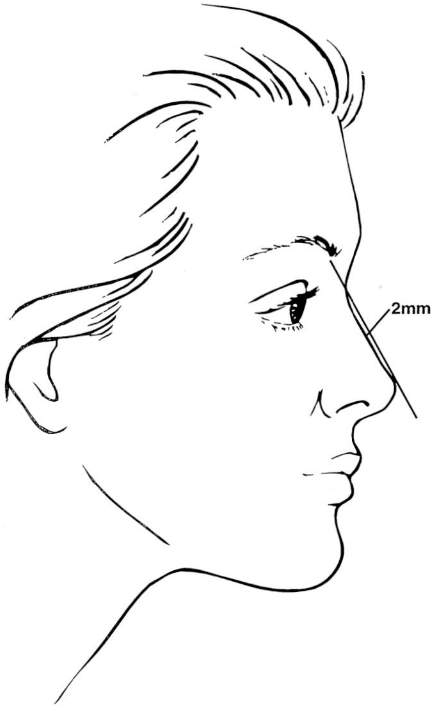

Figure 17. Nasal dorsum.

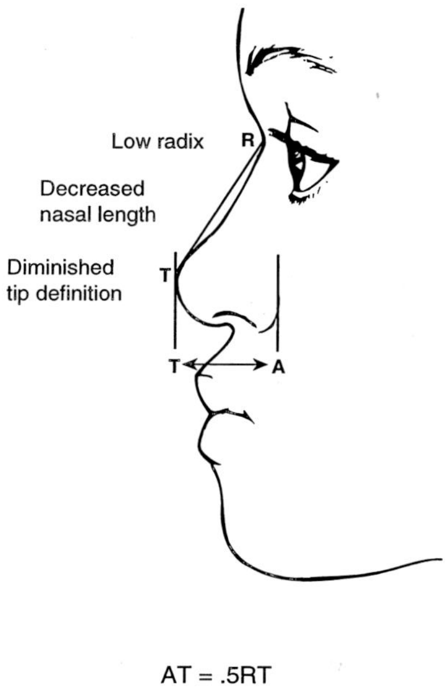

Figure 19. Nasal assessment in the African American, Hispanic, and Asian.

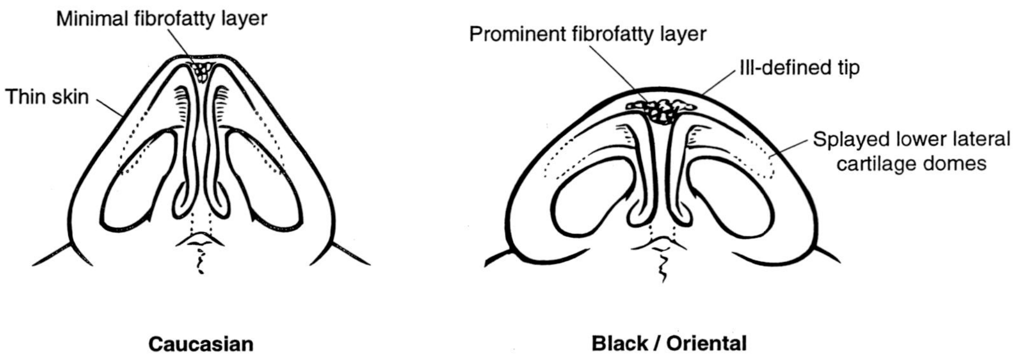

Figure 20. Thick fibrofatty layer obscuring tip definition.

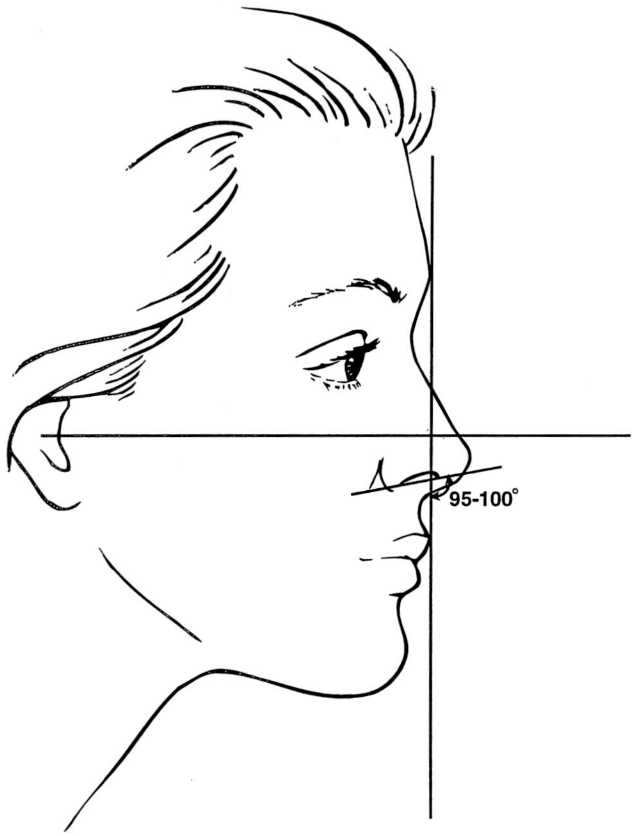

Figure 21. Nasolabial angle.

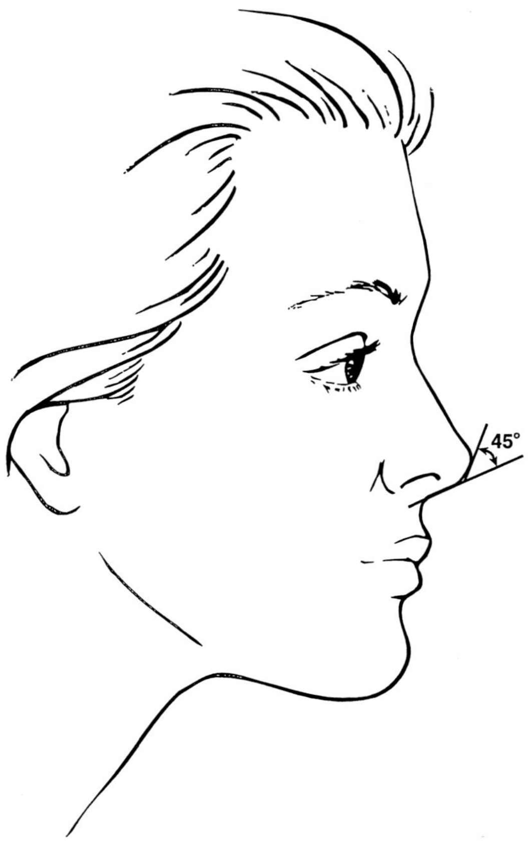

Figure 22. Columellar–labial angle.

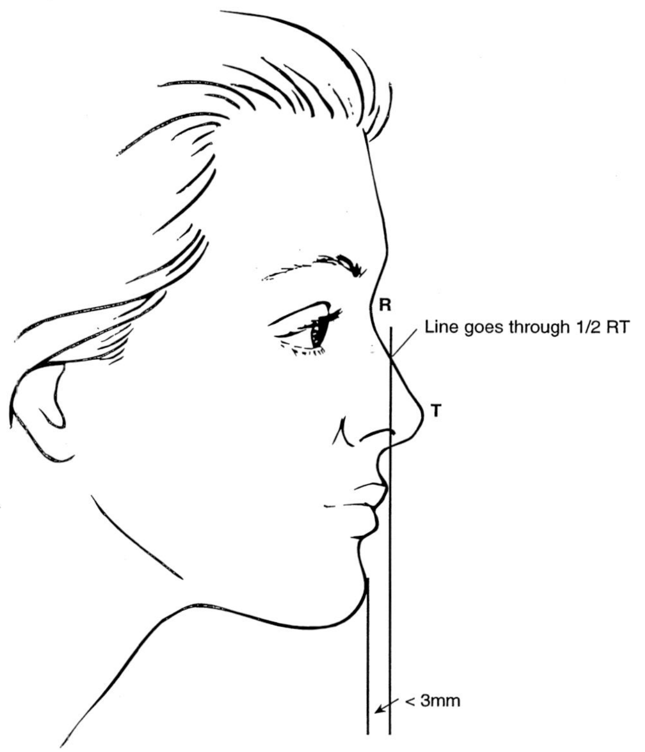

Figure 23. Aesthetic relationship of lip and chin complex.

Americans. Diastosis of the lower lateral cartilage at the tip, along with thick skin and a thick fibrofatty subcutaneous layer above the lower lateral cartilage, obscure nasal tip definition (Fig. 20) (7,8).

In addition to evaluating nasal tip projection and the dorsum of the nose, one should also assess the degree of supratip break. A slight supratip break gives the nose more definition and distinguishes the dorsum from the tip. This is preferable in women but not in men.

One next determines the degree of tip rotation. A straight line is drawn through the most anterior and posterior edges of the nostril (Fig. 21). The nasolabial angle is formed between this line and the plumb line. In women this angle is between 95 and 100°, while in men 90–95° is preferable. The nasolabial angle is contrasted with the columellar–labial angle, which is formed at the junction of the columella and upper lip (5,6). This angle should be ~45° in Caucasians, Castillians, and Middle Easterners but is much more acute in Blacks, Hispanics, and Asians (Fig. 22) (7,8). A prominent caudal septum creates increased fullness in this area and can give the illusion of increased rotation even though the nasolabial angle is within normal limits.

Finally one examines the relationship between the lip and chin. The upper lip should project 2 mm more than the lower lip. In women the chin is slightly posterior to the lower lip (2–3 mm), while in men the chin is more prominent (Fig. 23) (6). Asians frequently possess a deficiency of the jaw line and chin projection along with a prominence in the mandibular angles and the malar width. This creates a fragile balance that must be appreciated during aesthetic evaluation (7).

CONCLUSIONS

When evaluating a patient for facial aesthetic surgery and rhinoplasty, it is essential to consider the entire dentofacial unit. Grecian principles of balance and harmony with respect to the nose, upper and lower lip, and chin should be recognized. The most important step is to define the ideal nasal length specific to the facial proportions of the patient. Once defined, the ideal nasal length becomes the basis for calculations of the radix, tip, and chin projection.

Aesthetic surgery in non-Caucasians is distinct and requires a solid sense of what constitutes ethnic facial aesthetics. With this in mind, one must also recognize the aesthetic objectives in ethnic rhinoplasty patients. This most often includes a desire to look more like the accepted standard of beauty and a desire for a more attractive nose that retains its ethnic character.

REFERENCES

1. Farkas LG, Hreczko TA, Deutsch CA. Objective assessment of standard nostril types—a morphometric study. *Ann Plast Surg* 1983;11:381.
2. Romm S. Art, love, and facial beauty. *Clin Plast Surg* 1987;14:579.
3. Romm S. *Dynamics of beauty: The changing face of beauty*. St. Louis: Mosby, 1992.
4. Farkas LG, Kolar JL. Anthropometrics and art in aesthetics of women's faces. *Clin Plast Surg* 1987;14:599.
5. Gunter JP, Rohrich RJ. Facial analysis for the rhinoplasty patient. Presented at 11th Annual Dallas Rhinoplasty Symposium, Dallas, TX, 1994.
6. Rohrich RJ, Sheen JP. *Secondary rhinoplasy. Reoperative plastic surgery*. St. Louis: Quality Medical, 1994:1–110.
7. Flowers RJ. Rhinoplasty in Oriental patients: repair of the East Asian nose. In: Daniel RK, ed. *Rhinoplasty aesthetic plastic surgery*. 2nd ed. Boston: Little, Brown, 1993.
8. Rohrich RJ, Daniel RK, Gunter JP, Sheen JH, Tebbetts JB. Nasal augmentation. *Perspect Plast Surg* 1990;4:15.
9. Byrd HS, Hobar PC. Rhinoplasty: a practical guide for surgical planning. *Plast Reconstr Surg* 1993;91:642.
10. Gunter JP, Rohrich RJ. Lengthening the aesthetically short nose. *Plast Reconstr Surg* 1989;83:793.
11. Gunter JP, Rohrich RJ. Augmentation rhinoplasty—a new concept in dorsal onlay grafting. *Plast Reconstr Surg* 1990;86:39.
12. Gunter JP, Rohrich RJ. The importance of alar-columellar relationship. Presented at 11th Annual Dallas Rhinoplasty Symposium, Dallas, TX, 1994.
13. Gunter JP, Rohrich RJ. External approach for secondary rhinoplasty. *Plast Reconstr Surg* 1987;80:161.
14. Rohrich RJ. The black rhinoplasty. In: Daniel RK, ed. *Rhinoplasty aesthetic plastic surgery*. 2nd ed. Boston: Little, Brown, 1993.

SECTION III

Skin Care for People of Color

Ethnic Considerations in Facial Aesthetic Surgery, edited by W. Earle Matory, Jr.
Lippincott–Raven Publishers, Philadelphia © 1998.

9

Skin Care

Editor's Commentary

W. Earle Matory, Jr.

> We should all know that diversity makes for a rich tapestry, and we must understand that all the threads of the tapestry are equal in value no matter what their color.
> — Maya Angelou

Excessive thickening of the stratum corneum is a key contribution to many skin ailments in patients of any hue. Excessive build-up of pyknotic and horny cells contributes to the thickened, coarse, dull appearance of aging skin along with fine and dense rhytids. Accumulation of desquamating cells within pilosebaceous ducts and glands results in acne, pseudofolliculitis barbi, and hydradenitis suppurativa. Dyschromias including hypopigmentation and hyperpigmentation commonly display an uneven distribution of melanin within the epidermal layers. Strong consistency of these findings in ethnic skin presents challenges for the patient and for the skin caretaker. These challenges are compounded by the high degree of sensitivity of ethnic skin to the sun, medications, make-ups, and deodorants.

Desquamating agents like alpha-hydroxy acids (AHAs) and isotretinoin (Retin A) can be used to effectively address each of the most common concerns for the skin in patients of color: aging, occlusive pilosebaceous disease, and dyschromias. Thus, one must develop an armory of agents and procedures along with options to address ethnic skin. Crucial elements include desquamators, moisturizers, and pigment neutralizers.

W. E. Matory, Jr.: A New You Plastic Surgery Medical Group, Irvine, California 92714

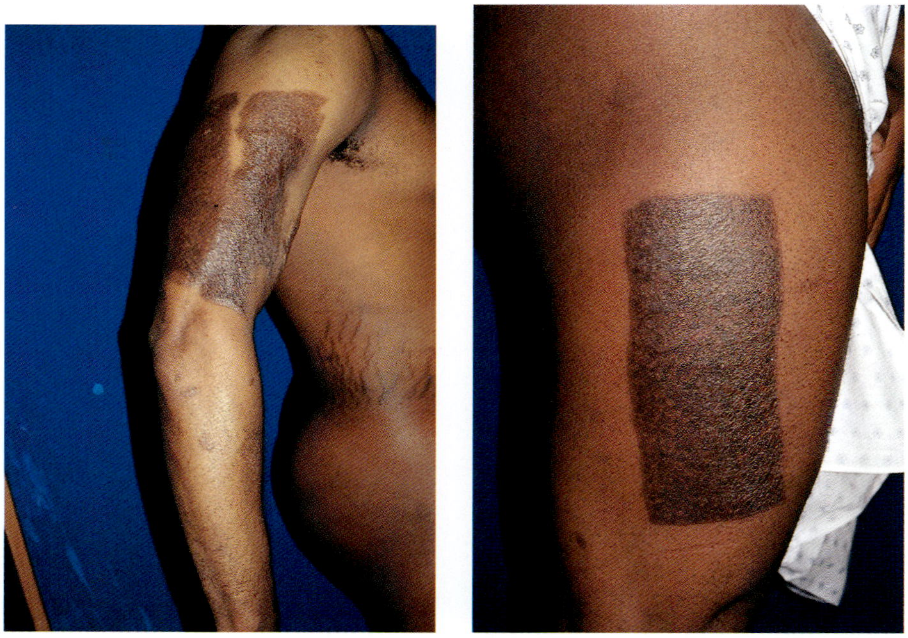

A B

Figure 1. Post-inflammatory hyperpigmentation after donor harvest **(A)** and after split-thickness grafting **(B)**. This process is caused by a combination of hemosiderin and melanin deposition.

IMPACT OF AGING ON THE SKIN

The Aging Process

Photoaging, or damage caused by the sun, is responsible for 95% of the visible signs of aging. The first signs of aging are noticed at age 20 when a few creases occur at the corners of the eyes and/or mouth. Every day sun exposure begins in infancy and continues throughout life, gradually progressing to epidermal and dermal damage. Early on, the skin feels drier and lacks luster and fine lines begin. The overall texture of the skin is less smooth and soft. These changes occur primarily in the epidermis as a result of the accumulation of dead cells within the stratum corneum. Epidermal cellular growth becomes erratic, and the rate of normal stratum corneum decreases. Individuals of color are less likely to form rhytids, but have the same or greater degrees of facial fat and muscle dislocation due to gravitational effects and loss of elasticity.

Microscopic findings show that epidermal cells become enlarged and irregular. Melanocytes vary in density, with fluctuations up to 10–20% per decade, resulting in skin darkening or unevenness (Fig. 1). The dermis thins and collagen fibers become more brittle. Elastin, which contributes a youthful tension and spring within the skin, diminishes in strength and number. Under-protection and abnormal production of collagen and elastin lead to sagging skin, particularly in locations where gravitational forces are significant, e.g., the nasolabial fold and the submental area. The combination of these microscopic changes results in a thinning of the non-keratodic epidermal and the dermal layers, along with susceptibility of the skin to infection, dryness, other environmental changes, and cancer. Melanin concentration minimizes but does no eliminate these solar and temporal effects on the skin. Skin looseness and rhytidosis are noted to a lesser degree.

Cutaneous Aging in Individuals of Color

Many of the visible signs of aging that occur in the Caucasian occur one or two decades later in the Asian, Hispanic, African American, Asian Indian, and American Indian. Very rarely do you see crow's feet at the corner of the eyes or extra skin at the corner of the mouth or in the pre-auricular area. Fine wrinkles of the face occur less commonly, except in the smoker. Nasal skin may lengthen as osteocartilaginous support diminishes. Upper lid skin laxity may be moderate, while lower skin laxity is minimal. Creases along the lower lid tend to be associated with lax muscle and ligamentous support rather than secondary to excess skin. Lipstick bleed is noted frequently in the individual of color, particularly in the lower lip, which tends to evert significantly, as it does in the Caucasian (for further details see Chapter 11).

People of color do tan! Ultraviolet A rays inflict damage on the skin along with hyperpigmentation. Dyschromias as well as exacerbated acne are the most common effects following extended sun exposure. Ultraviolet B-inflicted skin cancers, however, are less commonly noted. Ultraviolet C rays, highly toxic to human, plant, and animal life, are primarily absorbed by the ozone layer. Patients of color must be instructed regarding sun protection against each of the ultraviolet rays. Aluminum-based sun blocks along with umbrellas, hats, long-sleeved shirts, and 180° ultraviolet-protective sunglasses are essential for proper skin protection.

Travel and climactic changes affect the skin. Airline and automobile travel act as strong skin desiccants. As a result pores fill with desquamating skin that is adherent, lacking the humidifying component. Climactic changes, i.e., travel from a cold to a hot environment or vice versa, contribute to dryness, oiliness, and sweatiness. Smog additionally results in an accumulation of products within the pores.

Occupational exposures to substances including harsh chemicals, hair and nail treatments, dishwashing detergents, abrasive cleansers, pesticides, and herbicides contribute to dryness and irritation in addition to toxic reactions. Computer screens or excessive sun exposure may result in eye strain or squinting, contributing to periorbital wrinkling.

SKIN DISCOLORATION (DYSCHROMIAS)

Society defines one of the most important aspects of attractiveness to be smooth, even skin tone. Darkened and lightened areas of the face often result from the effects of acne, aging, wind, sun, and chicken pox, to name a few of the culprits. Patches of hypo- and hyperpigmented skin catch the eye easily and are interpreted as unhealthy, ugly, painful, contagious, or in some cultures simply socially unacceptable. Color of the skin is primarily dictated by three pigments: hemoglobin, melanin, and carotene. Any varied or irregular distribution of any one of these pigments results in dyschromia. Common dyschromias include post-inflammatory hyperpigmentation, telangiectasia, and rosacea.

Post-Inflammatory Hyperpigmentation

This is the typical response to healing in pigmented skin (Fig. 1). It is a common outcome following minor or major trauma, acne, chicken pox, razor bumps, hormonal changes, or aging/sun exposure. Any precipitating factors like acne or folliculitis must be under control prior to addressing the hyperpigmentation. Post-inflammatory hyperpigmentation is the most common dyschromia encountered by the plastic surgeon. Hormonal influences like pregnancy and oral contraceptives may exacerbate spontaneous hyperpigmentation, i.e., melasma/chloasma, as well as dyschromias that follow acne or other inflammatory lesions. Frequently used antibiotics like tetracycline and erythromycin precipitate hyperpigmentation. Because there are so many factors influencing skin tone and color, the surgeon must ensure that patients are aware that there are no guarantees associated with non-surgical and surgical skin-lightening modalities.

Correcting Dyschromias

Patients should be advised regarding the strong hyperpigmenting effects of ultraviolet exposure. They should be aware that this exposure may be exacerbated on overcast days, even though the sun may not be visible. Scented aftershaves and spray colognes on any sun-exposed areas should be avoided to limit dark spot precipitation.

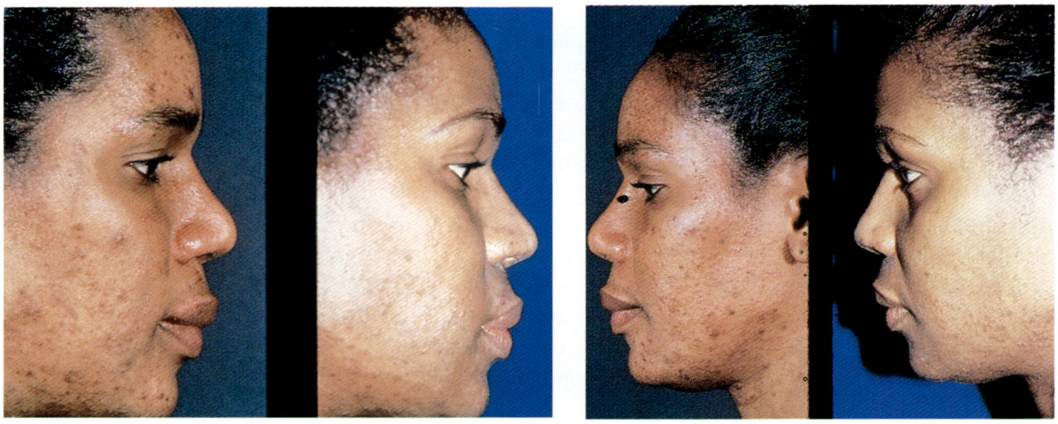

Figure 2. Post-inflammatory hyperpigmentation secondary to acne and electrolysis along with oral tetracycline responding well to cessation of tetracycline home treatment with glycolic acid 10% and a series of six glycolic peels 70–80%. Concomitant treatment with hydroquinone 4% was applied to areas of hyperpigmentation. Incidental rhinoplasty.

Skin care should begin by cleansing with an exfoliant and rinsable cleanser appropriate for the patient's skin type. Hydroquinine 2–4% and/or kojic acid solution is then applied (Fig. 2). After 5 min of penetration, sun block with a sun protection factor of 15 is then used followed by any desired make-up. A combination of agents is most effective in reducing hyperpigmentation. Hydroquinone, kojic acid, and AHAs work in an additive fashion to lighten darkened areas. Retin A also potentiates the hypopigmenting effectiveness of each of these compounds. The Nd-Yag laser dramatically reduces melanin concentration within the basal layer.

Kojic acid is a safe and effective skin lightener that has a very solid reputation in parts of Asia where hydroquinine use is not allowed. In this country, kojic acid which is derived from the fermentation of starch and sugar and is used as a precursor in the production of malt flavor and other flavorants in the food industry. The Japanese discovered the value of kojic acid as a skin lightener in food industry laborers. Because of its mildly antibiotic properties, it is particularly useful in the treatment of hyperpigmentation that often accompanies acne conditions.

Kojic acid is blended with other natural ingredients, all of which are the most recent arrivals on the depigmenting scene: Niacinamide is an enzyme co-factor in the vitamin B group and inhibits melanogenesis, glabridin and glabrene are the depigmenter components of licorice root, and hematein is the logwood extract that interrupts melanogenesis.

Kolite cream also contains licorice essential oil, witch hazel, and cross-linked fatty acids from sunflower seeds and safflower seeds for a very moisturizing, non-oily, non-comedogenic base (Fig. 3).

Kolite can be used with unlimited frequency. However, one must wear sunblock during the day. This product may be used for spot treatments or regionally depending on the nature of the dyschromia. It should be applied to the involved area and thoroughly massaged into the skin. It may be used on any part of the body, including face and neck. There are no contraindications, and compliance is satisfactory.

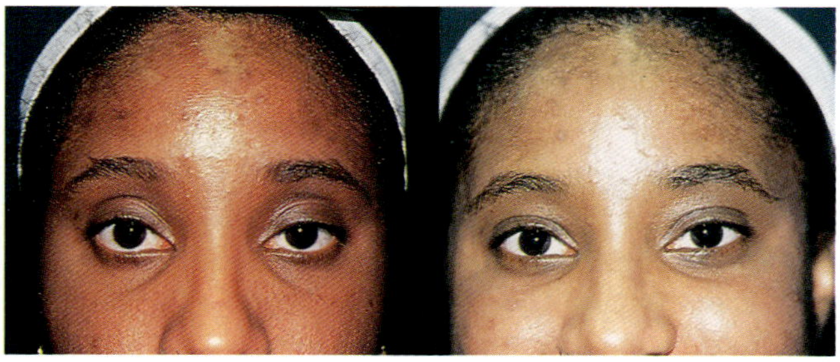

Figure 3. Post-inflammatory hyperpigmentation due to acne softened by 10% glycolic home treatment and kojic acid.

Optimizing Success

1. Treat any causative condition, e.g., acne or razor bumps, prior to starting a color correction program.
2. Encourage follow-ups with your aesthetician every 4 weeks.
3. Encourage refills well in advance, so that supplies are adequate.
4. Be aware of all medications that your patient is taking whether prescribed or over the counter. Note that some medications may worsen hyperpigmentation or dyschromia or may result in an additive or exacerbated side effect. Common offenders are tetracycline and erythromycin.
5. Test skin for allergy to hydroquinine prior to applying it. Tests should be applied for 3 days in a hidden location. Avoid esther and methyl esther compounds, the most common allergens.
6. If skin becomes irritated, stop all active products (lighteners, glycolic acid, Retin A) for 1 day. Advise the patient not to stop the sunscreens and facial cleansers. Encourage follow-up appointments if irritation persists.
7. We recommend a light glycolic or lactic acid peel 50–70% every 1–4 weeks. Advise patients that if they see an improvement, they should still continue to use the products until the physician has assessed the pigmentary changes.
8. Nd-Yag laser provides a more rapidly effective modality for countering hyperpigmentation. Scabbing resolves within 5–7 days. Ongoing skin treatment as noted helps to expedite the return of uniform skin tones and repigmentation.

ACNE AND OILY SKIN

Sebaceous glands and follicles are constantly shedding the keratinic layer. The sun, wind, dryness, and medications that diminish the production of sebum contribute to congestion of cutaneous pores. Adhesion of the desquamation products within the pores leads to ductal occlusion. The naturally occurring bacteria of the skin, *Propionibacterium acne*, ingest sebum, which is ultimately excreted as an inflammatory fatty acid byproduct. These desquamation products accumulate at the pore aperture. Aeration and sun exposure cause a darkening of these desquamating byproducts, resulting in blackheads (Fig. 4). Closed comedones are caused by pores that are plugged proximal to the pore aperture without resultant dilation of the follicle. Long-term (months) ductal occlusion results in papule, pustule, nodule, or cyst formation. Acute bacterial proliferation or eruption of the pore contents within the dermal bed results in an acutely inflamed lesion or abscess. The progression of a papule into an abscess may occur within 24–36 h unless decompression is effected using some of the modalities described in the subsequent treatment section. Peri-comedone inflammation results in ultimate dermal atrophy and fibrocyte proliferation, with subdermal contracture causing ice-pick scarring. Discoloration with hypo- or hyperpigmentation usually accompanies this chronic process in individuals of color (Fig. 5).

Management of acne requires the identification and elimination of causative factors, continuous cleansing of skin, desquamation products, control of inflammation, and prevention of long-term scarring and discoloration (Figs. 6–8). The most successful way to control acne is to arm the patient with information.

Causative Factors

Many daily activities contribute to the development of acute and chronic acne. The key component to successful treatment is a dramatic change in lifestyle.

1. Stress. Stress is the most consistent factor leading to breakout periods. The physical stress of long or night shift work, exam periods, marital distress, as well as social or societal pressures of Western civilization all contribute to mental and physical strain. Harsh economic times play an almost universal role in the complexities of daily living.

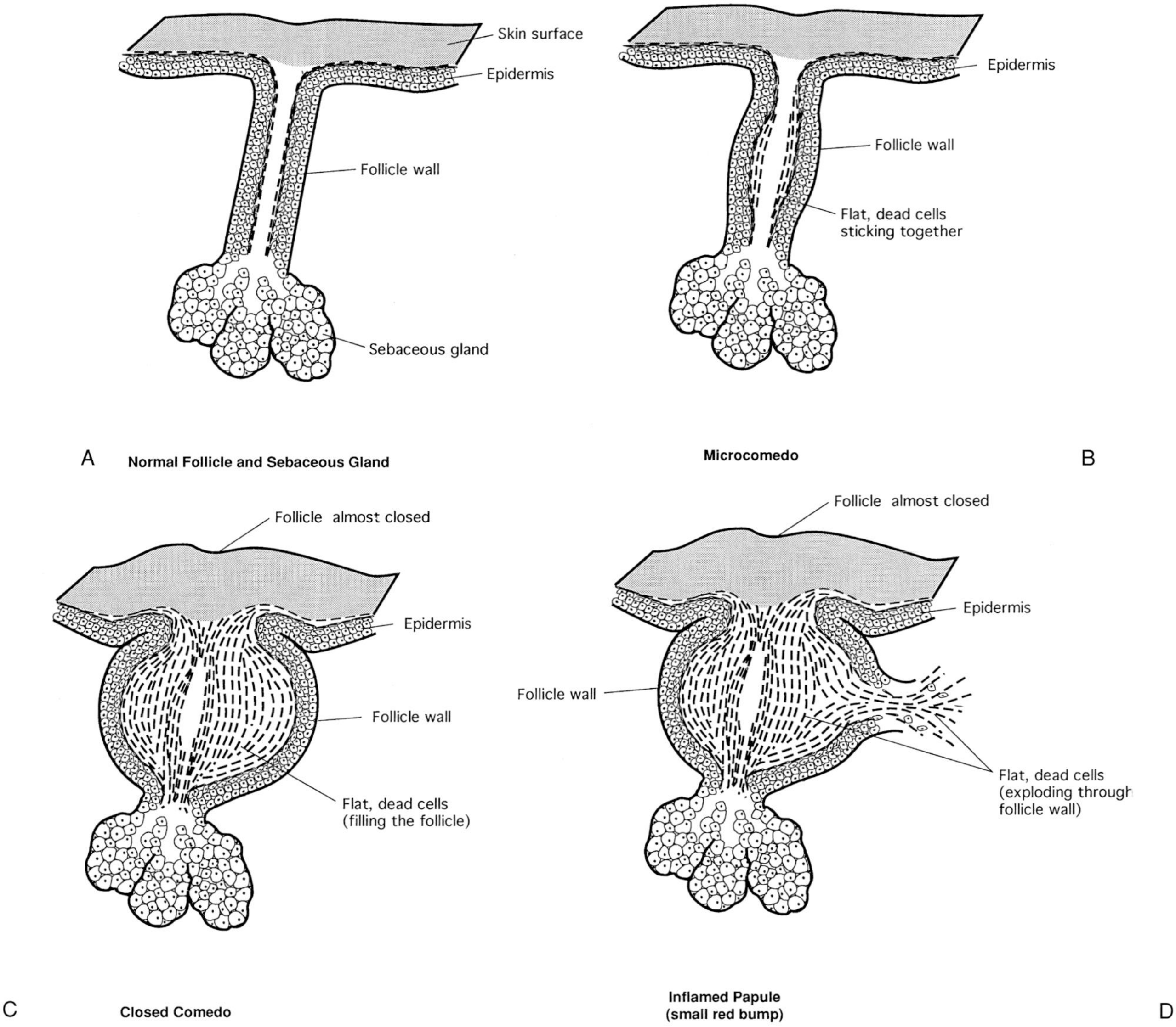

Figure 4. Pathogenesis of acne and oily skin.

2. Lack of sleep. The night shift, sleepless nights, or overworking make it next to impossible to clear one's face. Recommend a good night s sleep daily for at least 7 or 8 hours

3. Cosmetics. One-third of adults develop reactions to cosmetics or clothing. Fabric softeners like Cling-Free, Bounce, and Snuggle are frequent culprits. Comedogenic ingredients cause microcomedones that may ultimately become more visible and troublesome. Patients with extensive involvement in the back or chest should be queried regarding the use of these products. One should avoid animal, vegetable, and mineral oils. Beware of oil-free claims by manufacturers as these may contain synthetic oils including isoprophyl myristrate, red dyes, stearic acid, cetyl alcohol, sodium laurel sulfate, and laureth-4 and other animal or vegetable oils that can be highly comedogenic. Check the ingredients!

4. Picking. Physical manipulation of the skin is one of the most consistent characteristics of human nature. This process dramatically increases inflammation and prolongs or exacerbates acne sequelae. Patients must understand that picking will not only prolong acne lesion but will also worsen scarring.

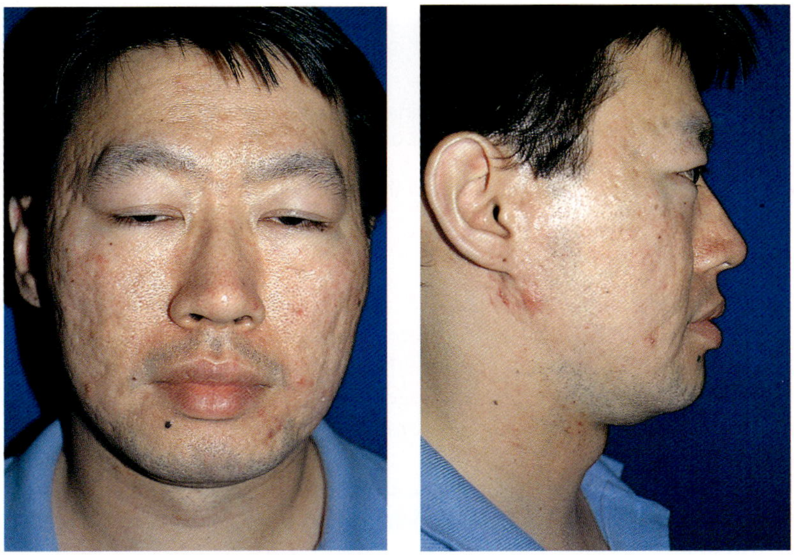

Figure 5. Glandular occlusive disease is common among Asian, Hispanic, American Indian, and African races. It is often diffuse with many stages of activity, acute, subacute, postinflammatory hyperpigmentation, ice-pick scarring, facial pitting, and hyper- and hypopigmentation.

5. Hormonal changes. High levels of progesterone that occur just prior to menstruation, along with cravings for salty or fatty foods, make the pre-menstrual period a common time for acne flare-up. For similar reasons, the first 3 months of pregnancy and the first 90 days after delivery can be devastating. Low-estrogen birth control pills like Ovral, Lo-Ovral, Loestrin, Norlestrin, and Norinyl commonly precipitate new lesions. Demulan 1/35 and Ortho-Novum 1/35 are less problematic. Testosterone along with associated salt cravings contribute to acne flare-ups in the adolescent and in the older male.

6. Diet. Iodide, ingested most commonly with salt, is by far the most significant dietetic factor. Fast foods or cooking styles from the Far East (seaweed, soy sauce, monosodium glutamate), South/Central America, Africa, or the Caribbean tend to be heavily salted and iodide concentrated. Sushi wrapped in seaweed and tortilla chips are prime examples. Frozen foods and vitamin supplements often contain significant doses of iodine.

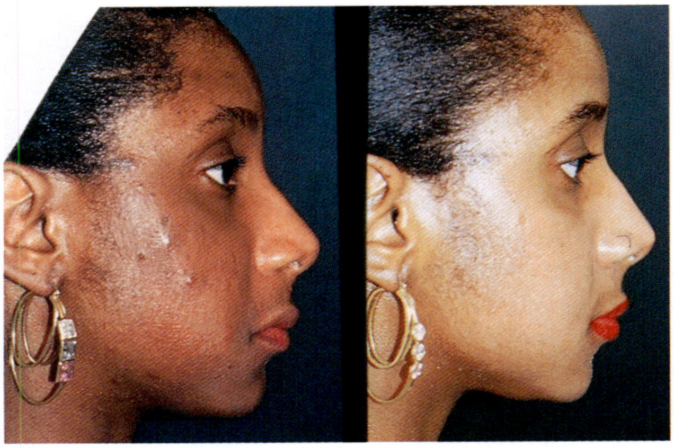

Figure 6. This result was achieved with elimination of hair pomade, use of benzoyl peroxide for acute lesions along with glycolic acid 10%, hydroquinone, and topical clindamycin.

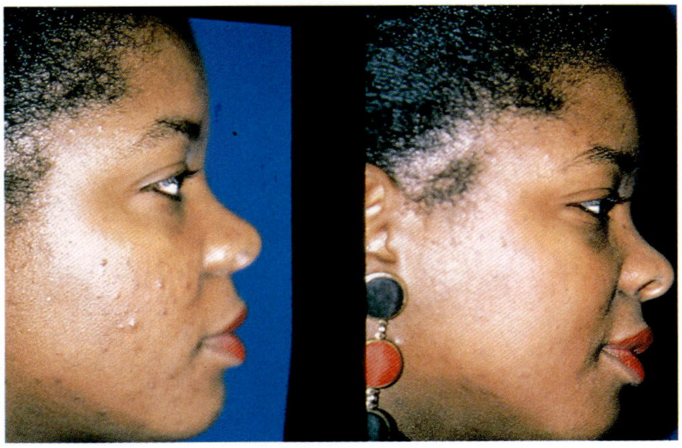

Figure 7. This student followed instructions to gain control of her study and sleep hours, along with elimination of comedogenic make-up and the treatment regimen used in Fig. 6.

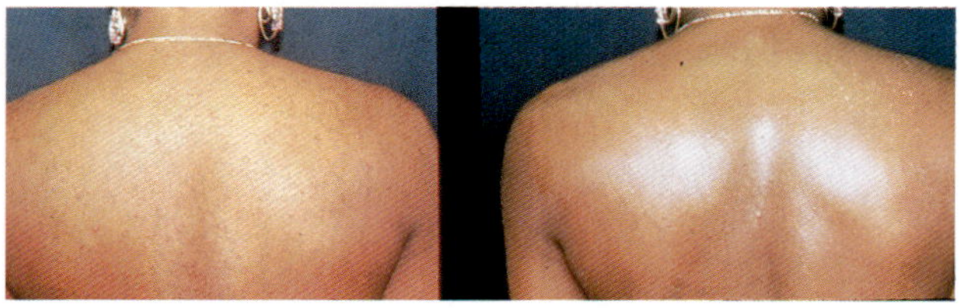

Figure 8. Elimination of irritating wool sleep wear and low-estrogen birth control concomitant with the treatment plan outlined in Fig. 6 along with serial 70% glycolic peel yielded this outcome on the chest and back.

Fat is a significant component of the U.S. diet including fast foods, cheese, processed foods, frozen foods, and dairy products. Sweets, particularly chocolate, may also be sugar and fat laden. Stir-frys in peanut oil are filled with salt, fat, and testosterone, and peanuts themselves are commonly ingested comedogenics. While the scientific evidence supporting dietary contributions to comedogenesis may be in question, individual dietary adjustments are usually very effective.

7. Weather. Ultraviolet exposure increases cell turnover along with an accumulation of dead skin that may clog pores. As noted, sun may exacerbate color changes in the skin, dark spots, and associated inflammatory response. Climate variations like travel from a cold to a tropical climate or any dramatic change in temperature and moisture may precipitate pustule formation. U.S. soldiers that traveled to Vietnam or to the Mediterranean Gulf were commonly faced with severe skin reactivity. Conversely, Chinese, Cambodians, or Jamaicans coming to the United States frequently incur the same problem. U.S.-born citizens may experience seasonal variations to breakouts as well.

8. Medications/chemicals (acne medicamentosa). Seizure medications like Dilantin are particularly troublesome. Steroids taken in any form can be a problem. The weight lifter looking for a body boost may pump up his pectoralis muscles, but he may also develop disfiguring comedones. Other inciting agents include lithium, danazol, danacrin, marijuana, cocaine, and amphetamines. Exposure to industrial chemicals and oils (tar and asphalt) may result in work-related blemishes.

9. Pressure/friction (acne mechanica). White collar workers and teenage Romeos continuously rest the phone on the side of the face. Eyeglasses may fit improperly, particularly in individuals of color who have a flattened nasal bridge. Baseball caps, headbands, and non-cotton workout gear cause irritation. As a result, pressure points develop on the nose, cheeks, or ears, causing associated blackheads.

10. Travel. The dissipation of the earth's ozone layer has resulted in a dramatic increase in the harshness of sun and wind exposure. Travel tends to increase exposure to our changing environment. The dryness of airplane, automobile, or train ventilation systems further contributes to dead skin accumulation and a progressive accumulation within cutaneous pores.

OTHER PILOSEBACEOUS OCCLUSIVE DISEASES

Pseudofolliculitis Barbae

The inflammatory foreign body reaction of ingrown hairs progresses to follicular occlusion. As a result perifollicular papules and micro- and macroabscesses form (Fig. 9). Proliferation of the hair follicle contributes to nodules that may be of significant size. Pseudofolliculitis is precipitated by the shaving habits of the African American, Asian, Hispanic or Caucasian who has susceptible dense and/or curved hair follicles (Fig. 10) that become entrapped based on poor shaving habits. Abrasions or small cuts on the skin caused by shaving with dull razors, too close a cut from electrical razors, and poor cleansing of the face are common precipitating factors (Fig. 11).

A similar process occurs in the nape of the neck and/or scalp (Fig. 12) particularly after the scraping/cutting effect of a straight razor (Fig. 13). This process was a common practice in the U.S. Military, resulting in lifelong problems for many U.S. veterans. The strong

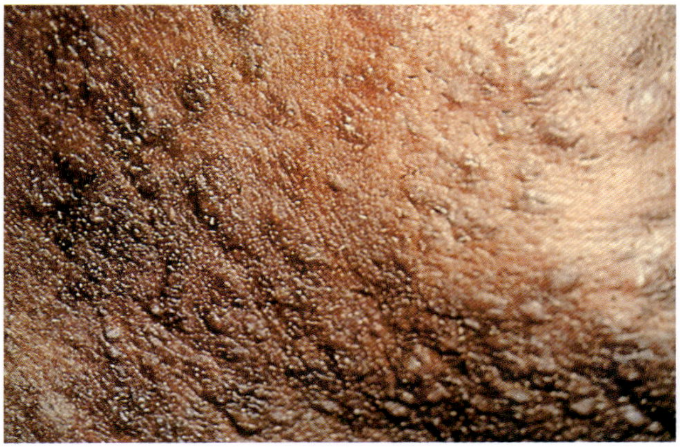

Figure 9. Perifollicular papules and micro/macroabscesses from an inflammatory reaction to occluded follicles and ingrown hair.

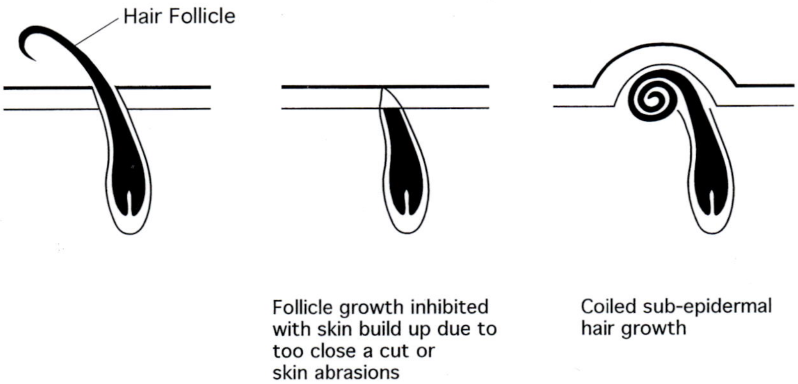

Figure 10. Pathogenesis of pseudofolliculitis barbae.

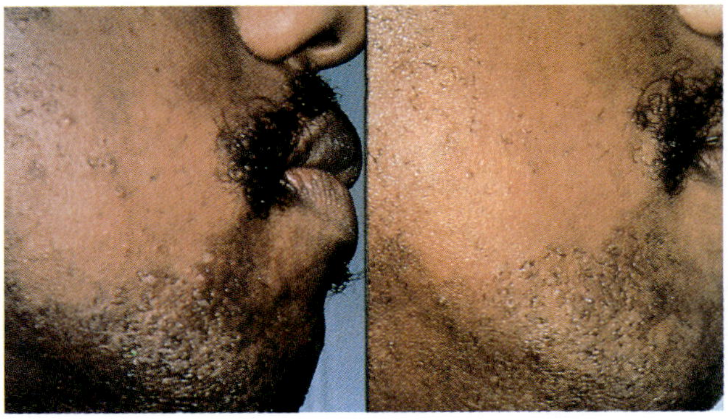

Figure 11. Control of pseudofolliculitis is optimized with daily shaving with a fresh razor, avoidance of an electric razor (too close a cut) and dull razors, and the use of a glycolic acid 10% cleansing program augmented with hydroquinone, benzoyl peroxide, and topical antibiotics.

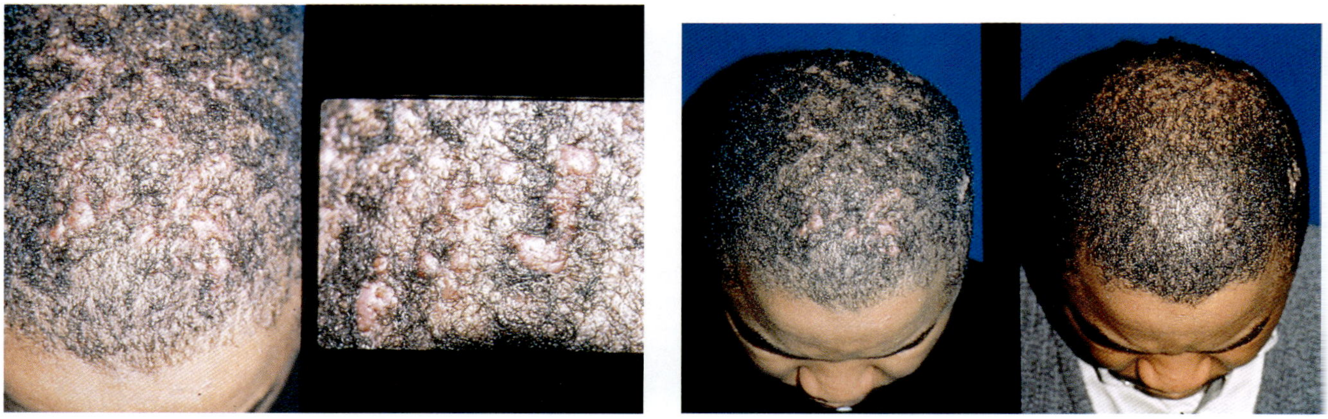

Figure 12. Pseudofolliculitis of the entire scalp is best managed by the regimen outlined in Fig. 11. Shaving must be avoided.

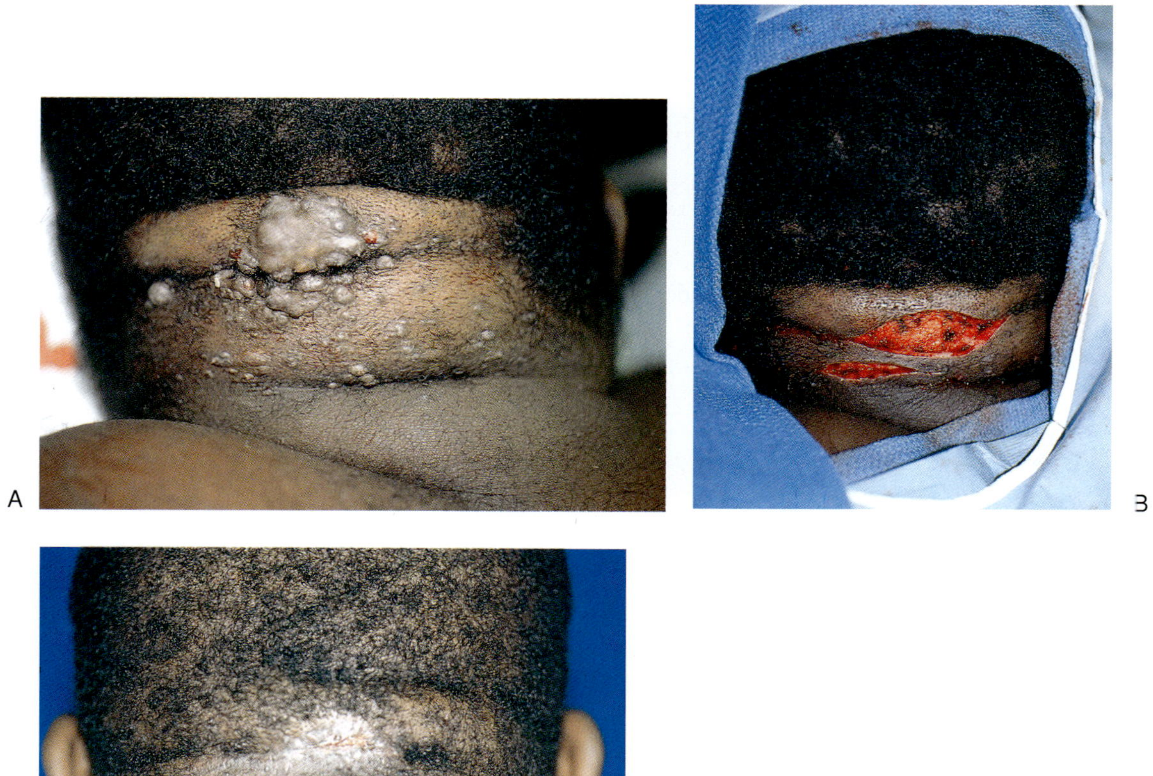

Figure 13. Pseudofolliculitis nuchae **(A)** is best managed by excision of densely involved areas **(B)** followed by healing of secondary intent **(C)**.

A

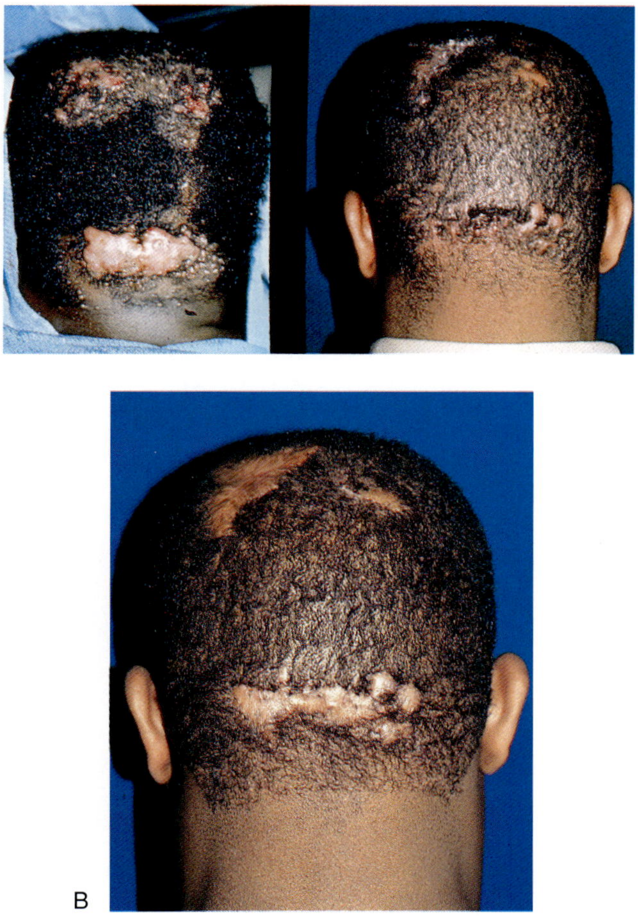

B

Figure 14. Acne kelordalis **(A)** occasionally hypertrophy develops after excision, noted in this patient 5 months after excision **(B)**. Intralesional injection with triamcinolone 40 mg/ml expedited resolution in the postoperative view at 2 years. At this point scar reduction procedures can be attempted.

degrees of bacterial contamination and the propensity for recurrent folliculitis are best managed by wide excision and healing by secondary intent (Fig. 14).

Hidradenitis Suppurativa

Hidradenitis suppurativa is a chronic cicatrizing suppurative disorder of any area of the body that bears apocrine glands. Over 60% of individuals have a genetic component often associated with a single gene. Hormonal contributions are confirmed by worsening with estrogen, progesterone, or androgen ingestion, the failure of hidradenitis to develop before puberty, and the decline in disease activity after menopause.

The magnitude of social, economic, psychiatric, and medical sequelae of this disease is not well appreciated. Inability to wear deodorant, resultant poor hygiene, frequent hospitalizations/surgery, and pain each contribute to major alterations in lifestyle. Involvement of the scalp, perifolliculitis capitis abscendens et suffodiens (dissecting cellulitis of the scalp), and recurrent abscesses of the vertex and occiput are particularly disfiguring and desocializing (Fig. 15). Each of these occlusive pilosebaceous diseases responds well to adjunctive treatment modalities outlined below.

Diffuse involvement of the perineum or axilla is managed with excision to but not involving fascia followed by healing of secondary intent. Various well vascularized local and

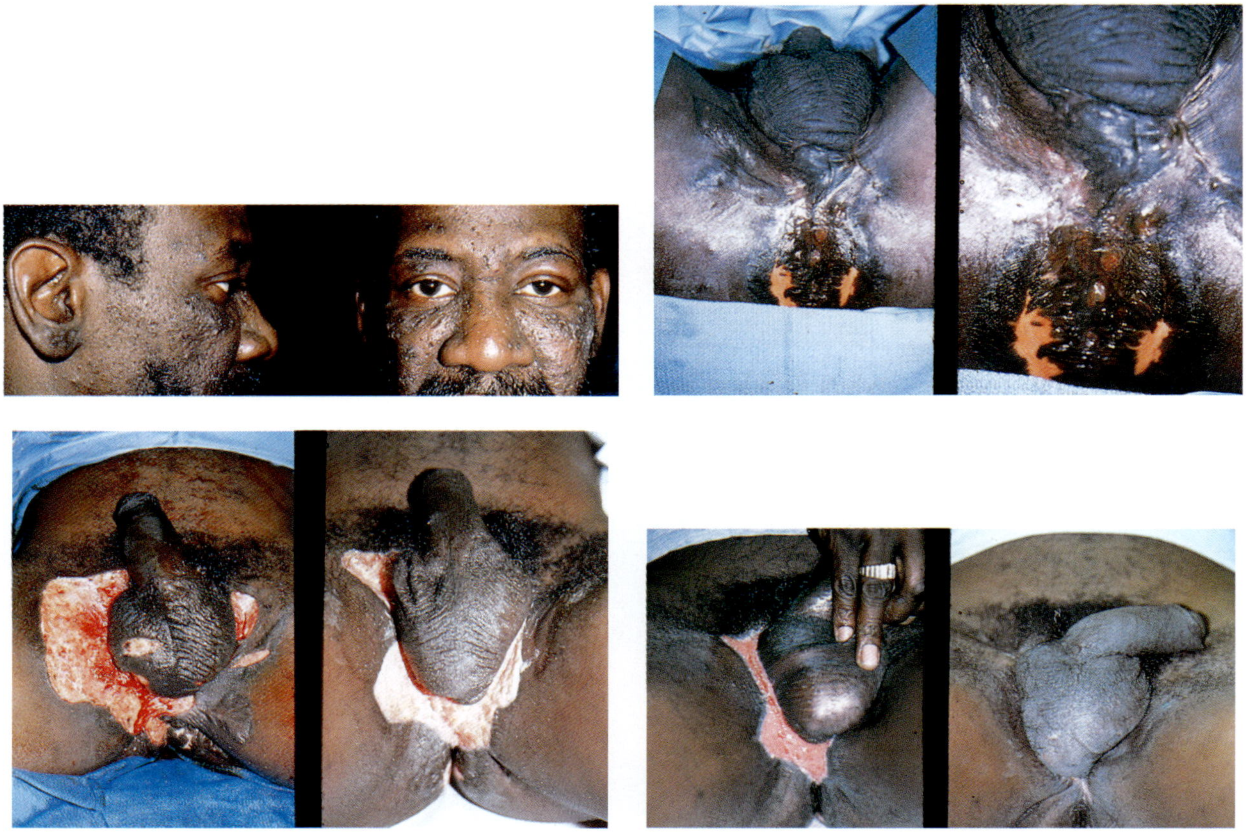

Figure 15. Ethnic males have a propensity for diffuse pilosebaceous occlusion including pseudofolliculitis, chronic cystic acne **(A)** and hidradenitis sappurativa, nuchal, scalp, axillary, chest, back, groin, and anus. Surgical, systemic, and topical treatment are necessary for therapeutic control. **B:** Groin and anal hidradenitis were problematic for the patient. **C:** Immediately following wide resection to fascia. **D:** After healing by secondary intent at 6–8 weeks. Isotretinoin, glycolic acid treatment (10–20%), glycolic peels (70–80%), benzoyl peroxide (2.5–10%), and sulfur masks.

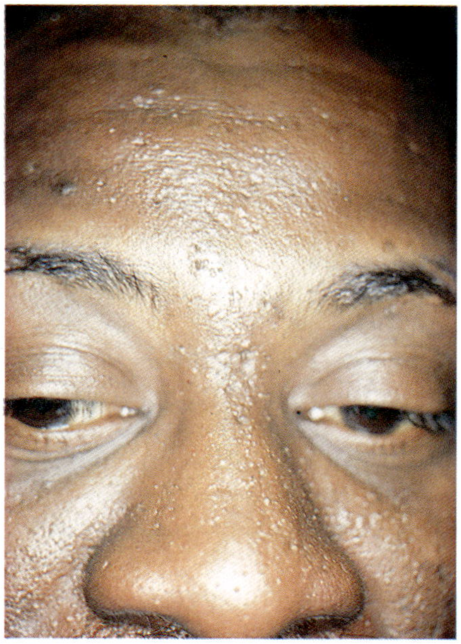

Figure 16. Milrasis after dermatorasion. Thick oily skin of the nose and T-zone increases the likelihood of developing various pilosebaceous conditions that may require care perioperatively. Preoperative treatment of these conditions optimizes postoperative sequelae.

regional flaps (e.g., split latissimus, split pectoralis) can be alternatively used to cover the axilla or face. Perineal motion and high degrees of contamination limit flap effectiveness in the groin and complicate wound healing.

It is not unusual for patients, especially the ethnic male, to have facial, nuchal, axillary, chest, back, perineal, and/or anal pilosebaceous occlusive disease (Fig. 16). Pre- and post-surgical support should include AHAs, tretmoin, isotretinois, benzoyl peroxide, and sulfur masks. These are all effective adjuncts to maintenance and control of the debilitating disease.

OTHER PILOSEBACEOUS OCCLUSIVE DISORDERS

The following pathologies are far more common in patients with thick oily skin (Fig. 16).

Syringomas. Tiny white nodules similar to closed comedones usually become most prominent during adolescence.

Milia. Tiny nodules similar to closed comedones are small keratinaceous cysts surrounded by stratified keratinizing epithelium. In that they have no openings, they are true cysts, not comedones.

Rosacea. Commonly seen in oily skin and mimicking acne vulgaris. The erythemidous background commonly involves the nose and infraorbital area unlike acne vulgaris.

Adenoma sebaceum. White telangiectatic papules on the nose, nasolabial fold, and cheeks are often solid connective tissue nevoid growths that have no association with follicles. Many patients may have associated neurological symptoms.

Rhinophyma. Long-existing rosacea presents with a grotesque hyperplasia of sebaceous glands in connective tissue of the nose. Pathognomonic for rosacea are papules noted on a erythematous cutaneous background.

Drug reaction. Acute onset of acne, extensive involvement, unusual locations, or other signs of systemic drug toxicity may be noted.

TREATMENT MODALITIES

Prime modes of non-surgical treatment involve skin cleansing and desquamation of keratotic accumulation. Isotretinoin in doses of 2 mg/kg/day for as long as 2 years has had marginal success in 30–50% of patients with active disease. Conversely, isotretinoin or tretinoic acid in combination with AHAs has proven to be very effective in my hands. The inflammation associated with subacute and chronically inflamed lesions can be significantly lessened with these modalities. Anti-androgen (ethinyloestradiol/levonorgestrel) combinations have proven to be effective in females. Side effects noted in males preclude their use.

Persistent folliculitis may require operative decompression of the cysts or abscesses. Use of an 11 scalpel tip to allow external follicular growth works very effectively. Many patients may require decompression every 3–12 months.

Alpha-hydroxy Acids

The use of AHAs dates back to Egypt, when Cleopatra and other women of this era bathed in sour milk (lactic acid) and applied red wine to their faces (tartaric acid). AHAs are decarboxylated acids of fruits and foods, e.g., malic acid from apples, tartaric acid from grapes, lactic acid from sour milk, and citric acid from citrus fruit. The smaller molecular size of glycolic acid, derived from sugar cane, allows the highest degree of skin penetration by any of the AHAs. Van Scott has patented the use of a number of alpha-hydroxy agents in the United States and several foreign countries. The patents are relatively all-inclusive including the use of AHAs as well as their reactionary byproducts.

The effectiveness of AHAs appears to be related to its action in decreasing cellular adherence within the stratum corneum. So excessive build-up of dead skin cells is minimized

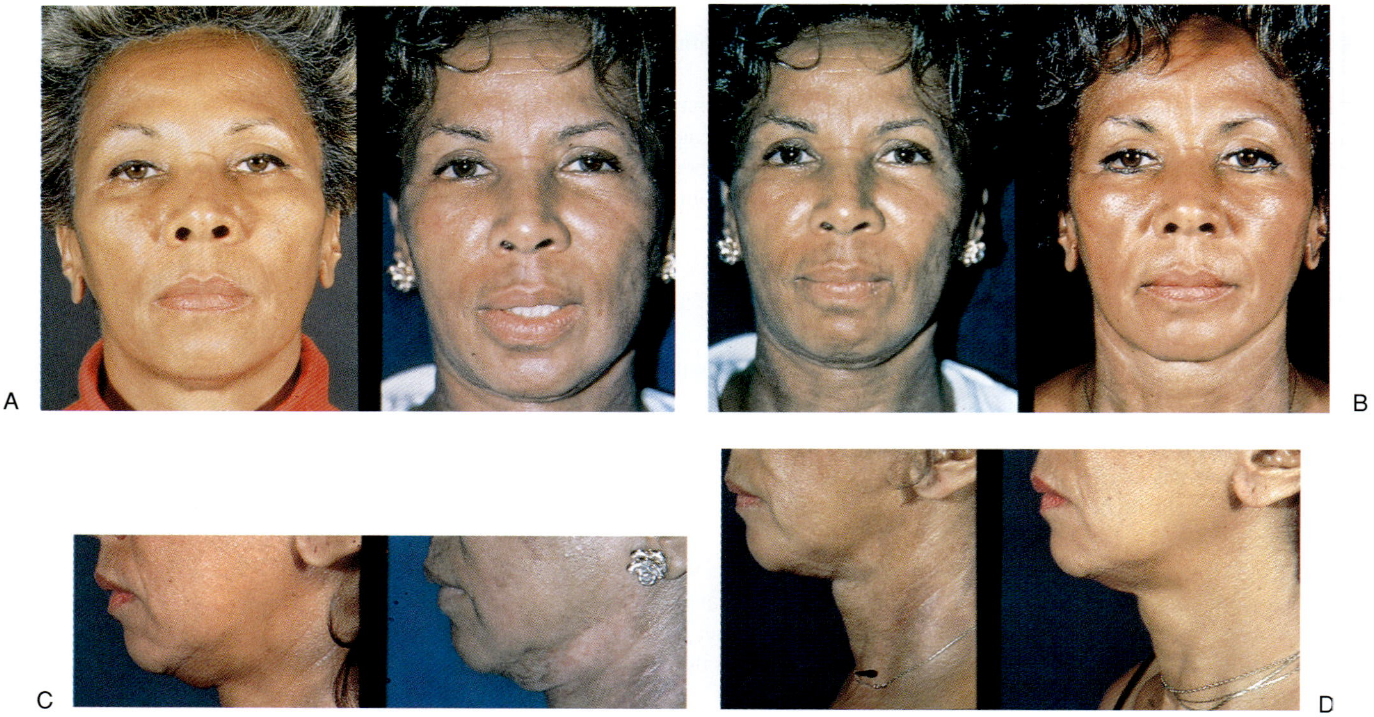

Figure 17. A–B: Trichloroacetic acid peels 17–35% can be used in the individual of color. Pigmentary return is prolonged and spotty with color changes noted pre-operatively 1, 2, and 72 months following trichloroacetic acid 35%, with complete color return, usually at 3–6 months. **C–D:** The return of skin color in the neck after trichloroacetic acid peel is slower and less consistent as demonstrated at 0, 1, 2, and 12 months following trichloroacetic acid 35%. Medium-depth peels of the neck are not advised in patients of color.

as a result of the sloughing that occurs. A dramatic smoothing of skin, lessening of fine lines, and improved skin texture, hydration, softness, and youthful glow are observed (Fig. 17). The actions of AHAs diminish follicular build-up in acne-prone skin, hydradenitis suppurativa, rosacea, and pseudofolliculitis barbae. Cellular turnover also expedites the resolution of hyperpigmentation (Figs. 18 and 19).

Administration

Ten percent glycolic acid is the most effective dosing used at home on a daily basis. Our patients are advised to start on an every-third-day basis and progress to a daily basis. This minimizes skin irritation and diminishes scabbing. The patient with sensitive skin will benefit from lactic acid, which acts more slowly but is less problematic.

The natural build-up of oils and various skin products has been significantly lessened within a 4- to 6-week period. This is followed by concentrated peels utilizing alpha-hydroxy agents, trichloracetic acid, or phenol. In people of color, the medium or deep peels take longer for the even return of skin pigmentation. Medium and deep peels may also result in irregular pigmentation of the skin and are thus not advised.

A number of other products promote the effectiveness of AHAs.

Adjunctive Products

Isotretinoin (Retin A/Accutane)

These vitamin A derivatives are effective desquamators of the epidermis. In addition, isotretoin penetrates the dermis, resulting in some regeneration of elastin. Of note, while

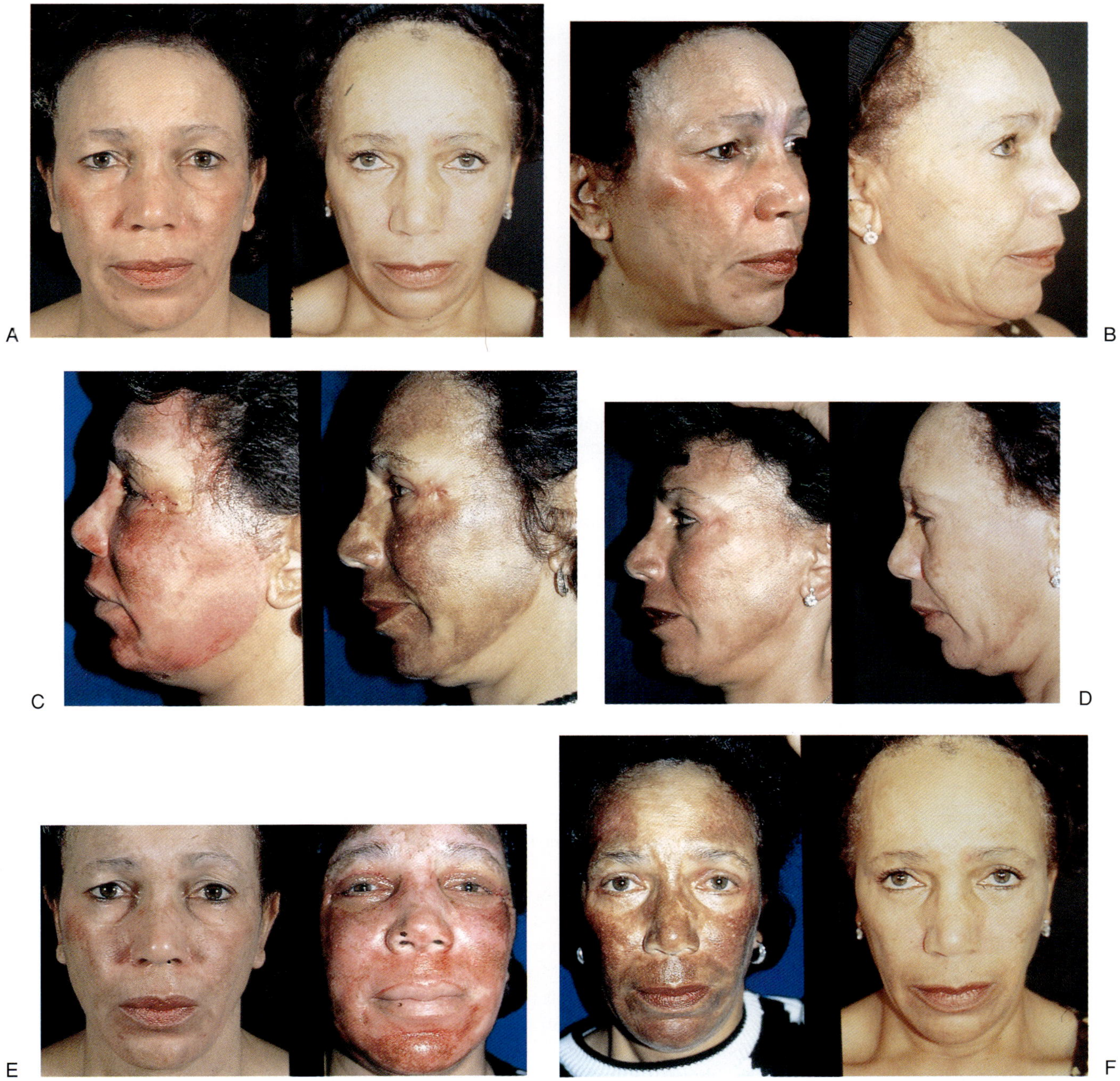

Figure 18. A–F: Melasma in the fair-skinned patient responds well to medium-depth trichloroacetic acid 35% as depicted pre-operatively and at 12 months post-operatively *(above left and right)*. Stages of recovery are shown at 3, 30, 60, and 90 days in the lateral view (C and D) and at 0, 2, 14, and 120 days in the frontal view (E and F).

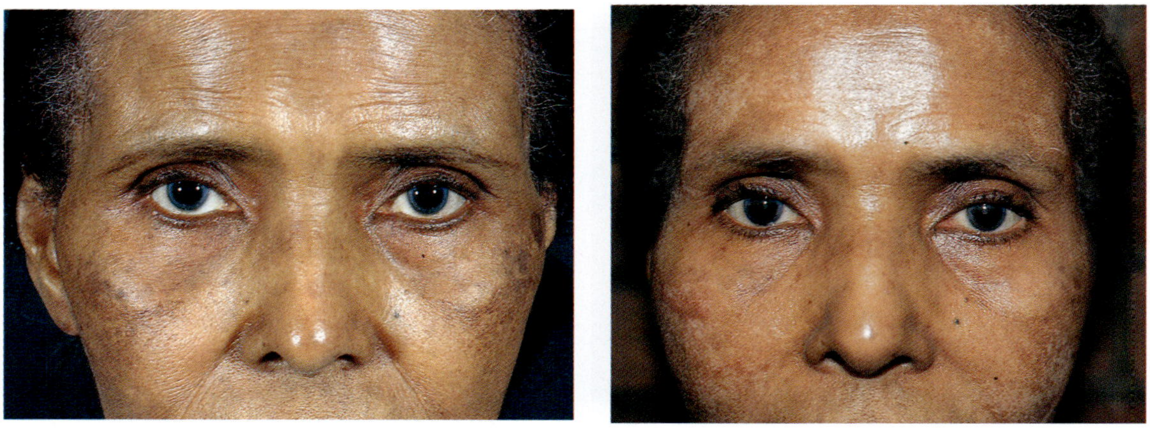

A B

Figure 19. A–B: Melasma in the medium or darkly pigmented individual also responds to medium-depth peel but may leave patchy hypopigmentation as shown before and 36 months after trichloroacetic acid 35%. A lower trichloroacetic acid peel 17% or Nd-Yag laser is likely to yield a more select lightening of melasma in the more pigmented patient.

Retin A is a readily simple and readily available derivative of vitamin A, only Ortho Pharmaceutical, a subsidiary of Johnson & Johnson, can legally manufacture Retin A until the patent expires. In our experience, we have found that when Retin A is used in pigmented skin, there is a sallowness and lightening of the skin. When higher concentrations of AHAs or other medium and deep peels are performed, pigmentary return is slow or irregular. Permanent discoloration has been noted in a few patients. For these reasons, we recommend that Retin A be used with discretion in individuals of color.

Skin Lighteners

Hydroquinone and kojic acid along with glycolic acid are useful agents in lightening hyperpigmentation that is commonly seen in the patient of color. In addition, hydroquinone and kojic acid also augment the effectiveness of AHAs and Retin A in rejuvenating the skin.

These agents are applied nightly. Kojic acid and hydroquinone may be found in combination from a number of vendors and have proven to be the most effective skin-lightening regimen. Areas of irritation may be noted, particularly when various substrates are combined with hydroquinone. Most preparations are alcohol based or in an oil-based cream. Excessive drying may result from the alcohol, or a greasy feel may be noted with the oil preparation. Water-based gel tends to be more palatable. The alcohol- or oil-based cream formulas may have irritating components (see Table 1). By scrutinizing your product line, you can limit the irritating skin reactions that frequent currently used skin care regimens.

Table 1. *Product ingredients to avoid*

Cocoa butter	Isopropyl palmitate
Coconut butter	Isostearyl isostearate
Corn oil	Myristyl lactate
Hydrogenated vegetable oil	Myristyl alcohol
Soybean oil	Isocetyl alcohol
Shark liver oil	Oleyl alcohol
Cottonseed oil	Cetearyl alcohol
Acetylated lanolin alcohol	Wheat germ glyceride
PEG-16, lanolin	Laureth-4
Caprylic, lauric, myristic, or stearic acid	Steareth-10
Cetyl acetate	Oleth-3
Isopropyl myristate	

Hyaluronic Acid

Antioxidants like vitamin C and E further augment the effectiveness of the AHAs. Hyaluronic acid, along with antioxidants, heighten penetration and lessen the irritation that often accompanies AHAs.

Benzoyl Peroxide 1–10%

Benzoyl peroxide propels peroxide into the occluded anaerobic environment of sebaceous gland, this allowing the release of oxygen. Acne caused by *Propionibacterium*, an anaerobic organism, is effectively eliminated with the use of benzoyl peroxide. Benzoyl peroxide is an excellent adjunct in the management of pilosebaceous occlusive disease, whether it be acne, pseudofolliculitis barbae, hidradenitis suppurativa, or rosacea.

One should note a number of considerations regarding the use of benzoyl peroxide:

1. Skin desiccation is a natural sequela of aeration of the skin. Aggressive moisturization is the key.
2. To be effective, benzoyl peroxide must be applied continuously. Patients may note improvement with initial application, but benzoyl peroxide must be applied several times daily for ongoing effectiveness.
3. Tolerance of the skin to benzoyl peroxide is gradual. One should start with lower concentrations applied to active or subacute lesions. As the skin tolerance is increased, prolonged application and increasing doses to 10% will optimize pilosebaceous control.
4. Avoid products that have any of the irritating components that are listed in Table 1, particularly isopropyl myristate, isopropyl palmitate, sodium lauryl sulfate, and laureth-4.
5. Avoid eye irritation by using cotton swabs to apply it to lesions close to the eyes. Redness, itching, and conjunctivitis may result otherwise.
6. Many preparations have a gritty feel. We have been pleased with a micronized form of benzoyl peroxide that is non-comedogenic and less desiccating (MD Formulations Benzoyl Peroxide).
7. Avoid photosensitizing medications (see Table 2). These medications will heighten the effect of sun exposure in lightening or darkening the skin, particularly in individuals of color.

Antibiotics

Systemic or oral antibiotics have little effectiveness in addressing cutaneous infections. Because of the associated heightening of skin sensitivity, we advise that these products not be used in patients with any skin type, but particularly in individuals of color:

Antibiotics. Topical antibiotics including clindamycin and erythromycin can be used in the patient with chronic cystic acne, acne vulgaris, hydradenitis, or pseudofolliculitis barbae.

Antiviral agents. Herpes I and II may be brought under control using Zovirax 400 mg taken by mouth six times daily. Topical Zovirax will diminish pruritus and irritation.

Table 2. *Photosensitizing medications to avoid: "Sun exposure will lighten or darken your skin"*

Antibiotics	Anti-depressants	Diuretics
Tetracycline	Elavil	Lasix
Vibramycin	Norpramin	Diuril/Hydrodiuril
Sulfonamides	Tranquilizers	Diabetic
Griseofulvin	Librium	Tolbutamide (Orinase)
Minocycline	Thorazine	Chlorpropamide (Diabinese)
Anti-fungals	Navane	Anti-psoriatics
	Haldol	Psoralen

Moisturizers. Skin emollients are a key component of any skin treatment regimen. Each of the agents that are used has a desiccating effect on the skin. Post-peel regimens are augmented with the use of phospholipid combinations that enhance penetration of the emollient.

VITILIGO: A RAPID AND EFFECTIVE TECHNIQUE TO EVEN SKIN TONES

"The light and dark areas of my face make me look like a leopard! It started with a spot on my nose. Now it's everywhere—my eyelids, cheeks, neck, arms, back, and chest." "People stare. I don't go out. I've lost two jobs."

Over 20 million in the United States and upward of 100 million world-wide suffer from pale discolored patches of skin, a phenomenon commonly referred to as vitiligo (Fig. 20). Often confused with leprosy, vitiligo is not infectious. It is, however, perceived as an ailment, often resulting in fear and avoidance. The extent of involvement worsens with age, almost uniformly leading to psychological, social, and economic disparity. Vitiligo may develop following elective surgery in the heavily pigmented skin. Some knowledge of hyperpigmenting conditions is therefore appropriate for the cosmetic surgeon (Fig. 21).

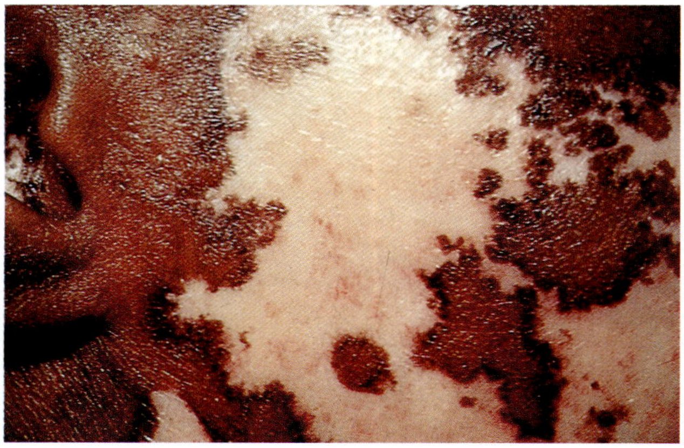

Figure 20. Vitiligo. Ghostly, spotty white patches develop spontaneously, following a trauma or after elective surgery in patients of color.

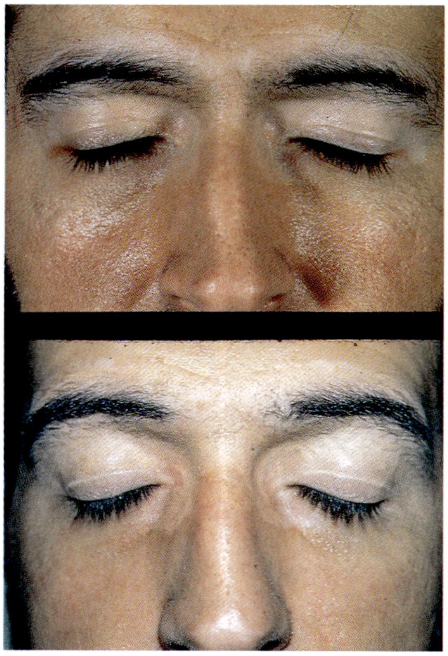

A

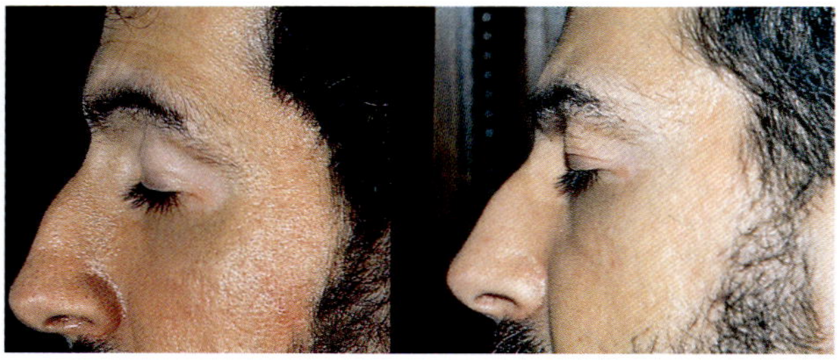

B

Figure 21. Vitiligo of the upper **(A)** and lower **(B)** lid addressed using dermal pigmentation.

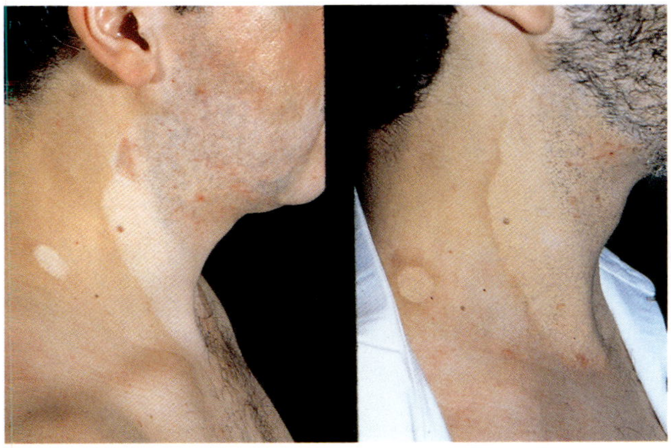

Figure 22. The limitations of currently available techniques for dermal pigmentation are demonstrated (after dermal pigmentation). New areas of hypopigmentation may necessitate additional treatment; currently used pigments do not provide ideal color match especially in the ethnic patient; there are natural variations in pigment color throughout the body, e.g., the anterior versus medial neck or the medial upper lid versus lateral lid skin.

Why Does Vitiligo Occur?

A common affliction among the Greeks and the Asian Indian, records date the presence of vitiligo as early as 1400 B.C.E. From the centers of Africa to the pillars of Rome, vitiligo has heaped its misery on many. Inherited, post-injury, and unknown factors contribute to a paucity of melanin pigment and melanocyte death, robbing the skin of its color. The white patches tend to merge with time, often yielding a ghostly or spotty appearance that is considered a physical disfigurement (Fig. 22). In fact, vitiligo is commonly misinterpreted as an infectious disease like leprosy. Cosmetic cover-ups and agents that increase the skin's sunburn reaction (psoralens) are cumbersome and time consuming and have varied response. These products have frustrated thousands of vitiligo sufferers.

Other Conditions That Lighten the Skin

Lupus erythematosis is a chronic inflammatory disorder that may be present in 6–12% of individuals of color. The condition when confined to the skin, Discoid lupus erythematosis, is typified by red thickened plaques located on sun-exposed areas. In dark-skinned individuals, central areas of hypopigmentation (lightened) and telangiectasia are highly visible and disfiguring. Only 5% of those with discoid lupus develop systemic disease, or systemic lupus erythematosis. The sun is the most common precipitating factor (Fig. 15). A number of other conditions cause light spots on the skin, including lupus, pityriasis alba, psoriasis, and tinea versicolor.

Great News for Vitiligo Sufferers!

Dye impregnation (dermal tattooing) provides and excellent, often long-term evening of the skin tone. The skin is numbed with a skin cream (tetracaine–adrenaline–cocaine mixture). Dye is selected to closely match the surrounding skin. In that many of these patients have varied tone or multiethnic backgrounds and shades, multiple colors may need to be mixed. A pencil-like instrument with multiple tiny needles is then used to impregnate the deep layer of the skin (dermis) with dye (Fig. 21). By angling the pencil both perpendicularly and obliquely, skin tones can be made more uniform (Fig. 22).

Multiple Treatments

Skin pigment and tones within the skin are constantly changing. The difficulties of matching the varied colors of an individual's skin and addressing these changes require that corrective surgery involve more than one procedure. Optimal results are achieved with two to four treatments to each area (Fig. 23).

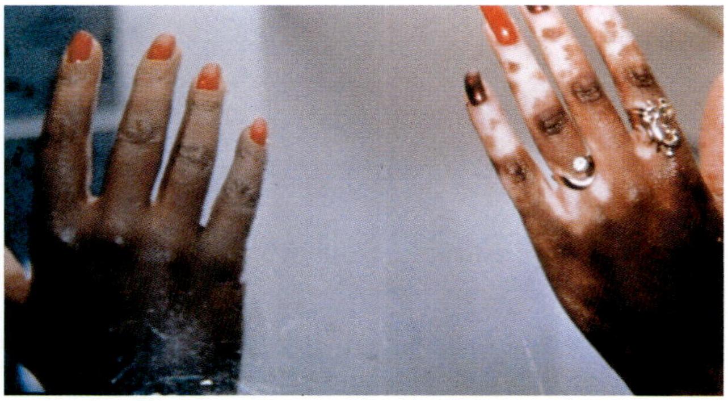

Figure 23. Vitiligo of the hand represents a high treatment priority to minimize social isolations that occur due to fears that this disease is contagious. Sophisticated make-up application and/or dermal pigmentation represent excellent treatment options.

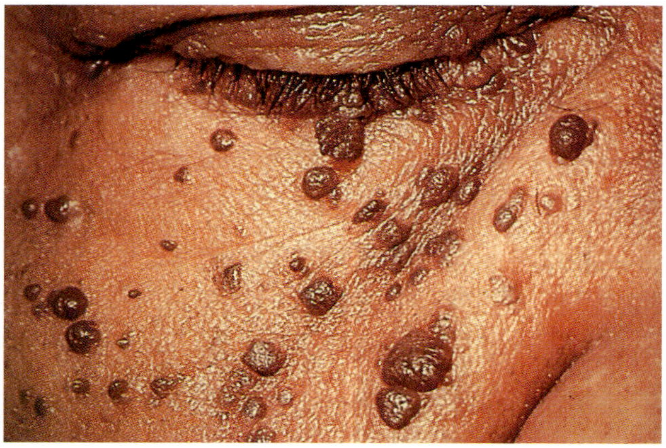

Figure 24. Dermatosis papulosa (nigricens) consists of darkly pigmented lesions that occur on the face, neck, chest back, and groin.

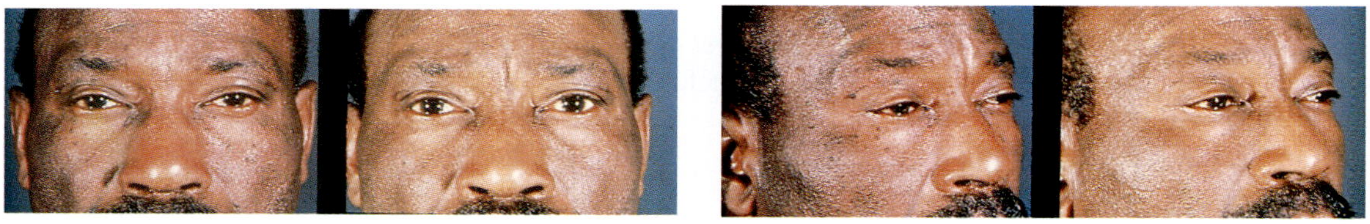

Figure 25. Dermatosis papulosa (nigricens) is most easily addressed using ophthalmic electrocautery if under local anesthesia with or without sedation. Initial post-operative hypopigmentation is followed by hyperpigmentation with return of neutral pigmentation within 3–4 months.

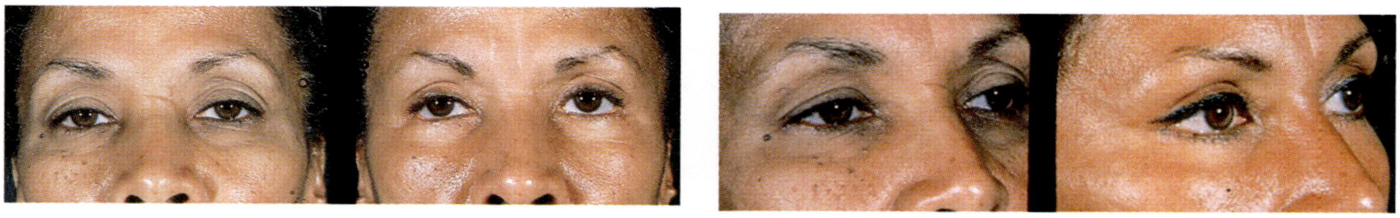

Figure 26. One year following cauterization of dermatosis papulosa (nigricens), malar fat injection, and quadrilateral blepharoplasty.

Risks

Risks are few. However, any surgical procedure may serve to exacerbate lightening of the surrounding skin. This technique is so gentle that we have not seen any progression of vitiligo following dermal tattooing.

Touch-Up Surgery

New skin color is retained for 2–10 years, depending on the type of dye. When fading occurs, simple touch-up procedures can enhance or adjust skin tone. Dermal pigmentation is an effective and safe method for softening the miseries of vitiligo.

SKIN TAGS (DERMATOSIS PAPULOSA)

Darkly pigmented raised lesions from the skin can begin to appear at puberty, on the face, neck, chest, and back (Fig. 24). Dermatosis papulosa increases in number with age, often seeming to consume the face and neck (Fig. 25). Tags may occur in family members and may interfere with eyelid movement or with necklace or bra fit (Fig. 26). Electrocautery and freezing are very effective methods of eradicating dermatosis papulosa.

Ethnic Considerations in Facial Aesthetic Surgery, edited by W. Earle Matory, Jr.
Lippincott–Raven Publishers, Philadelphia © 1998.

10

Skin Care for Patients of Color

Kathryn Leverette and Yolanda L. Moore

Beauty is only skin deep.
— Proverb

The complexities of care for the highly sensitive skin of individuals of color present immense challenges to the plastic surgeon and aesthetician.

While darker skin is often thicker, oilier, more elastic, and less prone to the effects of aging and photo damage, it is particularly sensitive to acne and other environmental elements. Reactions to dairy, seafood, and citrus are more common and often more extensive than in the Caucasian. The darker complexion can make it more difficult to recognize generalized erythema and irritation and patient complaint or comment may become your best gauge.

One of the most troubling concerns for people of color is that of hyperpigmentation. Virtually all skin disorders may lead to pigmentary change. In addition, the deterioration of our earth's ozone layer is causing an increasing number of serious cases of sun damage, skin cancer, and uneven facial skin tone.

Many patients are sensitive or highly allergic to substances such as hydroquinone, a drug approved by the Food and Drug Administration (FDA) for use in cosmetic and pharmaceutical topicals to inhibit the overproduction of melanin. Darker skin may be sensitive to commonly used chemical and enzyme peels, topical acne therapies (e.g., benzoyl peroxide), resorcinol or Retin A, soaps, fabric softeners, scented products, sun exposure, and abrasive scrubs. We suggest a 3-day patch test placed on the side of the neck to determine sensitivity when introducing a new product to a sensitive-skinned patient.

PROCEED WITH CAUTION

As a rule of thumb, clinical treatment should be geared toward sensitive skin until the clinician understands the individual skin responsiveness.

K. Leverette and Y. L. Moore: The Solutions Center, Oakland, California 94606

Disorders that commonly affect patients of color are acne, melasma (chloasma), post-inflammatory hyperpigmentation, ashen skin, razor bumps (pseudofolliculitis barbae), occipital scalp disorder (acne keloiditis), keratosis pilaris, flesh moles (dermatosis papulosa nigra), deodorant bumps (hydradenitis suppurativa), pomade acne, Mongolian spots, dark circles around the eyes, hypopigmentation (vitiligo), tinea versicolor fungus, seborrheic conditions, and keloid and hypertrophic scarring from any cause.

Acne sufferers of color are often "mismanaged" with the commonly prescribed treatments such as oral generic antibiotics, Accutane, and Retin A. Each agent can cause photosensitivity and hyperpigmentation and can be devastating on darker skin. Topical acne treatment should involve the conservative and gradual use of benzoyl peroxide, alpha-hydroxy acids (AHAs) (especially glycolic acid), and oil-free sunblock. The care of an experienced skin care specialist is crucial. Inexperienced clinicians have a tendency to utilize ineffective or problematic treatments, e.g., the use of blood lancets to extract comedones on darker skin. A safer bet is the "two-step" extraction method that is preferable for the keloid-prone patient. This technique utilizes a five- to seven-diopter magnifying lamp. An ultra-fine needle tip to dilates the follicle for a minute or two, followed by a sterile extra-fine Miltex Shamberg extractor to evacuate the lesion.

DECIPHERING SKIN PROBLEMS

Dark skin can appear dry, but oftentimes it is simply a case of oily or combination skin accompanied by a keratinized dehydrated condition commonly referred to as "ashy skin." It is characterized by a grayish appearance due to the accumulation of the dead, scaly, uppermost layers of the epidermis.

Though commonly seen on the face, the most severely affected areas seem to be the elbows, hands, feet, and knees. It is most noticeable shortly after bathing when the outermost layer of the skin (stratum corneum) has dried. Ashy skin sufferers are compelled to lubricate these areas with rich, oily products that only temporarily relieve the tight, dry feeling. These products mat down the dead cells under a layer of emollient. Therapeutic efforts should be aimed at gentle exfoliation with a loofah or natural bristle body brush and keratolytic body lotions containing glycolic and/or lactic acid. Generous hydration adds moisture-building factors as opposed to layers of oil.

Cosmetic complaints by women of color generally run from acne and dark spots to make-up problems and uneven facial skin tone. Scalp disturbances are frequent, including seborrhea, dandruff, and alopecia (from hot combs, tight braids, and lye relaxers).

Each disorder must be addressed by the practitioner by carefully questioning about probable cause: past treatments, medications, sensitivities, allergic reactions, sun exposure, and lifestyle.

THE MAKE-UP MYTH

The key to addressing the post-operative and/or the daily make-up needs for people of color lies in using golden tones and natural lighting. The common belief promulgated by "color analysts" that most or all Blacks are "winters" with cool-toned skin must be dispelled. While some women of color definitely possess cool undertones and can wear fuchsia-, burgundy-, magenta-, and blue-based make-up, the vast majority of women of color look best and feel most comfortable in warm and golden earth tones such as copper, rust, brown, coral, olive, and warm reds.

Custom foundation or camouflage cover creams should never be blended or matched in artificial light. The result could be equally problematic in choosing and purchasing make-up under department store fluorescent lighting. One may make a substantial investment in products, only to find the colors "too pink" or otherwise inappropriate after leaving the store.

Take-home products should include gentle cleansers, exfoliating masks and gels, oil-free moisturizers, and sunblocks. Topicals containing active ingredients should be allergy tested and prescribed when needed, and regular follow-up visits are helpful to monitor results and potential side effects.

Hair products should be checked for comedogenic ingredients such as cocoa butter, isopropyl myristate, coconut oil, and vitamin E that can cause pomade acne, the stubborn breakouts that appear on the forehead and hairline.

EXPERIENCED ELECTROLYSIS

Genetics, age, and hormonal imbalance can cause some women to experience unwanted hair growth. Unwanted hair is frequently observed on the lower half of the face and neck and/or chest, especially in the chin area. This entity is especially common in women of color. One should work only with electrologists who are experienced in working on darker skin and who employ the "blend method" of electrology. To avoid folliculitis and irritation, anti-bacterial and cortisone products are often necessary along with diligent use of a sunblock to prevent hyperpigmentation. Because "hair bumps" can create an inflammatory and/or itching response, picking and scratching must be discouraged. Electrology treatments and concomitant skin care supervision should be performed regularly to minimize post-treatment inflammation or hyperpigmentation.

HYPERPIGMENTATION

Of the many skin disorders that affect the darker races, hyperpigmentation or dark spots is the most frequent complaint. Virtually all dermatologic problems and clinical procedures lead to hyperpigmentation. Hormonal and post-inflammatory hyperpigmentation may develop as a result of acne, razor bumps, melasma, chemical irritation, friction, electrolysis, allergy, overuse of abrasives, certain medications and hormones, chicken pox, sunburn, insect bites, trauma, surgical procedures, and chemical peels. These are but a few of the offending mechanisms.

Hormonal and post-inflammatory hyperpigmentation can be treated effectively through innovative treatments involving light glycolic acid peels, topical AHAs in formulations containing hydroquinone, which is the only FDA-approved skin lightener, and kojic acid, a botanical skin-lightening agent from Japan, along with the diligent use of a non-greasy sunblock suited to skin type.

The keys to controlling hyperpigmentation include having a complete medical history that notes certain lifestyle issues. Hormones, pregnancy, unchecked acne flare-ups, picking, sun exposure, overscrubbing, eczema, and sensitivities to hydroquinone and glycolic acid and inappropriate chemical peeling procedures are only a few of the many factors that can make or break any skin-lightening program. All causative factors must be brought under control before pigmentation problems can be resolved.

Kojic acid and ascorbic acid are welcome developments for patients allergic or sensitive to hydroquinone. Like hydroquinone, they can be combined with glycolic acid, whose small molecule acts as a carrier to the target tissues. Unlike hydroquinone, they have a low incidence of adverse reactions. Hydroquinone is currently being scrutinized by the FDA for long-term safety and for allegations that it may cause the severe skin disorder exogenous ochronosis. Another concern regarding hydroquinone is the mislabeling by some manufacturers who fail to provide ample precautions about too much sun, the need for daily sunblock, and the risks of severe inflammation due to allergic reactions.

The practitioner and patient should discuss past hydroquinone usage and reactions and stress serious suncare and clinic procedures such as light glycolic acid peels to boost results. Diligent daily use of a sunblock is an absolute must because passive sun exposure, such as riding in a car, poses the greatest risk. Many patients of color mistakenly feel that they do not need to use a sunblock for intermittent sun exposure because they do not sunburn. This is fallacy! The same or greater precautions against sun exposure are appropriate for individuals of color.

SERIOUS SUNCARE FOR PEOPLE OF COLOR

Dark skin can be as susceptible as lighter skin to the ravages of too much sun, including elastosis, wrinkling, hyperpigmentation, keratoses, malignancies, and uneven skin tone. Often, a patient of color will say, "I'm not trying to get a tan, or I never burn." Yet, unintentional day-to-day sun exposure damages darker skin the most.

As the ozone diminishes, people of color need to protect their skin any time they are exposed (Table 1). Sun exposure that occurs while riding a bus, driving a car, jogging outdoors, walking down the street, or working in the garden is the most dangerous. When going outdoors, even for a short time, patients must apply sunblock to all exposed skin. A high sun protection factor (SPF) is necessary at all times, even on dark skin, to block the increasingly hazardous rays. Hourly applications are indicated when patients are exposed to either direct sunlight and overcast skies and after swimming or perspiring, even if the product is labeled waterproof or water resistant.

To be absorbed into the epidermis, chemical sunscreen agents must be applied no less than 30 min prior to sun exposure. People of color should not neglect the backs of the hands, forearms, and neck as these areas tend to darken quickly, especially on the driver side. Patients should also be counseled to wear fleece-lined latex gloves for dishwashing to avoid chemical irritation that often results in hyperpigmentation on the backs of the hands, dramatically worsened while driving in the sun, or by irritated hands gripping the steering wheel.

For women, foundations that contain sunscreens usually provide too little protection. Most contain minimal sunscreen ingredients because the higher SPFs dilute the coverage. The exceptions are camouflage cover creams used to hide skin abnormalities. Most contain titanium dioxide and dense pigment, can be completely opaque, physically block the sun, and are usually waterproof and sweatproof when applied correctly and set with fixing powder.

There is a proliferation of professional and over-the-counter suncare products, and many contain ingredients that can cause stinging and allergic reactions on sensitive skin. Avoid prescribing sunscreens that contain paraaminobenzoic acid and high levels of benzophenone, oxybenzone, and padimate O if skin is sensitive or if the patient uses Retin A or Accutane. Effective and non-irritating sunblock ingredients for more sensitive skins include lower levels of benzophenone, octyl methoxycinnamate, menthyl anthranilate, octyl salicylate, and titanium dioxide.

Sunblocks must be user-friendly and selected according to skin type and product comedogenicity. Heavy creams, such as those containing tropical oils, can aggravate acne and do not encourage daily compliance since they tend to appear greasy. Oily-skinned patients should use water, aloe vera, and/or alcohol-based gels, while those with normal to dry skin should use non-comedogenic, hydrating lotions.

Table 1. *Lifestyle tips for patients of color: fading dark spots faster*

1. Avoid the sun; never skip sunblock, even on cloudy days.
2. Obtain prescription noncomedogenic waterproof sunblock for outdoor exercise.
3. Apply sunblock a full 30 min before exposure.
4. Wear 100% ultraviolet-protected sunglasses whenever outdoors.
5. Tint car windows to the legal limit to help diffuse intense sun.
6. Treat acne or razor bumps with modalities appropriate to ethnicity.
7. Avoid applying scented aftershaves or cologne to sun-exposed body parts.
8. Order refills of active topicals in advance to avoid having to start over, slowly weaning the skin back onto potent products.
9. Treat overdried, irritated skin by skipping a day or two of all "active" products, using only cortisone cream and sunblock until the symptoms subside.
10. In the absence of irritation, superficial exfoliating procedures with glycolic acid done every 2 wks will help therapeutic products penetrate better, if serious suncare compliance is followed.
11. Follow-up visits should be held monthly to re-evaluate treatment.
12. Do not scrub off dead skin cells if peeling or flaking accompanies treatment with Retin A or acid-based skin lighteners; use a sulfur clay mask after cleansing for "passive" exfoliation.

People of color with sensitive skin should not use SPFs higher than 20 unless the product contains only chemical-free titanium dioxide, which often needs to be custom-tinted with make-up pigments to blend with darker skin. High levels of sunblock chemicals can be irritating on almost anyone, especially in the eye area. Even though they may offer more protection, the ingredients combined to provide all that SPF coverage are potentially irritating.

For lips and the eye area, there are waterproof, emollient sunscreen balms available that provide more moisture and protection than products for the cheek and forehead areas. The eyes and orbital eye area should not really be an issue because they should always be covered by 100% ultraviolet-protected sunglasses when outdoors. Glasses and sunglasses can be coated for prescribed ultraviolet protection at an optometrist's office.

IF TOO MUCH SUN ALREADY SHOWS

If the hands, face, and other areas have already darkened from everyday sun exposure, prescribe skin-lightening products that contain glycolic acid and hydroquinone and/or kojic acid. If fade creams have not been used in the past, perform a 4-day patch test (using a very thin coat) on the side of the neck and the inside of the elbow to test for hydroquinone allergy. Then, have patients apply lighteners sparingly to the entire affected area every other night at first, building up to nightly use on non-irritated skin. Counsel patients to apply an ultra-thin coat, rub into the skin thoroughly, and not to attempt to dot acid-based lighteners onto dark spots. This can cause stinging, peeling, scabbing, irritation, and darker and larger lesions, with lighter halos surrounding the spots. Have patients apply sunblock suited to skin type to all sun-exposed skin and reapply as directed. This preventive regimen, if followed diligently, results in smoother, healthier, younger-looking, even-toned skin. Glycolic acid office procedures can boost the homecare program and are recommended every 2–4 weeks.

Pregnancy, oral antibiotics (especially tetracycline and minocycline), blood pressure medications, diuretics, hormone replacement, contraceptives, and retinoic acids are a few of the drugs that can cause moderate to severe sun sensitivity on virtually anyone, especially people of color. Extra care must be taken to avoid all unnecessary sun exposure and to reapply potent sunblock regularly.

ACNE IN PEOPLE OF COLOR

Acne is a genetic disease of the follicular epithelium; i.e., dead skin cells stick together and sludge within skin pores. We know that acne originated in Europe. It is much less common in areas where European colonization was non-existent and where co-mingling between European settlers and natives was infrequent. Acne is less common among Japanese who shun intermarriage. In contrast, the Spaniards occupied the Philippines for centuries, making acne prevalent in the the Filipino culture.

Because ethnic skin is so diverse and the aggravating factors of acne so very important, a thorough intake consultation is vital. Addressing the issues of medical history, genetics, past acne treatment, skin care habits, diet, and other lifestyle issues. Aggravating factors of acne include:

1. Stress is the major acne aggravator for all acne sufferers. It is largely a Western problem, compounded by work pressures and city life. Take, for example, the young Black professional striving to prove himself; the Korean single mother raising her children alone; a low-income Hispanic student struggling to maintain the grades and the scholarship she so desperately needs; the new immigrant from Southeast Asia who faces economic hardship, a language barrier, and alien American customs. Then there is the physical stress of night shift employment and inadequate sleep common to each scenario.
2. Sun exposure severely damages the glandular follicle, causing premature aging, skin cancer, and solar acne later in life. In addition, sunlight exacerbates the hyperpigmentation that afflicts the vast majority of ethnic acne sufferers.

3. Hormone levels fluctuate with the seasons, reaching their highest peak around October, a common timing for acne breakouts.

4. Climate plays a major role. When a U.S. tourist visits a humid tropical island or U.S soldiers travel to the tropics, each may develop tropical acne, a severe, painful, and scarring condition secondary to hot, humid weather. However, the opposite is also true of immigrants from the tropics. While they enjoy near-perfect skin in their native land, they become severely afflicted after a few months in the United States, probably due to the climate change, stress, and the Western lifestyle.

5. Pressure/friction or acne mechanica afflicts athletes who wear baseball caps, helmets, headbands, non-cotton workout gear, etc. White-collar workers and teenage Romeos may use the telephone exclusively on one side of the face, causing friction and acne flare-ups, similar to fiddler's acne. Those who wear ill-fitting eyeglasses, particularly Asians who can be hard to fit because of a flattened nasal bridge, are prone to acne mechanica on the nose, between the eyes, and on the upper cheeks.

6. Patients must be cautioned that picking and tampering with the skin can worsen the disorder, causing larger lesions that are slow to heal and more likely to hyperpigment.

7. Industrial chemicals and oils can aggravate acne, as can fluorocarbons, cutting oils, chlorine, and humidity in the workplace.

8. Diet can be a problem for any acne patient who lives in the West. Salty foods containing iodides are a frequent culprit. In addition, many people of color, based on their stressful lifestyles, frequent fast-food restaurants, which are noted for their use of iodized salt. The Asian diet is also high in iodides: seaweed, soy sauce, monosodium glutamate, seafood sauces, and shellfish, coupled with stir-frying in peanut oil (which also contains acne-generating hormones), can be incriminated. Sushi wrapped in seaweed and salty tortilla chips are consistent ethnic food troublemakers. Vitamin and mineral supplements and health food store seasonings often contain high amounts of iodized salt, sea salt, and kelp.

9. Certain drugs can incite acne. Corticosteroids (topical, systemic, and illegal), oral contraceptives, lithium, Danazol, Danacrin, Dilantin, cold and flu medications containing bromides, marijuana, cocaine, and amphetamines, to name a few, can aggravate acne.

10. Menstrual cycles exacerbate acne flare-ups due to high levels of progesterone that occur before the onset of menses and due to pre-menstrual stress along with cravings for iodide-rich foods.

11. The first trimester of pregnancy as well as the 60–90 days after birth can be devastating. Concomitant economic pressure, hormonal changes, and lack of sleep can make matters worse.

12. Low-estrogen pills can be acne aggravators. The buzz word "low dose" can sometimes mean high androgen, which increases sebum production.

13. Acne cosmetica afflicts one-third of U.S. women. Comedogenic ingredients cause microcomedones to form deep in the follicle, which later results in larger acne lesions. Be aware that "oil-free" claims often mean no animal, vegetable, or mineral oil. Synthetic oil is classified as a fatty acid; thus, an "oil-free" claim is legal. Synthetic oils such as isopropyl myristate and its chemical cousins, C and D red dyes in blushers and powders, stearic acid, cetyl alcohol, sodium lauryl sulfate, and laureth 4 are only a few of the known acne generators. Hair products, body care products, and pomades often contain cocoa butter, coconut oil, vitamin E, and other aggressive oils and fatty acids, which are just as risky for those who are acne-prone. Fabric softeners, especially the sheets thrown in the dryer, can induce acne or dermatitis on virtually anyone.

GLOBAL ACNE CARE: TREATMENT MODALITIES FOR PATIENTS OF COLOR

The Homecare System

A daily system of anti-bacterial and exfoliating treatment is paramount to the control of ethnic acne (Table 2). True control simply means that no physical sign of the disease is visi-

Table 2. *Suggested home treatment regimen*

Daytime
1. Use rinsable cleanser suited to skin type. Not every acne patient has oily skin.
2. Apply a non-oily gel-based bleaching lotion (glycolic acid/hydroquinone) to hyperpigmented spots and allow it to dry a couple of minutes.
3. Apply a full-spectrum non-comedogenic sunblock, suited to skin type. Remind the patient that sun exposure can aggravate acne and darken hyperpigmentation.
4. Custom-blend oil-free foundations in the office to match skin tone and to help cover acute acne lesions. Blushers should be made with carmine and iron oxide pigments other than D and C red dyes, which are coal tar derivatives and known acne aggravators.

Evening
1. The evening routine begins with cleansing followed by an anti-inflammatory sulfur-based clay mask.
2. The active acne lesions are then iced for 2–5 min, which reduces inflammation and allows benzoyl peroxide to penetrate better.
3. Benzoyl peroxide is then applied over the entire affected area, avoiding the eye area. Use 10% benzoyl peroxide gels for moderate to severe acne.

ble in its active stage. Since acne is a treatable disorder with no permanent cure, adult acne sufferers will most likely be tied to a non-comedogenic home regimen for life, whether or not they continue clinical acne treatment on a regular basis. For acne patients to achieve total clearing of active acne, the discontinuation of home treatment and positive lifestyle changes amounts to skin care suicide. Retention hyperkeratosis (i.e., dead skin cells building up and sticking together in the follicle) is the chronic condition common to genetically prone individuals. If the patient (a) does not adhere to a diligent daily care system that reduces corneocyte cohesion, interferes with retention hyperkeratosis, and kills bacteria, and (b) does not make permanent lifestyle changes, visible signs of the disease will begin to reappear almost immediately.

For our purposes, we will simplify matters by forming four large ethnic categories: Black, Hispanic, Asian, and Mediterranean. Certain people fit the profile of more than one racial or ethnic group. Here is where a wealth of practical clinical experience, diligent patient supervision, and lots of questions as to past acne treatment and the reactions to various medications will help the practitioner determine the best course of treatment. For example, an individual of mixed parentage that includes Black should be treated as such at first because of the predominant sensitivity of Black skin. Filipino Caucasians should be treated moderately at first and aggressively as treatment progresses because Filipino skin is usually extremely tough. To generalize, place Black skin as ultra-sensitive, Caucasian and Mediterranean skin somewhere in the middle, with Asian and non-Black Hispanic skin being resistive by comparison. Your judgment will become refined with experience.

About Antibiotics

If the patient requested a definition of acne, it would read something like this: Acne is a genetic disease evolving from retention hyperkeratosis of the follicular epithelium. If we are dealing with a follicular disorder, why flood the body with antibiotics so that a tiny amount ends up in the pore killing only a fraction of the bacteria? This treatment would not reduce retention hyperkeratosis. Topical penetrating antibiotics are far more rational as well as more effective. On darker skin, the use of anti-bacterial and keratolytic topicals such as benzoyl peroxide sulfur and AHA gels formulated with salicylic acid are preferential treatments. In addition, there are many side effects of oral antibiotics that include, most notably, severe sun sensitivity that leads to severe hyperpigmentation.

Isotretinoin (Accutane)

Isotretinoin (Accutane) is an extremely potent systemic retinoid used in the treatment of severe or recalcitrant cystic acne. This vitamin A derivative functions by turning off sebaceous glandular activity and keratinization. Side effects are frequent and varied, including severe birth defects, severe sun sensitivity, changes in glucose levels, diabetes, kidney malfunction, severe dry and peeling skin, chapped lips, gum inflammation and bleeding, permanent hair loss, aching joints, nausea and vomiting, hyperostosis and arthralgias, headaches, blurred vision, conjunctivitis, cheilitis, rectal bleeding, and digestive disturbances. The side effect of severe photosensitivity and hyperpigmentation is a significant concern for patients of color. Obviously, regular pregnancy testing, foolproof birth control, and blood tests for liver and kidney function and glucose levels are mandatory. Patients should be advised not to take vitamin supplements to avoid additive effects of vitamin A derivatives.

Unfortunately, more and more patients with lesser grades of acne are casually being prescribed Accutane. Of note is that isotretinoin does not work for all types of recalcitrant acne. Especially with darker skin pigments, cystic acne may clear within one or more cycles of isotretinoin treatment, only to have the condition return within months of cessation of the drug. When doses and/or frequency are increased, cystic acne may come under control, but an oily Grade II non-inflamed acne or angry Grade III pustular acne may progress. Because of the lesser degree of effectiveness in individuals of color and the increased risk of permanent photosensitivity and hyperpigmentation, isotretinoin should be considered a last resort, subsequent to exploration of all other modalities.

Tretinoin (Retin A)

Tretinoin (Retin A) is an effective topical keratolytic whose exact mode of action is unknown. A number of anti-comedogenic activities have been described, including decreased microcomedone formation, diminished cohesiveness of follicular epithelial cells, and stimulation of mitosis, and cell turnover of epithelial (follicular) cells, resulting in comedone extrusion. The safety and efficacy of the long-term use for acne or for aging have not been established.

The gel and liquid formulas are helpful in the treatment of non-inflammatory Grades I and II of acne vulgaris and chronic cystic acne. The liquid form is most effective and may, as a result, induce local irritation that responds well to brief cessation of product application and topical 1% corticosteroid and aloe vera (Alocort). The cream, on the other hand, is oily and loaded with comedogenics like isopropyl myristate and stearic acid. Irritation that may be induced by any form of Retin A is minimized by graduating the frequency and the dose of product to build up skin tolerance.

Limitations of tretinoin are as follows: (a) There is no anti-bacterial capability. Topical anti-bacterials, along with benzoyl peroxide, e.g., clindamycin (Cleocin T) and erythromycin (Emgel), are beneficial supplements to acne care. (b) Photosensitivity that is induced by Retin A may inflict severe hyperpigmentation in individuals of color. Protective precautions against sun exposure must be stringent and constant. Oral or systemic antibiotics may also contribute to photosensitivity-induced hyperpigmentation. (c) Hypopigmentation or a graying of the skin may result from prolonged tretinoin therapy and sun protection. These reservations, along with the lesser complexity of alpha-hydroxy agents, limit our use of Retin A in pigmented individuals.

Alpha-Hydroxy Acids

These non-toxic fruit acids, especially glycolic acid, are far more gentle than Retin A, especially for ethnic acne. AHAs are comparably effective in reducing hyperkeratosis and excessive flaking and in fading hyperpigmentation. Fewer adverse side effects are noted with AHAs than Retin A, i.e., excessive flaking, redness, blotchiness, irritation, hyperpigmentation, and photosensitivity. AHAs are proving to be a mainline treatment for acne, discoloration, and aging for individuals of color. AHAs also have a lower price tag and wider availability through direct dispensing. High-concentration chemical peels that allow prompt return to work are safe for people of color. Homecare products are available in gels, lotions, and creams, in strengths ranging from 4 to 18%. The oil-free varieties are more appropriate for acne and can be introduced in a thin application every other night and with a gradual progression to twice-daily usage. Glycolic acid gels can be effectively worn under benzoyl peroxide at night and under sunblock during the day. When formulated with salicylic acid, glycolic acid gels are even more effective.

Benzoyl Peroxide

Benzoyl peroxide penetrates the follicle and releases oxygen, thus killing the common infective agent, *Propionibacterium acnes*, an anaerobic bacteria. It also causes desirable desquamation similar to Retin A and the AHAs, thus loosening acne impactions. Benzoyl peroxide worn on the skin for a long enough time each day will continue to peel within the follicle, retard bacteria overgrowth, and thus keep new impactions from forming.

The skin becomes accustomed to low concentrations of benzoyl peroxide, rendering it less effective. In turn, any benzoyl peroxide medication strong enough to clear acne and keep it clear is too strong to be tolerated overnight for most patients early in the treatment process, especially for the patient of color. Benzoyl peroxide should be introduced very gradually, slowly building up to all-night usage. Temporary darkening of the skin that occurs in those of color using benzoyl peroxide is also lessened by initiating treatment slowly. The stronger 10% water-based benzoyl peroxide gels are preferable to moisturizing versions in that they do not contain oils or moisturizers that impede the action of benzoyl peroxide.

Guidelines for benzoyl peroxide therapy categorized according to ethnic skin type and ethnic background:

African American/Black skin. Black skin can be ultra-sensitive, so begin with no more than 10–15 min for the first 3 days and gradually increase the wearing time. Black acne patients must be cautioned to avoid abrasive scrubs. Warning: Benzoyl peroxide can temporarily hyperpigment black skin, so a very conservative schedule must be followed to slowly increase to overnight usage.

Hispanic skin. Be slightly more aggressive on Hispanic skin unless the patient has recent African heritage. Some Puerto Ricans, Cubans, and Panamanians have skin that is highly sensitive, comparable with that of the African American.

Asian skin. Start with 30 min of benzoyl peroxide on Asians and double the wearing time every 3 days.

Mediterranean skin. This category includes Arabs, Israelis, Iranians, Russian Jews, Greeks, Italians, European Spaniards, Asian Indians, and other olive-skinned people of color. Proceed in a fashion similar to that used for Hispanic skin, but be aware that redness can be encountered on fairer-skinned individuals.

Some patients either become sensitive to benzoyl peroxide, fit into more than one ethnic category, or do not respond to benzoyl peroxide therapy. Other anti-bacterial keratolytic topicals, such as sulfur, resorcinol, or salicylic acid, may be introduced. By gradually increasing keratolytic topicals and monitoring patient progress, clearing can often be achieved within 2 months without discomfort, excessive scaling, etc., which often accompany most unsupervised acne therapy. Of note, a detailed patient intake form will make the practitioner aware of known allergies and past use of these products.

Once benzoyl peroxide medication is tolerated the entire night for 2 weeks, medication may be worn for an additional 4 h in the evening. After another week or two, benzoyl peroxide may be fortified with a small amount of finely crushed U.S.P. flowers of sulfur. If total clearing is still not achieved, lifestyle issues should be re-examined and evaluated during regularly scheduled office visits. Alternatively one may prescribe a less opaque benzoyl peroxide gel or an AHA gel with salicylic acid for daytime use and gradually increase the strength of glycolic gel topicals. Office procedures, including acne facials, single-coat Jessner's, and glycolic acid peels, are performed on recalcitrant cases.

RAZOR BUMPS (PSEUDOFOLLICULITIS BARBAE)

Pseudofolliculitis barbae (razor bumps) is a constant grievance for African American, Hispanic, and some Caucasian men and women who shave, tweeze, or use depilatories. Caused by stiff hair and a curved follicle, whiskers curl, growing back into the skin or follicle. The resulting inflammation, or "bumping up," creates painful, pus- and hair-filled lesions that swell, itch, and blanket the affected area. As the initial phase "heals," the ingrown hair burrows under layers of dead skin cells that often darken, causing the entire lower face and neck to become pitted with hyperpigmentation or "shadowing." This annoying, chronic condition persists until hair removal ceases altogether or when an altered shaving regimen is selected. The best shaving alternatives are barber's clippers or using a single-edge blade passed once in the direction of the hair growth.

The aesthetic and medical aesthetic market is flooded with exfoliating scrubs and anti-bacterial keratolytic topicals to help stop this "bumping up" altogether. Swelling, burning, and itching can be alleviated by temporary use of professional products containing aloe vera and hydrocortisone (Alocort). Hyperpigmentation is handled by the skin-lightening combinations of glycolic acid with hydroquinone and/or kojic acid accompanied by diligent use of sunblock and sun avoidance.

Glycolic acid and enzyme peeling treatments should involve a skilled professional who may also release trapped hairs with a fine-gauge needle (not blood lancets) but only on non–keloid formers. The frequent desquamation caused by these approaches helps to dissolve the build-up of dead skin cells and allows anti-bacterial topicals to penetrate better.

DARK CIRCLES UNDER THE EYES

The cause of darkening skin in the orbital eye area can often be uncovered in the initial consultation. Common causes are listed in Table 3.

In cases where genetics is the culprit, a warm-toned, opaque, corrective cover cream is the only real answer. Since some cover creams tend to cause a dry appearance and accentuate undereye wrinkles, the camouflage product can be blended with about one-sixth oil-free moisturizer on a metal palette, applied gently around the eyes, and then spread with a make-up sponge. It is set with a micro-milled loose setting powder.

Certain aspects of the patient's lifestyle, including too little sleep, sleep disorders, frequent air travel, crossing time zones, and night shift employment with interrupted sleep during the day, cause dark circles. Changing sleep habits to no less than an uninterrupted 7 h a night will help relieve symptoms.

Topical exfoliants such as benzoyl peroxide, glycolic acid, trichloroacetic acid, and resorcinol, as well as environmental irritants, can cause temporary darkening in the orbital eye area on some patients when applied too close to the eye. Using eye creams simultaneously with acne medications can cause them to migrate through moisturizers into the delicate tissues surrounding the eyes, resulting in inflammation and hyperpigmentation. Long-term use of potent fluorinated corticosteroids in the eye area may also lead to darkening and swelling.

Appropriate patient selection techniques, careful application of potentially irritating topicals below the orbital eye area, and avoidance of eye creams during acne therapy will minimize irritation.

Hyperpigmentation accompanied by itching and mild peeling can be caused by frosted eye shadows, contaminated mascara, products containing D and C red dyes, perfumes, and

Table 3. *Common causes of darkened skin in the periorbital area*

Heredity	Contact dermatitis
Lack of sleep	Chronic allergies
Chemical irritation	Sun exposure

constant rubbing. Switching to hypoallergenic matte eye shadows, avoiding red dyes and scented products, and changing mascara every 3 months or more often brings almost immediate relief. A mild hydrocortisone cream should be used until the dermatitis disappears, within a few days at most.

Out-of-control allergies cause dark circles, even in children. Many anti-histamines are accompanied by unpleasant side effects and daytime drowsiness, causing allergy sufferers to be inconsistent with their treatment. In addition to removing the irritants causing the allergies, control can be achieved by a sympathetic, progressive allergist who can prescribe one of the newer highly effective anti-histamines that lack drowsy side effects or a steroid nasal spray, which works on swollen nasal tissues without entering the bloodstream.

Sunscreens and skin lighteners are often applied to the face, and not the eye area, thus completely leaving this area darker than the adjacent skin. Patients should be advised to wear 100% ultraviolet protection eyewear when outdoors for any length of time.

ACNE KELOIDITIS

Acne keloiditis often appears in the Black and Hispanic scalp after a close haircut (usually a razor cut). Shorter hairstyles and a lack of barber shop sanitation can incite this disorder. This entity often progresses to a chronic, disfiguring condition causing local infections, ingrown hairs, hypertrophic scarring, and permanent hair loss in severe cases.

Occurring primarily in the occipital scalp area and on the neck, traditional medical treatment has involved little more than oral antibiotic and corticosteroid injections with disappointing results. This all-too-common disorder can be well managed by an alert clinician.

The patient should be advised to forgo closely cropped hairstyles and to stop wearing unwashed headgear, such as baseball caps, often used to hide the problem. Allowing the hair to grow out, using an anti-bacterial wash twice a day, and applying a clear AHA gel or lotion during the day and a potent anti-bacterial acne medication such as benzoyl peroxide with sulfur at night can help clear a mild to moderate case in a few weeks.

Stubborn or severe cases can benefit from potent weekly glycolic acid peels or multiple-coat Jessner's procedures and referral to a physician for a course of oral minocycline and a series of corticosteroid injections into the larger lesions. In recalcitrant cases, surgery is sometimes performed to excise the entire problem area in the often futile hope of leaving a hairline scar at the base of the scalp that may be hidden under the hair. Unfortunately, the patient who is prone to acne keloiditis is often prone to hypertrophic scarring. The common post-surgical outcome is a thick, disfiguring, cigar-shaped scar. Early detection and effective non-surgical treatment are the keys to controlling acne keloiditis.

PRE-OPERATIVE AND POST-OPERATIVE SKIN CARE

Prior to cosmetic surgery, the patient's skin must be free of comedones, papules, pustules, and nodules. A series of cleansing, exfoliating facial treatments is advisable to evacuate comedones, drain inflamed pustules, and remove sebaceous filament. Prior to dermabrasion, it is mandatory to have comedones removed and pustular lesions under complete control to minimize the risk of scarring. For patients of color, scar potential and skin tone must always be taken into careful consideration and a patch test performed to enable the surgeon to predict probable results. In aesthetic plastic surgery, the patient's goals are usually subjective and surgical improvement does not guarantee patient satisfaction. Prior to resurfacing chemical peels, patient selection and choice of the peeling solution are equally crucial and a conservative, supervised 4- to 8-week program of Retin A and AHA may be indicated to prepare the skin for an even peel result. Obviously, due to skin sensitivities, the possibility of patient non-compliance and the risk of hyperpigmentation, possible inflammation, and photosensitivity, the patient must be gradually and conservatively weaned onto these pre-peel topicals. Sun avoidance and daily use of full-spectrum sunblock are mandatory, and patients must be carefully selected and monitored on a regular basis.

Post-operative care involves several important phases for patients of color. Post-operative cleansing and facial treatments must be gentle, non-abrasive, appropriate for skin type, and undertaken with the approval of the surgeon. Gentle, exfoliating AHA shampoos and cleansers can help alleviate tightness, keratinized build-up, and itching on the face and scalp during the healing process, though special care must be taken to keep these cleansers away from peeled or dermabraded skin until approved by the surgeon. Chemical-free tinted titanium dioxide sunblock creams can help moisturize and protect the the skin from sun, wind, and environmental pollutants without irritation. Protective post-peel balms must be anhydrous, emollient, and occlusive and should contain lipids and hydrocortisone to help relieve itching and tightness and discourage picking of newly peeling dermabraded skin. Contrary to common practice, aesthetic rehabilitation (with the exception of trauma and burn injury) should be scheduled pre-operatively and must include expertly matched medical make-up (cover creams), image and color consulting, and a make-over appropriate to patient ethnicity. Cover cream shades are more easily chosen to match golden olive and darker skin tones in natural daylight during the pre-operative consultation when the patient is more receptive to the instructions, color choices, and advice of the make-up therapist. With the surgeon's approval, the second consultation and make-up lesson can be scheduled ~1 week post-operatively. The patient will then have a few days to practice camouflage techniques and updated make-up tricks before returning to the workplace. The medical aesthetician's role is vital at this point, by helping address patient concerns about appearance the healing process, appropriate skin care maintenance, and suncare. Sensitivity, empathy and experience with skin care geared to ethnicity, including treatment techniques and make-up appropriate for patients of color, are vital factors in choosing the professionals to work closely with your cosmetic surgery patients during the pre- and post-operative periods.

All too often, hypertrophic scarring, whether an expected complication or not, can become a problem. In my own practice, I gradually developed a post-operative regimen that can be both efficacious and preventative if the patient is open-minded, cooperative, and compliant. I always discuss the risks and likelihood of abnormal scarring and plan all strategies with the surgeon and patient in advance. I patch test the patient pre-operatively (twice daily for 3–5 days) for allergy or sensitivity to aloe vera, hydroquinone, kojic acid, low percentages of glycolic acid, micellized vitamin E, allantoin, deproteinized hemodialysate, epidermal growth factor, biological DNA, vitamin K, paraben preservatives, sunscreening agents, and other ingredients. I request a prescription from the surgeon for a supply of silicone gel or clear silicone sheeting and a Jobst pressure garment, hood or mask, if indicated to help prevent hypertrophic scarring. Immediately after the operation, I custom-blend a gel serum that may contain whole leaf aloe vera (with the alloin irritant removed), epidermal growth factor, biological DNA, vitamin K, and allantoin, to which I add micellized vitamin E (processed so the oil molecule is reduced to a water-soluble, more absorbable form) and 5% deproteinized hemodialysate. Deproteinized hemodialysate works by improving the utilization of oxygen and nutrients to help return reversibly damaged tissue to a normal state. Vitamin K has been shown to alleviate bruising and erythema and may or may not be indicated. Allantoin is a natural healing agent derived from comfrey and a soothing, non-irritating preservative. Aloe vera, appropriately grown and processed, is penetrating, hemostatic (reduces bleeding topically and below the surface), anti-inflammatory, and anti-pruritic and promotes healing. Aloe vera is also bactericidal and fungicidal when used in high concentrations, though some patients may experience stinging and may not be able to tolerate it. In these cases, aloe vera is simply removed from the recipe. Epidermal growth factor, known to incite cellular proliferation and promote healing, exhibits a growth-stimulating effect on epidermal and epithelial cells, especially when combined with small amounts of DHEA, a powerful androgen. DNA, a natural polymer derived from salmon milt, crosses the epidermal layers to the deeper tissues and has been used post-operatively for decades in Europe for wound-healing and scar-reducing purposes. Micellized vitamin E, bioavailable to the skin because of the small size, has been shown to effectively reduce scar formation when used within a limited window of time before permanent scars are formed.

With the surgeon's approval, a version of this alcohol-free, irritant-free gel serum is mixed and applied generously to the incision, dermabrasion, or chemical peel site and reapplied hourly. If abnormal scarring is either a high-risk factor or a definite given, the site should be covered with a non-stick dressing to be changed every 2 h after reapplication of gel serum. Silicone gel or sheeting is applied over the dressing and the pre-measured pressure appliance is worn over the silicone up to 22 h/day post-operatively. Later, daily wearing time may be reduced to 16 h/day for a minimum of 9 months to a year. Based on results and patient compliance, pressure appliances and silicone sheeting (worn over the appropriate topicals) may still be indicated. They should be worn consistently at bedtime and discontinued only with the surgeon's consent. A series of triamcinolone injections into the site may or may not be indicated at various intervals during the post-operative period to help flatten or prevent hypertrophic scarring. Sun avoidance and chemical-free sunblock are mandatory, even under silicone sheeting, which is sometimes worn alone during the day. Immediately post-operatively, the surgeon generally prescribes a short-term antibiotic and medication for pain management and may suggest a long-term holistic nutritional regimen consisting of a balanced diet, zinc picolinate, buffered sago palm–derived vitamin C with bioflavanoid complex, micellized micro-nutrients, and anti-oxidants including Pycnogenol, vitamins A and E, beta-carotene, *Arnica montana*, and possibly other vitamins, minerals, and natural anti-inflammatories. As healing progresses, a new custom cream topical may be applied over the original serum (under the dressing, silicone sheeting, and pressure appliance). This anti-inflammatory cream can contain aloe vera, hydrocortisone, epidermal growth factor, DNA, deproteinized hemodialysate, vitamin K, micellized vitamin E, zinc, and allantoin, or a combination of these. The penetrating and anti-inflammatory properties of aloe vera make it possible to use a lower percentage of hydrocortisone. This concoction helps speed healing, reduces erythema and edema, moisturizes the site, and prevents the inevitable itching that comes with the territory. In addition, micellized vitamin E, silicone sheeting, and pressure appliances, though cumbersome and claustrophobic, help prevent and/or reduce hypertrophic or keloid scarring dramatically, block the sun, and keep the patient from scratching and tampering with incisions and scabs. Later, the cream topical may again be altered to contain a low percentage of AHA, especially glycolic acid (which acts as a vehicle to carry hydroquinone and other ingredients to the target tissues), hydroquinone, kojic acid, ascorbic acid (an anti-oxidant that prolongs the shelf life of hydroquinone), and allantoin, applied over a coat of micellized vitamin E.

As the skin becomes adjusted to the AHA, the percentage should be re-evaluated and increased gradually and applied more sparingly to avoid irritation. A dressing may still be indicated to protect silicone gel, which disintegrates after a few daily washings. Clear silicone sheeting such as SIL-K is transparent and washable, lasts indefinitely, and eventually makes dressings unnecessary. Full-spectrum sunblock must be worn whenever the patient is exposed to any sunlight at all, even if silicone sheeting covers the site. With the surgeon's approval, in the absence of irritation, weekly or biweekly glycolic acid office procedures help smooth out scar tissue and loosen comedones and milia that often appear on peeled and dermabraded skin and along incision lines, where follicles have been temporarily or permanently disrupted. Glycolic acid also exfoliates epidermal layers to allow for superior and even absorption or healing agents and skin lighteners, the amelioration of dyschromia following chemoabrasion and dermabrasion, and the gradual reduction of the discoloration and thickness of incision scars.

KERATOSIS PILARIS

One of the most annoying skin disorders is the stubborn genetic condition known as keratosis pilaris. It is characterized by thousands of hard, non-inflammatory keratin plugs covering the hair follicles, making the skin rough and pebbled, both in appearance and in feel. On Blacks, Hispanics, and Asians, keratosis pilaris can resemble thousands of blackheads blanketing the skin.

The areas most commonly affected are the backs of the arms, the front and sides of the upper legs, the buttocks, and the cheeks of small children. Pilaris is certainly not limited to those areas. This disorder is worsened dramatically by picking and scratching, which induce secondary infection. The resulting sores heal slowly and scar or hyperpigment, mimicking burned-out acne. The risk of hyperpigmentation due to picking runs high in these ethnic groups.

While there is no lasting cure for keratosis pilaris, consistent home management can keep the bumpy symptoms in check. Twice-daily gentle use of an abrasive sponge, loofah, or natural bristle body brush with a sulfur or benzoyl acne soap will solve the problem. Daily application of keratolytic topicals is highly effective, e.g., sulfur/resorcinol lotion, 10% benzoyl peroxide 12–15%, glycolic gel or lotion, the stronger Retin A formulations, and prescription-strength Lac-Hydrin (12% lactic acid). Since February 1989, many insurance companies have stopped covering Retin A prescriptions for adult patients over 26 years of age. The vast amounts needed to keep keratosis pilaris under long-term control make its use financially prohibitive.

Since keratosis pilaris most frequently affects the upper arms and thighs, topical exfoliants may be used somewhat aggressively, though strengths and application schedules should be evaluated and varied according to the skin sensitivity of the affected body part.

For inflamed conditions, cleansers and topicals should contain benzoyl peroxide and/or sulfur that are both anti-bacterial and keratolytic. A note of caution: Test for benzoyl allergy and inform patients that it bleaches fabric and must not be worn if one expects to perspire or be exposed to the sun. Glycolic/hydroquinone mixtures should also be allergy tested before use on hyperpigmented skin. While sulfur may be odorless in its container, it can mix poorly with the body chemistry of some patients and may impart a most unpleasant odor.

An odorless topical AHA (glycolic and/or lactic) can be applied in a thin coat during the day and will not harm fabric. For non-inflammatory and for post-inflammatory cases, AHA topicals can be applied twice daily. While the glycolic exfoliates the build-up of keratin the hydroquinone helps the glycolic to penetrate, thus inhibiting overproduction of melanin.

Treating children should be left to highly experienced practitioners and should be approached conservatively. Gentle use of a mild exfoliating soap and the supervised application of a 2.5% benzoyl peroxide following an allergy test should prove adequate and effective.

All patients should adhere to sun protective skin care, especially when hyperpigmentation is present. Side effects of this treatment program for keratosis pilaris include temporary dryness, mild peeling and itching, and the presence of darker dry patches, all of which subside as the skin becomes acclimated to the active agents.

Excessively rough manual exfoliation and picking should be discouraged. Glycolic procedures performed in the office can be useful in stubborn cases. Home treatments must be continued permanently to prevent symptoms from recurring.

TINEA VERSICOLOR

Tinea versicolor is a chronic, asymptomatic, superficial infection characterized by scaly, hyperpigmented, macular patches. The fungus itself produces azaleic acid that interferes with melanin production in affected areas and may be additionally cytotoxic to the melanocytes. Patches range in color from light to dark pink to tan. Although the name suggests a variety of colors, the hue of all patches is about the same in any one patient. The areas involved usually lie between the chin and the waist, on the trunk and arms, and sometimes to the wrist. Facial involvement is rare except in Blacks. Patients are bothered mostly by the appearance, although the rash may be pruritic, especially during times of perspiration. Involved untreated areas are usually hypopigmented patches that are lighter than the surrounding skin. A Wood lamp will intensify pigmentary changes and will define the extent and margins. Infected areas appear orange under fluorescence.

Tinea versicolor is caused by the organism *Pityrosporon orbiculare*. It is seen mostly in young adults living in temperate climates and accounts for ~5% of all fungal infections. The fine scales of tinea versicolor are teeming with hyphae and spores.

Factors predisposing a clinical infection include (a) pregnancy, (b) genetic predisposition, (c) immunosupresssion of any sort, (d) high plasma cortisol (i.e., patients taking corticosteroids), and (e) a warm and humid climate. Tinea versicolor infections persist for years due to inadequate treatment or re-infection.

Tinea versicolor is treated in a variety of ways, most of which will prove successful if used diligently for a prolonged period of time. Though infection can be resolved, re-infection is all too common, and pigmentary changes can take months to resolve. Persistent lesions demand biopsy to rule out an alternative diagnosis including malignancy. Most topical methods are messy, tedious, frustrating, and time consuming. Patients give up, preferring to live with the disease rather than undergo the treatment.

Evening application of the following anti-fungal preparations is followed by an exfoliating bath. Treatment products include the following:

Zinc pyrithione (Head and Shoulders, Danex, Zincon, DHS-Zinc) applied 10 min nightly for 14 days.

Selenium sulfide suspension (Exsel, Selsun, Iosil) applied nightly and allowed to dry on the skin for 10 min for 14 consecutive days, with a 5- to 10-min application on alternate nights for another 14 days.

Sodium hyposulfite 25% applied to lesions twice a day for 14 days.

Tinver lotion (25% sodium thiosulfate, 1% salicylic acid, 10% alcohol) applied to lesions twice a day for 14 days.

Anti-fungal creams such as clotrimazole (Lotrimin), miconazole (Monistat-Derm), holoprogin (Halotex), and tolnaftate (Tinactin) preparations applied to lesions twice a day for 14 days.

Retinoic acid (Retin A) applied twice a day for 2 weeks will cure tinea versicolor and help to resolve the pigmentary changes. This modality may be expensive unless there is insurance coverage.

Oral ketoconazole (Nizural), taken in doses of 200 mg daily for up to 25 days, will lead to a 78–90% cure rate. A single 400-mg dose is equally if not more effective. Nizural is a broad-spectrum anti-fungal imidazole that is useful in the management of many chronic fungal infections.

DERMATOSIS PAPULOSA NIGRA (FLESH MOLES)

Dermatosis papulosa nigra, sometimes called "flesh moles," afflict about one-third of African Americans, with significant aesthetic concern. Dermatosis papulosa nigra runs in families and are found predominantly in persons of African descent, though they have also been reported in Mexicans, Asians, and other dark-skinned people.

They begin to appear at puberty and increase mainly during pregnancy and with age especially, between the ages of 30 and 50 years, tapering off by the late fifties. After age 60, it is uncommon to acquire new dermatoses papulosa nigra, though old ones tend to grow larger to look like pigmented skin tags. Female Blacks are more commonly affected in the United States. In Africa males present most commonly with dermatosis papulosa nigra.

To the untrained eye, dermatosis papulosa nigra and moles may seem indistinguishable. Under the microscope, however, moles have specific nevus cells, while dermatosis papulosa nigra does not. Furthermore, moles extend into the deeper dermal layers, while dermatoses papulosa nigra are merely a dark thickening of the epidermis. Varying between 1 and 3 mm in size, dermatoses papulosa nigra are evenly distributed throughout the face, neck, upper torso, and back and are most concentrated in the malar area.

Other mole-related skin conditions affecting Blacks, though less common than dermatosis papulosa nigra, include the following:

1. Skin tags, or flesh-colored benign moles, are usually larger than dermatoses papulosa nigra and are usually located under the arms and breasts, in the neck area, and in other folds or creases of the body.
2. Seborrheic keratoses are related to dermatosis papulosa nigra but are usually larger, darker, and more irregular and corrugated. These keratoses are not pedunculated.

3. Warts may look like cauliflower spots on the skin and are viral in origin. Recurrent growth is a common sequela.

These areas become irritated dependent on location, i.e., by wearing glasses or clothing, shaving, bathing, etc. Options for removal include electrocauterization, direct excision, and freezing with liquid nitrogen. Temporary mild to severe hyperpigmentation may occur following removal.

Though these skin conditions are rarely cause for concern, any pigmented lesion should be evaluated by a physician. Rapid growth, color changes, irregular shape or borders, bleeding, irritation, or ulceration may indicate malignancy. While melanoma is infrequent, its incidence in the U.S.A. is increasing in all populations.

PRE-OPERATIVE AND POST-OPERATIVE SKIN CARE

Prior to any cosmetic surgery, the skin of any patient, especially those of color, should be as free of acute, subacute, and chronic inflammatory lesions and hyperpigmentation as possible. A number of peri-operative factors contribute to inflammation of the skin, including surgical insult, topical adhesives, tape, and dressings, to name a few. This is particularly true for nasal surgery. The subacute acne lesion or sebum-laden pores of the nasal tip may become acutely inflamed or may contribute to chronic tip edema. Any resultant or exacerbated inflammatory response may prolong healing, worsen scarring, and routinely induce post-inflammatory hyperpigmentation.

A short series of cleansing and exfoliating facial treatments is advisable to evacuate comedones and remove sebaceous filament from follicles. Prior to dermabrasion it is especially important to have all comedones removed and acne lesions under total control to minimize the risk of scarring. At this point, patient selection is crucial and the type of scarring and skin tone must be taken into careful consideration. Prior to peels, a 4- to 8-week program of Retin A in the evening and an AHA topical treatment during the day will prepare the skin surface for an even peel application. Due to skin sensitivities, hyperpigmentation, possible inflammation, and photosensitivity, clients should be gradually introduced to these products. Sun avoidance and daily use of a full-spectrum sunblock are mandatory.

Post-operative care involves three important components. (a) Cleansing and facial treatments must be gentle, non-abrasive, and appropriate for the skin type and should be undertaken only on the approval of the surgeon. Gentle shampoos and cleansers can keep the patient comfortable and alleviate tightness, build-up, and itching on the face and scalp that commonly occur during the healing process. Chemical-free titanium dioxide-based sunblocks will moisturize and protect the skin from sun, wind, and environmental pollutants without irritation. (b) We suggest a sun post-peel balm that is anhydrous, emollient, and occlusive. Balms contain lipids, chemical-free sunblock, and hydrocortisone that soothe, protect, and relieve itching on freshly-peeled or dermabraded skin. (c) Aesthetic rehabilitation includes make-up (cover creams), image and color consulting, and a make-over. Each should be planned during the pre-operative period. Cover creams are more easily matched to skin tone prior to surgery. The patient will be more receptive to the initial consultation and the advice of the therapist. With the surgeon's approval, the second consultation and a make-up lesson can be scheduled ~1 week post-operatively. The patient will thus have a few days to practice camouflage techniques and special cover-up maneuvers before returning to the workplace. A few weeks later, light glycolic acid peels, suncare, and skin lighteners can be used to relieve any post-operative discoloration. The aesthetician is a key component to an expeditious and problem-free return to the workplace. The aesthetician's role is also vital in addressing patient concerns about appearance, the healing process, and appropriate skin care maintenance and suncare. Experience with skincare concepts, techniques, and make-up on patients of color is vital in choosing the appropriate professionals to handle these patients during the post-operative period.

ETHNIC CONSIDERATIONS FOR MICROPIGMENTATION PROCEDURES

Special considerations must be entertained when performing micropigmentation procedures on ethnic skin. The inevitable probability of hyperpigmentation, and in some cases an inclination to hypertrophic scarring, require a thorough patient evaluation and specialized operative approaches.

Depending on the type of micropigmentation procedure performed, resultant hyperpigmentation may enhance the end result. For instance, permanent eyeliner procedures resulting in hyperpigmentation at the site of trauma may give the eyeliner a more subtle and softer appearance. The implantation of dark-colored pigment and the body's natural response to hyperpigment can create a more natural look that cannot be duplicated when coloring lighter skin. Anecdotally, dye pigments seem to be retained longer with a lesser degree of fading.

While hyperpigmentation and bruising are common after micropigmentation, hypertrophic scarring is rare. The risk of abnormal scarring, on the other hand, may be increased by deep dermal needle penetration or by excessive abrasion.

For people of color, micropigmentation procedures should be approached with caution. Only through pigment color patch testing, technical experience, and an in-depth knowledge of different skin types will the risk of hyperpigmentation and scarring be minimized.

Micropigmentation Modality for Vitiligo

Vitiligo is an acquired depigmenting condition of unknown cause that results in uneven skin coloring, often manifesting as skin areas completely void of pigment. For individuals of color, this condition is more common and the loss of pigment is more visible and pronounced. As a result, social, psychological, and economic well-being are often compromised.

The most accepted treatment modalities for vitiligo include phototherapy with PUVA or PUVASOL, topical and intralesional steroids, phenylalanine, topical fluorouracil, and transplantation of in vitro cultured epidermis. These therapeutic measures often require long-lasting treatment programs and commitments that may be challenging to even the most patient of individuals. One of the newest and most effective forms of therapy is micropigmentation. Micropigmentation provides options for areas that have been resistant to other treatment measures.

Non-allergenic oxide pigment colors are custom-blended to match skin color. Color match is difficult because of varied pigmentation as a result of vitiligo as well as the many shade variations that are present on any body part. Currently used pigments do not perfectly match skin tones in any ethnic group. On the other hand, immediate and sometimes permanent improvement is consistently achieved for the vitiligo sufferer.

The potential risk of uneven pigmentation must be understood. Caution should be taken whenever pigmenting areas close to the normal tissue. Precise punctures with minimal abrasion will minimize post-surgical hyperpigmentation. Micropigmentation for patients of color has proven to be a successful, safe, and effective form of therapy.

RECOMMENDED READING

Arch Dermatol 1982;118.

Brody. *Chemical peeling*. Chicago: Mosby Year Book, 1992.

Brown GL, Nanney LB, Griffen J, et al. Enhancement of wound healing by topical treatment with epidermal growth factor. *N Engl J Med* 1989;321:76.

Coats. The silent healer: history, chemistry, uses of aloe vera.

Cowen R. Speeding up wound healing the epidermal growth factor way (epidermal growth factor). *Sci News* 1989; 136:39.

Cunliffe. *Acne, clinical features of acne, side effects of acne therapy; treatment of acne, scars*. Martin Dunitz Year Book Medical Publishers.

Dalle P. Skin photosensitizing agents and the role of reactive oxygen species in photoaging. *J Photochem Photobiol* 1992.
Epstein, Ernst. Common skin disorders. 3rd ed. 1988. Physician's desk reference.
Falabella R, Escobar C, Correro I. Transplantation of in vitro cultured epidermis bearing melanocytes for repigmenting vitiligo. *J Am Acad Dermatol* 1989;21:257–264.
Fulton. *Step by step guide to clearing acne*. 1978.
Hardy M. The biology of scar formatin. *Physical Ther* 1989;69:1014.
ICMAD. *Simplified guide to cosmetic labeling*. ICMAD, War Congress, Bethesda, MD, 1989.
Marikovsky M, Breuing K, Liu PY, et al. Appearance of hepatin-binding epidermal growth factor in wound fluid as a response to injury. *Proc Natl Acad Sci USA* 1993;90:3889.
Montyna C. Architecture of black and white facial skin. *J Am Acad Dermatol* 1991;24:929–927.
Montagra C, Prota, Kenney. *Black skin structure and function*. Academic Press, 1993.
Ortho Dermatological Division. Patient instruction sheet. 1985.
Physician's desk reference.
Rackett, Rothe, Grant-Kels. Diet and dermatology: the role of dietary manipulation in prevention and treatment of cutaneous disorders. *J Am Acad Dermatol* 1993;29:447–461.
Roche Laboratories. Accutane (isotretinoin). In severe recalcitrant cystic acne, used to advertise benefits, contraindication, patient selection and side effects. *Dermatol Nurs* 1994.
Rusting R. Skin deep: a recombinant growth factor hastens wound healing (epidermal growth factor). *Sci Am* 1989;261:38.
Salerno. Anti-oxidants and anti-aging: zinc required for DNA synthesis . . . wound healing. *Ad Dermatol News* 1992;2:1–5.
Sauer. *Manual of skin diseases*. Philadelphia: Lippincott.
Sauer, Gordon. *Manual of skin disorders*. 5th ed. 1986.
VanScott, Yu. Alpha hydroxy acids: therapeutic potentials. *Can J Dermatol* 1989;108–112.
VanScott, Yu. Procedure for use in clinical practice. *Cutis* 1989;222–228.

Ethnic Considerations in Facial Aesthetic Surgery, edited by W. Earle Matory, Jr.
Lippincott–Raven Publishers, Philadelphia © 1998.

11

Skin Care for People of Color

Rebat M. Halder and
Sharon E. Bridgeman-Shah

ACNE VULGARIS

Acne vulgaris is one of the most common chronic diseases that affects virtually all individuals at some time in their life. It affects ~17 million individuals in the United States, making it the most commonly treated cutaneous disorder (1). This appears to hold true across racial lines as suggested by Halder et al., who found acne vulgaris to be the most common dermatosis encountered in Black patients in private practice (2). Peak incidence for this disease occurs in the teenage age group, but middle-aged individuals, particularly women, can also be affected (1).

Acne can be non-inflammatory or inflammatory (3). Non-inflammatory acne refers to comedonal acne, which is characterized mainly by whiteheads (closed comedones) and blackheads (open comedones). Inflammatory acne is characterized by papules, pustules, and in the more severe forms nodules and/or cysts. The severe nodulocystic form of acne is significantly less prevalent in Blacks than in Whites (4,5). When it does occur in Blacks it is confined mostly to the face. Pomade acne, a predominantly non-inflammatory comedonal form seen as a result of hair-grooming agents, is seen almost exclusively in Blacks (6). Post-inflammatory hyperpigmentation commonly occurs at the site of resolved acneic lesions in Black skin and can be cosmetically distressing, often leading to social problems.

R. M. Halder and S. E. Bridgeman-Shah: Department of Dermatology, Howard University College of Medicine, Washington, D.C.

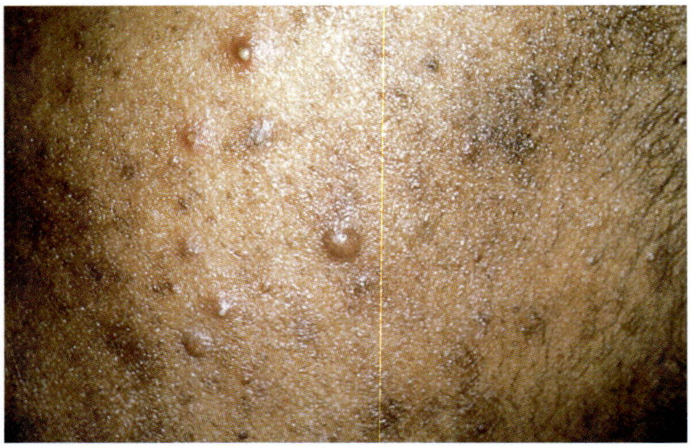

Figure 1. Acne vulgaris with pustules, papules, and post-inflammatory hyperpigmentation.

This hyperpigmentation occurs as a result of the exaggerated response of the melanocytes in Black skin produced by inflammatory reactions or trauma (Fig. 1).

Acne vulgaris is a disorder of the pilosebaceous follicles, primarily those on the face, neck, and upper trunk. Four etiologic factors have been identified in the pathogenesis of acne (3,7): (a) overproduction of sebum usually as a result of androgenic influence on sebaceous glands, (b) hyperkeratosis of the pilosebaceous duct, (c) proliferation of *Propionibacterium acnes (P. acnes)* within the follicles, and (d) production of inflammation in response to elaborated bacterial products and sebum.

Sebum production is increased in acne patients, and the quantity of sebum produced usually correlates with the severity of the condition (7,8). Moreover, the substantial reduction of sebum secretion usually results in decreased activity of the disease. In one study, Pochi and Strauss failed to disclose any significant differences between the sebaceous glands of Blacks and Whites.

Hypercornification of the follicular epithelium occurs in acneic skin with resulting blockage of the polisebaceous duct (6). Plewig and Kligman have suggested that Black skin is prone to hyperkeratosis and as such Blacks may be highly susceptible to comedone formation (6).

P. acnes, a component of normal skin flora, has been found in increased quantities on the skin of acne-prone individuals even before the onset of puberty (9).

There have been no reports thus far of quantitative differences of *P. acnes* between the races. The anaerobic environment produced by the blocked duct with resultant retained sebum is ideal for proliferation of the bacteria. The eventual rupture of micromedones and extrusion of their contents (sebum, free fatty acids liberated by *P. acnes*, keratin, hair, and enzymes) into the dermis result in an inflammatory response that can be very severe as seen in the nodulocystic form of acne vulgaris (3).

Treatment of acne is similar for all races. Physicians need to be sympathetic counselors focusing on strong patient–doctor relationship to ensure maximum compliance. A number of therapeutic agents are currently available for treating acne. Usually a combination of pharmacologic agents is used. The most commonly used topical medications include antibiotics, benzoyl peroxide, and retinoic acid (Retin A). Caution should be exercised when using benzoyl peroxide and Retin A on Black skin because of the risk of irritation with resulting post-inflammatory hyperpigmentation. Systemic agents include antibiotics and isotretinoin (Accutane), which is reserved for severe recalcitrant forms of nodulocystic acne. The less frequently used agents include corticosteroids (used intralesionally for severe inflammatory response seen in nodulocystic acne), birth control pills, topical salicylic acid, and spironolactone. Combination therapy is usually necessary for individualized care and optimum results.

Tetracycline, minocycline, and erythromycin are some of the oral agents used for treating acne. Topical antibiotics including erythromycin and clindamycin have fewer systemic side effects than oral antibiotics when used for acne, but the concentration of antibiotic in the follicle is also less with the topical formulations (3). Erythromycin may cause gastrointestinal upset; tetracycline has reduced efficacy when taken with dairy products and as such should be taken on an empty stomach. Tetracyclines also have the added possible phototoxic side effect (10). There is a risk of pseudomembranous enterocolitis when using clindamycin even in its topical form (11).

Retinoic acid (Retin A) and salicylic acid are the two topical keratolytic agents used in the treatment of acne vulgaris. Retin A, a vitamin A derivative, is the most effective topical comedolytic agent and is recommended for most forms of acne (3,12). Patients should be given detailed instructions on proper usage and side effects of Retin A. Sun sensitivity is associated with Retin A treatment. Patients should also be made aware of the likelihood of skin irritation within the first 2 weeks of application of this medication, especially when applied on wet skin. Some patients will experience a flare of their acne within the first month of therapy, but if they can get past this period, they will begin to see the benefits of this medication. For patients with sensitive skin, every other night or even less frequent application may be initially necessary with increasingly frequent applications as tolerance permits. Topical medications containing salicylic acid are helpful adjuncts in treating acne vulgaris (3). Salicylic acid is often used by patients unable to tolerate the irritation caused by Retin A.

Isotretinoin (Accutane) is a systemic medication reserved for severe recalcitrant nodulocystic acne (3,13). The exact mechanism of action in this disorder is unknown, but the isotretinoin decreases the size of sebaceous glands, rate of sebum production, and quantity of *P. acnes* and has both anti-keratolytic and anti-inflammatory effects. Side effects include dry mucous membranes, headaches, pseudotumor cerebri, inflammatory bowel disease, increase in levels of triglycerides, and teratogenicity. It is because of the teratogenic potential that Accutane should be cautiously prescribed for females of child-bearing age. If the medication is used in this group of individuals, serum pregnancy tests are required before initiating therapy and each month for the duration of therapy. Female patients also need to use at least two different methods of birth control for the period of time on this medication.

Adjunctive therapy using intralesional corticosteroids may be used to decrease the inflammation in nodulocystic acne. There is a risk of cutaneous hypopigmentation at the site of injection, particularly in Black patients, and atrophy of overlying skin. Comedone extraction is also useful for treating the non-inflammatory lesions. It is simple and may prevent patients using their fingers to pick at lesions. Cyst drainage is helpful when it applies. This procedure speeds healing but may result in scar formation. Varying concentrations of hydroquinone can be used to help fade the resulting post-inflammatory hyperpigmentation that occurs very frequently in Black acneic skin, but there is a risk of ochronosis with long-term usage (14).

In the treatment of acne vulgaris, surgery is usually reserved for scars once active lesions resolve. Punch grafting and collagen implantation are surgical modes of therapy found to be useful for acne vulgaris (15,16). Although chemical peels, cryosurgery, and dermabrasion have been found to be useful in the treatment of acne vulgaris, these modalities should be cautiously used in Black patients because of the possibility of adverse pigmentary disturbances (16). The risks for patients undergoing surgical excision of scars include the routine risks of basic surgery. Collagen implantation should not be attempted prior to pre-testing patients for sensitivity to the bovine collagen used (3).

PSEUDOFOLLICULITIS BARBAE

Pseudofolliculitis barbae, or razor bumps, the term most frequently used by laypersons, is a common, distressing, chronic problem seen almost exclusively in Black men as a result of shaving (Fig. 2) (17). Prevalence ranges from 45 to 83% among this population (17,18,19). In the past this condition has been responsible for racial tensions in the military because of the requirement for a clean-shaven face (17,19). In civilian life pseudofolliculitis barbae also causes tensions in occupations that require a clean-shaven appearance such as police and fire departments, food services employees, and flight attendants (17). The etiology of pseudofolliculitis barbae is a foreign body inflammatory reaction surrounding an ingrown hair. The condition is also seen in women who shave their axillary and pubic regions (17).

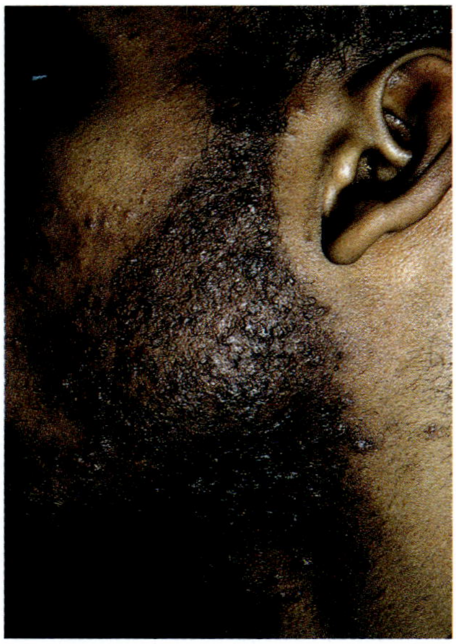

Figure 2. Pseudofolliculitis barbae showing ingrown hairs, papules, and post-inflammatory hyperpigmentation in beard areas.

Structural differences account for behavioral differences among hairs of different races. The kinky hair seen frequently in Blacks has an elliptical, flattened appearance on cross section, whereas the hairs of Asians and Whites are round and oval, respectively. It is this basic difference that accounts for the increase in prevalence of pseudofolliculitis barbae in Blacks (17).

Two major mechanisms are involved in the pathogenesis of pseudofolliculitis barbae: extrafollicular and transfollulicular penetration (17,20). In extrafollicular penetration, hair growing out of the follicle and shaved develops a sharp, pointed, flattened top that, because of its natural curl, is able to repenetrate the epidermis with subsequent progression to the dermis, as the hair grows. Once the hair enters the dermis, a foreign body inflammatory response is initiated. Strauss and Kligman pointed out that the beard hair in Blacks initially grows parallel to the skin surface for a brief period and when cut at an oblique angle forms an exaggeratedly pointed tip that easily penetrates the skin (21). Pinkus described the phenomenon of loop hair: As a hair grows out of the skin in the extrafollicular pathway, it forms an arc or loop when it reenters the skin, with the loop increasing in size as the hair grows (17,22).

Transfollicular penetration usually results from improper shaving technique such as pulling the skin taut and the use of razors that lift hairs prior to cutting, resulting in retraction of the cut hair with a pointed tip below the skin surface. The sharp tips pierce the follicular wall and enter the dermis, causing the inflammatory reaction.

Patients affected with pseudofolliculitis barbae cannot aim to have a smooth, close shave (22). Moreover, there are no cures for this condition, and treatments that offer relief for one individual may not necessarily do so for another. Treatment of pseudofolliculitis barbae aims to prevent transfollicular penetration by allowing the hair to reach the follicular opening and then to prevent loop formation with resulting extrafollicular penetration. The following are recommendations for therapy:

1. Cessation of shaving, if possible. This is often impractical and may be even out of the question for some individuals.
2. Maintenance of hairs at an optimum length of 0.5–1 mm to prevent both modes of penetration. This can be obtained using triple O electric clippers (17,20).
3. Chemical depilatories containing calcium thioglycolate have been advocated by several authors (17,21). These may be irritating but patients can try twice-weekly or every-other-day regimens.
4. Use of a foil-guarded manual razor developed for treatment of pseudofolliculitis barbae (17,23). This razor has a single-edged, polymer-coated, stainless-steel blade with a ser-

rated foil guard covering approximately one-third of its cutting edge. It prevents close shaves and transfollicular penetration.

5. Manual freeing of ingrown hairs is an adjunctive measure that is often used (17).

6. Topical retinoic acid by itself or used in combination with topical corticosteroids has also been tried for this condition and may be of some benefit. Irritation can occur as a side effect of tretinoin (17,24).

7. Shaving only in the direction of hair growth and not against the grain is strongly suggested (17).

8. Topical application of glycolic acids has been found to be helpful in some cases (25).

9. Epilation, which has been recommended as a cure for pseudofolliculitis barbae, should be avoided in Blacks. Electrolysis produces poor results because the hairs and follicles of Blacks are curved and it is virtually impossible to destroy the hair root with the available straight electrolysis needles (17). Also, x-ray epilation may result in severe hyperpigmentation in Blacks (17).

HIDRADENITIS SUPPURATIVA

Hidradenitis suppurativa is a chronic, inflammatory, cutaneous disorder that affects the axillary and anogenital regions in genetically predisposed individuals (26). The disease may also rarely affect the areolae of and region between the breasts, periumbilical area, and nape of the neck (27). Obesity and tropical climate are also thought to be predisposing factors for development of this condition. There is no racial predilection in hidradenitis suppurativa (26,28). Individuals affected with severe disease sometimes experience disabling discomfort and can suffer compromise of their social life.

Some patients have disease restricted to one area of the body with little progression to severe disease. Other cases can remit spontaneously, and still others may have almost complete involvement of apocrine gland-bearing areas. Acute disease may present with pruritus and hyperhidrosis and few lesions that are often infected with *Staphylococcus aureus*. Chronic hidradenitis suppurativa manifests as suppurative abscesses and is characterized by remissions and relapses. As the disease extends into subcutaneous tissue, persistent suppuration with sinus tract formation occurs.

Hidradenitis suppurativa is thought to result from poral occlusion with subsequent dilation of the apocrine gland followed by severe inflammation in a much similar fashion as occurs with acne vulgaris (26). In individuals prone to the keratinous plugging of the apocrine duct, there is extension from an infected gland to adjacent ones (26,29). As infection progresses, eventual fibrosis and sinus tract formation occur with continued suppuration. There appears to be some hormonal influence as evidenced by the greater frequency of flares during the second half of the menstrual cycle (26). Treatment of hidradenitis suppurativa usually consists of combined medical and surgical management.

Medical management includes the following:

1. Basic hygienic practices, with use of anti-bacterials and complete drying, and the wearing of loose clothing are simple measures that can be of much benefit (26).
2. Topical or oral antibiotics (penicillin, erythromycin, or tetracycline) are part of standard therapy used to decrease bacterial load (26).
3. Mild topical or intralesional corticosteroids may be useful adjuncts (26).
4. Acitretin, a new systemic retinoid, has also been reported to be effective (30).

Risks of these therapies include the side effects of the medications used as previously described under acne vulgaris treatment.

Surgical management includes the following:

1. Incision and drainage of individual lesions. This is a temporizing method of treatment and abscesses commonly recur (26).
2. Surgical excision of sinus tracts once infection has been treated by antibiotics (26).
3. Exteriorization and diathermy of lesions (26).

4. Complete excision of axillary and perineal skin with skin grafts and flaps for reconstruction. This is the only true method for preventing recurrence (26).

Risks of surgical management include the standard risks of any surgery.

KELOIDS

Keloids are benign dermal tumors that may arise de novo or, as is more frequently the case, in response to injury. The tendency to form keloids appears to be inherited, but the exact mode of inheritance remains unclear (31). It is well known that the skin of Blacks and Asians leaves more prominent scars than the skin of Whites and shows a greater tendency toward keloid formation (32).

These tumors are usually easily recognized by clinicians, especially those that occur on the earlobes occurring as a result of ear piercing or those along surgical incisions. The lesions appear as firm, flesh-colored to reddish brown tumors with discrete but irregular borders (Fig. 3). Patients may complain of tenderness on palpation or pruritus of the skin overlying the keloids. It can be difficult to distinguish keloids from hypertrophic scars, but keloids will often extend beyond the boundary of the original wound, invading surrounding normal skin (15). In contrast, hypertrophic scars, however large, are confined to the area of tissue damaged by the original injury (32).

Keloids can occur on any part of the body but most commonly are seen on the chest, shoulders, and earlobes. They are rarely located on the fact, palms, and soles. Spontaneous keloid formation, though rare, arises most commonly on the midchest and is seen more often in Blacks (15).

Keloids represent a deranged mechanism of healing. There have been several theories of the etiology of these tumors (31). In most patients, preceding trauma is the only provoking factor (31). Post-surgical keloids have been said to occur as a result of increased skin tension in scars (31). Cutting across Langer lines with subsequent increased skin tension has also been suggested as causative (31,33). Some other factors suggested to be contributory have been infection and hormonal influences. Histologically, keloids characteristically show excessive, randomly arranged collagen that has a glossy, slightly refractile appearance, mucinous ground substance, few fibroblasts, and no foreign body reaction (15,31,32).

Keloids are difficult to treat, often requiring long-term therapy. They also tend to recur. As a rule, prevention is the best option. Known keloid-prone individuals should refrain from having non-essential cosmetic surgical procedures, and all surgical wounds should be closed with minimal tension following relaxed skin tension lines as far as possible. For keloid formers, Kelly suggests that pressure gradient elastic garments or apparatus to apply pressure be worn for ~4–6 months after major skin trauma or surgical procedures (15,31).

Once keloids have formed, therapeutic options are varied and include the following:

1. Keloidectomy with or without intralesional corticosteroids injected into the resulting surgical scar to decrease chances of recurrence (31).

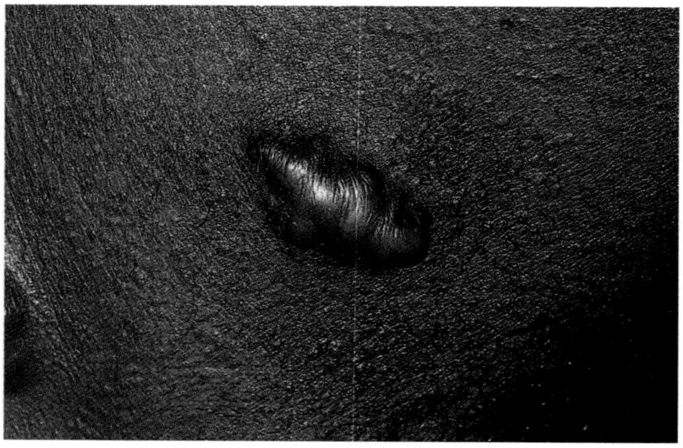

Figure 3. Keloid resulting from trauma showing a firm, flesh-colored to red tumor.

2. Intralesional corticosteroid injections using triamcinolone every 3–4 weeks (31).
3. Topical application of potent corticosteroids or the use of corticosteroid impregnated tape (31).
4. Cryosurgery (15).
5. CO_2 laser and Nd:YAG laser (15,31,34).
6. Topical application of retinoic acid in combination with a potent topical steroid (31,35).
7. Promising investigational agents including intralesional interferon, collagenase, interleukin-1, and tumor necrosis factor.

CHEMICAL PEELS

Chemical peels are currently being used for a number of conditions, including acne scarring, removing wrinkles, treating keratoses, and correcting uneven pigmentation of the skin. Phenol and trichloroacetic acid peels have been used in Black patients. As these are deeper peels, the results have often been unfavorable due to the labile response of melanocytes to these agents in Blacks (15). Marked post-inflammatory hyperpigmentation and hypopigmentation can result. Phenol and trichloracetic acid peels can also cause keloids and hypertrophic scarring. The more superficial peels such as the alpha-hydroxy acids (AHAs) have the potential of causing post-inflammatory hyperpigmentation in Blacks (15). A lighter peel using lower concentrations of AHAs should be used in Blacks (15).

VARIATIONS IN NORMAL SKIN PIGMENTATION

Post-inflammatory hyperpigmentation can be an extremely devastating condition for Black patients. In a study of Black patients who visited private practice dermatologists in Washington, D.C., the third most common diagnosis was disorder of pigmentation other than vitiligo (2). The majority of these patients had a diagnosis of post-inflammatory hyperpigmentation. Grimes found that many Black patients were concerned more about removal of ugly dark spots than about resolving the underlying skin condition such as comedones, papules, pustules, or eczema (16). The significance and psychosocial impact of post-inflammatory hyperpigmentation are very high.

Post-inflammatory hyperpigmentation is a result of an exaggerated labile response of melanocytes in Blacks to cutaneous injury (16). Inflammatory skin diseases cause the release of peptides in the skin that alter the activity of melanocytes (16). This can result in an increase in number and size of epidermal melanocytes, or it may result in pigmentary incontinence, that is, the deposition of pigment in the upper dermis. Inflammatory disorders of the skin such as eczema and papulosquamous and vesiculobullous disorders can cause post-inflammatory hyperpigmentation. In Blacks, pityriasis rosea and lichen planus are frequently associated with post-inflammatory hyperpigmentation, so these should initially be treated aggressively. Topical agents such as retinoic acid and benzoyl peroxide are also causes of post-inflammatory hyperpigmentation in Blacks (Fig. 4) (16).

The treatment of post-inflammatory hyperpigmentation consists of the use of hydroquinone-containing bleaching preparations; however, these are effective primarily for more superficial or epidermal hyperpigmentation. Epidermal hyperpigmentation is detected by intensification of the pigmented area of skin by Wood's light examination.

Post-inflammatory hypopigmentation is also the result of the exaggerated labile responsiveness of melanocytes in Blacks to cutaneous injury (16). This condition is also common and can be significant in Black patients because of the contrast between normally pigmented skin and light areas. The same diseases that cause post-inflammatory hyperpigmentation can also be responsible for causing post-inflammatory hypopigmentation in Blacks. In addition, other causes include potent topical corticosteroids, intralesional steroids, cryotherapy, dermabrasion, and chemical peels (16). Thus, these should be used carefully in Black patients. The treatment for post-inflammatory hypopigmentation is to wait for gradual pigmentation to return, which may take from 6 to 12 months. The patient must be reassured that some pigmentation may eventually return. Cosmetic cover-ups can be used and psoralens combined with UVA light (PUVA) may have to be used to help hasten repigmentation.

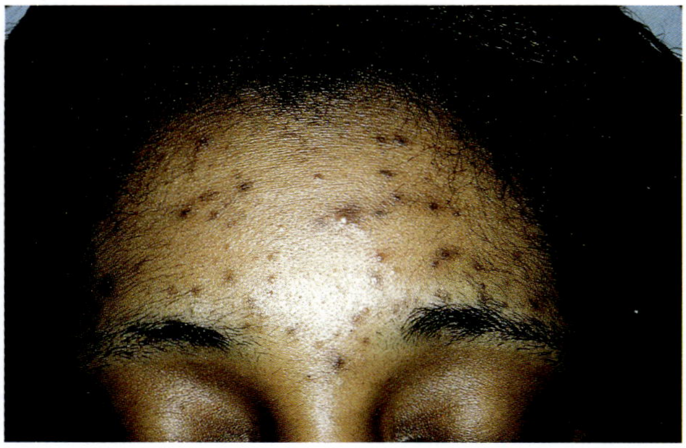

Figure 4. Post-inflammatory hyperpigmentation due to acne vulgaris showing darkly pigmented macules.

VITILIGO

Vitiligo is an acquired idiopathic, sometimes familial depigmentation disorder of skin characterized by milk white macules that occur anywhere on the skin and tend to enlarge over time (Fig. 5). Common sites of initial involvement include the perioral and periorbital areas of the face, hands, feet, elbows, and knees as well as the genitals and perianal area. Microscopically, affected skin is characterized by a total absence of melanocytes. Vitiligo is associated with an increased incidence of systemic autoimmune and/or endocrine diseases as well as systemic immunologic abnormalities (36). The mechanism of pigment cell destruction continues to elude investigators; however, an autoimmune hypothesis is currently favored (36).

The incidence of vitiligo is ~1–2% of the population worldwide, affecting all races and sexes equally (36). However, because of the stark contrast that occurs between depigmented skin and normally pigmented skin, the psychological effects of this disease can be extremely devastating, particularly in darker-skinned races such as Blacks. Patients with vitiligo have low self-esteem (37,38). They are subject to rude remarks by strangers and often describe embarrassing episodes such as others hesitating to shake their hands.

Because of the psychological problems associated with vitiligo, it should be treated if possible. Unfortunately, no cure is available for vitiligo as the cause is not yet known. There are, however, treatments to which variable percentages of patients with vitiligo will respond (39). For limited areas of vitiligo, particularly in the face, cosmetics can be very useful, particularly products such as Dermablend and CoverMark. These are not waterproof, however. Vegetable stains such as Vitadye and Dyoderm can also be used. Topical steroid therapy is sometimes effective in repigmenting areas of vitiligo. Low-, mid-, and high-potency preparations have been used. High-potency steroids work best but should be used for limited periods of time to avoid adverse side effects that they may cause. Children should be given low- to mid-potency steroids. One of the major treatments for vitiligo is the use of

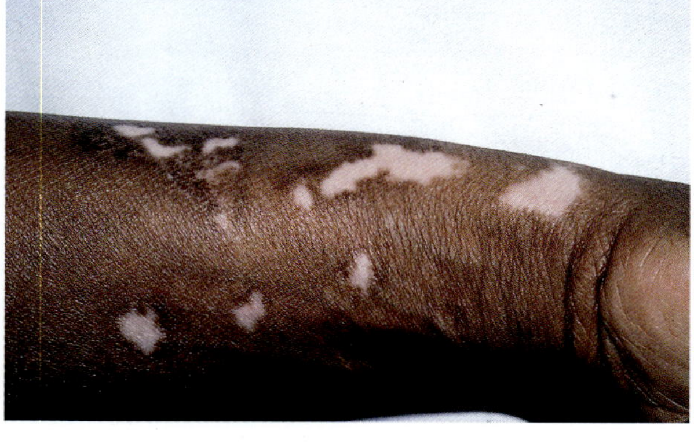

Figure 5. Vitiligo showing depigmented white areas of skin with angular borders.

psoralen photochemotherapy (PUVA). This is available as two forms, topical PUVA for <20% body surface involvement and oral PUVA for more extensive disease. PUVA therapy should be administered only by those who are familiar with this form of therapy because of potential side effects, which include blistering and burning of the skin. Some data suggest that PUVA may be involved in the formation of cataracts, alteration of cutaneous immunity, and skin cancer formation (39).

Therapy for lesions that are non-responsive to medical therapy includes surgical techniques such as autologous epidermal mini-punch grafts for the treatment of small macules (39,40). Such grafts may produce cobblestoning and spotty repigmentation or the development of koebnerization of the vitiligo into the donor sites. Infection may occur at the donor or recipient sites.

Micropigmentation (tattooing) involves the microsurgical placement of iron oxide pigment into the dermis of vitiliginous skin to replace the color in that area (41). It is difficult to match perfectly the pigment of the surrounding area. Pigment in the dermis tends to fade, and the Tyndall effect often alters the color. Micropigmentation works best for the lip area, especially for individuals with dark skin. Tattooing of the lips may induce episodes of herpes simplex.

The technique of autologous melanocyte transplants involves harvesting melanocytes from a small area of pigmented skin from the patient and expanding the melanocytes in cell culture. The cultures melanocytes are transplanted into vitiliginous skin. This technique requires a laboratory experienced in melanocyte cell culture. At present, the application of this technique is limited to small macules because of the difficulty of obtaining large numbers of melanocytes from cell culture (39).

Depigmentation or removal of remaining pigmentation can be considered in patients who have >50% cutaneous involvement and who have been recalcitrant to repigmentation (39). For some individuals with extremely disfiguring vitiligo on the face who are not desirous of or willing to attempt repigmentation, depigmentation may be considered as an initial therapy. It also may be the first therapeutic option for patients with vitiligo so extensive that repigmentation is highly unlikely. Depigmentation should be considered permanent and irreversible. Although patients on occasion do regain some areas of color and repigmentation, this is not to be expected.

REFERENCES

1. Yonkosky DM, Pochi PE. Acne vulgaris in childhood: pathogenesis and management. *Dermatol Clin* 1986;4:127–136.
2. Halder RM, Grimes PE, McLaurin CI, Kress MA, Kenney JA Jr. Incidence of common dermatoses in a predominantly Black dermatologic practice. *Cutis* 1983;32:388–390.
3. Pochi PE, Quan M. *Acne vulgaris.* Kansas City: Family Physician Monograph, 1991:1–24.
4. Wilkins JW, Voorhees JJ. Prevalence of nodulocystic acne in white and negro males. *Arch Dermatol* 1970;102:631–634.
5. Kelly AP, Sampson DD. Recalcitrant nodulocystic acne in Black Americans: treatment with isotretinoin. *J Natl Med Assoc* 1987;79:126–170.
6. Plewig G, Kligman AM. *Acne and rosacea.* 2nd ed. New York: Springer-Verlag, 1993:375.
7. Pugliese PT. Physiology of the skin: biology of acneic skin. *Skin Inc.,* 1992;X:31–38.
8. Pochi PE, Strauss JS. Sebaceous gland activity in black skin. *Dermatol Clin* 1988;6:349–351.
9. Leyden JJ, McGinley KJ, Mills OH, Kligman AM. Age related changes in the resident bacterial flora of the human face. *J Invest Dermatol* 1975;65:379–381.
10. Pochi PE. Management of refractory acne. *Hosp Pract* 1985;20:73–82.
11. Cleocin T. *Physicans' desk reference.* 48th ed. Montvale, NJ: Medical Econ Data Prod Co., 1994:2403.
12. Leyden JJ, Shalita AR. Rational therapy for acne vulgaris: an update on topical treatment. *J Am Acad Dermatol* 1986;15:907–914.
13. Pochi PE, Ceilley RI, Coskey RJ, et al. Guidelines for prescribing isotretinoin (Accutane) in the treatment of female acne patients of childbearing potential. *J Am Acad Dermatol* 1988;19:920.
14. Grimes PE, Davis LT. Cosmetics in blacks. *Dermatol Clin* 1991;9:53–68.
15. Grimes PE, Hunt SG. Considerations for cosmetic surgery in the black population. *Clin Plast Surg* 1993;20:27–34.
16. Grimes PE, Stockton T. Pigmentary disorders in blacks. *Dermatol Clin* 1988;6:221–281.
17. Halder RM. Pseudofolliculitis barbae and related disorders. *Dermatol Clin* 1988;6:407–411.
18. Alexander AM, Delph WI. Pseudofolliculitis barbae in the military: a medical, administrative and social problem. *J Natl Med Assoc* 1974;66:459–464.

19. Brauner GJ, Flandermeyer KL. Pseudofolliculitis barbae. Medical consequences of interracial friction in the US Army. *Cutis* 1979;23:61–66.
20. Brauner GJ, Flandermeyer KL. Pseudofolliculitis 2: treatment. *Int J Dermatol* 1977;16:520–525.
21. Strauss JS, Kligman AM. Pseudofolliculitis of the beard. *Arch Dermatol* 1956;74:533–542.
22. Pinkus H. Chronic scarring pseudofolliculitis of the Negro beard. *Arch Dermatol* 1943;47:782–792.
23. Alexander AM. Evaluation of foil-guarded shaver in the management of pseudofolliculitis barbae. *Cutis* 1981;27:534–542.
24. Kligman AM, Mills OH. Pseudofolliculitis of the beard and topically applied tretinoin. *Arch Dermatol* 1973;107:551–552.
25. Perricone NV. Treatment of pseudofolliculitis barbae with topical glycolic acid. A report of two studies. *Cutis* 1993;52:232–235.
26. Banerjee AK. Surgical treatment of hidradenitis suppurativa. *Br J Surg* 1992;79:863–866.
27. Cutting KF, Thomas F. Lasting relief from a distressing condition surgical intervention in hidradenitis suppurativa. *Prof Nurse* 1992;8:106–112.
28. Wiltz O, Schoeltz DJ, Murray JJ, Roberts PL, Coller JA, Veidenheimer MC. Perianal hidradenitis suppurativa. The Lahey Clinic experience. *Dis Colon Rectum* 1990;33:731–734.
29. Yu CC, Cook MG. Hidradenitis suppurativa: a disease of follicular epithelium rather than apocrine glands. *Br J Dermatol* 1990;122:763–769.
30. Hogan DJ, Light MJ. Successful treatment of hidradenitis suppurative with acitretin. *J Am Acad Dermatol* 1988;19:355–356.
31. Kelly AP. Keloids. *Dermatol Clin* 1988;6:413–424.
32. Muir IFK. On the nature of keloid and hypertrophic scars. *Br J Plast Surg* 1990;43:61–69.
33. Flin MH. The biological basis of Langer's lines. In: Longacre JJ, ed. *The ultrastructure of collagen*. Springfield: Thomas, 1976:132–140.
34. Abergel RP, Dwyer RM, Meeker CA, et al. Laser treatment of keloids: a clinical trial and an in vitro study with Nd:YAG laser. *Lasers Surg Med* 1984;4:291.
35. Janssen DeLimpens AMP. The local treatment of hypertrophic scars and keloids with retinoic acid. *Br J Dermatol* 1980;103:319.
36. Mosher DB, Fitzpatrick TB, Hori Y, Ortonne JP. Disorders of melanocytes. In: Fitzpatrick TB, Eisen AZ, Wolff K, Freedberg IM, Austen KF, eds. *Dermatology in general medicine*. 1993:903–995.
37. Porter JR, Beuf AH. Racial variation in reaction to physical stigma: a study of degree of disturbance by vitiligo among black and white patients. *J Health Soc Behav* 1991;32:192–204.
38. Porter JR, Beuf AH, Lerner AB, Nordlund JJ. Psychosocial effect of vitiligo: a comparison of vitiligo patients with normal control subjects, with psoriasis patients, and with patients with other pigmentary disorders. *J Am Acad Dermatol* 1986;15:220–224.
39. Nordlund JJ, Halder RM, Grimes PE. Management of vitiligo. *Dermatol Clin* 1993;11:27–33.
40. Falabella R. Treatment of localized vitiligo by autologus minigrafting. *Arch Dermatol* 1988;124:1649–1655.
41. Halder RM, Pham HN, Breadon JY, Johnson BA. Micropigmentation for the treatment of vitiligo. *J Dermatol Surg Oncol* 1989;15:1092–1098.

SECTION IV

The Aging Patient

Ethnic Considerations in Facial Aesthetic Surgery, edited by W. Earle Matory, Jr.
Lippincott–Raven Publishers, Philadelphia © 1998.

12

Aging in People of Color

W. Earle Matory, Jr.

All would live long, but none would be old.
— Benjamin Franklin

Aging in the more darkly pigmented races is less apparent and occurs at a later age. Many of the components found in aging of the fairer races are absent as demonstrated by the 63-year-old woman who is of African American, American Indian, and Portuguese descent shown in Fig. 1. Serial photographs of a model are shown over a 50-year span (Fig. 2). Note the changes that have occurred from ages 19 to 25 to 35 to 45 with rather dramatic sequelae of aging demonstrated in the comparison at age 19 vs. age 58. Many of the same phenomena are illustrated in the man shown in Fig. 3 at ages 20, 27, 35, and 50 with notable differences seen in comparing age 20 and age 60.

Each of these patients illustrates consistencies in the aging process that have been noted in our review of 400 models, male and female, in serial decades of life (Table 1A, B). Note the paucity of fine lines of the face, including crow's feet, lip lines, and fine periorbital and perioral wrinkles. Brow ptosis seems to occur to a lesser degree and a decade later in life than in the Caucasian. Moderate excesses of upper lid skin are noted as age increases, while lower lid skin does not increase to a great degree. In a fashion temporally and physically similar to that in the Caucasian, malar fat pads tend to sag toward the nasolabial fold. The latter contributes to increased proptosis and infraorbital shadowing. Excess pre-auricular skin is minimized; however, there is a descent of the submusculoaponeurotic layer (SMAS) contributing to increased jowl formation and mandibullary/submental fat and muscle accumulation. Thus, the cutaneous changes of aging seem to be more subtle and less prominent than those noted in the deeper layers, the SMAS, fatty, and muscular layers. Each of these findings was confirmed in our observation of (a) serial decades (a series of individuals in each decade of life), (b) serial photographs spanning 20–50 years, and (c) generations of the same family.

W. E. Matory, Jr.: A New You Plastic Surgery Medical Group, Irvine, California 92714

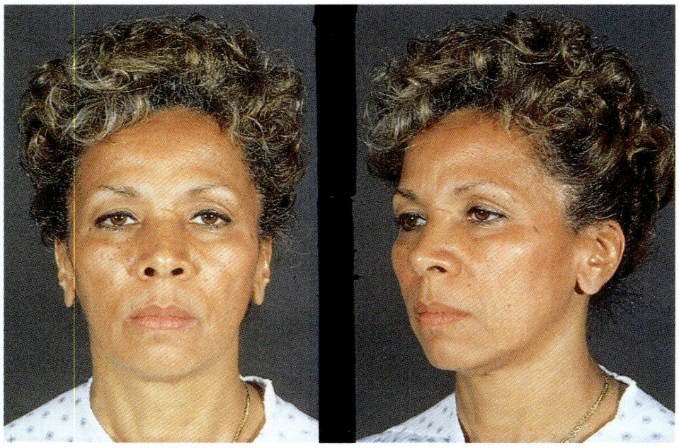

Figure 1. This 63-year-old woman demonstrates a paucity of many of the classic signs of aging, including forehead, periorbital, and perioral skin laxity. These and other signs of aging noted in the Caucasian are seen far less commonly or at a later age in the African American, Hispanic, and Asian patient.

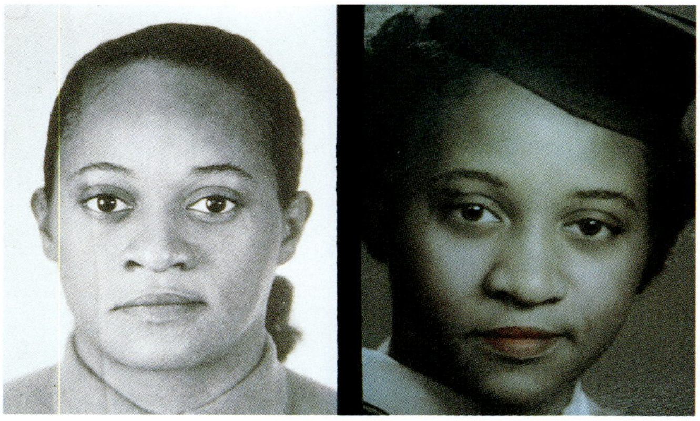

A

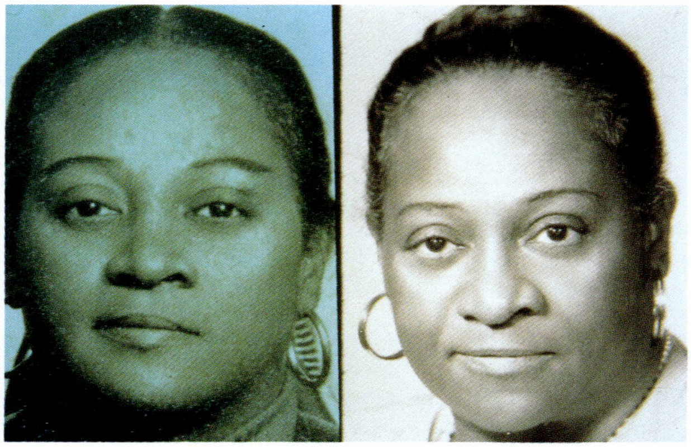

B

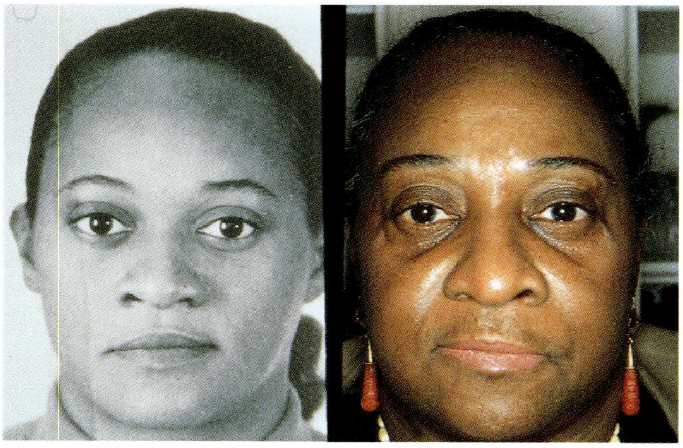

C

Figure 2. Serial photographs are shown of the same African American woman at ages 19 and 25 **(A)**, ages 35 and 45 **(B)**, and ages 19 and 55 **(C)**.

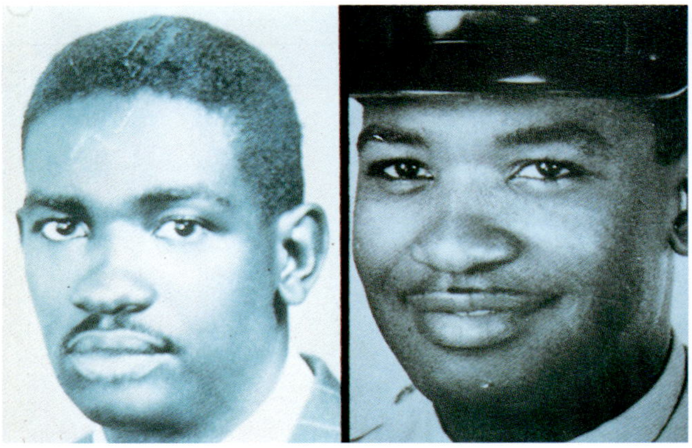
A

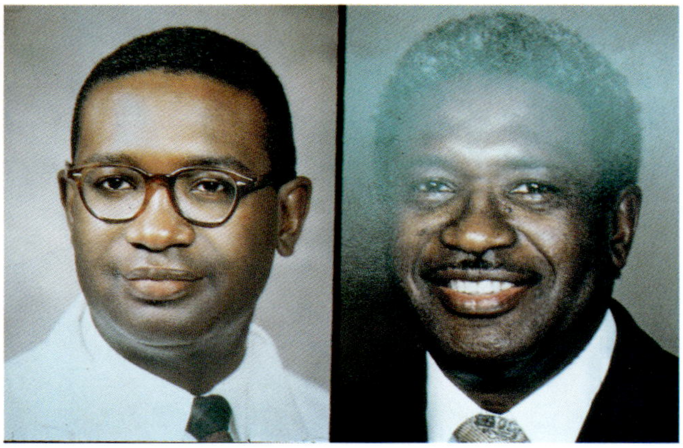
B

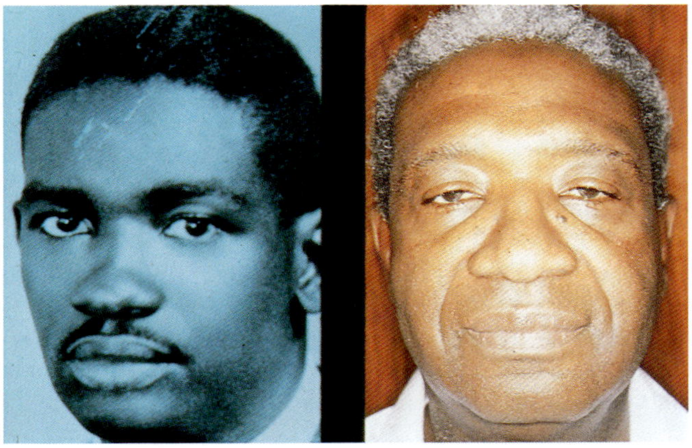
C

Figure 3. Serial photographs are shown of the same African American man at ages 20 and 28 **(A)**, ages 35 and 50 **(B)**, and ages 20 and 55 **(C)**. Note the mild brow ptosis, descent of malar fat with loss of malar prominence and infraorbital shadowing.

Table 1. *A. Aging in the African American female*

Serial decades (No. = 25 per age group)			40–50	50–60	Over 60
Malar	Flattening	$p < 0.05$	13 (50%)	18 (72%)	19 (74%)
Nasolabial fold	Prominence	$p < 0.05$	16 (64%)	20 (78%)	22 (86%)
Lips	Protuberance	$p < 0.05$	9 (36%)	15 (58%)	19 (74%)
	Mucosal show		8 (32%)	14 (54%)	15 (58%)
Nose	Lengthening		3 (12%)	5 (18%)	9 (34%)
	Oily tip		8 (32%)	11 (44%)	12 (48%)
Chin	Recession	$p < 0.05$	11 (44%)	17 (66%)	15 (58%)
Neck	Submental skin laxity		10 (40%)	18 (72%)	22 (88%)
	Excess fat		9 (38%)	19 (76%)	21 (84%)
Scalp	Male pattern		1 (2%)	1 (2%)	1 (4%)
Hair loss	Temporal	$p < 0.05$	11 (42%)	9 (36%)	17 (66%)
Forehead	Brow ptosis		5 (18%)	6 (24%)	10 (38%)
	Furrows Frontal	$p < 0.05$	2 (8%)	5 (20%)	7 (26%)
	Glabella		3 (10%)	4 (14%)	6 (22%)
Eyelid	Upper Moderate laxity		8 (32%)	15 (58%)	24 (94%)
	Lower Minimal laxity		16 (64%)	18 (72%)	20 (78%)
	Scleral show		9 (36%)	16 (62%)	19 (74%)

Table 1. *B. Aging in the African American male*

Serial decades (No. = 160 per age group)		40–50	50–60	Over 60
Malar	Flattening	56	74	92
Nasolabial fold	Prominence	68	84	98
Lips	Protuberance	64	76	80
	Mucosal show	38	46	54
Nose	Lengthening	32	46	72
	Oily tip	44	48	54
Chin	Recession	46	42	44
Neck	Submental skin laxity	52	68	86
	Excess fat	46	72	84
Scalp	Male pattern	36	42	40
Hair loss	Temporal	10	12	14
Eyebrow	Lateral alopecia	22	28	36
Forehead	Brow ptosis	16	38	46
	Furrows Frontal	8	12	26
	Glabella	32	44	68
Eyelid	Upper Moderate laxity	22	40	76
	Lower Minimal laxity	70	84	92
	Scleral show	44	56	74

Microscopic evaluation of aging in the African American is illustrated in Fig. 4. The hematoxylin and eosin stain demonstrates a 45-year-old's skin of the eyelid (Fig. 4, top) and nasolabial fold (Fig. 4, bottom). While there is some vacuolization of the basal area, there is little evidence of solar elastosis, skin wrinkling, or dermal atrophy. In Fig. 5, one notes pre-auricular skin in the Caucasian (above) and in the African American (below). Both of these 60-year-old patients had a strong history of sun exposure. In contrast to the African American, note the marked solar elastosis, skin wrinkling, and dermal atrophy in the Caucasian.

In the following sections, we will review commonly noted changes in each area of the face.

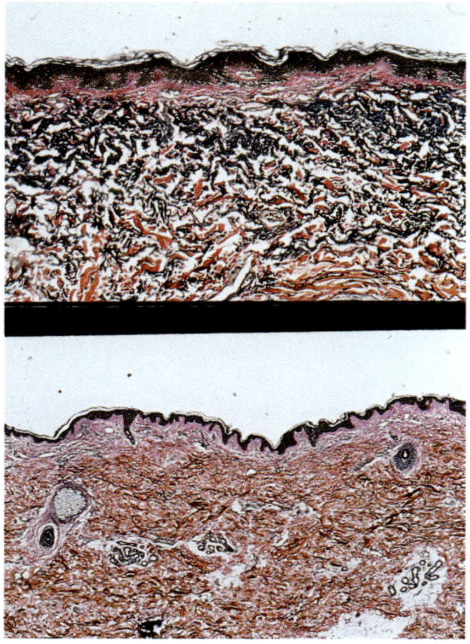

Figure 4. Hematoxylin and eosin stains were performed on pre-auricular skin *(top)* and upper eyelid skin *(bottom)*. Note the paucity of facial elastosis and rhytidosis.

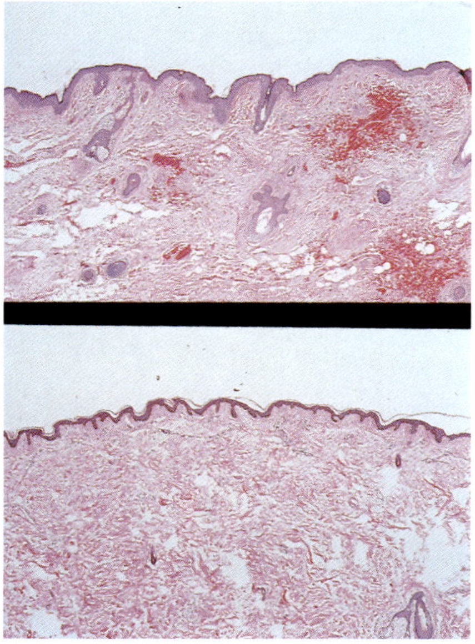

Figure 5. In comparing Caucasian skin in the pre-auricular area *(top)* and skin in the medium-pigmented African American or Hispanic *(bottom)*, the latter presents far less rhytidosis, telangiectasia, and elastosis. Subdermal atrophy is also noted to a lesser degree in the African American, Asian, and

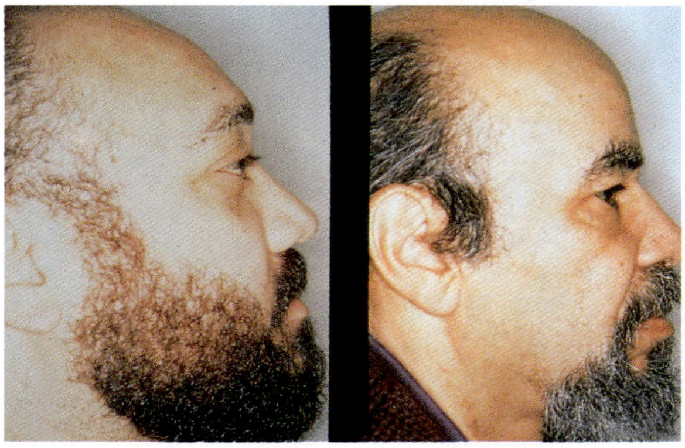

Figure 6. Frontal and temporal alopecia are common in the African American man. Temporal alopecia begins at age 30 and peaks in the 50s.

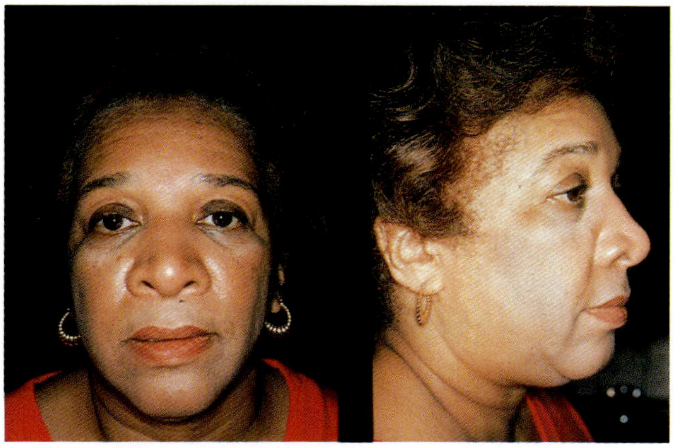

Figure 7. Temporal alopecia occurred to some degree in over 50% of the Hispanic and African American women in this study, beginning at age 30 and peaking at age 50–60.

SCALP

Frontal and temporal alopecia are commonly noted in the African American male (Fig. 6). With strong family history, the onset may be as early as age 30. In the female, varying degrees of temporal alopecia were almost uniform in the African American and less so in the Asian and Hispanic, being first noted at age 35–40 (Fig. 7). This progresses by age 60, at which point hair pieces and extensions are frequently used. Follicle growth in the African American is distinct from that in the Caucasian (Fig. 8). With oblique angulation of the follicle in the Caucasian roots, the punch biopsy should be angled parallel to the follicle (i.e., obliquely). In the African American, the punch should once again be parallel to the follicle, which is in a direction perpendicular to the skin. This minimizes trauma to the hair follicle and optimizes graft take.

PERIORBITAL AREA

Proptosis is a common finding in most African Americans and is also seen in many Hispanic and Asian individuals. Malar hypoplasia seems to play a vital role in causing the moderate disproportion of the orbital contents and the overlying soft tissue coverage (Fig. 9). Proptosis is frequently noted at birth and is well represented by cultural and artistic depictions of the African American, Asian, and Hispanic (Fig. 10). Figure 11 demonstrates common findings associated with aging, including laxity of the forehead, malar, and peri-

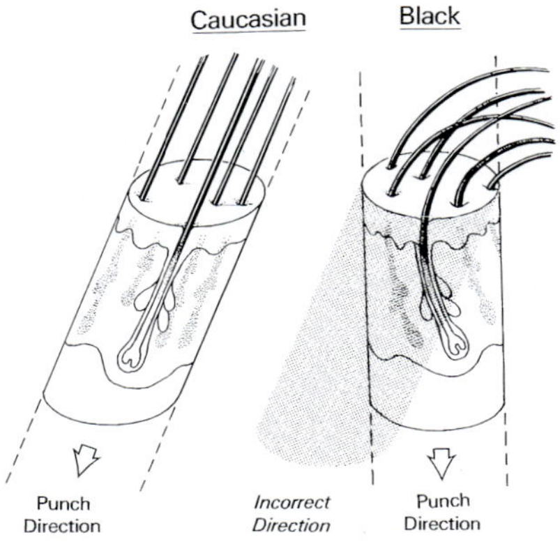

Figure 8. Hair growth in the Caucasian is oblique in contrast to that in the African American and some Hispanics, perpendicular to the skin. Ideal punch direction for graft harvesting should be oriented differently in each ethnic patient to maximize follicle preservation.

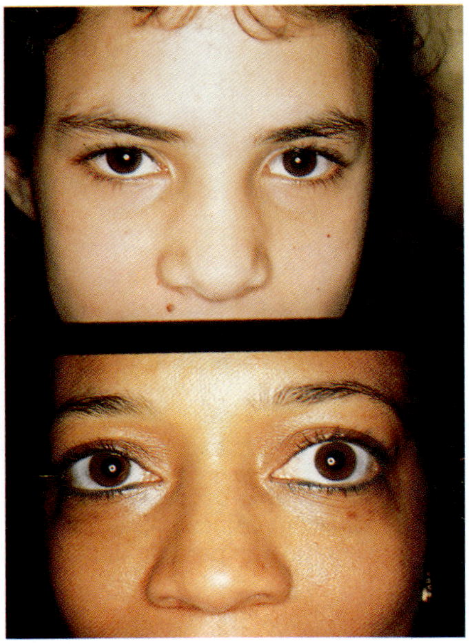

Figure 9. Proptosis is very common in the African American, Asian, and Hispanic. Visibility of proptosis increases with aging as the soft tissue cover of skin, fat, and muscle descend toward the nasolabial fold.

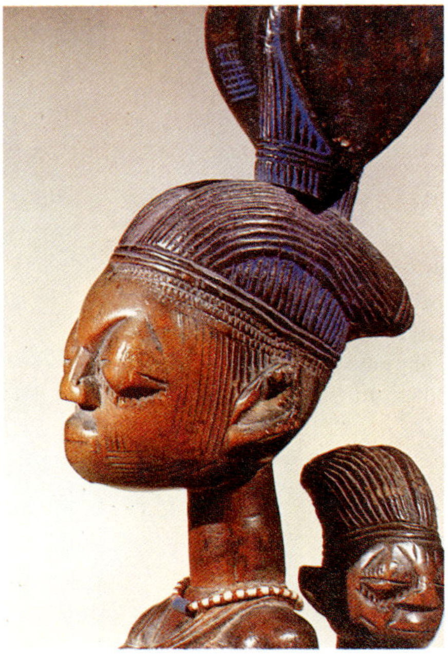

Figure 10. The commonality of proptosis is perhaps best illustrated by many African, Hispanic, and Asian art pieces.

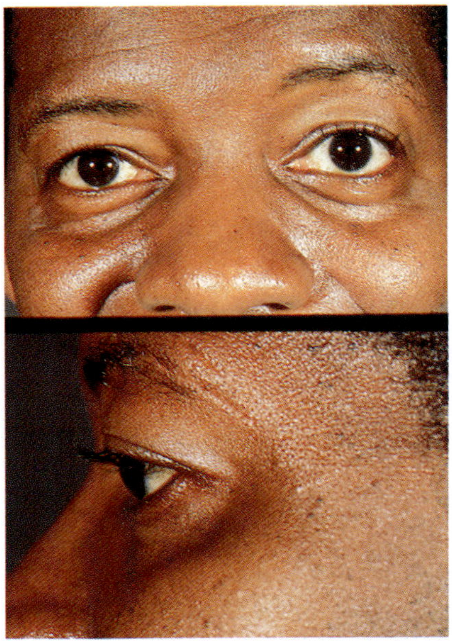

Figure 11. Proptosis in this man is exacerbated by lower skin laxity, weak snap response, and bilateral asymmetric descent of malar fat pads. Bulging upper eyelid fat is noted in the medial and middle compartments as well as lateral fat prominence just below the orbital rim.

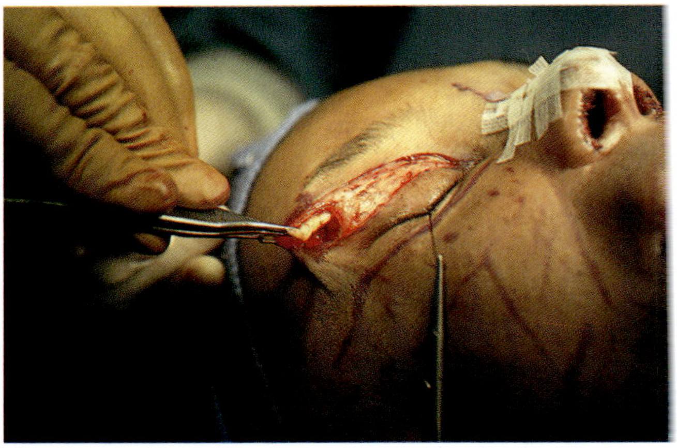

Figure 12. The lateral fat pad should be routinely resected or repositioned when present.

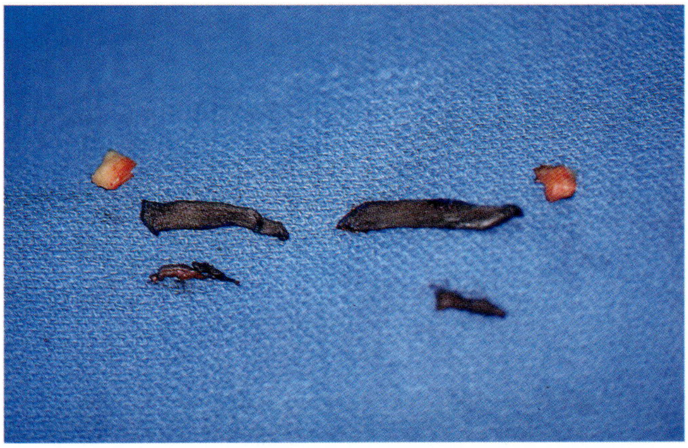

Figure 13. Moderate skin resection of the upper lids concomitant with minimal skin resection on the lower lids is a most appropriate maneuver. There is very little excess skin of the lower lids and over-resection will surely result in ectropion. Lateral resection of 3–4 mm of vertical width is maximal.

oral areas, asymmetrical brow ptosis, moderate excesses of upper lid skin, with minimal excess lower lid skin. Malar fat and descent contribute to prominence of the nasolabial fold and concomitant shadowing along the infraorbital rim. Scleral show is almost always seen in the presence of proptosis. Medial and upper fat pads tend to be notable with a sizable lateral component as depicted in Fig. 12. Skin resected from the upper lids may range from 8 to 15 mm in vertical width versus from 2 to 3 mm in the lower lid (Fig. 13). Upper lid hooding and fat eventration have been addressed in this 53-year-old woman in a similar fashion (Fig. 14). In Fig. 15, this 63-year-old woman underwent a moderate upper lid excision of excess skin, transconjunctival fat removal of the lower, scar revision of the nasal dorsum, and cauterization of periorbital skin tags, shown at 28 months.

A two- to three-pack/day history of cigarette smoking contributed to exaggerated periorbital aging in the 60-year-old woman shown in Fig. 16. Note the extensive hooding with visual field obstruction along with malar sag, crow's feet, and increased prominence of frontal and frown lines. A 2-cm vertical width of upper lid skin and 5 mm of lower lid skin were excised along with fat removal from all upper and lower lid compartments. The results are shown 18 months later (Fig. 16).

As aging progresses, so does lid laxity, scleral show, and accompanying symptoms like epiphora. Lower lid laxity with a weak snap test are frequently noted (Fig. 17). Lid-

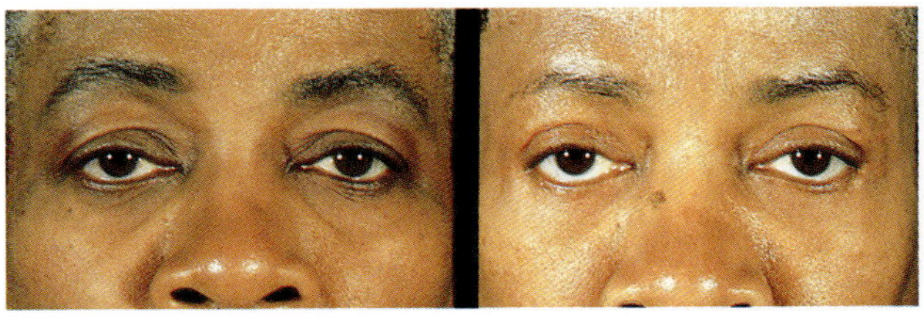

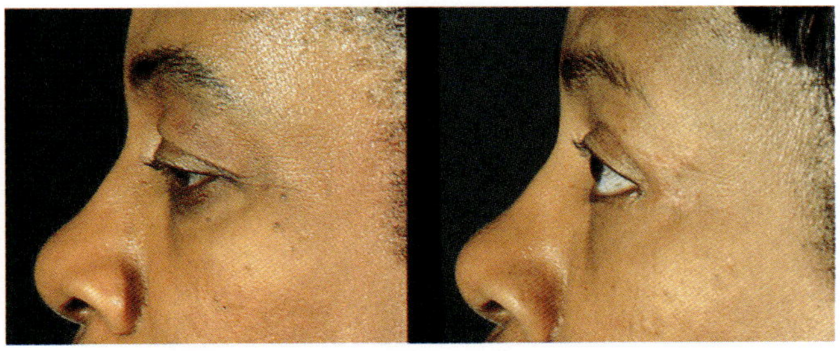

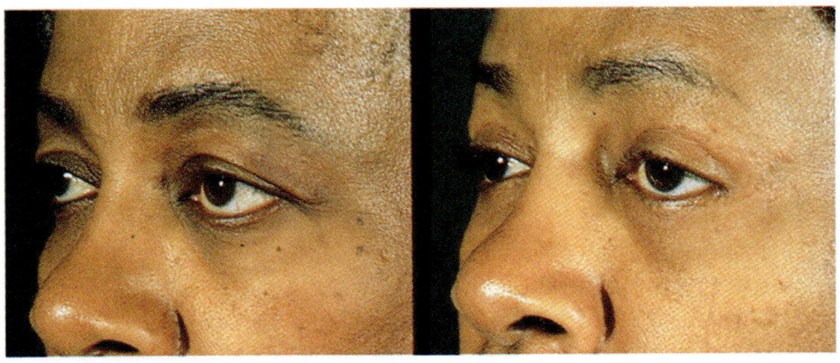

Figure 14. Moderate upper lid skin resection and minimal lower lid skin resection without fat pad removal. Results are shown 14 months after blepharoplasty.

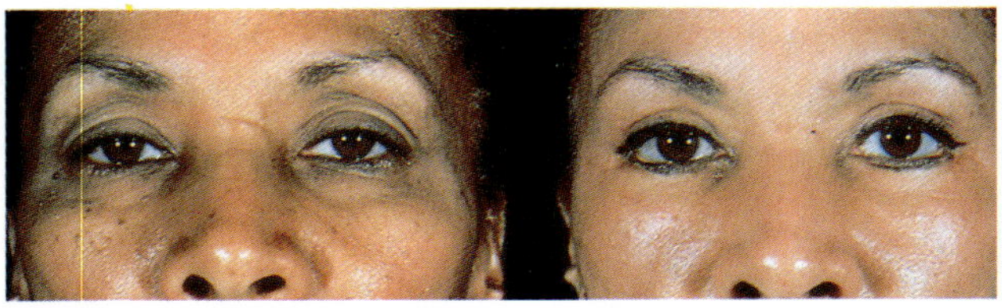

Figure 15. Removal of moderate upper lid skin, no upper or lower fat resection, minimal lower lid skin, along with scar revision of the nasal dorsum and cauterization of skin tags. Results are shown 18 months after surgery.

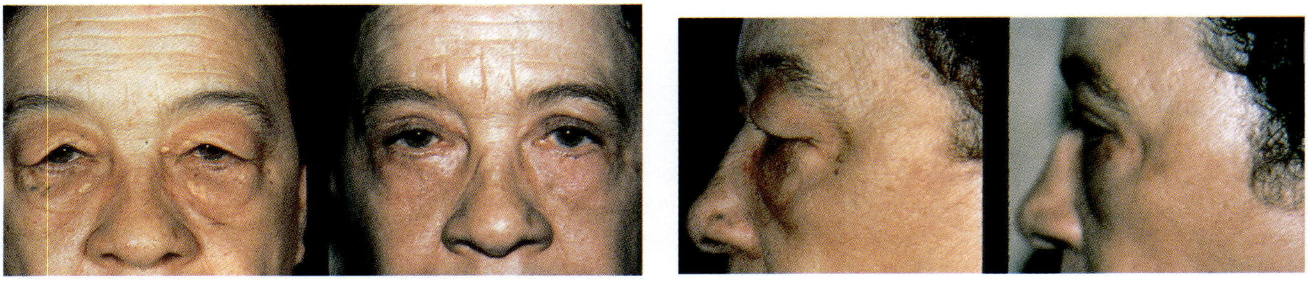

Figure 16. A two- to three-pack/day cigarette smoker demonstrates marked dermatochalasis with upper lid hooding and visual field obstruction. There is bilateral upper lid ptosis as well as epiphora and 2 mm of scleral show. Schirmer's test 18/20. A 6 × 2.5–cm resection of skin of the upper lid and a 4 × 0.6–cm resection of skin of the lower lid along with lateral canthoplasty (dermal pennant) yielded this outcome at 24 months.

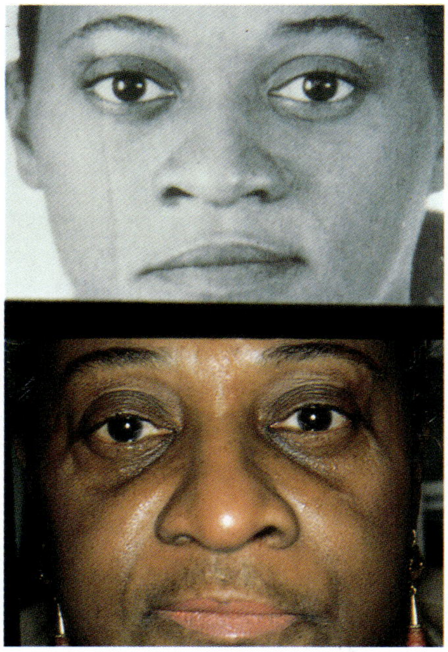

Figure 17. This 19-year-old shown at age 55 demonstrated the progression of periorbital aging with proptosis contributing to lower lid laxity, scleral show, and epiphora.

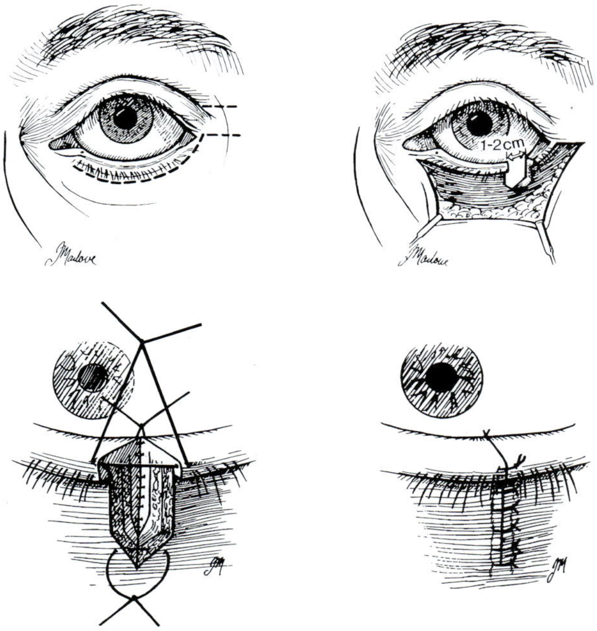

Figure 18. Lower lid laxity can be addressed by resection techniques only when the lower lid circumference is adequate to cover the globe at the lower limbus. Tarsal wedge resection shaped as an inverted house can be completed with a layered closure.

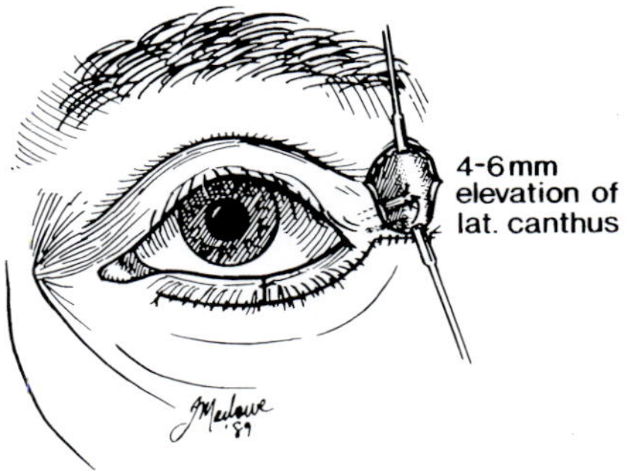

Figure 19. Repositioning of the lateral canthus 2–6 mm cephalad or use of a dermal pennant technique may be preferable or may, when indicated, be performed in conjunction with a tarsal wedge resection.

tightening procedures as illustrated in Figs. 18 and 19 are beneficial. Tarsal wedge resection is useful when tightening of the lid does not result in increase scleral show. The circumference of the lid must be adequate to cover the globe. If the horizontal length of the lid is excessive, a tarsal wedge resection can be performed in an inverted house resection. This resection optimizes lid approximation after closure.

Resuspension of the lateral canthus provides a more functional lid cover and more effectively diminishes scleral show (Fig. 19). Dermal pennant techniques can also be useful in this regard. Figure 20 presents a patient 14 months following excision of upper lid skin, removal of fat from the medial mental and lateral fat pads, and lower lid lateral canthoplasty.

Permanent lash liner can also highlight the periorbital area. Dermal pigmentation in the African American and Hispanic patient should use black pigment, in distinct contrast to the strict avoidance of black in the Caucasian (Fig. 21). In the Hispanic patient, requests are

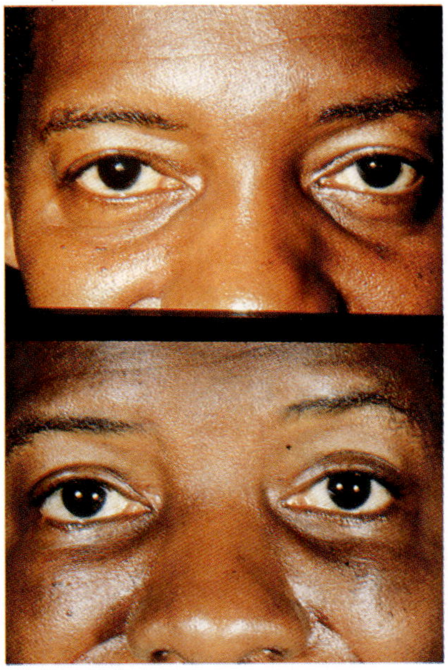

Figure 20. Results are shown following a moderate resection of upper lid skin, minimal resection of the lower lid skin, and malar augmentation using Silastic implant. Tarsal wedge resection was also completed along with lateral canthoplasty to minimize lid retraction.

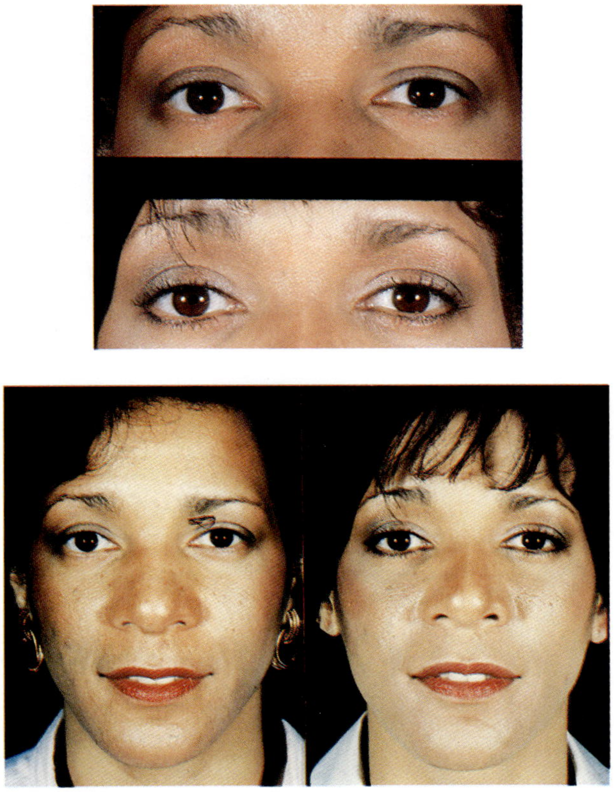

Figure 21. Permanent lash liner is a nice adjunct in addressing the periorbita. Black and very dark brown are colors of choice in the African American and Hispanic.

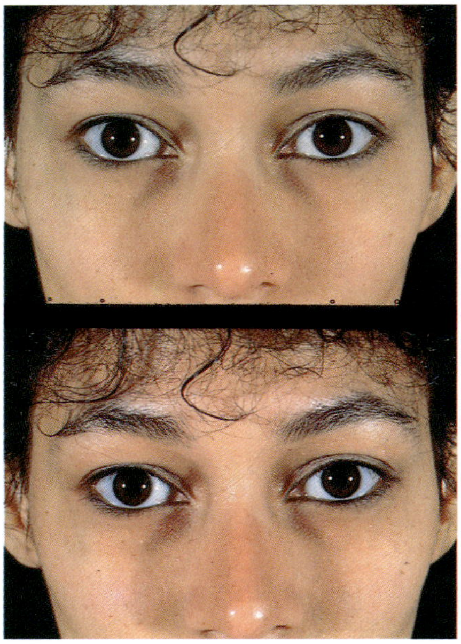

Figure 22. Patients may request highly stylized, trendy placement of lash liner. One should lean toward more conservative placement, leaving desired style adjustments to daily make-up application by the patient.

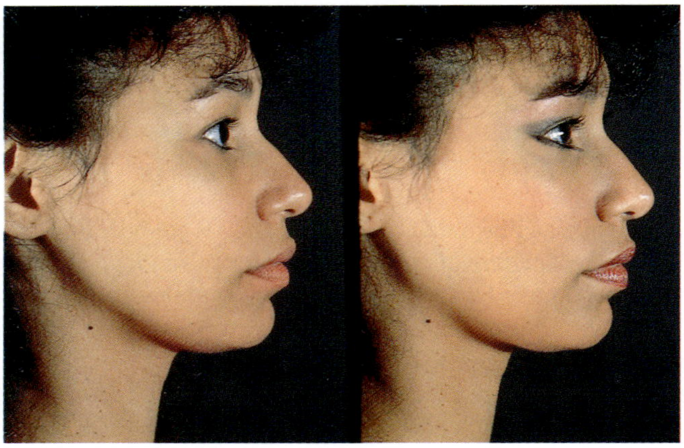

frequently made for highly stylized lash liner. In general it is preferable to use a conservative placement technique in light of the frequently changing styles (Fig. 22). The latter can be adjusted as desired by the patient with personalized application.

DESCENT OF THE MALAR FAT PAD

Malar fat contributes to increased fullness of the nasolabial fold and the subsequent weakness of the infraorbital area. These findings are noted in serial generations of the same family (Fig. 23, left) and in serial decades (Fig. 23, right). The goals therefore in African American, Asian, and Hispanic malarplasty are resuspension of the malar fat pad and promotion of malar prominence with alloplastic or autologous malar augmentation. Our early experience (Fig. 24) utilized Proplast and silastic implants that softened the infraorbital shadowing in most instances (Fig. 25). This was reasonably effective; however, the paucity of the soft tissue overlying the infraorbital rim in light of the gravitational descent of the malar fat pad resulted in occasional visibility of the superior pole of the prosthesis (Fig. 26).

We now feel that resuspension of the malar fat pad with or without autologous fat grafting of the malar prominence yields consistent malar rejuvenation with minimal deformity and optimal cosmesis (Fig. 27).

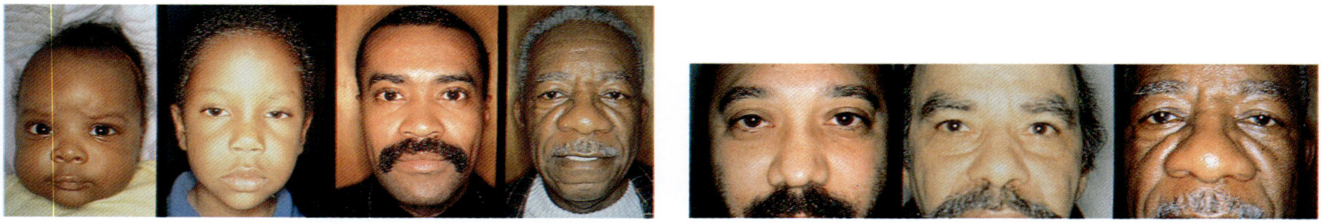

Figure 23. Progressive prominence of the nasolabial fold with aging is noted in serial generations, ages 1, 10, 38, and 60 *(left)* and serial decades, ages 38, 55, and 60 *(right)*.

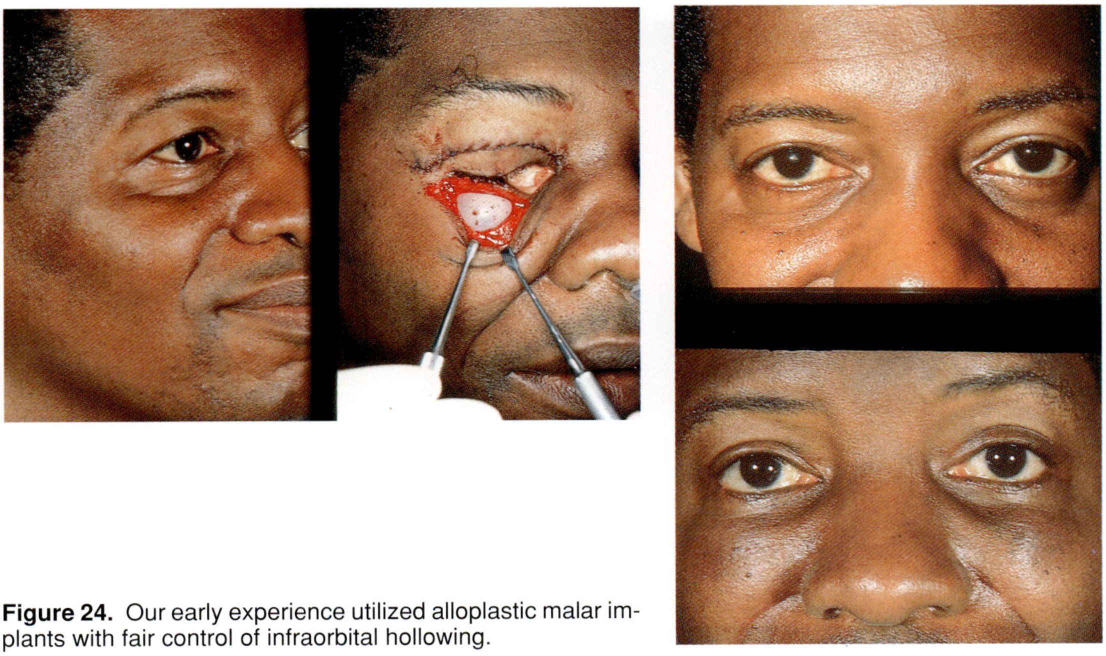

Figure 24. Our early experience utilized alloplastic malar implants with fair control of infraorbital hollowing.

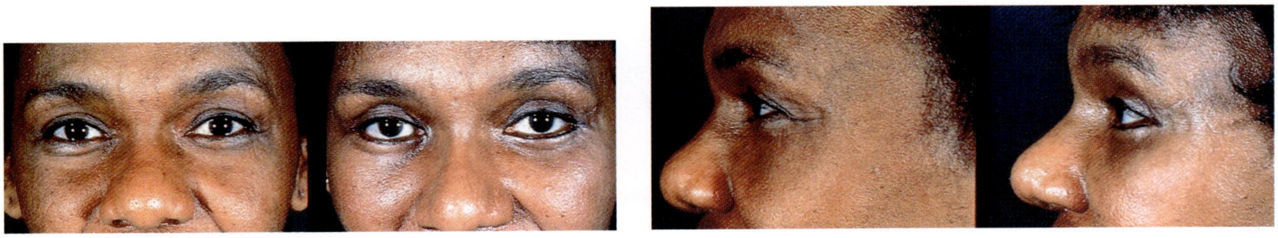

Figure 25. Upper and lower lid blepharoplasty and dorsal augmentation rhinoplasty (with autologous rib) and Silastic malar augmentation were completed in this 54-year-old woman.

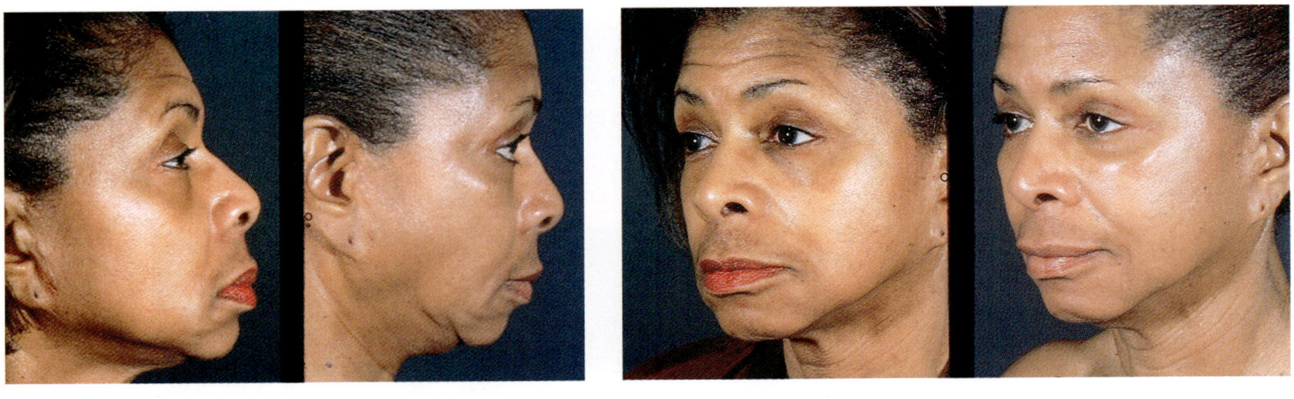

Figure 26. We no longer use alloplastic malar implants in this population because of the frequent visibility of the upper edge of the implant. With descent of the malar fat pad, there is very little soft tissue to cover the implant.

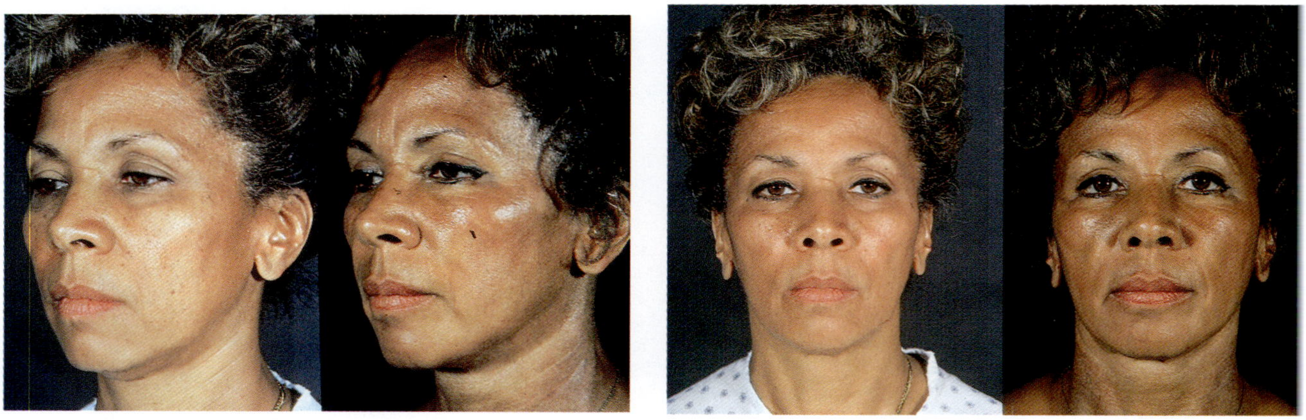

Figure 27. We prefer the use of malar fat resuspension to the temporal fascia or, if deemed appropriate by the patient, injection of autologous fat to supplement the malar prominence. In this patient, 15 cc of fat was added to the malar fat pad; the patient is shown 24 months after augmentation.

THE NASOLABIAL FOLD

Serial generations illustrate progressive prominence of the nasolabial fold (Fig. 28). Increased prominence of the fold is also noted in comparing photographs of a 20-year-old and the same patient at 55 years old (Fig. 29). Resuspension of the malar fat pad (to the lateral orbital rim or to the temporal fascia) through an infraorbital or pre-auricular incision tends to be the most effective way to restore the malar fat and to soften the nasolabial fold. A direct excision of the nasolabial fold has also been utilized very effectively (Fig. 30) with results shown in Fig. 31.

The occasional thin man may be concerned about the lack of subcutaneous fat in the jaw and temporal areas. The patient in shown in Fig. 32 demonstrates the result 14 months after autologous fat injection of the jaw, malar, and temporal areas.

THE LATERAL FACE AND NECK

While there is a paucity of pre-auricular skin excess, the prominence of jowling and submental and lower facial fatty fullness along with prominent platysmal banding are common findings in the African American, Asian, and Hispanic face after the age of 40. Fat prominence is most commonly noted at ages 30–45 at which point muscle laxity becomes more obvious (Fig. 33). A resultant lower facial fullness contributes to roundness of the face. Suction lipectomy is the most effective technique for submental and lower facial fullness in the younger (under age 40) patient (Fig. 34).

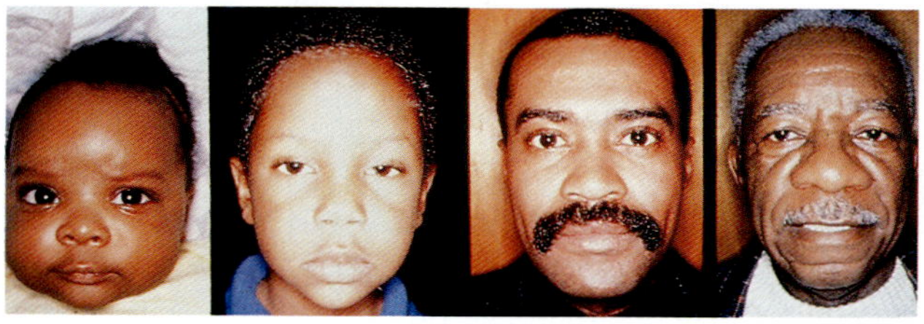

Figure 28. Progressive prominence of the nasolabial folds is illustrated in serial generations, ages 1, 10, 38, and 60.

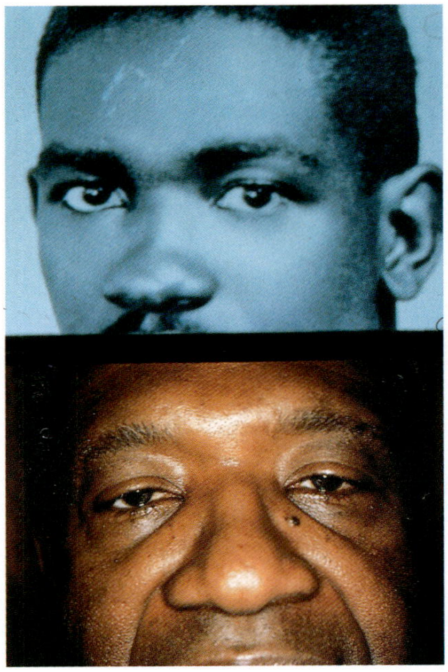

Figure 29. Note the dominance of facial aging centering on the nasolabial fold in this 55-year-old in comparison with his photograph at age 19.

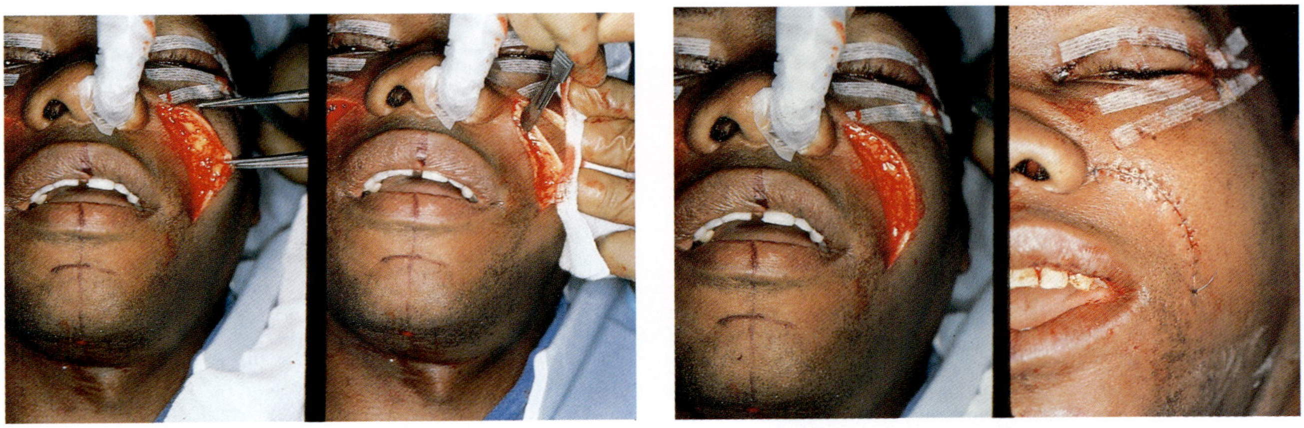

Figure 30. While suction lipectomy can be used to soften the nasolabial fold, contour irregularities are common. In our early experience, dramatic improvements have been accomplished with direct excision and layered closure.

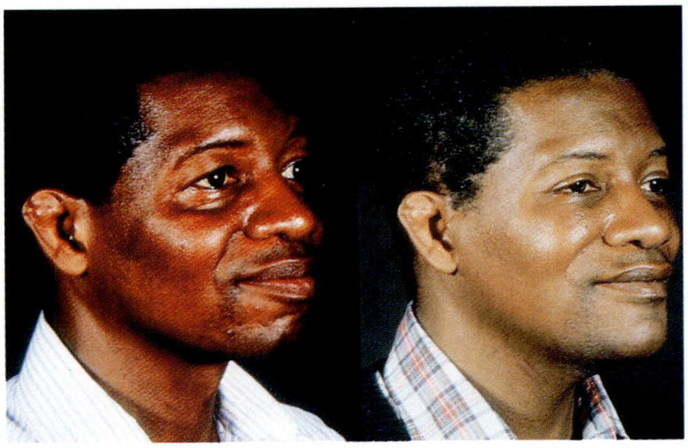

Figure 31. The patient in Fig. 30 is shown 18 months after nasolabial fold resection along with malar augmentation using a silastic implant.

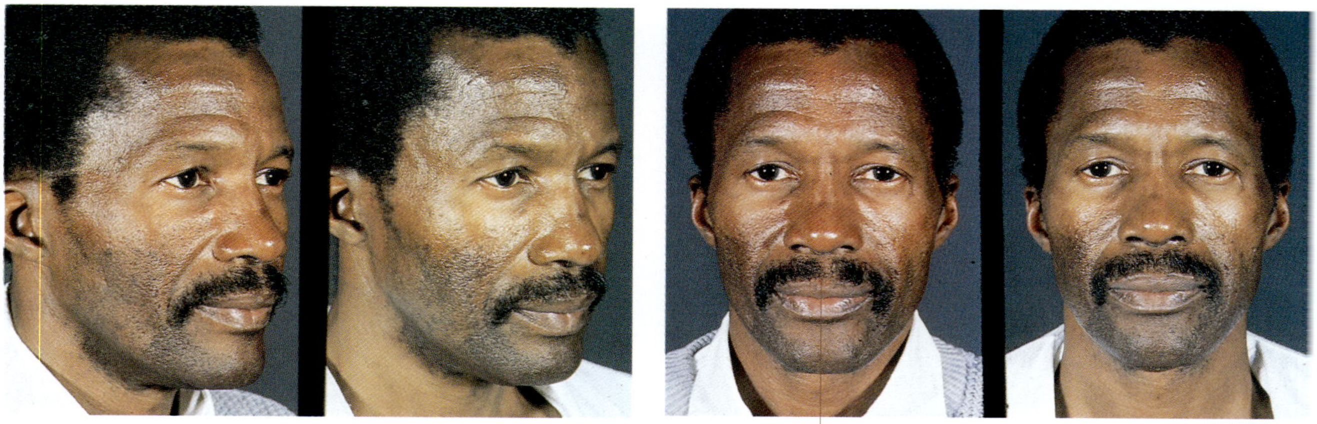

Figure 32. The occasional patient may present with a paucity of soft tissue in various facial areas, e.g., in this patient, the jowl and temporal areas. Autologous fat injection was used to add fullness to these areas as seen 22 months after injection.

A

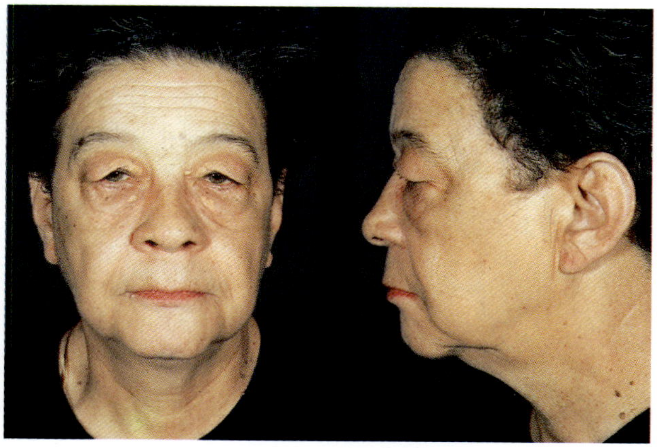

B

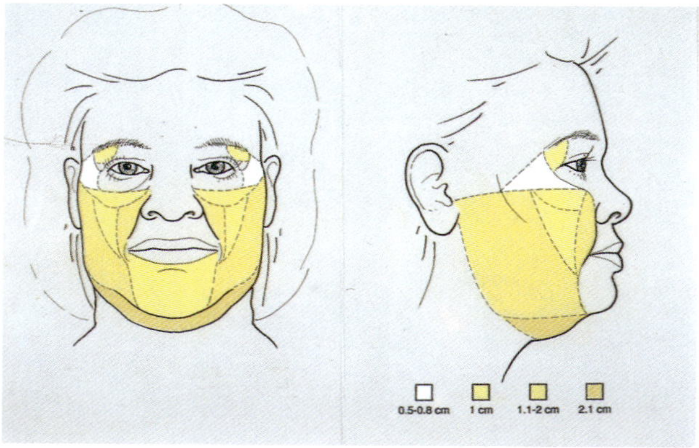

C

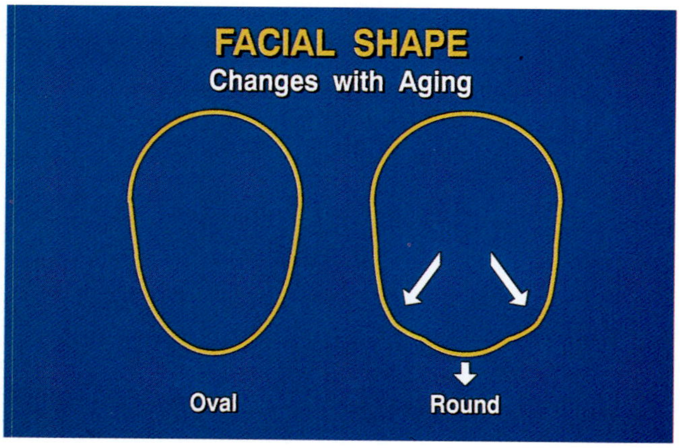

Figure 33. Descent of the malar and jowl fat pads along with increased submental fullness **(A)** contribute to an increased fullness of the lower face **(B)** and a resultant roundness of the aging face **(C)**.

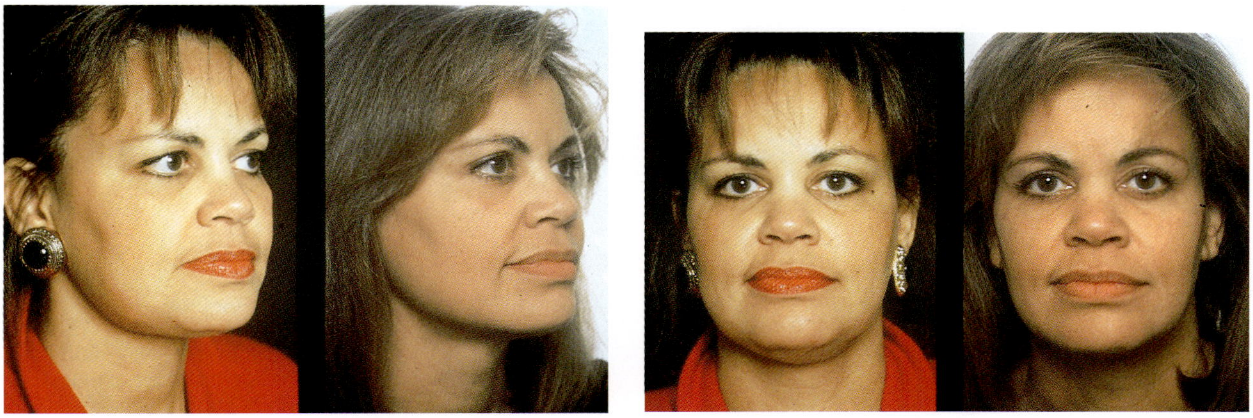

Figure 34. In the younger patient (younger than 40 years), submental and mandibular suction-assisted lipectomy can be utilized to soften the submental fullness in the lower third of the face and upper neck.

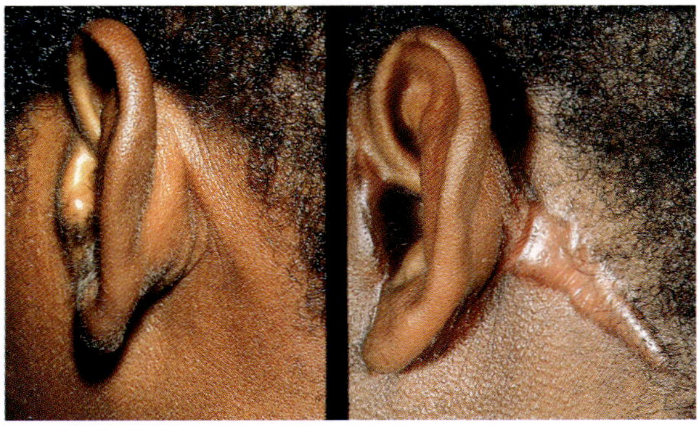

A

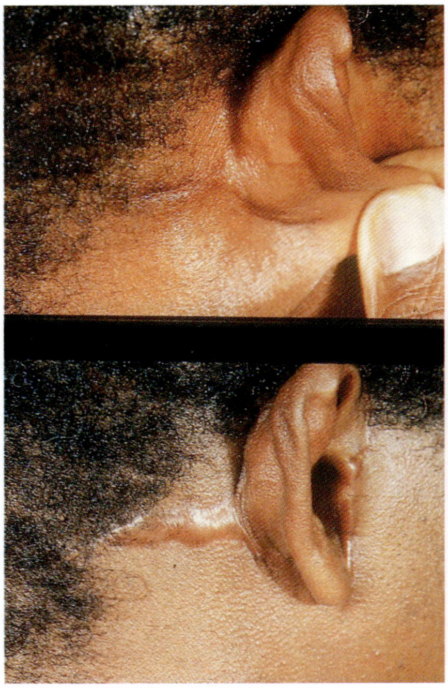

B

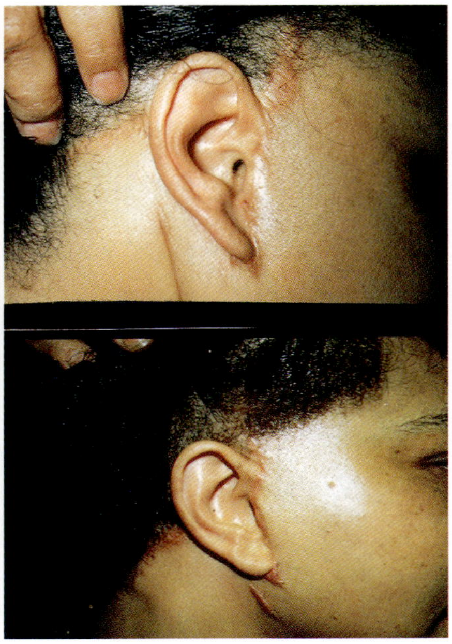

C

Figure 35. As aging progresses, facelift techniques may be necessary **(A)**. Traditional facelift incisions in the African American, Hispanic, and Asian commonly result in hypertrophic scarring **(B)**. When test incisions are used as a method of predicting the likelihood of post-auricular scarring after a facelift, skin tension can predictably increase the tendency for hypertrophic or keloid scarring following rhytidectomy **(C)**. This was a patient from an outside medical center after rhytidectomy using Dexon sutures for closure. She is shown 6 months after rhytidectomy with persistent suture irritation and inflammation in pre- and post-auricular locations.

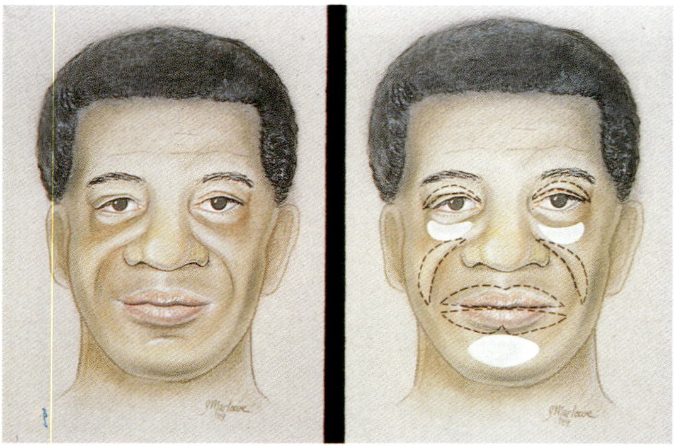

Figure 36. Another alternative is to use malar and chin augmentation along with direct excision of the nasolabial fold as a method of facial rejuvenation in people of color.

In those patients for whom rhytidectomy is deemed appropriate, one must be cautious about the post-auricular incisions, which have a strong tendency to hypertrophy or keloid (Fig. 35, top). The thickness of the mastoid dermis appears to be a contributing factor. Tension in this area is another contributor as demonstrated in Fig. 35 (lower left). This photograph demonstrates a test incision that has healed with minimally widened scarring. Following rhytidectomy in the same patient, note scar widening 10 months later, suggesting that tension may be a contributing factor. In Fig. 35 (lower right), a patient underwent rhytidectomy by another surgeon who used Dexon subdermal sutures. Suture reactivity was considerable, as noted 8 months following the procedure.

Pre- and post-auricular vertical incisions tend to heal with minimal thickening or widening in contrast to mastoid sutures. We therefore recommend that one avoid the standard rhytidectomy incision in patients of color whenever possible. In most instances the primary contributions to aging in this population include infraorbital shadowing and a prominence of the nasolabial fold with fullness of the submental area with or without chin hypoplasia (Fig. 36). These findings can be more directly addressed with malar fat repositioning with or without malar augmentation, chin augmentation, and submental suction-assisted lipectomy (Figs. 37–39). When jowling and mandibular skin laxity are present along with platysmal banding, a mini-facelift with or without submental plication can be performed. The mini-lift (Fig. 40) involves an incision beginning at the sideburn extending into a post-tragal position crossing anterior to the earlobe and then progressing 5 mm above the post-

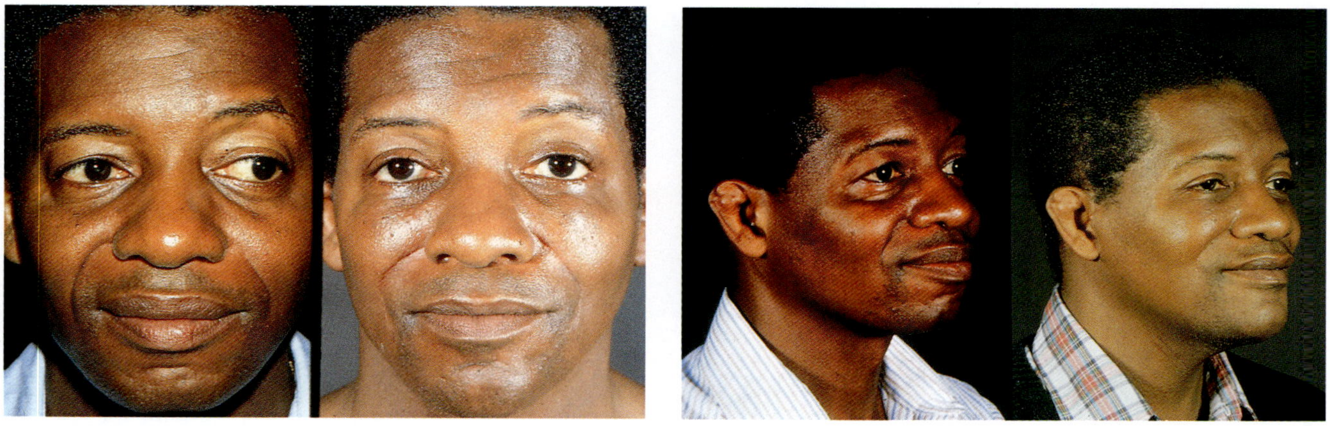

Figure 37. This 53-year-old man underwent malar and chin augmentation along with direct excision of the nasolabial fold, lip reduction, and upper and lower blepharoplasty with lateral canthoplasty.

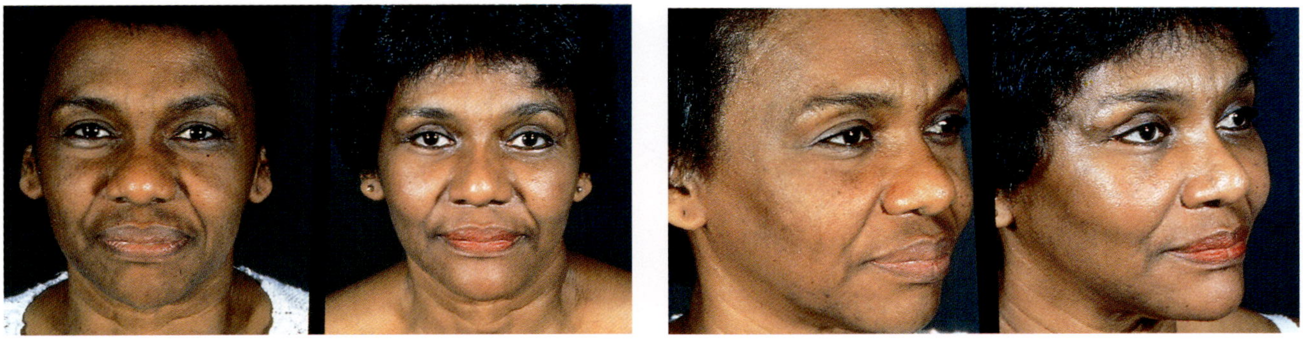

Figure 38. This patient underwent upper and lower blepharoplasty, malar augmentation, direct excision of the nasolabial fold, and Silastic chin augmentation with submental suction-assisted lipectomy.

auricular sulcus. The latter results in subsequent positioning of the scar in the sulcus as opposed to lying in a more visible area. A separate incision, 3 mm posterior to the post-auricular hairline and parallel to the hairline, is made for additional neck contouring. A submental stab incision is used if suction alone is necessary. This can easily be extended to perform direct fat resection and or platysmal plication, if desired. These incisions allow full access and undermining of the entire face and neck. I prefer a subcutaneous dissection in all planes fully mobilizing the malar fat pad to the nasolabial fold and suspending it to the temporal fascia. An oblique strip of SMAS is resected from the earlobe to the lateral canthus, measuring ~1–1.5 cm × 6 cm in vertical length. The SMAS is reapproximated using a running 3-0 Proline. Platysma anterior to the sternocleidomastoid is secured to the mastoid fascia using a 3-0 polypropylene suture. A small strip of medial platysmal muscle can be resected followed by double-layer plication of the platysma using a running 3-0 polypropylene. Excess skin is resected in the pre- and post-auricular and scalp incisions, leaving no points of tension. Interrupted vicryl sutures are used to approximate the pinna, the pre-auricular fascia, and dermis of the skin flaps to minimize tension on the skin closures. Post-auricular sutures are used to approximate the dermis of the post-auricular skin, post-auricular fascia, and mastoid skin. The latter prevents movement of the incision and tension following skin approximation. Skin staples are used to approximate the post-auricular incision after resection of a 1- to 1.5-cm-wide strip of hair-bearing scalp.

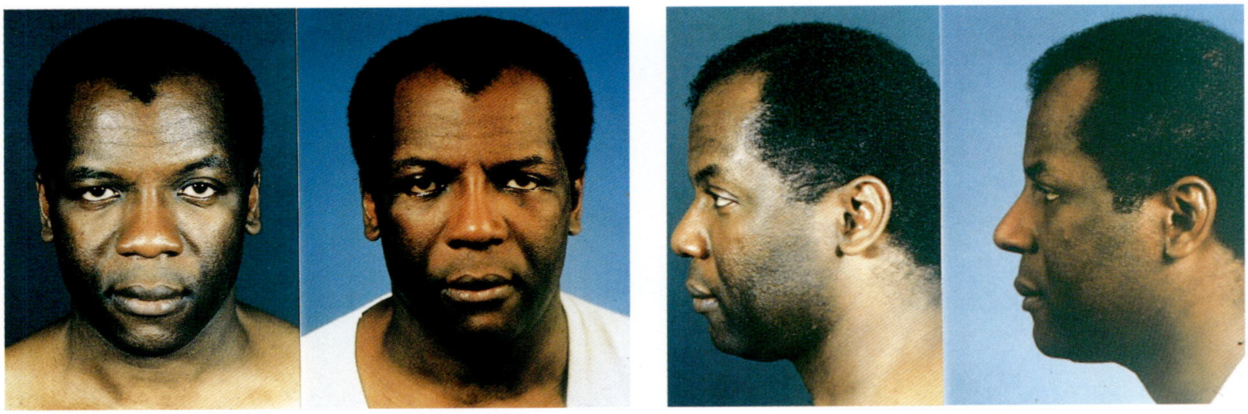

Figure 39. This 45-year-old man underwent dorsal nasal augmentation and M-strut tip enhancement with malar and chin implantation, submental suction-assisted lipectomy, and direct excision of the nasolabial fold. Results are shown at 16 months.

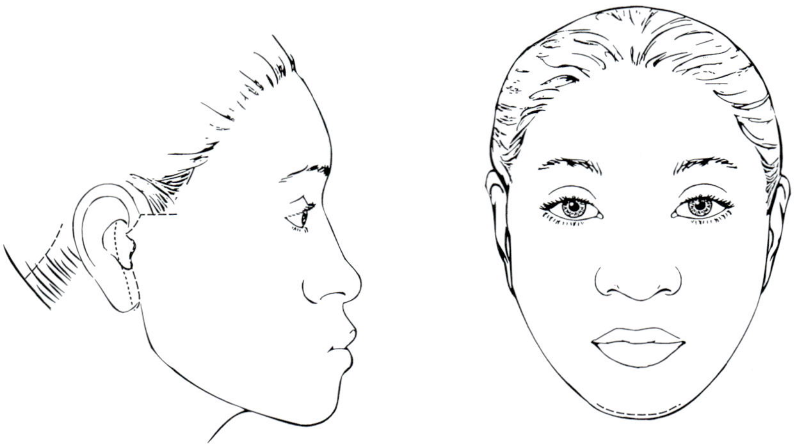

Figure 40. When rhytidectomy is indicated by significant jowl and submental fullness and/or platysmal banding, we suggest using a mini-rhytidectomy incision. A transverse incision begins at the sideburn and extends in a retrotragal fashion to and along the retroauricular sulcus. A separate incision 4 cm posterior to the hairline is made. Submental stab or 4-cm-long incision can be utilized for submental contouring with liposuction or platysmal plication, respectively. This technique eliminates the portion of the rhytidectomy incision that is most likely to develop hypertrophic or keloid scarring.

THE LIPS

Anterior and vertical dimensions of the lip progress with aging. Common presentations in many African Americans, Hispanics, Asians, and the occasional Caucasian include full upper and lower lips with pink vermilion show (Fig. 41). Mucosal laxity progresses, often contributing to cheilitis/drtying (Fig. 42). These findings increase from age 30 to 40 and peak after age 50–60.

Mucosal reduction must take into account the dental relationships. Overbite and open bite deformities are commonly noted and contribute to labial hypertrophy. Orthodontics is advised strongly but not always selected. Mucosal resection is optimized by removing an ellipse anterior to the sulcus (Fig. 43) measuring from 8 to 15 mm in vertical width. Prior to actually resecting, undermining should be completed, and then the amount of mucosa to be resected is determined by trial and error, cutting, and temporary placement of sutures. This more conservative approach will diminish the likelihood of over-resection and subse-

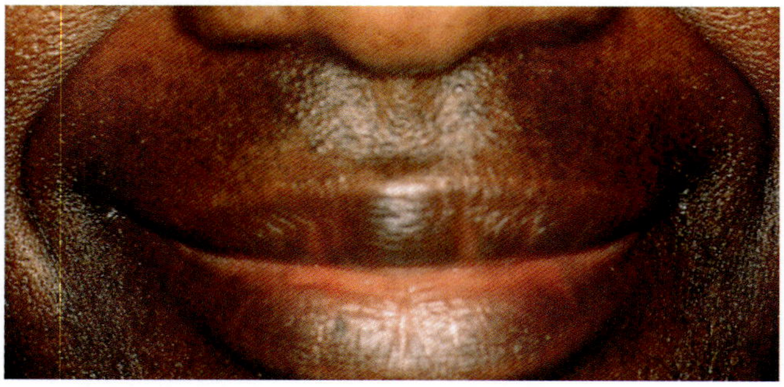

Figure 41. Common complaints in African Americans, Hispanics, and some Asians about the lips are referable to increased labial prominence and anterior projection along with pink vermilion show.

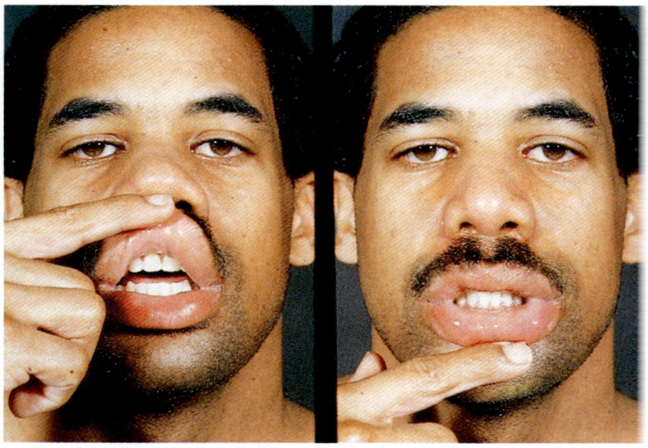

Figure 42. Mucosal laxity increases with aging and may frequently be associated with mucosal cysts and cheilitis.

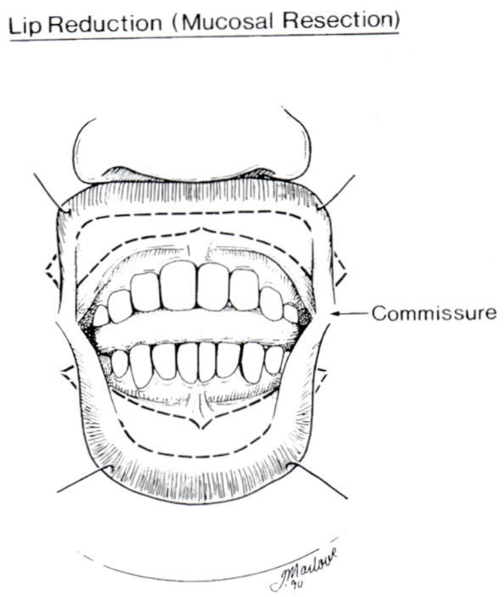

Figure 43. Mucosal resection can best be performed by resecting an ellipse of mucosa just anterior to the alveolar sulcus extending just lateral to the commissure. Undermining should be performed prior to resection. Once this is completed, the amount of mucosa can be determined by trial-and-error placement with temporary sutures prior to mucosal resection. The latter technique minimizes post-reduction labial incompetence.

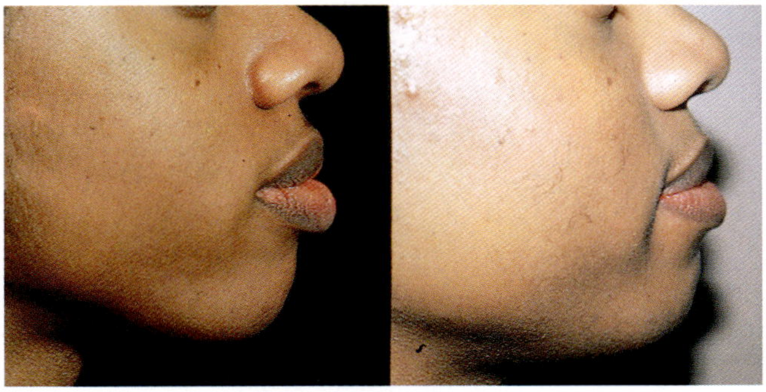

Figure 44. The patient is shown after resection of a 12 × 63–mm strip from her upper lip and a 15 × 63–mm strip from the lower lip.

quent labial incompetence. In the patient shown in Fig. 44, 9 mm × 6.3 mm was removed from the upper lip and 15 mm × 63 mm from the lower lip.

SUMMARY

The distribution of the characteristics of aging in the African American is presented in Tables 2–4. While many findings are consistent with those in the fairer races, the predominance of certain characteristics of aging is best managed by an armamentarium of surgical approaches.

Table 2. *Aging in the African American female*

Generations		Child	Parent	Grandparent
Malar	Flattening	6	1	14
Nasolabial fold	Prominence	4	10	12
Lips	Protuberance	6	13	14
	Mucosal show	2	9	13
Nose	Lengthening	0	4	13
	Oily tip	0	9	12
Chin	Recession	7	8	11
Neck	Submental skin laxity	0	9	13
	Excess fat	0	7	14
Scalp	Male pattern	0	1	3
Hair loss	Temporal	0	8	9
Eyebrow	Lateral alopecia	0	0	3
Forehead	Brow ptosis	0	5	7
	Furrows Frontal	0	3	4
	Glabella	0	6	9
Eyelid	Upper Moderate laxity	5	13	14
	Lower Minimal laxity	15	15	14
	Scleral show	6	12	11

No. = 15

Table 3. *Aging in the African American male*

Generations		Child	Parent	Grandparent
Malar	Flattening	4	6	8
Nasolabial fold	Prominence	2	5	7
Lips	Protuberance	3	6	7
	Mucosal show	1	5	6
Nose	Lengthening	0	2	4
	Oily tip	0	4	5
Chin	Recession	4	3	5
Neck	Submental skin laxity	0	4	6
	Excess fat	0	3	7
Scalp	Male pattern	0	2	4
Hair loss	Temporal	0	1	3
Eyebrow	Lateral alopecia	0	0	1
Forehead	Brow ptosis	0	2	4
	Furrows Frontal	0	1	3
	Glabella	0	4	6
Eyelid	Upper Moderate laxity	2	6	8
	Lower Minimal laxity	8	8	7
	Scleral show	5	6	7

No. = 8

Table 4. *Aging in the African American*

Serial photographs		Female (No. = 18)	Male (No. = 12)
Malar	Flattening	16	10
Nasolabial fold	Prominence	14	11
Lips	Protuberance	11	9
	Mucosal show	9	6
Nose	Lengthening	17	10
	Oily tip	7	7
Chin	Recession	8	6
Neck	Submental skin laxity	15	9
	Excess fat	16	11
Scalp	Male pattern	1	7
Hair loss	Temporal	14	4
Eyebrow	Lateral alopecia	3	8
Forehead	Brow ptosis	4	4
	Furrows Frontal	6	5
	Glabella	8	8
Eyelid	Upper Moderate laxity	18	11
	Lower Minimal laxity	13	10
	Scleral show	15	11

RECOMMENDED READING

Matory WE Jr, Falces E. Non-Caucasian rhinoplasty: a 16-year experience. *Plast Reconstr Surg* 1986;2:239.

Matory WE Jr. Special problems in the Black face. In: *Current therapy in plastic and reconstructive surgery.* Philadelphia: Decker, 1988:470–477.

SECTION V

Abnormal Scarring

Ethnic Considerations in Facial Aesthetic Surgery, edited by W. Earle Matory, Jr.
Lippincott–Raven Publishers, Philadelphia © 1998.

13

Abnormal Scarring

Editor's Commentary

W. Earle Matory, Jr.

COMMON CAUSES

Abnormal or keloid scarring in Caucasians and non-Caucasians rarely occurs following properly performed elective surgery. Problem scarring is most often a reaction to some inflammatory insult to the dermis as opposed to an elective atraumatic and appropriately aligned wound closure. Frequently, reactive material of some sort plays a contributing role, e.g., an imbedded foreign body or highly reactive sutures [chromic, silk, polyglycolic acid (Dexon)]. Wound closure that is compromised by tension, hematoma, repetitive trauma, allergic reaction, ischemic or crush injury, or tissue malalignment may additionally incite hyperactive scar production (Fig. 1).

CONTRIBUTING FACTORS FOR KELOID OCCURRENCE

A thickened dermis, as is found on the post-auricular area, earlobe, upper arm, back, neck, chest, and abdomen, is a key contributing factor to keloid formation (Fig. 2). Pre- and post-auricular incisions frequently heal with hypertrophy and hyperpigmentation. Dermal thickness and increased mobility frequently noted in these areas contribute to wound separation and incisional hematomas and/or seromas (Fig. 3). Resultant inflammatory reaction induces keloid/hypertrophic scar formation (Fig. 4).

Foreign body, suture materials, infection, excessive wound tension, hematoma, and other factors that prolong the inflammatory response will incite excessive collagen production and will diminish collagenase activity, thus promoting abnormal scarring.

W. E. Matory, Jr.: A New You Plastic Surgery Medical Group, Irvine, California 92714

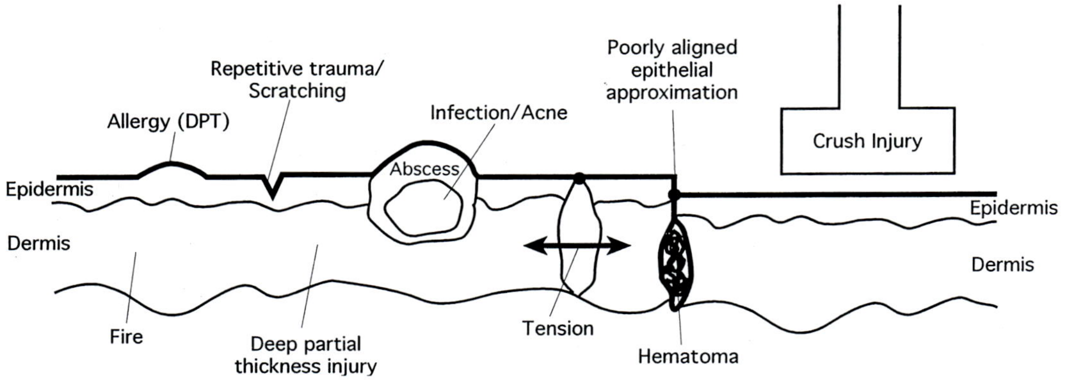

Figure 1. Causes of excessive scar formation.

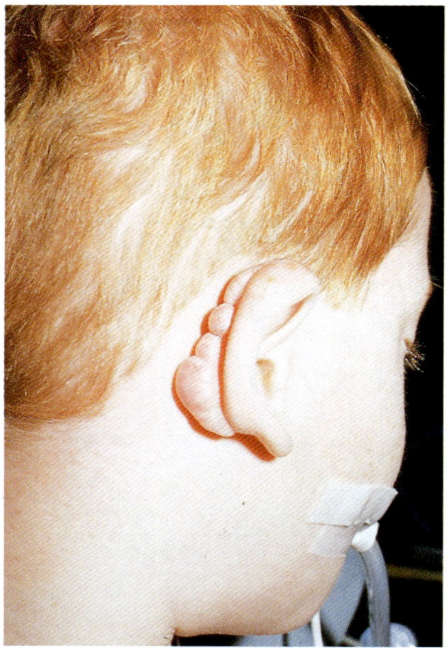

Figure 2. Keloid scarring on a Caucasian man 2 years after setback otoplasty, as shown, is more likely to occur when inflammatory entities are present in the wound (e.g., silk, chromic, polyglycolic acid). (Courtesy of Robert Ruberg, M.D.)

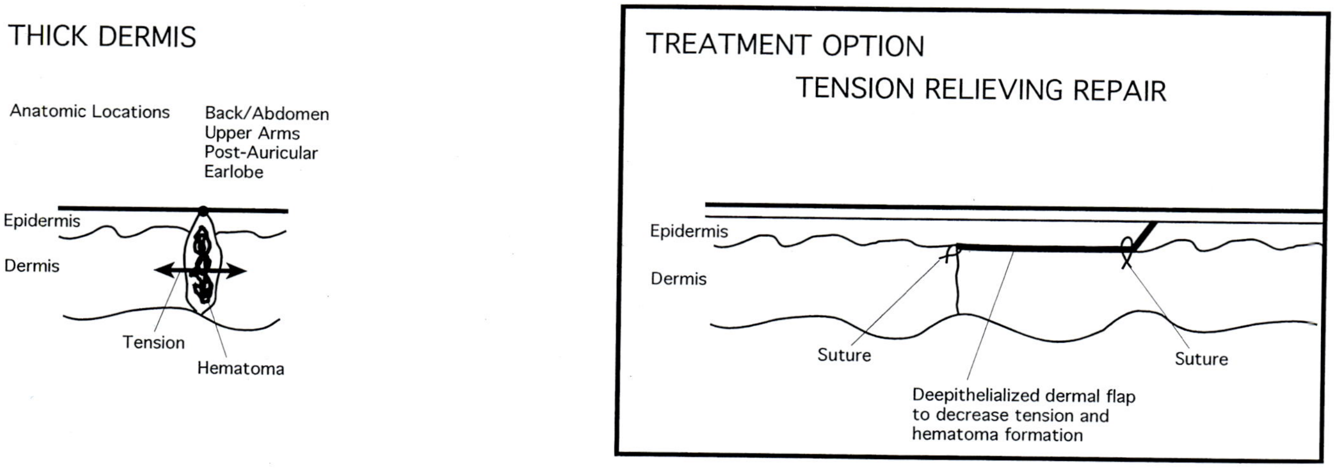

Figure 3. Pathogenesis of excessive scar formation.

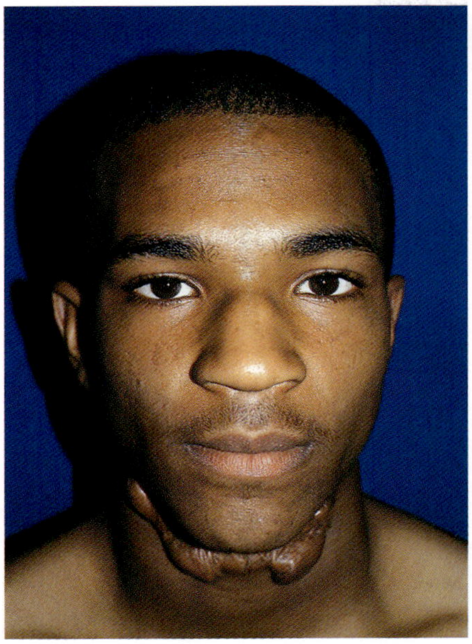

Figure 4. A keloid of the neck 7 years following excision of a thyroglossal duct cyst.

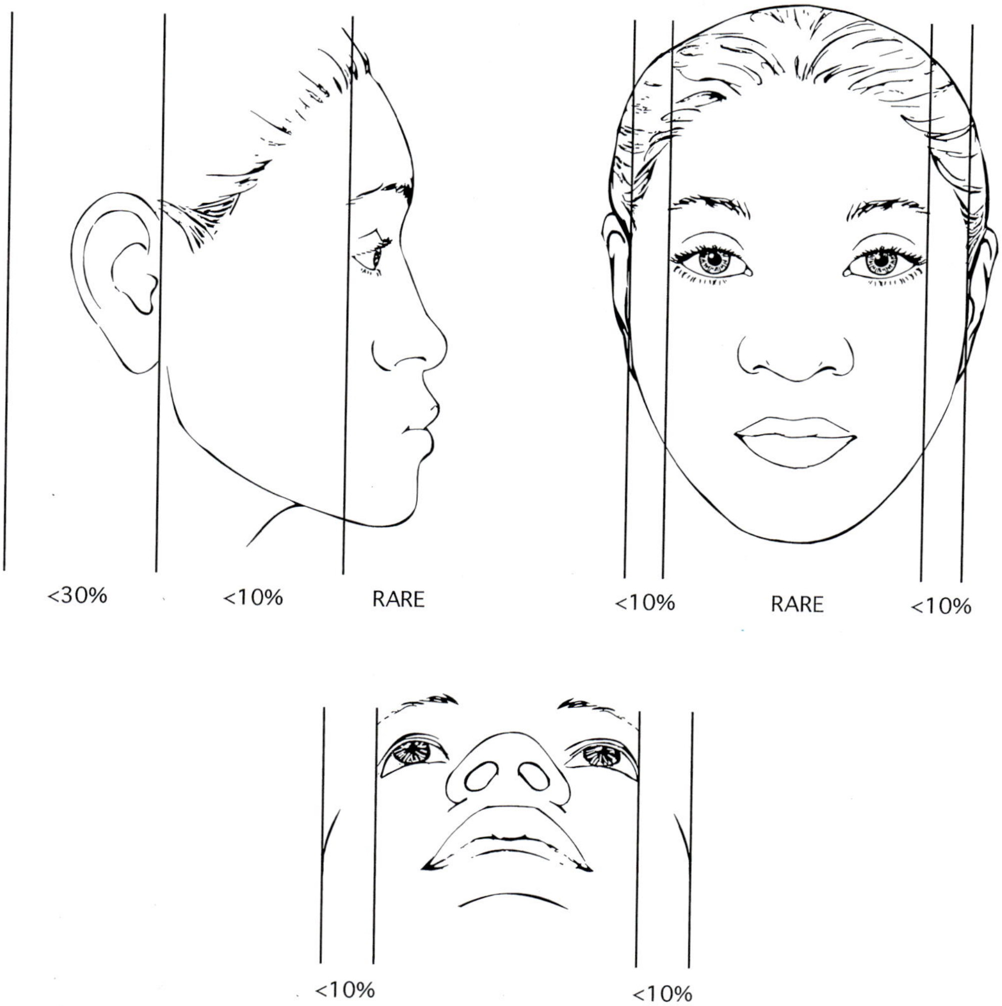

Figure 5. Incidence of keloid formation following elective incisions.

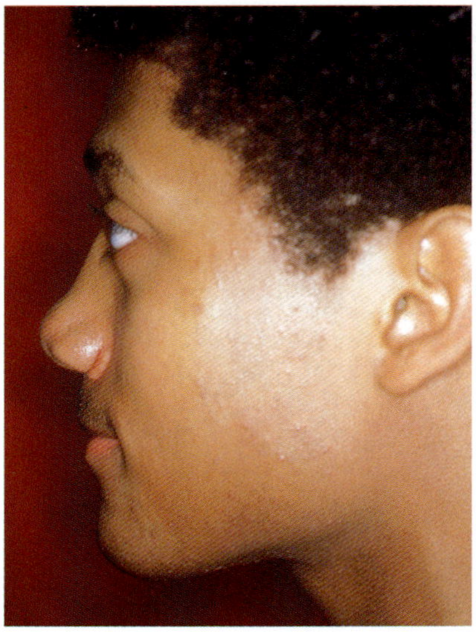

Figure 6. Hypertrophic scar. External incisions on the nose rarely form keloids. If Weir excisions are performed, the incision should preserve a 1- to 2-mm strip of the alar base to allow optimal skin approximation. (Courtesy of Patrick McMenamin, M.D.)

WHERE KELOIDS DO NOT OCCUR

In my experience of well over 10,000 elective surgical incisions on ethnic facial skin, keloid scars rarely develop on the central face, that is, from lateral canthus to lateral canthus (Fig. 5). Hypertrophic or abnormal scars may form as a result of imbedded foreign body, poor tissue alignment (Fig. 6), abrasions, burns, or crush injury. On the other hand, keloids may occur in the central face following severe trauma, e.g., untreated deep dermal burns or scarification techniques (that use imbedded foreign body to incite inflammation). Elective surgical incisions on the central face rarely, if ever, form hypertrophic or keloid scars.

TREATMENT AND PRACTICAL APPROACHES

Pruritus, burning, pain, redness, and continued growth suggest ongoing inflammatory response. Surgical intervention should be avoided during the acute or chronic inflammatory phase of scar formation or keloid development. Dermal reactivity can be diminished by the following:

Steroidal treatment
- Topical steroid. Avoid dermal atrophy by dosing with Telmovate cream 0.5% applied daily for 10 days; omit for 3 weeks, then repeat.
- Injectable glucocorticoid. Triamcinolone acetonide 40 mg/cc injected monthly for 6 months.
- Silastic material applied topically to abnormal scars.

Pressure dressings
- Compression earrings or garments worn 24 h/day.

This combination of modalities will lessen local inflammation, thus eliminating symptomatology and potentially limiting scar hypertrophy (Fig. 7).

SURGICAL TREATMENT

Once acute and subacute wound inflammation has been minimized, intralesional excision can effectively address keloid scarring. At the time of primary repair or when addressing the keloid, wound tension can be lessened or eliminated by using a deepithelialized dermal flap.

Post-auricular incisions following rhytidectomy have a strong tendency toward hypertrophy or keloid transition. Keloid recurrence may be noted as long as 2 or more years after surgical repair. Thus, one cannot be assured of successful revision of keloids prior to 24 months. Incisions should be preferentially placed on the concha, ~4–5 mm above the post-auricular sulcus. Subsequent closure with minimal tension will minimize the likelihood of scar deformity.

One can eliminate the horizontal component of the post-auricular incisions by utilizing the endoscope as described in Chapter 22. Exposure of the platysma anterior to the sternocleidomastoid is achieved by making an incision in the scalp posterior to the mastoid 3 cm within the hairline. This dissection requires particular attention to the location and preservation of the greater auricular and occipital nerves. With the optimal visualization provided by the endoscope, safety and sympathy of the dissection are maximized.

DEPRESSED SCARS

Flattening and hypopigmentation are common sequelae of post-traumatic and post-surgical injury. These are best managed with excision and reapproximation of dermal fat or fat grafts. The hyperpigmented scar can be reduced secondarily if desired (Fig. 8).

A

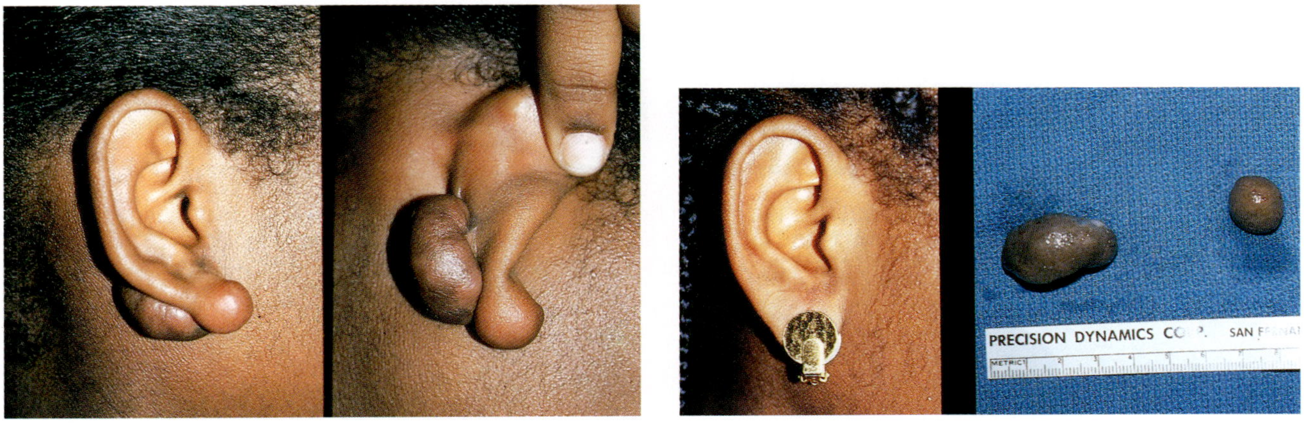

B

C

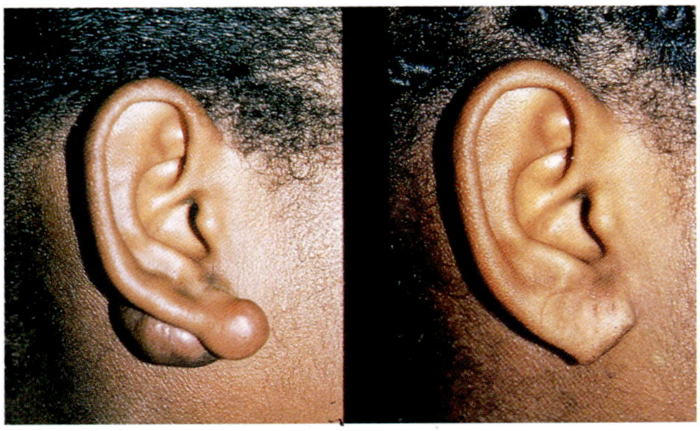

Figure 7. A keloid of the earlobe following ear piercing **(A)** was treated for 6 months with intralesional triamcinolone followed by intralesional excision and immediate application of compression earrings **(B)**. Results are shown 3 years after treatment **(C)**.

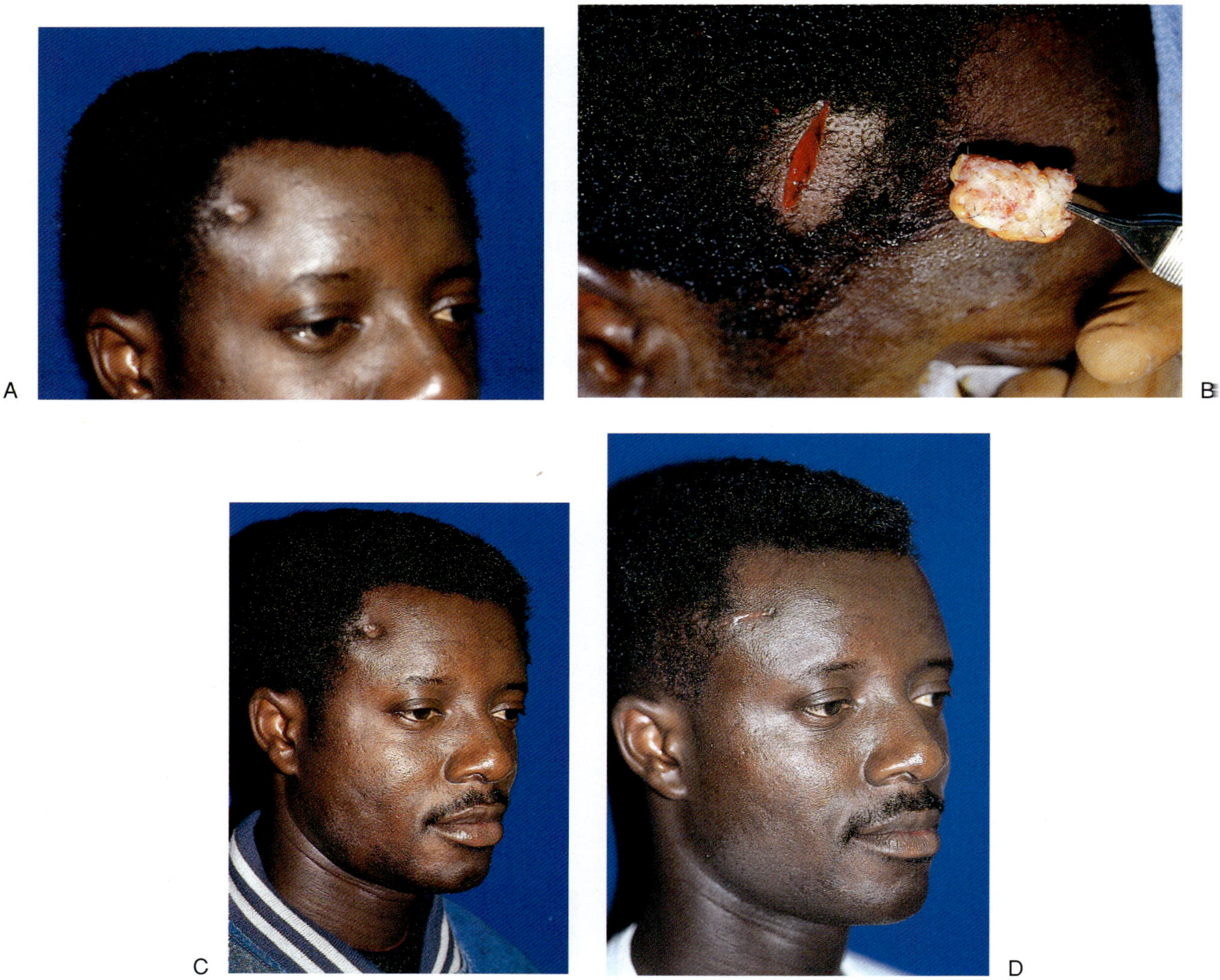

Figure 8. Flattening and hypopigmentation are common sequelae of trauma and elective surgery **(A and D)**. These are best managed with dermal fat or fat grafts **(B)**. The hypopigmented scar can be resected secondarily if desired **(C)**.

Ethnic Considerations in Facial Aesthetic Surgery, edited by W. Earle Matory, Jr.
Lippincott–Raven Publishers, Philadelphia © 1998.

14

Disorders of Excessive Scarring

Raphael C. Lee, Mary Capelli-Schellpfeffer, and Elton X. Tinsley

Basic Research is like shooting an arrow into the air and, where it lands, painting a target.
— Homer Adkins

The primary objective of cosmetic surgery is to create a more pleasing self-image for the patient. Many factors dictate the success of this effort, including the patient's wound-healing response. The primary objective may not be reached if surgery is complicated by excessive scar formation. Hypertrophic post-auricular facelift scars are a dreaded concern for the aesthetic surgeon. It is a generally held view that the degree of dermal scarring is correlated to skin pigmentation. Because of fear of hypertrophic or keloid scarring, cosmetic surgery is often denied to those of dark-skinned ethnic groups. Often that fear may not be warranted. In this chapter, we will review the many factors influencing scar formation, and we will discuss clinical and experimental therapeutic options for disorders of excessive scarring.

NORMAL WOUND HEALING

In principle, optimal scar formation should be coplanar with the skin surface, narrow and inconspicuous in color. In adult wound healing, both genetic and epigenetic factors that are often beyond the surgeon's control determine whether this goal is reached. Even in uncomplicated surgical procedures, these factors may occasionally result in tissue-deforming scars. All of the factors controlling wound healing are not yet known; however, the picture is already complex. In the context of this review, the most important known variables and

R. C. Lee, M. Capelli-Schellpfeffer, and E. X. Tinsley: Department of Surgery, University of Chicago, Chicago, Illinois 60637

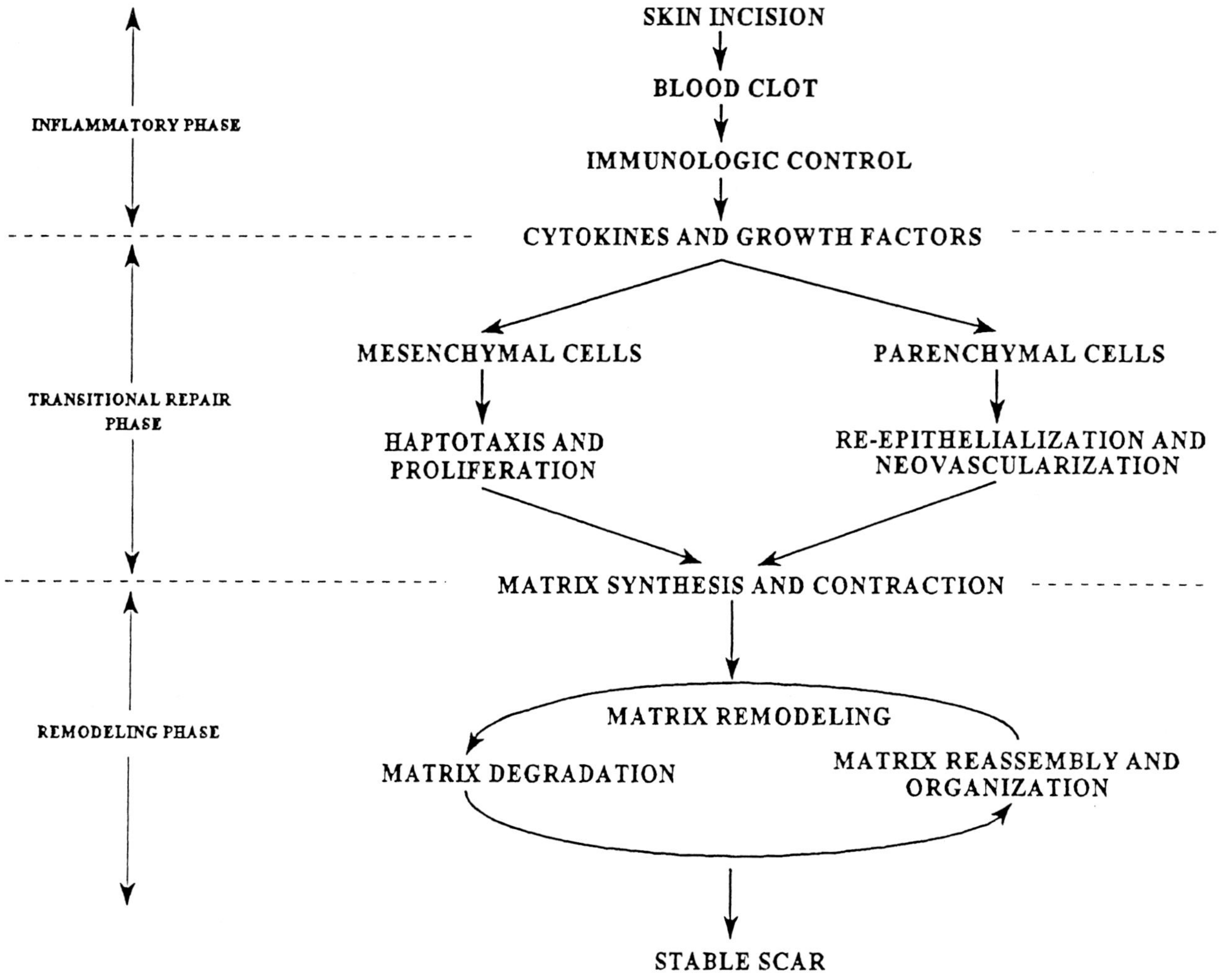

Figure 1. Simplified schema of the regulated cascade of cellular and biochemical events leading to wound healing by scar formation.

control mechanisms in the normal wound-healing cascade are noted (Fig. 1). This emphasizes the potential points of entry for the clinically regulable epigenetic factors that contribute to the development of excessive scars.

Processes responsible for wound healing can be organized conceptually into three phases based on the predominant biologic objective of the phase. There is considerable temporal overlap between these phases, which can be subdivided further. The duration of each phase depends on the conditions of the host, the wound, and the ambient environment. Because each phase of wound healing has a different primary objective, the biophysical signals that control each stage are somewhat different. Cells involved in wound healing must therefore be sensitive to the control signals generated during each phase.

The first stage of wound healing, which usually lasts 2–3 days, is called the inflammatory phase. Its principal objective is to remove damaged tissue or foreign debris from the wound and reestablish immunologic control. The inflammatory response is activated by cell injury and extravasation of blood constituents into the wound. An important biophysical signal during the inflammatory phase is established by the large concentration gradient of chemoattractants. Activated platelets and neutrophils release soluble mediators hat orchestrate subsequent events. Platelet products and the activated platelet surface are involved in establishing early hemostasis and recruiting cells to the site of injury. The release of soluble peptides such as platelet-derived growth factor, epidermal growth factor, and transforming growth factor from activated platelets sets up positive chemoattractant concentration gradients into the wound that guide the flow of incoming cellular traffic. This peptide signal induces neutrophil diapedesis through post-capillary venules and recruits tissue repair cells by haptotaxis.

Neutrophils remove microorganisms and establish the first line of defense against wound infection. Several of the potent soluble wound-healing mediators released in the inflammatory response are stimulators of collagen biosynthesis. Probably the most important of these mediators is interleukin-1 released by wound neutrophils. Interleukin-1 is a potent stimulator of collagen biosynthesis by fibroblasts. Prolonged inflammation can induce excessive wound fibrosis through this mechanism. Part of the neutrophil antimicrobial response is the release of microbiocidal peroxides and enzymes into the extracellular space, which adds to local tissue injury. Wound neutrophil content peaks during the inflammatory phase, after which it is replaced by tissue macrophages as the wound progresses into the repair phase. Heavy bacterial content or foreign bodies can act to prolong neutrophil recruitment with resultant prolonged inflammation, tissue damage, and edema that may delay or arrest the wound-healing sequence.

Later in the inflammatory phase, wound macrophages clear the wound of debris, senescent neutrophils, and any remaining microbes. Wound macrophages down-regulate acute inflammation by digesting the mediators of this phase. For example, the macrophage engulfs enzymes, large proteins, foreign bodies coated with complement, and antibodies by endocytosis. Macrophages also trigger tissue repair. As a result of the inflammatory phase, bacteria and debris are cleared from the wound and host immune controls are reestablished.

The second phase of wound healing, the transitional repair phase, usually begins as early as 72 h after wounding and continues for 3–6 weeks. In this phase, the primary wound-healing objective is to reestablish functional structural integrity to the injured tissue as soon as possible. Fibroblasts are principally responsible for this function. They are recruited into the damaged area over a self-organized fibronectin mesh. These cells rapidly synthesize a repair matrix consisting of collagen, elastin, glycosaminoglycans, glycoproteins, and other structural proteins to mechanically bridge the wound defect and provide a substrate for vascular and epidermal cell migration into the wound. Capillary loops develop to deliver the oxygen and nutrients necessary for the metabolic demands of wound closure. Fibroblasts rapidly proliferate and undergo a phenotypic change to express more contractile proteins. Phenotypically modulated fibroblasts, often referred to as myofibroblasts, generate mechanical tension in the extracellular matrix and contract the wound to reduce the wound dimensions.

Fibroblasts also produce proteolytic enzymes that degrade newly synthesized collagen and glycosaminoglycans and in doing so maintain a variable balance between synthesis and degradation processes. These proteolytic enzymes are synthesized and secreted in the zymogen form and are activated in the extracellular matrix. The enzymes' activation rate is controlled by the chemical conditions in the interstitial fluid where important regulatory factors are temperature, pH, and concentrations of enzyme inhibitors. The balance of synthesis and degradation is deterministic of the quality of wound repair. Extracellular matrix synthesis in normal wound healing is maximal for the first 21–28 days post-injury. During the first 3–4 weeks, the tensile strength of the wound increases in proportion to the concentration of collagen. Afterward the strength more gradually increases as extracellular matrix reorganization and cross-linking take place.

During the transitional repair phase, electrical current appears to also be an important biophysical control signal. Studies of mammalian wounds, including humans, have revealed the existence of transepidermal ionic currents. These currents are generated by amiloride-sensitive sodium pumps in the basal membrane of basal epidermal cells. Basal cells are ordinarily interconnected by tight junctions. Upon injury the nearest neighbor cell is lost, allowing current to flow. This current may guide basal cells across the wound. As the migrating cells cover the wound and contact each other, contact inhibition occurs, tight junctions are reestablished, and current flow is retarded. Current magnitude is a function of wound size and the ability of cells to generate current. Factors that inhibit wound healing such as ischemia and edema may do so by interfering with the ability of basal cells to generate current during the transitional repair phase of wound healing.

The transitional repair phase is followed by the proliferative phase of wound healing. Reepithelialization begins at 24 h. Basal epithelial cells from the surrounding wound edges migrate as a sheet of cells extending lamellipodia along the advancing edge. The stimulus for epithelial migration is thought to be loss of nearest neighbor to the wounding process. Intercellular contact inhibition down-regulates epithelial migration as the wound defect is closed. The more superficial epithelial layers and the deeper basement membrane layer develop after the initial basal layer has covered the wound. The wound is repigmented by migration of melanocytes from hair follicles.

With the mechanical connections to the surrounding tissues established, the proliferative phase gives away to the remodeling phase. Mechanical stress is the principal biophysical force that guides this final phase of wound healing. The collagen in the wound becomes more organized as the type III collagen laid down randomly in the early phases is replaced by type I collagen. During the remodeling phase of wound healing, cells within the scar direct the remodeling process according to the tissue mechanical stresses and other factors. The new collagen is organized in bundles, cross-linked and oriented in the same direction as this mechanical tension. Newly synthesized pro-collagen molecules are secreted into the extracellular matrix, while macrophages phagocytose and break down the existing extracellular matrix. The combination of fibroblasts and macrophages forms the basic processing unit to the remodeling phase. Glycosaminoglycans and other non-collagenous proteins important for early wound closure are removed from the wound. In time, continued intramolecular and intermolecular cross-linking occurs and the collagen bundles become more insoluble and more resistant to enzymatic degradation. The final tissue composition and architecture meet the strength requirements at that wound's specific location. The gain in tensile strength of the final wound will achieve only 70% of the strength of uninjured skin.

FACTORS RESPONSIBLE FOR EXCESSIVE SCAR FORMATION

Fundamentally, the diagnosis of too much (i.e., hypertrophic or excessive) scar is made by visual inspection and physical examination of the scar. If the scar forms a contour irregularity because it is thicker than the skin (Fig. 2), then it is commonly thought to be excessive. This qualitative approach often leads to miscommunication in the wound-healing literature.

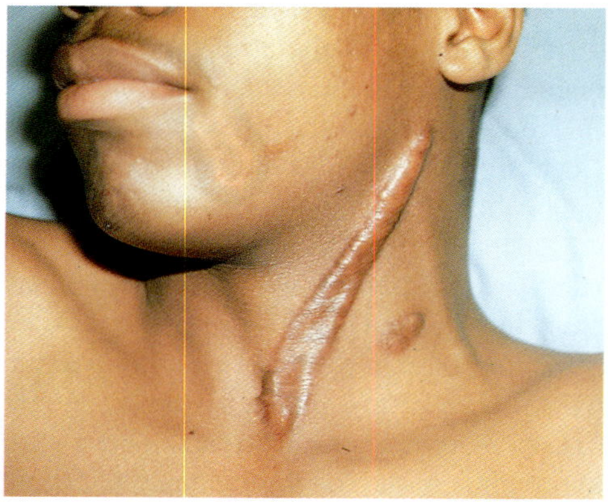

Figure 2. Lateral neck scars in a 19-year-old Black man. Note that the superior aspect of the medial scar is hypertrophic, while the lower aspect is just widened. The lateral scar is normal, which illustrates the importance of epigenetic influences on wound healing such as mechanical tension.

Table 1. *Common epigenetic causes of excessive scar formation*

Wound-healing phase	Epigenetic stimulus
Inflammatory	Hematoma or foreign body
	Infection or allergic reactions
	Edema
	Crush injury
	Deep partial-thickness wound
	Poorly aligned wound edges
	Repetitive trauma (scratching)
Transitional repair	Adolescence
	Pregnancy
	Lower skin temperature
	Endocrine disorders
	Adjacent or remote infections
	Neurofibromatosis
Remodeling	High skin tension
	Anatomic location
	Skin temperature

Why does excessive scar formation occur? Balanced scar formation and remodeling are essential to the development of an aesthetically acceptable scar. Disorders of excessive scar formation either represent too much formation or inhibited degradation tipping the balance toward biosynthesis of matrix. Circulating hormones, locally released cytokines, environmental conditions, the patient's immune status, and wound cell genetic programming are just a few of the variables that impact on the balance of scar synthesis and degradation. In general, factors that intensify or prolong inflammation, intensify the transitional repair phase, and/or change the balance of synthesis versus degradation in the remodeling phase lead to excessive formation of scar tissue. A few of the common epigenetic causes of excessive scar formation are listed in Table 1 according to the wound-healing phase in which they may primarily exert their influence. Hypertrophic (Fig. 2) and keloid (Fig. 3) scars are

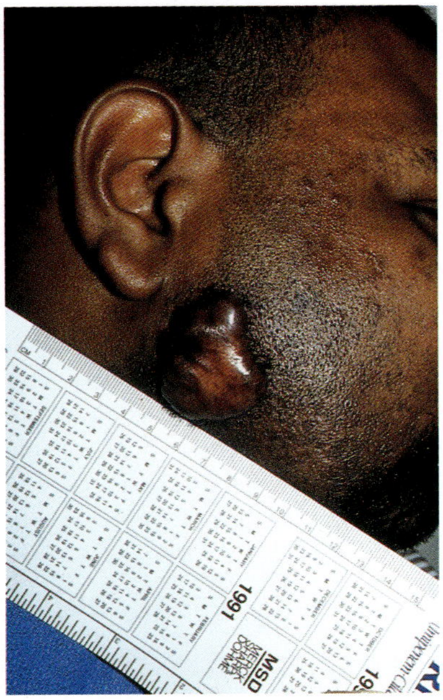

Figure 3. A 43-year-old Black man with adult-onset diabetes and with chronic supportive acne keloiditis of the face and neck of several years' duration. Inflammation is a powerful stimulator of scar formation.

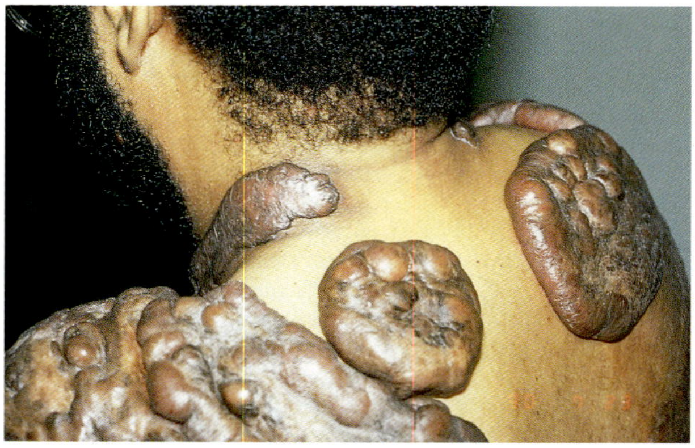

Figure 4. A 52-year-old Black man with true genetic keloid disease. Keloid scars are present over 20–30% of the body surface. Any skin break results in large scar formation. The factors that limit the extent of the scar growth are unknown.

two different types of disorders of excess scarring, respectively. These problems will be discussed in more detail later. The distinction between hypertrophy and keloid, although important, is not always easy to make. Wide disparities in the literature reflect this difficulty.

SKIN COLOR AND CUTANEOUS SCARRING

The precise role of the epidermis in regulating the wound-healing process remains to be determined despite the fact that the epidermis has long been recognized to be an important controlling factor. Skin pigmentation, a property of the epidermis, is generally thought to correlate with extent of scar formation. People with darker skin seem to manifest a higher rate of excessive scar formation. However, the influence of neither melanin nor melanocytes has been defined. While keloid scars are far more common in those of African descent, keloid formation can occur in members of any culture. The reported incidence of keloids in the general population ranges from a high of 16% in Zaire to a low of 0.09% in England. In the U.S. literature, the rate of keloid formation in Blacks is variously reported to be 5–15 more times likely than in Whites. In Hawaii keloids are five times more common in Chinese and three times more common in the Japanese than in the Caucasian population. These studies should be interpreted with caution. There is often considerable effort made in distinguishing and reporting scars as either being keloid or hypertrophic. Making the correct diagnosis requires detailed histopathologic study, often missing in these epidemiologic studies. In addition, fibroblasts from keloid patients are phenotypically distinct from normal and thus the disease is thought to be genetic in origin. True keloid disease (Fig. 4) can be found in different races but is not very common in any race. Dark skin is not essential for the diagnosis of keloid disease. Keloid scars are occasionally found in very fair-skinned, blond-haired patients. Thus, it seems more plausible that these reports correlating skin color with extent of scarring may be reflective of an epigenetic influence in all dermal scars rather than the probability of co-existence of the keloid phenotype.

CLINICAL MANIFESTATIONS OF EXCESS SCARRING

Hypertrophic Scars

Hypertrophic scarring results in overproduction of all components of the extracellular matrix, including cells, collagen, elastin, and proteoglycans. These histologic findings suggest that the normal control mechanisms that regulate the events of matrix formation and proliferation are persistent. Hypertrophic scars undergo spontaneous regression, which indicates that this scar can re-enter the late wound-healing phase of remodeling and scar maturation. Hypertrophic scars do not grossly invade normal surrounding tissues. These scars may achieve considerable size, causing significant spreading of the wound edges.

Scar hypertrophy is most likely following wound healing by secondary intention, particularly if it has required >3 weeks to achieve epithelial closure. Causes of local inflammation such as scratching, acne, hematoma, foreign body in the wound, or inaccurate wound closure also predispose to large scars. Systemic inflammation such as an infection at a remote site can also be influential. Large hypertrophic scar formation occurs more frequently among adolescents and during pregnancy, suggesting that hormonal growth factors are influential in wound healing. In the geriatric population, scar production is generally less.

The occurrence of hypertrophic scars is highest in body surface areas that are subjected to the highest dynamic skin tension. The notable exceptions are the load-bearing areas of the hands and feet. The anterior chest, shoulders, flexor surface of the extremities, and the anterior cervical triangles are the areas most commonly affected. Because skin tension is quite directional, as it relates to the direction of contraction of underlying muscles, the wound orientation in the skin is a factor of considerable importance. Scars oriented in the relaxed skin tension lines generally are smaller.

Chronic inflammation is a common cause of excessive scar formation. Examples include acne-related scars (Fig. 4), earring scars (Fig. 5), and scars in areas of repeated trauma. It is important to realize that large scars that form in response to prolonged inflammation are not necessarily keloid scars. This is best illustrated by the common earlobe keloid. While there is no doubt that patients with the keloid abnormality will produce large earlobe scars, the majority of common earlobe keloids occur in patients with normal scars elsewhere and therefore are probably best classified as inflammation-induced hypertrophic scars. In practice, it is most often possible to identify other scars in patients with earring-related earlobe keloids. If an identified scar has not been involved in repetitive trauma or inflammation, the behavior of these scars is probably more predictive of the response to controlled surgical wounding. The patient shown in Fig. 5 is a White girl who developed a hypervascular keloid of the right earlobe after a bee sting and two previous surgical resections of the scar.

Keloids etiologically related to acne and earring use result from chronic inflammation and are particularly troublesome because of facial disfigurement. Acne keloiditis is characterized by multiple foci of chronic suppurative skin appendage infections that break down into open wounds. They most frequently occur in the bearded region of the face (Fig. 4). Folliculitis with chronic drainage often responds to antibiotic therapy before definitive surgical resection. The earring keloid occurs in susceptible individuals as a result of chronic inflammation due to contact dermatitis. The industry standard for heavy metal contami-

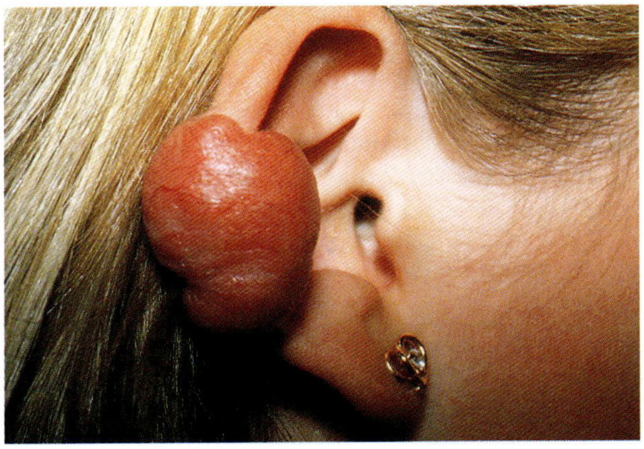

Figure 5. An 11-year-old White girl with a hypervascular keloid in the right earlobe caused by a bee sting at age 5. The lesion underwent a sudden increase in size at age 9 corresponding to accelerated body growth. The lesion was resected at that time and has rapidly recurred.

nants in earrings is five times higher than that which has been clinically proven to cause dermal irritation and inflammation (1 ppm chromium, nickel, and cobalt). For any treatment regimen to be successful, the inflammatory stimulus must be removed: Earring use should be discontinued for both pierced and clip-on style earrings when an earring keloid is treated.

It is with the population of patients with a history of earring- or acne-related keloids that there is the greatest uncertainty about the outcome of surgical incisions. As noted previously, very often normal scars can be identified on the patients in this group. While there may be increased responsiveness to inflammatory mediators, it is often possible to achieve normal scarring by following the surgical rules outlined later for avoiding excessive scar formation. While there may be increased risk of hypertrophic scar, this population should not be rejected out of hand for cosmetic surgery. If the patient fully understands the risk and has a significant cosmetic problem, then it may be wise to perform a small test incision. If scar hypertrophy begins in the test site, then it can be arrested early.

Keloid Scars

Keloid scarring has a very different behavior from hypertrophic scars. Keloid scars can best be characterized as locally invasive benign neoplastic scar tumor. The size of these scars is quite variable, and therein is the basis for confusion with hypertrophic scars. Compared with normal tissue, keloid scar is hypocellular and contains broad, poorly refractile, pale-staining bundles. The normal fine, fibrillar architecture is replaced by thick, irregularly branched, septal collagen bands. Keloids have been reported to be deficient in or devoid of lymphatics as well as elastic tissue. It has also been reported that keloids excised and grafted from high-tension areas to low-tension areas undergo atrophy. Keloid fibroblasts manifest a loss of normal feedback regulation of extracellular matrix production. Fibroblasts of keloid patients respond more vigorously to epidermal growth factor and transforming growth factor-beta, although the binding affinities and receptor densities for growth factors are the same for keloidal and normal cells. Thus, the abnormality is genetic. It was once thought that keloids were manifestations of infectious diseases. An article published in 1942 implicated tuberculosis as the cause; another article from that same year implicated syphilis. It is clear, however, that any condition that causes inflammation of the skin can cause keloid scarring in humans with the genetic abnormality. Keloid fibroblasts have a reduced growth factor requirement for stimulation and a prolonged cellular response. Age plays a role in keloid development as children and young adults are more commonly affected, and childhood keloids may undergo rapid growth during puberty. This suggests that growth factors and hormonal influences are involved. This finding is further supported by sudden increases in size and symptoms of keloids during pregnancy after years of apparent stability. Additionally, acromegalic patients may have an increased susceptibility. Keloids are only known to occur in humans.

Any break in the skin places that patient at risk for the development of this disorder. This is true except for certain privileged areas such as the eyelid skin and the skin of the palms and soles. Whether a keloid can arise spontaneously is unclear; however, the inciting injury can be so trivial as to be forgotten by the time a keloid develops. Keloids are known to arise after insect bites, childhood vaccinations, acne or herpes infections, as well as some other common skin lesions. Keloid scars will reach a specific size and remain that size for many years. What limits the local growth of these lesions is not known, but may relate to limitations in blood supply or nutrients.

Patients who form keloid scars present a major aesthetic surgical challenge. Cosmetic surgery is probably contraindicated. To achieve the aesthetically optimum result from reconstructive procedures requires interventions to prevent or reduce post-operative scarring.

MANAGEMENT OF EXCESSIVE SCARRING

The strategies to manage established scars or prevent excess scar formation depend on whether the patient forms keloids or hypertrophic scars. Making this distinction is impor tant and is very often done incorrectly. Except for rather extreme cases of keloid scarring, visual inspection is not adequate as a basis for diagnosis. Rather, the distinction can be made by histological criteria and/or consideration of the clinical history.

Surgery

In general, surgical excision alone is not an effective treatment. This therapy often results in recurrence to proportions greater than the initial excised scar. Particularly for keloid scars, surgery enters the patient into a vicious cycle of excision/recurrence with no apparent exit. Surgery combined with pharmacologic or radiation inhibition therapy is more successful. Patients who demonstrate a response to pre-operative intralesional medications have a higher success rate if this treatment is repeated post-operatively to prevent recurrence.

Garments and Coverings

Surface coverage with silicone sheeting or compression garments have been very effective in reducing hypertrophic scars, particularly for hypertrophic burn scars in the first year after injury (Fig. 6). The results with keloid scars are less encouraging. It was previously thought that continuous pressure influenced degradation of scar tissue and provided resistance to growth. However, surface coverage also increases skin temperature, which may be the primary mechanism. Type I collagenase activity against new collagen fibrils in the physiologic skin temperature range of 31–34°C has a very high activation energy (E_a = 101,050 kcal/mol) and therefore is very temperature sensitive. The temperature sensitivity approaches a 20-fold increase per degree centigrade. Raising the skin scar temperature by covering it with a gel sheet or elastic garment or down jacket will lead to less net scar formation. Type I collagenase is also the most abundant collagenase in scars, keloids, and normal skin. This enzyme is produced locally by granulocytes, macrophages, epithelial cells, and fibroblasts.

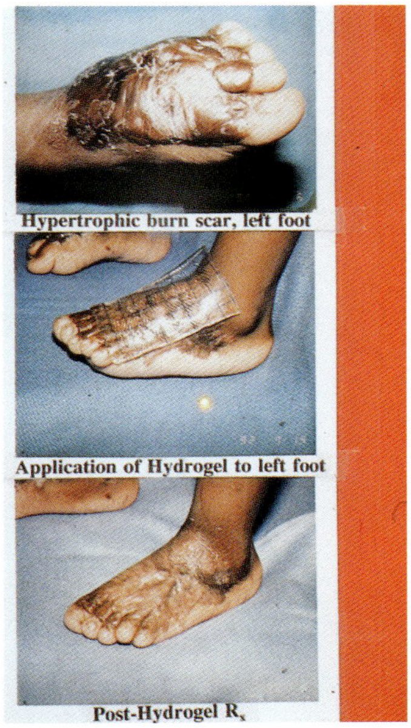

Figure 6. Scar softening, fading, and volume reduction occur. This effect can be produced by silicone and other materials as well. This response appears to be mediated by the physical consequences of surface coverage.

Steroids

Glucocorticoids, one of five major classes of steroids, are used to treat patients with hypertrophic scar or keloid. The commonly used glucocorticoids are hydrocortisone and triamcinolone acetonide. Although the mechanisms have not been fully elucidated, most reports support the hypothesis that steroids inhibit or decrease collagen biosynthesis in fibroblasts of normal human skin and keloids. Early studies of the effects of hydrocortisone could decrease collagen biosynthesis in normal human fibroblasts but not in keloid fibroblasts, but later the same group reported that hydrocortisone could inhibit collagen biosynthesis in keloid-derived fibroblasts but with patient-to-patient variation. This group also demonstrated that hydrocortisone could block the increasing rate of collagen biosynthesis induced by ascorbate treatment in normal human skin fibroblasts.

Triamcinolone acetonide, a fluorinated hydrocortisone derivative, has been shown to be more effective than the non-fluorinated hydrocortisone in the treatment of hypertrophic and keloid scars. In fact, triamcinolone is the most frequently used glucocorticoid in the treatment of hypertrophic and keloid scars. Triamcinolone has been shown to inhibit collagen biosynthesis in both keloid-derived and normal skin fibroblasts. Dexamethasone, another fluorinated hydrocortisone, inhibits collagen synthesis by decreasing the total cellular type I pro-collagen a1(I) mRNA and pro-collagen a2(I) mRNA. In addition to inhibitory effects on collagen synthesis, triamcinolone has been reported to increase collagen degradation. It has been shown that keloids treated by intralesional injection of triamcinolone have decreased levels of alpha-2-macroglobulin and alpha-1-antitrypsin, which are tissue inhibitors of metalloproteinases. The removal or inhibition of tissues inhibitors of metalloproteinases increases collagen degradation by collagenase. These studies have also revealed that the DNA content of keloids treated by intralesional injection of triamcinolone is reduced by 35% when compared with untreated lesions.

Calcium Antagonists

The strategy in treating excess scar is to induce collagenase production and increase enzymatic activity. We have noticed that the incorporation of [^{3}H]proline and [^{35}S]sulfate is retarded if fibroblast-populated collagen matrices have been treated with L-type voltage-gated calcium channel blockers such as verapamil or nifedipine. We have reported that 100 m*M* nifedipine reduces the incorporation of [^{35}S]sulfate and [^{3}H]proline by 60%. We have observed fibroblasts to change shape in response to calcium channel blockers. Intracellular actin filaments are depolymerized and the cells change from a stretched bipolar shape to a spherical shape. Verapamil induces fibrillar actin to aggregate within the cell without disrupting microtubules. We have applied indirect immunofluorescent techniques to study whether verapamil induced collagenase production by altering cell morphology.

In the clinical setting, intralesional verapamil has been effective for some patients with hypertrophic scars (Fig. 7). A very encouraging finding has been that some patients who had not responded to steroid treatment did respond to verapamil. Yet again there have been patients that did not respond to verapamil who did respond to stelazine, a commercial trifluoperazine. This agent is quite effective in treating earlobe keloids. Finally, a subset of patients exists that did not appear to respond to any of the agents used singly but did respond to alternating therapy of steroids and calcium channel blockers with 3-week intervals between treatments (Fig. 8). A comprehensive evaluation of calcium antagonists in treating excess scar is in progress (Fig. 9).

Radiation Therapy

The first keloid radiotherapy report appeared in the literature in 1906. It was not until 1981 that the technique was standardized. For keloids of the ear, 12–15 Gy in three to four fractions over 7–10 days is delivered. Recurrence rates with this regimen when begun

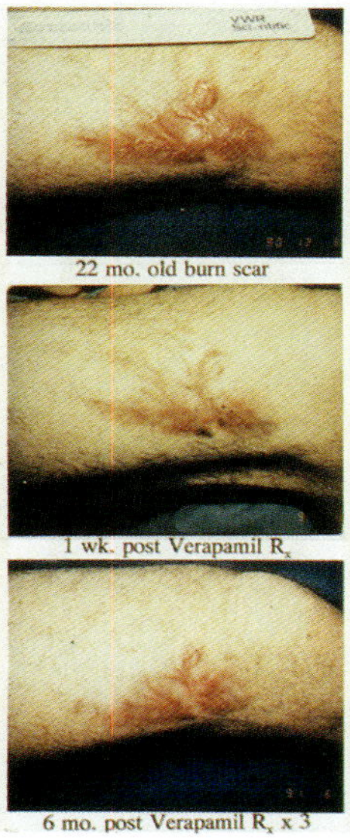

Figure 7. Photographs documenting the immediate response to intralesional verapamil injection in a stable 2-year-old burn scar on the right thigh of a 22-year-old man.

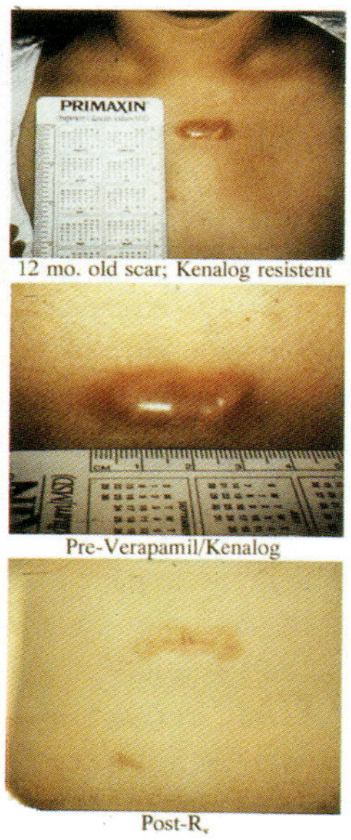

Figure 8. The response of a midsternal inflammation-induced keloid to alternating verapamil and triamcinolone injections as described in the text. This patient had previously failed to respond to triamcinolone or to verapamil therapy given alone.

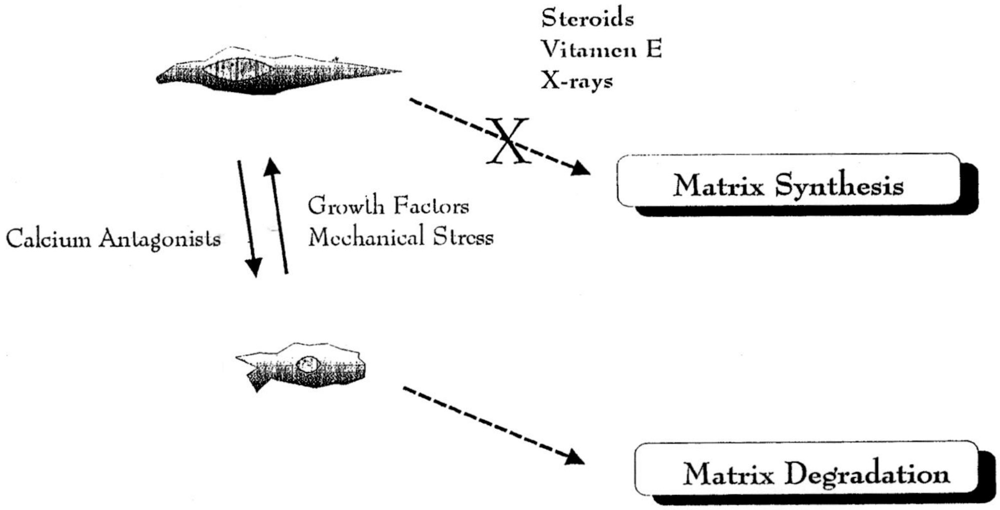

Figure 9. Conceptual schematic illustration of multimode drug therapy for control of scar. Agents that promote scar breakdown by inducing enzyme synthesis can be used in combination with drugs that inhibit extracellular matrix synthesis to achieve desired scar control.

within 1 week of surgical excision are extremely low (<1%). Most recurrences are due to the repeated trauma of repiercing the ears after initial keloid control. Most of the complications are cosmetic and related to skin color changes. The theoretical risk of inducing malignant transformation is of major concern. The neighboring ipsilateral thyroid lobe is particularly at risk. The risk/benefit ratio favors more conservative modalities in treating this benign disorder.

PRACTICAL METHODS TO AVOID EXCESS SCARRING

The ideal scar is flat and narrow and has a color identical to the surrounding skin. Precise adherence to the basic surgical principles and the rules that follow are important to achieve this result. Gentle handling of tissue to avoid cell injury is essential. Adequate incisions should be used to avoid substantial tugging or stretching of the skin. Incisions should be made with a sharp knife and carried through the skin in one pass. Multiple passes to incise through the skin will leave devascularized vertical tissue flaps in the wound. To maximally protect the epidermal barrier, the epidermis should not be handled with instruments. The dermis should be manipulated with fine sharp instruments and tension on closure should be minimized. Dermal closure eliminates dead space and supports the epidermis until the scar has gained adequate tensile strength. Suture technique is important. Suture methods that compromise circulation to the wound should be avoided. Monofilament sutures have the advantage of reducing inflammation. Use the smallest suture that will provide the necessary strength. Meticulous hemostasis should be achieved (drains will not substitute). The simplest closure is usually the best, and unnecessary incisions should be avoided. During reconstructive procedures, if the defect requires grafting or a flap, the results will be far superior to those obtained from closure under tension.

Incisions should be parallel to normal skin lines of tension, called relaxed skin tension lines or facial expression lines. A scar will widen when there is tension directed perpendicular to it. Undermining the skin minimizes this effect but does not eliminate it. Incisions made in the relaxed skin tension lines give a favorable result. Whenever possible, incisions should be hidden by hair or a natural barrier such as the submental or post-auricular regions. Natural junction lines such as the nasolabial fold, ear/cheek junction, or the eyelid folds are other hiding places.

The dressing is also important in minimizing scars. An important function of the dressing is immobilization. Immobilization reduces tissue inflammation and edema. In the East wound closure tapes are kept in place for 6–12 months post-operatively to reduce the scar volume. We prefer to use hydrocolloid wound dressings or silicone sheeting on the wound to accomplish this goal. Applied to the scars for 3–4 months, surface dressings will usually improve the scar's appearance, leaving it less conspicuous. Other agents such as triamcinolone and vitamin E creams may also be helpful if used appropriately.

SUMMARY

Careful patient selection, meticulous surgical technique, and an awareness of the control mechanisms involved in normal and abnormal wound healing can lead to optimal results and patient satisfaction. The occurrence of keloid or hypertrophic scar may cause hyperaesthesia, suppurative necrosis, contracture, and social isolation. Abnormal scars of the face, breast, or genital regions may cause sexual ostracism. All aspects of the patient's well-being may be attacked. It is therefore essential that the surgeon be apprised of developing techniques in the treatment of keloid and hypertrophic skin disorders. Additionally, unfounded fears based on myths regarding the etiology of excess scarring should be dispelled. Cosmetic surgery results are much better if these scars are avoided pre-operatively rather than treated post-operatively.

RECOMMENDED READING

Aggelar J, Frisch SM, Werb Z. Changes in cell shape correlate with collagenase gene expression in rabbit synovial fibroblasts. *J Cell Biol* 1984;98:1662–1671.

Ahn ST, Monafo WW, Mustoe TA. Topical silicone gel: a new treatment for hypertrophic scars. *Surgery* 1989;106:781–787.

Arnold HL, Franer FH. Keloids: etiology and management by excision and intensive prophylactic radiation. *Arch Dermatol* 1959;80:772.

Asboe-Hansen G. Hypertrophic scars and keloids: etiology, pathogenesis and dermatologic therapy. *Dermatologica* 1960;120:178.

Barker AT, Jaffe LF, Vanable JW. The blabrous epidermis of cavies contain a powerful battery. *Am J Physiol* 1982;242:R358–R366.

Bloom D. Heredity of keloids: review of the literature and report of a family with multiple keloids for 5 generations. *NY State J Med* 1956;56:511.

Borok TL, Bray M, Sinclair I, Plafker J, LaBirth L, Rollins C. Role of ionizing irradiation for 393 keloids. *Int J Radiat Oncol Biol Phys* 1988;15:865–870.

Canaday DJ, Lee RC. Scientific basis for clinical applications of electric fields in soft tissue repair. In: Brighton CT, Pollack SR, eds. *Electromagnetics in biology and medicine*. San Francisco: San Francisco Press. 1991:275–291.

Cheng JCY, Evans JH, Leung KS, Clark JA, Choy TTC, Leung PC. Pressure therapy in the treatment of post-burn hypertrophic scar—a critical look into its usefulness and fallacies by pressure monitoring. *Burns* 1984;10:154–163.

Cohen IK, Diegelmann RF. The biology of keloid and hypertrophic scar and influence of corticosteroids. *Clin Plast Surg* 1977;4:297–299.

Cohen IK, Diegelmann RF, Johnson ML. Effect of corticosteroids on collagen synthesis. *Surgery* 1977;82.

Cohen IK, McCoy BJ. The biology and control of surface overhearing. *World J Surg* 1980;4:289–295.

Cutroneo KR, Sterling KM, Shull S. Steroid hormone regulation of extracellular matrix proteins. In: Meecham A, ed. *Regulation of matrix accumulation*. Academic Press, 1986:119.

Darnell JE, Kerr IM, Stark GR. Jak-STAT pathways and transcriptional activation in response to IFNs and other extracellular signal proteins. *Science* 1994;264:1415–1421.

Davies DM. Scars, hypertrophic scars and keloids. *Br Med J* 1985;290:1056–1059.

Doong H, Myerov A, Lee RC. Calcium channel blockers depolymerize fibroblast actin to induce collagenase synthesis. *Surg Forum* 1993;44:738–740.

Enharnre A, Hammai H. Treatment of keloids with excision and postoperative x-ray irradiation. *Dermatologica* 1983;167:90–93.

Foulds LS, Barker AT. Human skin battery potentials and their possible role in wound healing. *Br J Dermatol* 1983;109:515–522.

Garb J, Stone MJ. Keloids: review of the literature and a report of eighty cases. *Am J Surg* 1942;58:315.

Jeffrey JJ. Collagen degradation. In: *Wound healing: biochemical and clinical aspects*. Philadelphia: Saunders, 1992:177–194.

Kelly AP. Keloids dermatology in black patients. *Dermatol Clin* 1988;6:413–424.

Ketchum LD, Robinson DW, Masters FW. Follow-up on treatment of hypertrophic scars and keloids with triamcinolone. *Plast Reconstr Surg* 1971;48:256–259.

Ketchum LD, Robinson DW, Masters FW. The treatment of hypertrophic scar, keloid and scar contracture by triamcinolone acetonide. *Plast Reconstr Surg* 1966;38:209.

Khaw PT, Doyle JW, Sherwood MB, Grierson 1, Schaltz G, McGorray S. Prolonged local tissue effects from 5-minute exposures to fluorouracil and mitomycin C. *Arch Ophthalmol* 1993;111:263–267.
Kischer CW. Comparative structure of hypertrophic scars and keloids. *Scan Electron Microsc* 1984;1:423.
Krieger LM, Pan F, Doong H, Lee RC. Thermal response of the epidermis to surface gels. *Surg Forum* 1993;44:738–740.
Larson DL, Abston S, Willis, et al. Contracture and scar formation in the burn patient. *Clin Plast Surg* 1974;1:653–656.
LeFore IC. Misconceptions regarding elective plastic surgery in the black patient. *J Natl Med Assoc* 1980;72:947–948.
Lee RC, Doong H, Jellema AF. The response of burn scars to intralesional verapamil. *Arch Surg* 1994;129:107–111.
Leibovich SJ, Ross R. The role of the macrophage in wound repair. *Am J Pathol* 1975;78:71–92.
Levy DS, Salter MM, Roth RE. Postoperative irradiation in the prevention of keloids. *AJR* 1976;127:509–510.
Linares HA, Larson DL. Elastic tissue and hypertrophic scars. *Burns* 1976;3:407.
McCauley RL, Chopra V, Ki YY, Hemdon DN, Robson MC. Altered cytokine production in black patients with keloids. *J Clin Immunol* 1992;12:300–308.
McCoy BJ, Diegelmann RF, Cohen IK. In vito inhibition of cell growth, collagen synthesis and prolyl hydroxylase activity by traimcinolone acetonide. *Proc Soc Exp Biol Med* 1980;163:216–222.
McGrath MH. Peptide growth factors and wound healing. *Clin Plast Surg* 1990;17:433–442.
Mercer NSG. Silicone gel in the treatment of keloid scars. *Br J Plast Surg* 1989;42:83–87.
Ng CL, Lee ST, Wong KL. Pressure garments in the prevention and treatment of keloids. *Ann Acad Med* 1983;12(suppl 2):430–435.
Ohmori S. Effectiveness of Silastic sheet coverage in the treatment of scar keloid (hypertrophic tissue). *Aesthet Plast Surg* 1988;12:95–99.
Peacock EE. *Wound repair*. Philadelphia: Saunders, 1984.
Perkins K, Davy RB, Wallis KA. Silicone gel. *Burns* 1982;9:201–204.
Pittet B, Rubbia-Brandt L, Desmaulière A, et al. Effect of τ-interferon on the clinical and biologic evolution of hypertrophic scars and Dupuytren's disease: An open pilot study. *Plast Reconstr Surg* 1994;93:1224–1235.
Placik VJ, Lewis VL. Immunologic association of keloids. *Surg Gynecol Obstet* 1992;175:185–193.
Rajnicek AB, Stump RF, Robinson KR. An endogenous sodium current may mediate wound healing in *Xenopus neurulae*. *Dev Biol* 1980;128:290–299.
Russell JD, Russel SB, Trupin MK. Differential effects of hydrocortisone on both growth and collagen metabolism of human fibroblasts from normal and keloid tissue. *J Cell Physiol* 1978;97:221.
Russell SB, Trupin W, Rodriguez-Eaton S, Russel JD, Trupin JS. Reduced growth factor requirement of keloid-derived fibroblasts may account for tumor growth. *Proc Natl Acad Sci USA* 1988;85:587–591.
Ryan GB, Cliff WJ, Gabbiani G, et al. Myofibroblasts in human ganulation tissue. *Hum Pathol* 1974;5:55.
Shamberger RC, Talbot TL, Tipton HW, Thibault LE, Brennan MF. The effect of ultrasonic and thermal treatment of wounds. *Plast Reconstr Surg* 1981;68:860–870.
Stenn KS, DePalma L. Re-epithelialization. In: Clark, Henson, eds. *The molecular and cellular biology of wound repair*. New York: Plenum Press, 1988.
Sterling KM, Harris MJ, Mitchell JJ, et al. Dexamethasone decreases the amounts of Type I procollagen mRNAs in vivo and in fibroblast cell cultures. *J Biol Chem* 1983;258:7644–7647.
Tredget EE, Shen YJ, Grace L, et al. Regulation of collagen synthesis and messenger RNA levels in normal and hypertrophic scar fibroblasts in vitro by interferon alpha-2b. *Wound Repair Regen* 1993;1:156–165.
Unemori EN, Werb Z. Reorganization of polymerized actin: a possible trigger for induction of procollagenase in fibroblasts cultured in and on collagen gels. *J Cell Biol* 1986;103:1021–1031.
Welgus HG, Jeffrey JJ, Eisen AZ. The collagen substrate specificity of human skin fibroblast collagenase. *J Biol Chem* 1981;256:9511–9515.
Wolff J. *The law of bone remodelling*. Marquet P, Furlong R, trans. Berlin: Springer-Verlag, 1986.

SECTION VI

The African American Patient

Ethnic Considerations in Facial Aesthetic Surgery, edited by W. Earle Matory, Jr.
Lippincott–Raven Publishers, Philadelphia © 1998.

15

The African American Patient

Editor's Commentary

W. Earle Matory, Jr.

In the African American, cosmetic surgery has gained increasing popularity over the last 15 years. Two major factors appear to be responsible. First, an increased economic prosperity has brought cosmetic surgery within reach. Second, well known black entertainers have made the results of plastic surgery widely apparent and accessible to individuals of color. The population of African Americans within the United States numbers ~50 million with an annual 7% increase. With this expanding population, we as plastic surgeons should anticipate seeing far more individuals of African American heritage in our practices. The two most common presentations for the African American seeking cosmetic surgery are rhinoplasty and correction of facial aging.

CULTURAL CONSIDERATIONS

The dominant influence of the European culture on individuals of color has historically been most prevalent in the African American. The pervasive images within the media identify attractive features as being blond, blue eyed, with fine and sculptured nasal and labial features. For centuries, efforts have been made by individuals of African American descent to become a part of the mainstream culture by adapting the mainstream ethnic features. To alter naturally curved hair, hair straightening has been commonly performed using heating irons and pomades.

Within the last 30 years, commensurate with improved economic stability, there have been a revitalization and appreciation for the African heritage. Most individuals presenting to my practice seek to improve their facial attractiveness with preservation of ethnic features. The vast majority of African American patients do not desire Caucasian features.

W. E. Matory, Jr.: A New You Plastic Surgery Medical Group, Irvine, California 92714

Ethnic Considerations in Facial Aesthetic Surgery, edited by W. Earle Matory, Jr.
Lippincott–Raven Publishers, Philadelphia © 1998.

16

Ethnic Considerations in the African American Patient

Fred J. Stucker

Restraint is the difference between a ham and an actor.
— Maurice Cottle

It would be presumptive as well as inappropriate to suggest a simple technique applicable to all or even a majority of African Americans seeking rhinoplasty. No one has advanced a procedure that can be universally adapted to and receive the endorsement of enough surgeons to even suggest a contribution in this area. A common technique, although I once offered one, is precluded by the diversity and variety of anatomical possibilities, the myriad of surgical suggestions, and more importantly the difficulty in defining and achieving an ideal result. The latter imposes the most insurmountable problem since "ideal" implies some universal potential for a perfect end result. In my view "ideal" means the optimum result considering the pre-operative anatomy, the skills of the operator, and the artistic talent to understand what is maximally achievable. The patient's perception of beauty and his/her desire for an ideal result combined with the above factors would render the cookbook approach unrealistic. The surgeon's concept of beauty, interpretations of the patient's wishes, and subsequent aesthetic surgical adaptation do surprisingly, in most instances, yield good results. The patient can further complicate this orchestration or surgical interpretation by limiting the surgeon, for instance, by not allowing an open rhinoplasty approach, or no external incisions, or perhaps refusing to permit a calvarial bone graft or harvesting ear or rib cartilage grafts. All of these factors prompted me to forsake my original position of utilizing a single rhinoplastic technique on the African American. Many more surgical techniques are available now than existed two decades ago.

F. J. Stucker: Department of Otolaryngology/Head and Neck Surgery, Louisiana State University Medical Center, Shreveport, Louisiana 71130-3932

PERSONAL THOUGHTS AND STRATEGIES

My involvement and interest in nasal surgery on Black patients span 25 years and include over 400 patients. This interest and enthusiasm remain essentially unchanged, but the same cannot be said for many of my earlier technical recommendations. I make no apology for these changes since advances and, it is hoped, progress dictate change. Evolutionary refinements are perhaps the most consistent aspect of most complicated surgical procedures. This is because sophisticated evolution in technical undertakings is relentless so that over a period of time these subtle changes may appear dramatic. So when I view my work over a long period, some early precepts and opinions bear little resemblance to what I subscribe to today. While it is true that today's literature does not suffer from a paucity of articles on this subject, 25 years ago ethnic considerations were essentially neglected. Although I now consider the topic of non-Caucasian rhinoplasty an extremely artificial one, this categorization identifies some of the most difficult nasal challenges that the rhinoplasty surgeon faces.

An undeniable truth is that we as surgeons repeatedly do only those procedures we know how to do. In the past, my personal recommendation for managing the African American nose was via a cartilage-splitting technique. At that time, I believed it was the maneuver of choice for most noses. Over the years, there has been an evolution in my approach to rhinoplasty, which now employs the technique that is the least radical of options available to convert or modify the unwanted feature. It has always struck me that a laudable goal in nasal surgery is to surgically violate only those tissues necessary to achieve the desired result and thus inflict as little trauma as possible. It appears just as obvious to me that if a technique does not allow reasonable accessibility to effect anatomic change, it should be discarded. There is a great deal of disagreement over the merits of various techniques. This debate is not likely to be resolved by this chapter, but some important observations relative to techniques warrant comment.

The single most destructive surgical maneuver in a routine rhinoplasty is severing the attachments between the upper lateral and lower lateral cartilages. These cartilages are always separated in both delivery and the cartilage-splitting techniques. However, this is avoided with the external rhinoplasty technique, but it is collectively the most traumatic technique of the commonly employed rhinoplasty approaches. It is paramount that the surgeon consider all of these factors prior to deciding which procedure is used so that the most propitious method is always employed.

Because of one's experience, an argument will ensue defending or criticizing a technique whenever applied to a particular nose. The reader may be interested in the divergence of my current and earlier philosophy when applied to African American rhinoplasty. My first publication on the non-Caucasian rhinoplasty was prior to any personal experience in using the external rhinoplasty, calvarial bone grafting, or tip grafts, which are essential to the armamentarium of today's experienced rhinoplastic surgeon. Few rhinoplastic surgeons routinely advocated or commonly employed any of these techniques two decades ago. The reader may be more inclined to appreciate the author's recommendations of today versus the pragmatic doctrine of earlier writings.

I believe that achieving the best aesthetic nose is possible without routinely utilizing the recommended geometric angles and various measurements. These rather well promulgated guidelines to create ideal symmetry create confusion and have little clinical usefulness. It is not uncommon that a rather unattractive nose may deviate little from the ideal angle and measurements. In routine clinical practice, the surgeon's aesthetic sense is a far better predictor of beauty. Some believe that since many experts recommend standardized surgical techniques, it follows we should standardize the end product. The capriciousness of both patient and surgeon leads me to believe an erector set approach is unwise. All successful rhinoplasty surgeons can intuitively recognize an unacceptable, unpleasant-appearing nose and, it is hoped, an ideal one as well. A nose is not so much a feature of beauty but one that enhances or harmonizes with a beautiful or handsome face. The nose, however, possesses the strong potential to detract from facial harmony. To modify its size and shape so as to better harmonize with the face is the fundamental justification for most cosmetic rhinoplasties. An appreciation of beauty is an essential attribute for success by a rhinoplasty surgeon. This gift cannot be replaced by a ruler and protractor. The angles and measurements are useful guides but can be misleading in the routine rhinoplasty on an African American. Some limits that can be achieved are absolute, such as tip projection. This then limits or dictates other parameters such as dorsal height. This in turn impacts absolutely on the nasofrontal angle. It stands to reason that it is optimum to have all these measurements ideal, but it is far superior to possess harmony with perhaps none of them ideal.

Thus, one should avoid forcing a nasal reconstruction into the ideal parameters when there is no prospect of achieving it or it may result in a bizarre appearance if one succeeds. An acceptable aesthetic compromise is a patient with apparent anatomic relationships. Futile overcorrection to achieve an ideal will inevitably yield a disaster. This recognition of complex relationships and the interdependence of the surgical modification are the subtle difference between the success and failure with rhinoplasty surgery. Inexperienced surgeons' rigid attempts to achieve standards to guide them will routinely lead to patient dissatisfaction.

PSYCHOSOCIAL CONSIDERATIONS

On balance there are far more common factors than differences when comparing rhinoplasties among the races. There are, however, some unique ethnic features that are valuable to point out.

I reviewed 100 consecutive records of pre-operative African American patients and 100 Caucasians. Their complaints relative to perceived deformities and defects were supplemented by analysis of the pre-operative photos. Specific areas and sites for surgical correction were noted. Although many Caucasians possessed similar deformities to those commonly identified in Blacks and vice versa, there were distinct ethnic differences. A major difference is that the Caucasian presenting for nasal surgery possessed fewer and perceived fewer deformities than did the African American. The African American complaints and observed deformities versus those of the Caucasians were present in a ratio of approximately two to one. The surgeon had fewer areas to correct or modify in Caucasian patients. This may be simplistically stated, "The African American patient is more of a surgical challenge." I believe this is absolutely true.

The most notable difference in the interview between White and Black patients considering nasal surgery is the answer to the query, "What specifically do you not like about your nose?" Or, put another way, "What specifically would you like changed given that it is possible to modify that feature?" The most common responses by Caucasian patients are as follows, in decreasing order of frequency: (a) hump deformity; (b) tip deformity; (c) nasal obstruction; (d) crooked nose; (e) nostril deformity; (f) depressed dorsum, saddle; (g) nasolabial problem; (h) weak chin. The eight most common defects in both races were compared in Table 1.

The Black patient's most common physical findings in the order of decreasing frequency were as follows: (a) tip is too big, fleshy (broad, flat); (b) base (alae) too broad; (c) nostrils

Table 1. *Common physical findings in patients requesting rhinoplasty*

	African American	Caucasian
Bulbous, amorphous tip	81	19
Wide alar flare	71	16
Round or horizontal nostrils	64	7
Short columella	63	13
Wide bony dorsum	59	17
Acute nasolabial angle	59	27
Depressed dorsum	56	11
Hump deformity	19	88
Total	472	198

Table 2. *Common complaints in patients requesting rhinoplasty*

	Caucasian	African American
Hump deformity	61	19
Tip deformity	53	81
Nasal obstruction	51	12
Crooked deviated nose	27	6
Nostril deformity	7	64
Saddle, depressed dorsum	11	56
Chin retrusion	13	9
Nasolabial angle deformity	8	59
Total	231	306

round; (d) columella short, tip depressed; (e) dorsum too wide; (f) nose too close to lip (nasolabial angle); (g) depressed dorsum; (h) hump deformity (see Table 2). Needless to say, these lists are editorially produced using my interpretation of the patients' complaints combined with the photos. It is wise to appreciate that the terms, defects, and deformities for any of these nasal characteristics are quite arbitrary and are quite useful for discussion purposes. However, most patients do not appreciate the term "deformity" for an anatomical characteristic, especially if it does not concern them or if they wish it to remain unaltered. Short of a candidate wishing an inappropriate or an incongruous change (in which case it is prudent not to proceed with the surgery), it is always wise to do only the modifications a patients desires, agrees upon, and fully understands.

Tables 1 and 2 demonstrate that the eight most common features of each race are distinctly at variance. More importantly, the White nasal candidates have an average of 2.42 items listed as opposed to 4.71 for the Black patients using only the 8 most common in each race. This comparison likely represents our society's concepts of beauty. These figures reinforce the impression that the usual Black rhinoplasty is a more difficult surgical challenge than is the Caucasian rhinoplasty not only because of numbers but also surgical complexity. Over the years my non-Caucasian patients have proved to be very appreciative in spite of less success in achieving an optimum result when compared with the long-term (10-year) results in my Caucasian patients. It is logical that difficult or challenging cases would not compare favorably with more routine ones. It is also quite likely that African Americans with minimal deformities do not seek surgery as do a significant number of Caucasians who possess relatively minor defects.

The thrust of this manuscript represents my thoughts and experience in surgically modifying nasal characteristics in African American patients over the last 25 years. Analyzing my early results prompted changes and attempts to achieve better long-term improvements. The most disappointing aspects of operating upon Black patients were relapses in the nasolabial angle, modifications of the alar bases, and difficulty in maintaining the initial improvement in tip projection.

TOPOGRAPHICAL ANATOMY

Common presenting symptoms or requests include refinement of broad fibrofatty tip, increasing tip projection, nostril orientation, narrowing alar bases, improving columellar length and shape, and opening the nasolabial angle. The width and projection of the dorsum are commonly addressed by augmentation.

The achieved tip projection dictates the degree of dorsal augmentation. The degree of tip projection results from a number of interrelated structural findings. There are many ways of describing the nasal tip in the African American: bulbous, flat, wide, fleshy, pendulous, depressed, etc. I believe that most patients wish a more elegant or sculptured tip. The anatomy that produces the wide, fleshy tip is thick skin and fibrofatty subcutaneous tissue over the tip. The underlying thin and frail lower lateral cartilages also contribute to an inelegant tip. Both medial and lateral crura are not only thinner, but they are shorter in their inferior and lateral extensions, contributing to a more rounded nostril. Superior and inferior columella flare accentuates the short columella as does the short flail medial crura and rudimentary or absent anterior nasal spine. It must be remembered that the refined, nicely sculptured tip will appear more projected than the broader or more bulbous one. Of note is that perception of increased projection occurs due to an actual as well as apparent physical lengthening. The weaker and more flail lower lateral cartilages, often seen in the African American, project poorly and would not support the ala if it were not for the thick fibrofatty jacket of skin. The round or ovoid nostrils with wide alar bases contribute to the actual as well as the apparent underprojection. The anterior maxillary spine is rudimentary or absent, which results in a poorly projected tip because the tip lacks a supportive foundation. A retrusion of the premaxilla, an inordinate anterior jutting of the maxillary teeth, and a generous outwardly rotated upper lip all collectively aggravate the apparent or perceived impression of inadequate tip projection. While underprojection is commonly apparent, it is more commonly real. Consequently the surgical correction of increasing tip projection must be addressed with actual increases as well as apparent improvements with camouflaging techniques.

SURGICAL DESCRIPTION

Correcting or improving these anatomical findings and their attended features is one of the more challenging aspects of the African American rhinoplasty. Nasal decortication or external rhinoplasty affords complete visualization of and access to the tissues responsible for the topographical features of the tip. No other technique provides the expanded view to allow soft tissue resection and cartilage modification with the use of incisions, resection, repositioning, and addition (free autogenous cartilage grafts). This approach need be employed in only those patients in whom all of the desired changes required outweigh the surgical trauma implicit in the external approach. Clearly most of the technical aspects can be achieved through closed techniques, and for years I advocated the latter in African American patients. It is, however, just infinitely easier to defat, mobilize, and medialize the lateral crura and place tip grafts in a much more expeditious maneuver and with greater precision when employing an open technique.

There are two basic variations of the transcolumellar incision that can be employed. In patients with no history of scar abnormalities, in whom the need for nasolabial exposure is not extensive and there is no need for columella lengthening, the routine inverted V transcolumellar incision is placed at the junction of the middle and upper third of the columella. The alternative V incision at the base of the columella routinely heals and will camouflage the scar in the natural crease (Fig. 1). The tip of the V that lies in the upper lip is

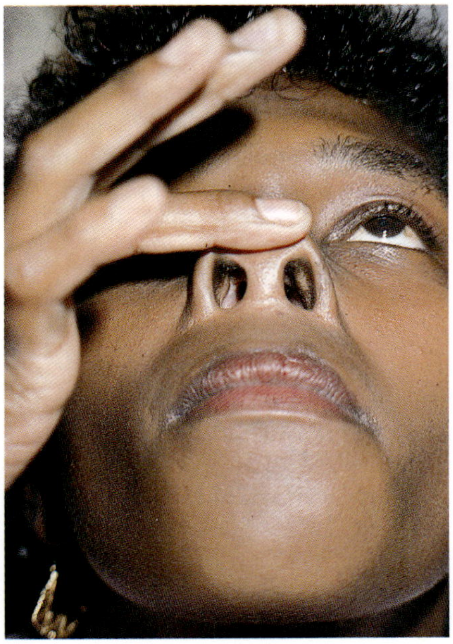

Figure 1. Demonstrates the acceptability of the base of columellar incision.

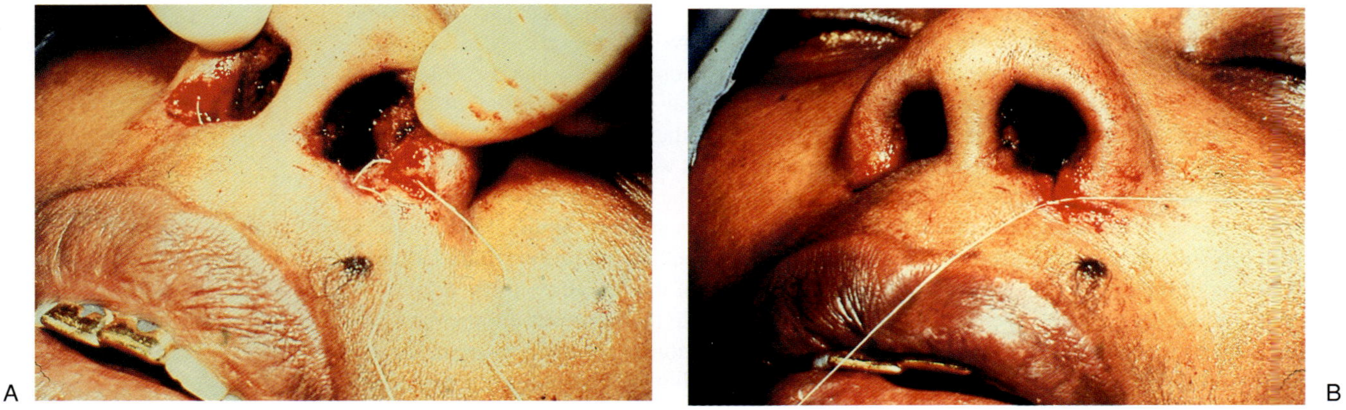

Figure 2. **A:** One suture passed beneath the columella with identical purchases in the alar base. **B:** Suture tied narrowing alar bases with one suture.

easily advanced superiorly to be utilized in lengthening the columella. More importantly, if the nasal spine region requires augmentation, this inferior transcolumellar incision affords unexcelled access. Experience with many hundreds of facial incisions in African American patients demonstrates that the camouflaging of facial scars is superior to that in Caucasians. Accurate closure with 6-0 non-reaction sutures produces excellent results. The exposure is accomplished by a transcolumellar incision connecting bilateral marginal incisions at the leading edge of the cartilage and decorticating the soft tissue just above the perichondrium. It is ironic that the open approach affords the only technique allowing accurate placement and fixation of a tip graft. Those vociferous advocates of the open approach perhaps do not always appreciate the creation of a subdermal scar lamina that often dictates the need for a tip graft to achieve the lost definition implicit in this technique.

There are other incisional approaches. Kabacher uses a columellar splitting combined with bilateral horizontal (sill) incisions. Santana employs a bilateral Caldwell-Luc-like incision connected across the midline. Then under direct vision he narrows the soft tissue attachment of the caudal nose across a widened pyriform aperture.

Most journal articles on this subject enumerate the many typical racial characteristics and the relationships of three-dimensional characteristics of the African nose (1–3). Santana narrows the widened alar bases with exposure of the pyriform aperture. He cleverly narrows the bases without alar base excisions by freeing the soft tissue attachments and fixing these more medially with a permanent suture. This is a novel and effective maneuver. Figure 2A demonstrates a technique through the more traditional alar base incisions utilizing a similar suture fixation.

In my experience, defatting as described by Romo and Shapiro (3) has not proved effective. It often results in irregularities and an artificial look. We no longer do any more than remove the fibrofatty tissue remaining over the skeletal cartilage following decortication in the subdermal plane. It has been suggested to use this tissue as a dorsal implant or augmentation. In my experience it is not likely to produce much effect in the short term and none in the long term.

SURGICAL TECHNIQUES FOR INCREASING TIP PROJECTION

Fundamental to improving tip projection is the sculpture or enhancement of tip definition. The surgical maneuvers for both are interrelated and will be discussed together.

Basic to modifying the tip and its projection is the utilization of autogenous graft material. Both availability and adaptability are important considerations, as is ease of harvesting. My preference is septal cartilage, which in my experience is commonly available. Severely deformed or previously operated septa in African Americans are unusual so looking elsewhere for autogenous cartilage graft material is rarely necessary. Of note, the septal cartilage in Blacks is quite thin, often measuring 1 mm in thickness in the midquadrangle cartilage region. It is prudent to harvest the septal graft interiorly along the floor where the width is thickest, usually 2–3 mm. Septal cartilage is ideal for fashioning a columella strut, a routine surgical step in increasing tip projection. The strut serves not only to stiffen the columellar support but also to provide length by straightening the superior and inferior flaring. This is accomplished with permanent buried mattress sutures. There is an actual as well as apparent improvement with this maneuver. Septal cartilage is also used to fashion the commonly employed tip (shield) graft to provide a refinement, so necessary in achieving definition in an amorphous tip. The resultant gain in tip projection is more apparent than real.

Another effective maneuver in improving tip projection is the use of a pedestal or plumping graft. Over the years I have employed autogenous cartilage, but my 5- to 10-year follow-up reveals that the initial gain results in relapses. Cartilage resorption is probably secondary to the motion and muscle action in this region. In my experience it is rare to see less than complete resorption of an autogenous cartilage graft in this region over 2 or 3 years. The initial effect is a significant improvement that prompted me to change graft material in the nasolabial angle. I have also employed autogenous bone, but the local availability and difficulty in fixation plus a similar experience with resorption prompted me to abandon this alternative. Materials that I have used as plumping grafts are Proplast (effective but was removed from the market), polyamide (not readily adapted to use in this region), Gortex (again difficult to adapt), and hydroxyapatite (quite promising). A pedestal graft not only actually increases tip projection but has the side benefit of opening an acute nasolabial angle to an aesthetically more pleasing one.

ALAR BASE SURGERY

Narrowing the alar base of the submental nasal triangle has the benefit of apparently increasing tip projection. This impression of a subtle thrust upward is entirely an illusion of improving projection or height. This maneuver is no panacea, and alar base resections must be carefully planned. In spite of some rather dogmatic suggestions, there is, in my view, no standard alar base incision or resection or technique that can routinely be employed to achieve an ideal result. Alar base surgery is fraught with misadventure and frequently may be meddlesome. Avoid alar base incisions that are placed in lateral to the alar crease. Incisions perpendicular to the cheek unquestionably lead to unacceptable scars. They widen due to the relentless action of facial muscles. If the dorsal height of the ala must be decreased with a full-thickness resection, the incision should be placed perpendicular to the ala and parallel to and ~ ½ mm superior to the alar crease. Facial dynamics will have no widening effect on such an incision. The majority of alar base incisions and/or resection for simple narrowing can be made in the floor, sill, or inferior alar crease and thus are easily camouflaged. On occasion I have utilized these incisions or resections to place permanent sutures from one side to the other to reinforce the narrowing of the bases with one permanent mattress suture (Fig. 2B). Gradual widening of the alar base after initial success is significant when patients are followed for 5–10 years.

TIP SURGERY

Management of the lower lateral cartilage in the African American is dictated by tip anatomy. The more the tip lacks definition, the more I am inclined to proceed with an external rhinoplasty. Although I do not believe that much can be gained by thinning the dermal layer of the skin, I routinely dissect and discard all the superficial fibrofatty tissue beneath the dermis. Skeletonizing or surgical attempts to thin the dermis can cause pigmentation changes that can persist up to 1 year (Fig. 3). The failure to provide long-term improvement is reason enough to avoid this maneuver. The external technique allows complete visualization of all architectural structures following meticulous skeletonization. A columellar strut is usually placed. If appropriate, the lateral crura can be medialized with

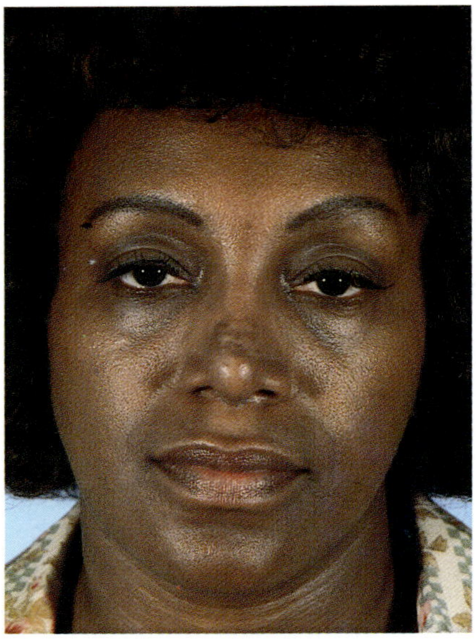

Figure 3. Pigmentation following defatting rhinoplasty at 7 months.

mattress suture fixation. By stealing the maximum of lateral crura without creating an unnatural look, increasing tip projection is realized. The lower lateral cartilage may be entirely freed during this step if necessary. The cephalic resection, vertical division, and horizontal resection may be done to achieve the desired result. The placement of tip graft is usually the final step in tip reconstruction. All of these techniques are reasonably safe because of the masking afforded by the thick fibrofatty skin covering.

MANAGEMENT OF THE DORSUM

Just as hump removal is one of the more common maneuvers in Caucasian rhinoplasty, augmentation is a rather routine feature in African American rhinoplasty.

In spite of these stereotypes, ~20% of African Americans are candidates for hump removal (Fig. 4), whereas nearly 50% require augmentation. It is my belief that since the caudal end of the nose is mobile, it should not routinely be augmented with a rigid implant. There are specific circumstances such as total nasal reconstruction where this tenet is legitimately ignored. There are also situations in which the only or the major area for augmentation is confined to the bony dorsum. In such instances (more common in Asians), a rigid implant such as a calvarial bone graft is quite appropriate.

The usual portion of the augmentation in African American patient extends over the bony cartilaginous dorsum. My recommendation for minor (<4 mm) dorsal depressions is that they be implanted with septal cartilage. For 25 years, I have had excellent success augmenting defects of >5 mm with a tightly rolled alloplastic mesh material. Mersilene mesh material is rolled to the desired diameter and is ideal for placement over the nasal dorsum. My early recommendation was to augment after performing medial and lateral osteotomies. My thinking was that the base could be narrowed and medial osteotomies produced a trough-like area for accommodating this implant. It became obvious that this routine step produced no benefit and that the osteotomies were to a large measure mettlesome. There is an occasional patient who benefits from the theoretical improvement of narrowing the base, but usually the augmentation creates an adequate illusion of a narrower base (Fig. 5). The markedly depressed nasal dorsum with an extremely wide base has no potential for improvement with osteotomies.

The tightly rolled mesh is sutured with a running 0000 nylon to prevent it from unwinding

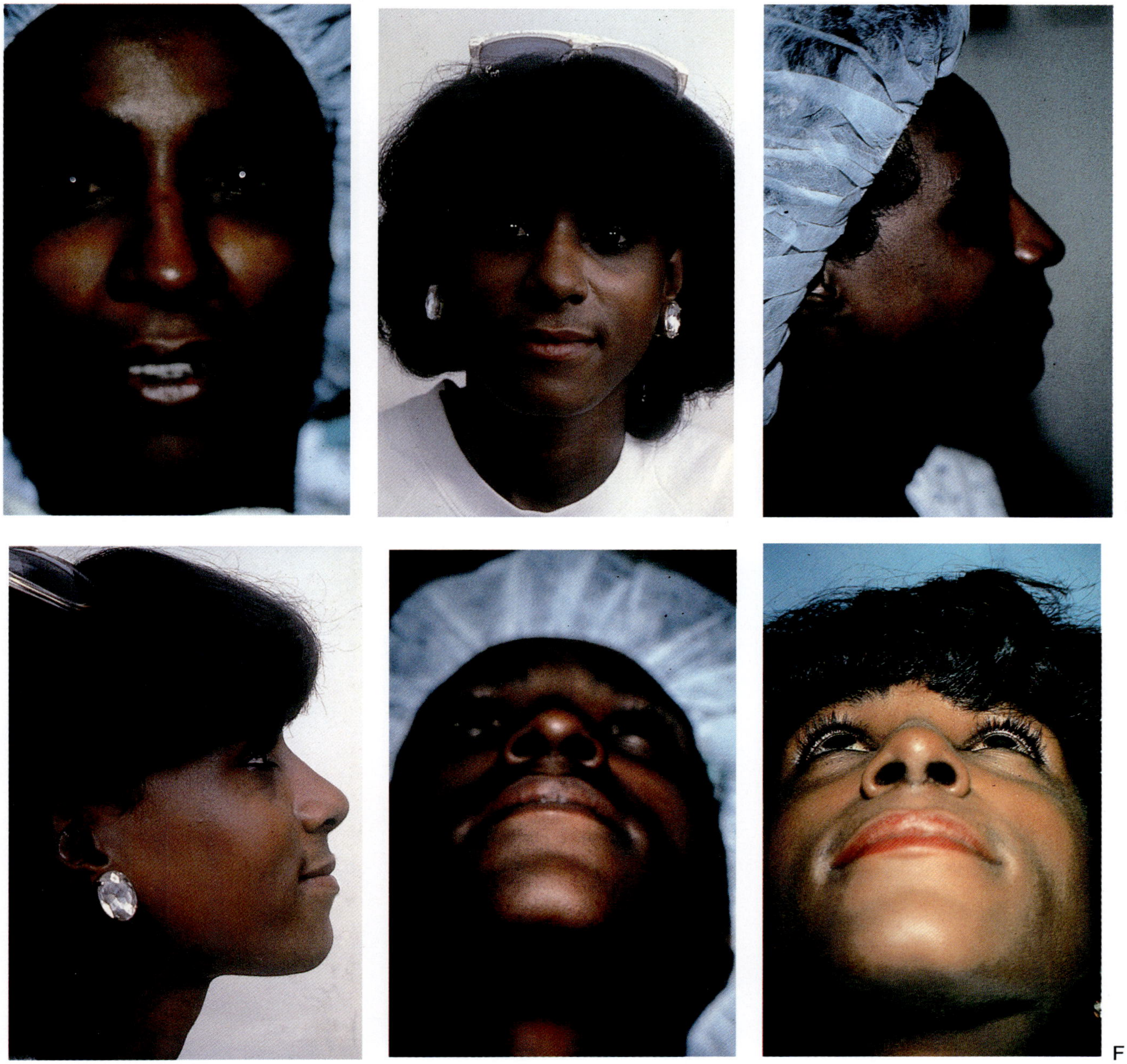

A, B C

D, E F

Figure 4. A: Pre-operative full face of Black American with hump deformity. **B:** Three years post-operatively, full face view. **C:** Pre-operative lateral view. **D:** Three years post-operatively, lateral view. **E:** Pre-operative submental view. **F:** Three years post-operatively, submental view.

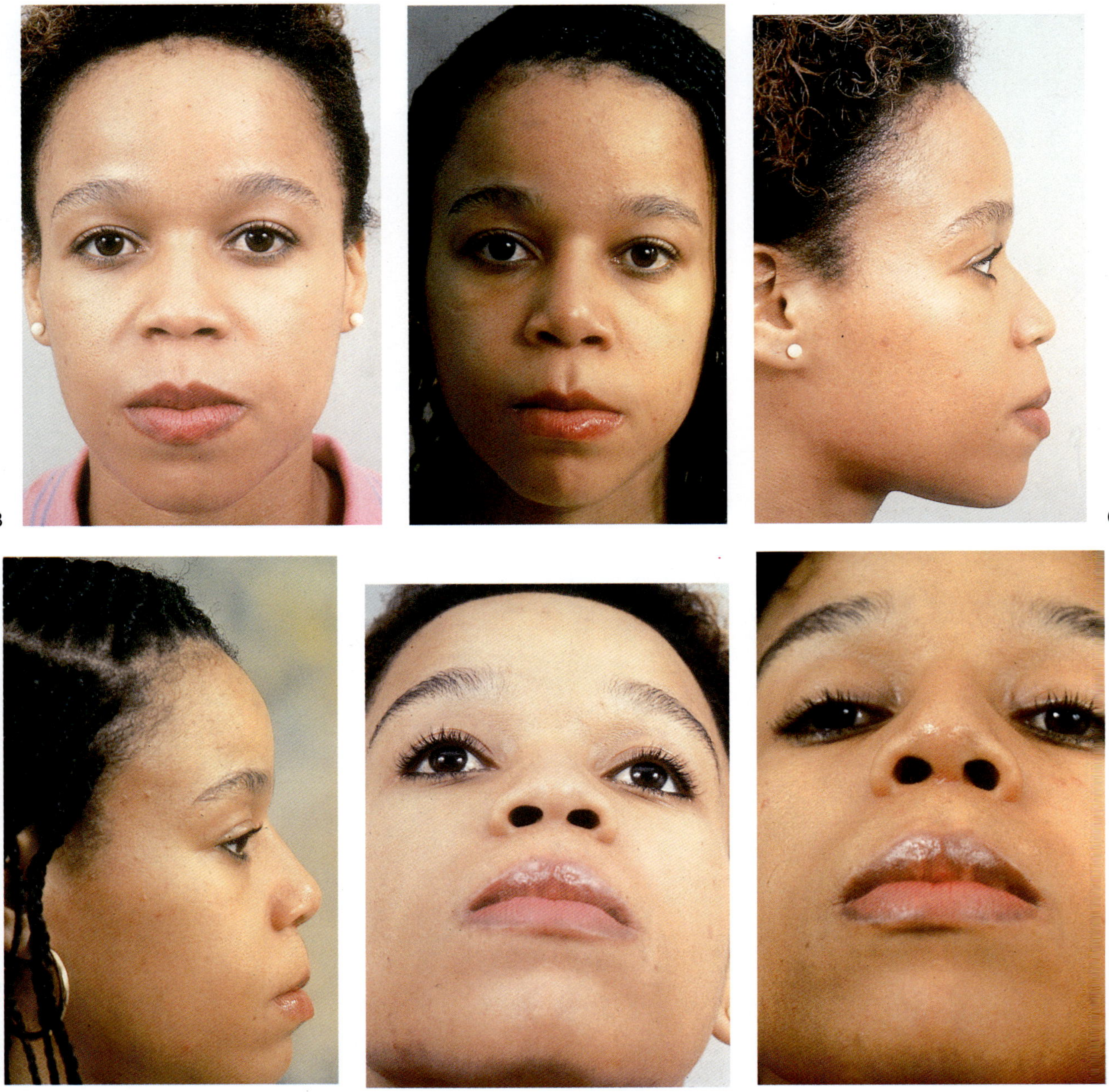

A, B C

D, E F

Figure 5. A: Pre-operative full face view of candidate for rhinoplasty. **B:** Two-year post-operative view demonstrating illusion of narrow alar base because of dorsal implant. Patient has also had plumping graft, columellar strut, and shield graft. **C:** Pre-operative lateral view. **D:** Two-year post-operative view. **E:** Pre-operative submental view. **F:** Two-year post-operative view.

A, B 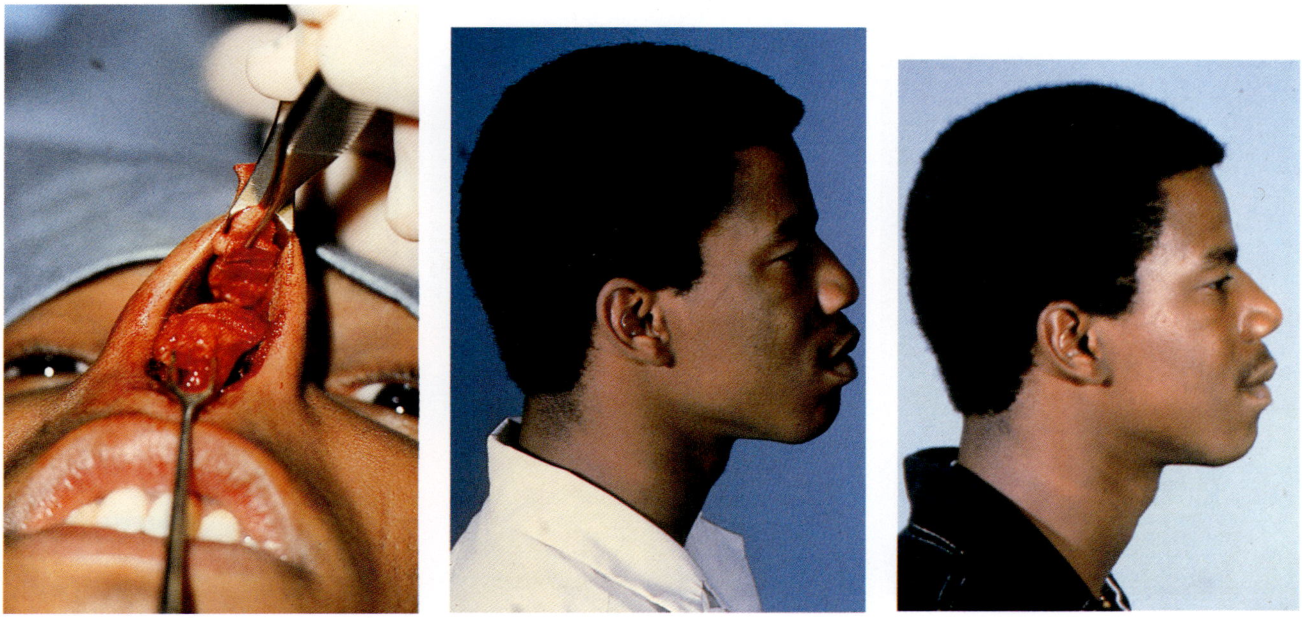 C

Figure 6. A: Intraoperative view of partial resection of rolled mesh after complete tissue incorporation. **B:** Pre-operative view of the patient in A prior to first surgery. **C:** One-year photograph following revision procedure.

and allows easily fashioning. The ends are tapered to fit precisely into the nasofrontal angle and cephalic to the tip cartilages. The importance of placing the rolled mesh on the nasal bone and beneath the soft tissue in the intercanthal region cannot be overemphasized. The implant will fibrose to the bony periosteum, and this serves (after fixation) to suspend the tip in a more rotated position. The lack of fixation and weight of solid implants will, by the action of gravity and the relentless stretch of aging tissue, result in tip ptosis. My experience with the rolled mesh first with polyamide and then Mersilene demonstrates that infection is extremely rare. I have lost only 5 in >400 nasal implants. Since soaking the mesh material with antibiotic solution, no infections have occurred and no implants have been lost in the most recent 162 cases. Three implants were removed because of patient unhappiness and two others have been modified by partial excision of portions of the implant (Fig. 6).

ADOLESCENT AND PEDIATRIC PATIENTS

Indications and types of surgery for the pediatric and adolescent African American patient parallel my philosophy for surgery in Caucasian youngsters. With an adolescent patient of adult or near adult proportions, the physical aspects and limitations are essentially like those in an adult. It must be remembered that the psychologic ramifications, however, can be profoundly different. Immature attitudes prompt a good deal of conservatism in the younger patient.

Pediatric patients are not routinely candidates for nasal surgery. As in Caucasian children, surgically correctable nasal airway problems are dealt with in a conservative manner. Septal deformities are infinitely less common in Black children than they are in African American adults when compared with Caucasians. The septum is addressed when obstruction warrants. Intervention must be directed with emphasis on preservation rather than resection. Acute nasal fractures are ideally reduced by closed techniques within the first week. If the dorsum and the septum cannot be aligned with closed methods, the bones are mobilized and aligned with a 2-mm osteotome forced along the fracture site. Hematomas, which are usually septal or alar, must be treated in a timely manner. The tissues around the

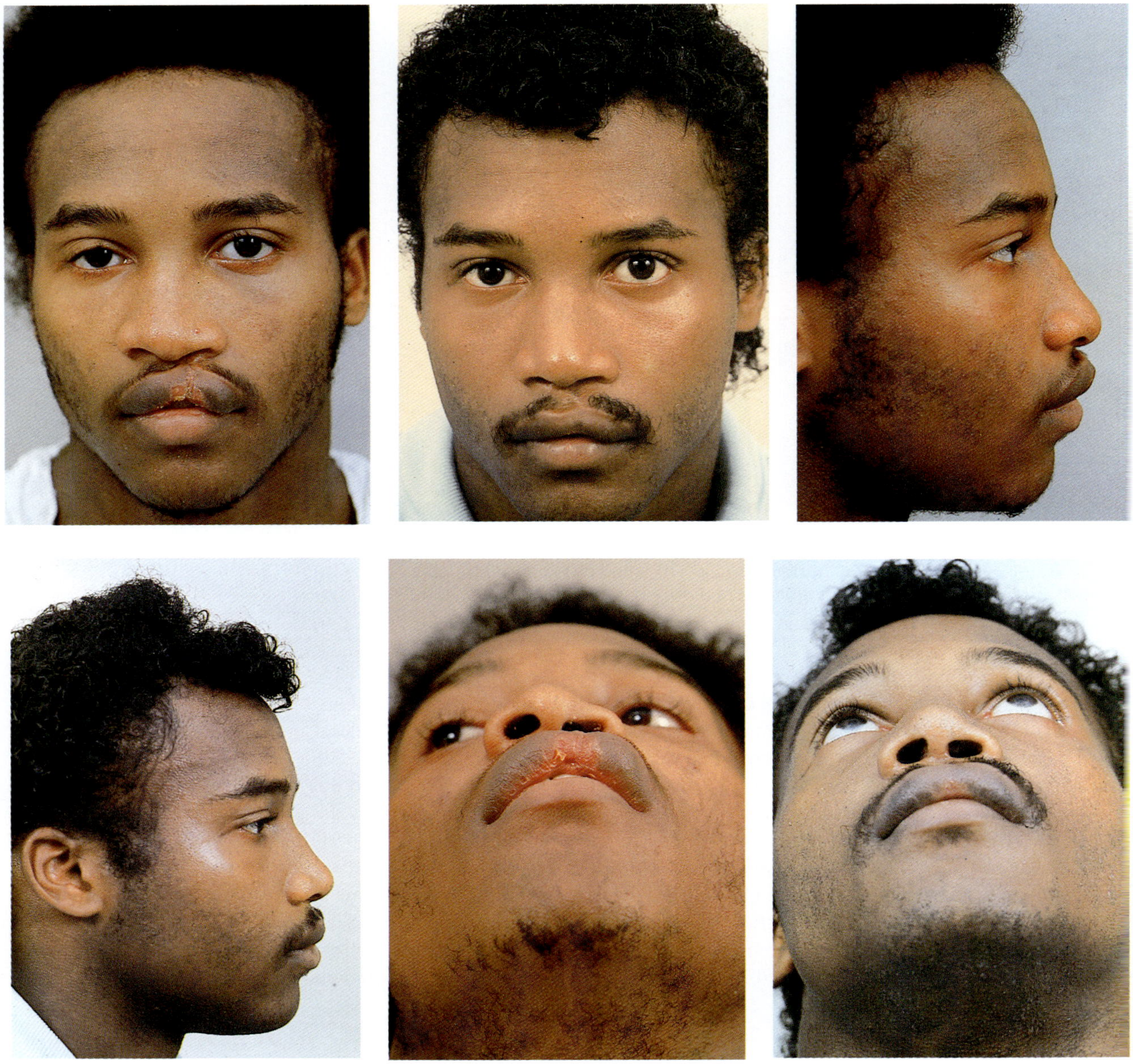

A, B C D, E F

Figure 7. A: Pre-operative view of 13-year-old. **B:** Six-year post-operative rhinoplasty, revision left lip surgery, and reduction cheiloplasty. **C:** Pre-operative submental view. **D:** Six-year submental view, same patient. **E:** Pre-operative lateral view. **F:** Six-year post-operative lateral view.

Table 4. *Maneuvers utilized in the respective 100 consecutive surgical patients of each race*

	African American (n = 100)	Caucasian (n = 100)
Columellar strut	92	9
Nasolabial implant	89	3
Tip graft	61	6
Alar base surgery	53	17
Augmentation	48	11
Lateral osteotomies	29	86
Hump resection	22	58
Meatoplasty	9	13
Septoplasty	6	58
Turbinate surgery	7	21

plasty are surgical accessibility, surgical modifications with minimal resection, and the use of autografts.

RECOMMENDED READING

Farkas L, Hreczko T, Deutsch C. Objective assessment of standard nostril types—a morphometric study. *Ann Plast Surg* 1983;11:381–389.

Kabaker SS. An approach to aesthetic rhinoplasty in the non-Caucasian nose. *Arch Otolaryngol* 1977;103: 451–467.

Kamer F, Parks M. A conservative management of the Negro nose. *Laryngoscope* 1975;85:551–558.

Matory WE Jr, Falces E. Non-Caucasian rhinoplasty: a 16-year experience. *Plast Reconstr Surg* 1986;77: 239–257.

McCurdy JA. Aesthetic rhinoplasty in the non-Caucasian. *J Dermatol Surg Oncol* 1986;12:38–44.

Meyer R. *Secondary and functional rhinoplasty: the difficult nose*. Orlando: Grune and Stratton, 1988.

Monasterio FO, Michelena J. The use of augmentation rhinoplasty techniques for the correction of the non-Caucasian nose. *Clin Plast Surg* 1988;15:57–72.

Ofodile FA, Bokhari FJ, Elliot C. The Black American nose. *Ann Plast Surg* 1993;31:209–219.

Romo T, Shapiro AL. Aesthetic reconstruction of the platyrhine nose. *Arch Otolaryngol Head Neck Surg* 1992; 118:837–841.

Santana PSM. Treatment of the Negroid nose without nasal alar excisions: a personal technique. *Ann Plast Surg* 1991;27:498–5078.

Stucker FJ. Non-Caucasian rhinoplasty and adjunctive reduction cheiloplasty. *Otolaryngol Clin North Am* 1987; 20:877–894.

Stucker FJ. A technique for the non-Caucasian nose. *Trans Pa Acad Ophthalmol Otolaryngol* 1976;82:417–422.

Ethnic Considerations in Facial Aesthetic Surgery, edited by W. Earle Matory, Jr.
Lippincott–Raven Publishers, Philadelphia © 1998.

17

Rhinoplasty in the African American Patient

W. Earle Matory, Jr.

Beauty—the adjustment of all parts proportionately so that one cannot add or subtract or change without impairing the harmony of the whole.
— Leon Battista Alberti

ANATOMIC CONSIDERATIONS

As outlined in the chapters identifying characteristics of beauty, there are wide variations in skin type and thickness and in bony and cartilaginous configurations of the nose. This is due to several factors, including country of origin and varying degrees of miscegenation. Some of the more challenging aspects of the anatomy of the African American nose are outlined. Note that each of these features is rarely present in every individual, but learning how to address each concern will make each operation a simpler one.

The skin of the nasal dorsum is thinnest at the radix bearing from 0.05 to 1 mm (Fig. 1). As the dorsal skin progresses inferiorly, the skin thickens, being thickest in the supratip and tip areas. The supratip may vary from 1 to 3 mm in thickness, with an underlying fibrofatty layer. Tip skin may be 1–5 mm in thickness. Thicker skin is often oily and sebaceous and associated with an increased incidence of cellulitis and miliasis following post-rhinoplasty splinting. For this reason, it is advisable for thicker-skinned patients to be treated prior to rhinoplasty with a combination of retinoic acid, hydroquinone, and alpha-hydroxy acids.

Beneath the thickened skin of the tip lies a broad, fan-shaped, thin, lower lateral cartilage. It is often bifid and bulbous due to a rounded curvature. Thickness of the alar skin along with an underlying fibrous layer further contributes to a broadness of the nose and a

W. E. Matory, Jr.: A New You Plastic Surgery Medical Group, Irvine, California 92714

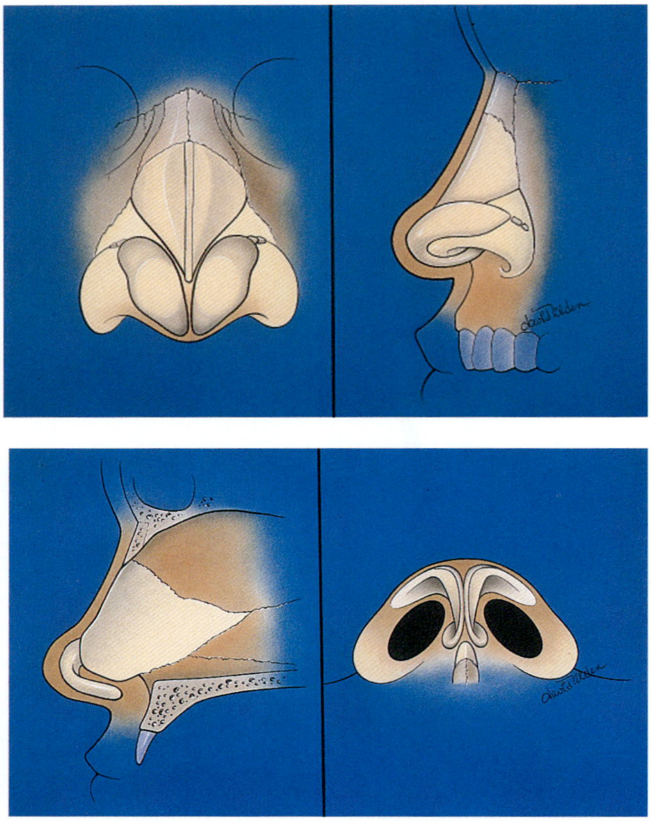

A

B

Figure 1. Nasal morphology. **A–B:** While wide variations in nasal configuration are noted in the African American, a number of commonly noted features may present challenges to the rhinoplasty surgeon. Skin is thinnest at the radix with maximal thickness up to 5–6 mm in the tip and supratip area. The strength of the underlying lower lateral cartilage is frequently unable to provide lifting support to the heavy tip skin. Along with the foreshortened columella and broad lower lateral cartilage, diastasis, and obtuse orientation of the genu, tip blunting and bifidity are often noted. Breadth of the nasal bridge is related to flared upper lateral cartilage and nasal bones, wide nasomaxillary suture lines, and diminished dorsal height. A broad prominent nasal tip and supratip may further exaggerate the deficit in height of the nasal dorsum. The medial footplate frequently does not anchor to the septum as it often does in the Caucasian, thus lessening tip support that is provided by the medial crura. Fixation of the medial footplate to the septum will strengthen tip support. Bifidity of the tip, the obtuse genu, and the foreshortened columella contribute horizontal oblong positioning of the nostrils, often accompanied by alar flaring. Septal cartilage is frequently short, 24–36 mm, concomitant with diminished nasal length. Thickness of the septum varies from patient to patient, ranging from 1 to 3 mm.

thickness of the tip. Alar attachment to the cheek tends to be wider set, often commensurate with broadly set eyes.

Dorsal width is influenced by broadly shaped and widely curved upper lateral cartilage and nasal bone. The septum tends to be short and not infrequently thin, making it a poor source for dorsal grafting and for tip support. In contrast to the Caucasian nose, the medial crura do not extend back to the septum; as a result, the nasal tip is supported by fibrous rather than cartilaginous connections. Overall thickness of the tip skin and progressive weakness of the cartilaginous and fibrous support allow the tip to drop, particularly in the aging African American.

HISTORICAL CONSIDERATIONS

Our initial experience in the African American was directed by the techniques of Josef and others as illustrated in Fig. 2. The approach advocated in the 1980s suggested the use of dorsal augmentation, lateral infracture, and lower lateral cartilage trimming along with a midcolumellar strut for tip enhancement. The latter, along with medial crural fixation, does lead to enhanced tip projection.

The major limitation in this approach is the cephalic rotation of the nasal tip and resultant foreshortening of the nose, which are an unfortunate sequelae for the African American nose (Fig. 3). A similar approach in a 30-year-old patient demonstrates the same phenomena (Fig. 4). In addition, cephalad rotation and nasal foreshortening contribute to an exaggerated supratip fullness as a result of the corrugation of supratip skin.

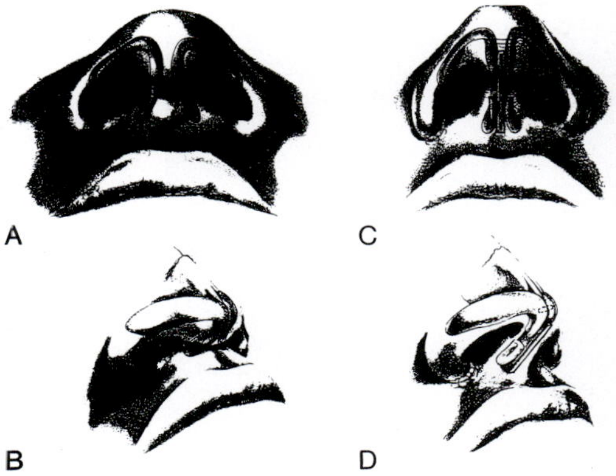

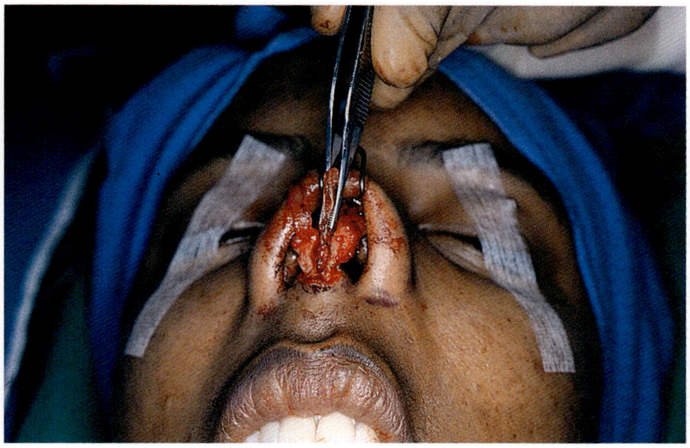

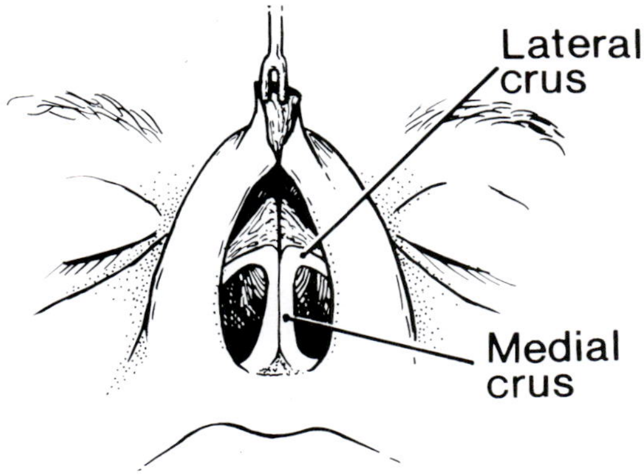

Figure 2. Medial crural fixation, previously advocated, is no longer advised, due to the resultant reduction in nasal length caused by the obligatory cephalad rotation that is effected by medial crural fixation.

TIP DEFATTING

During the 1970s and 1980s efforts were made to improve sculpturing of the nasal tip and supratip areas by defatting (Fig. 5). Aggressive resection of lower and lateral cartilage along with subdermal defatting may be beneficial only in the occasional patient. More often, these techniques result in significant post-operative edema lasting 18–24 months, countering the goals of tip refinement. More importantly, the problem of skin thickness has not been addressed using a subdermal defatting technique.

We therefore suggest that avoidance of aggressive defatting. If necessary, simple removal of fat that is adherent to the alar cartilage, once it has been exposed, is appropriate. Avoid subdermal defatting to minimize prolonged swelling. Tip defatting, particularly when used with the open technique, diminishes arterial and venous circulation of the tip and supratip area. Lymphatic congestion is also compromised, and as a result, swelling may persist for as long as 12–18 months. Some swelling may not resolve. While these techniques have been described as being effective in the past, the benefits achieved are far outweighed by the potential risk.

OPERATIVE TECHNIQUE

The choice of an external versus internal approach in the African American nose is perhaps best selected based on the surgeon's experience. Having been trained with the closed approach, I have used the open approach for ~8 years. Having the knowledge of both exposures, I prefer internal incisions. I explain to patients that we will try to perform the

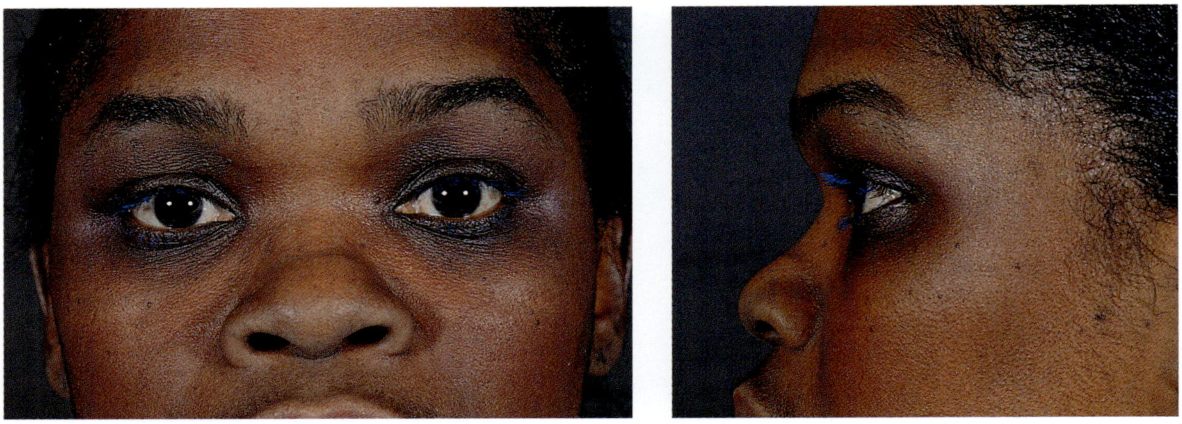

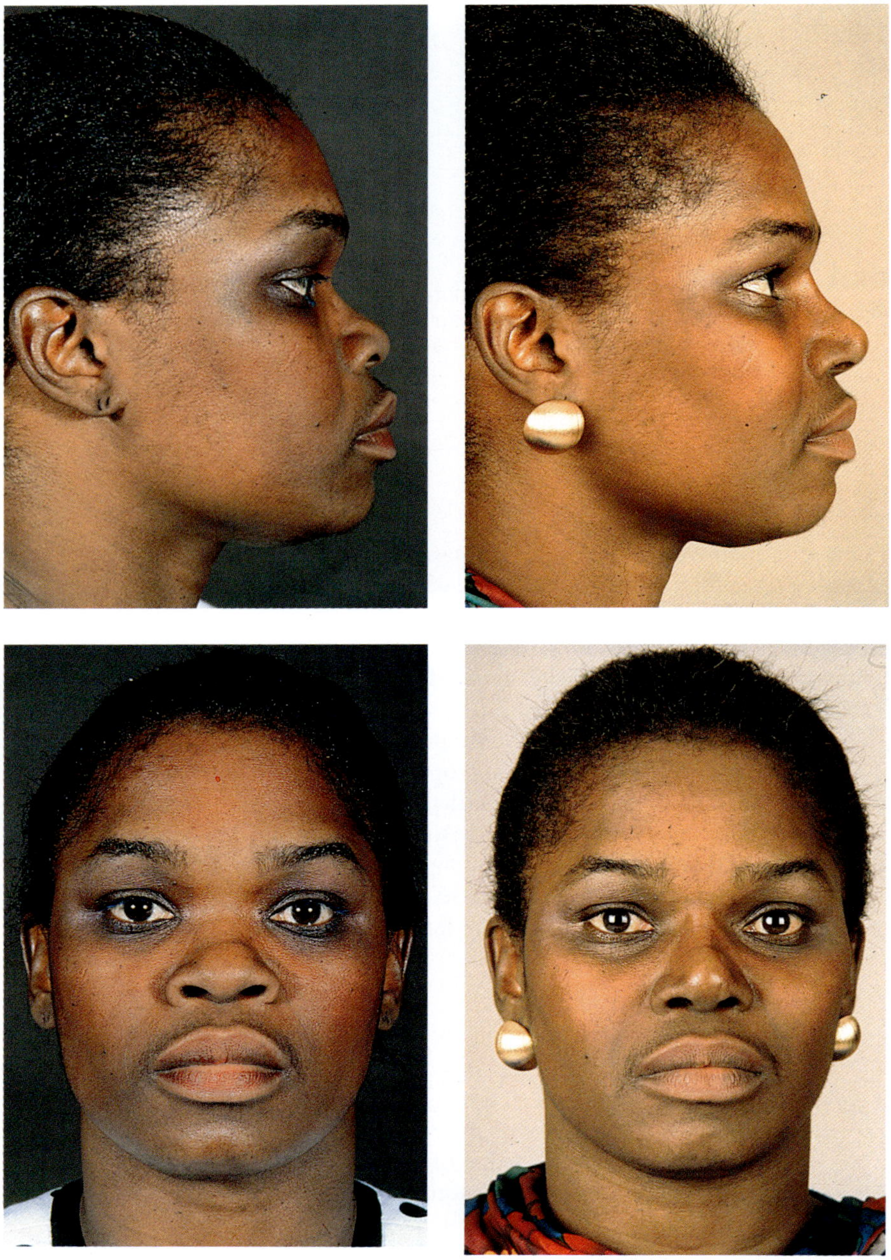

Figure 3. This 26-year-old woman presented for softening of her nasal tip and lessening of the width of her nasal bridge.

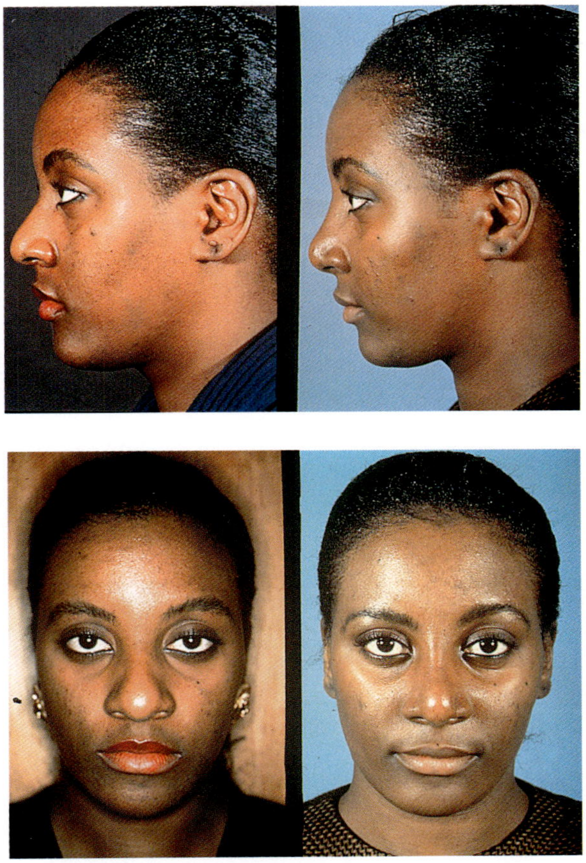

Figure 4. Midline position of the genu also compromises tip definition and increases supratip fullness as a result of cephalic rotation of the tip.

procedure without external incisions on the columella unless it becomes necessary to optimize the result. Thus, one is not obligated to adhere to one single approach.

Endonasal Approach

Infracartilaginous incisions optimize exposure to the lateral genu (Fig. 6A). A transfixion incision allows further mobilization of the crura (Fig. 6B). A separate intercartilaginous incision further mobilizes the lower lateral cartilage (Fig. 6C).

Cephalic Resection

With symmetrical exposure, cephalic resection can be optimized (Fig. 6D). In the female medial cephalic exposure may extend as far laterally as the extent of a bulbous curve. In males it is far more appropriate to be more conservative in limiting the amount of cephalic resection. Bulbosity may persist, but this is minimized with full-mobilization intercrurally and the subsequent medial rotation of the lateral crura.

Septal Harvest

A subperichondrial dissection is performed through the transfixion incision. Septal cartilage is harvested, preserving 5 mm dorsally and inferiorly. The thickness, shape, firmness,

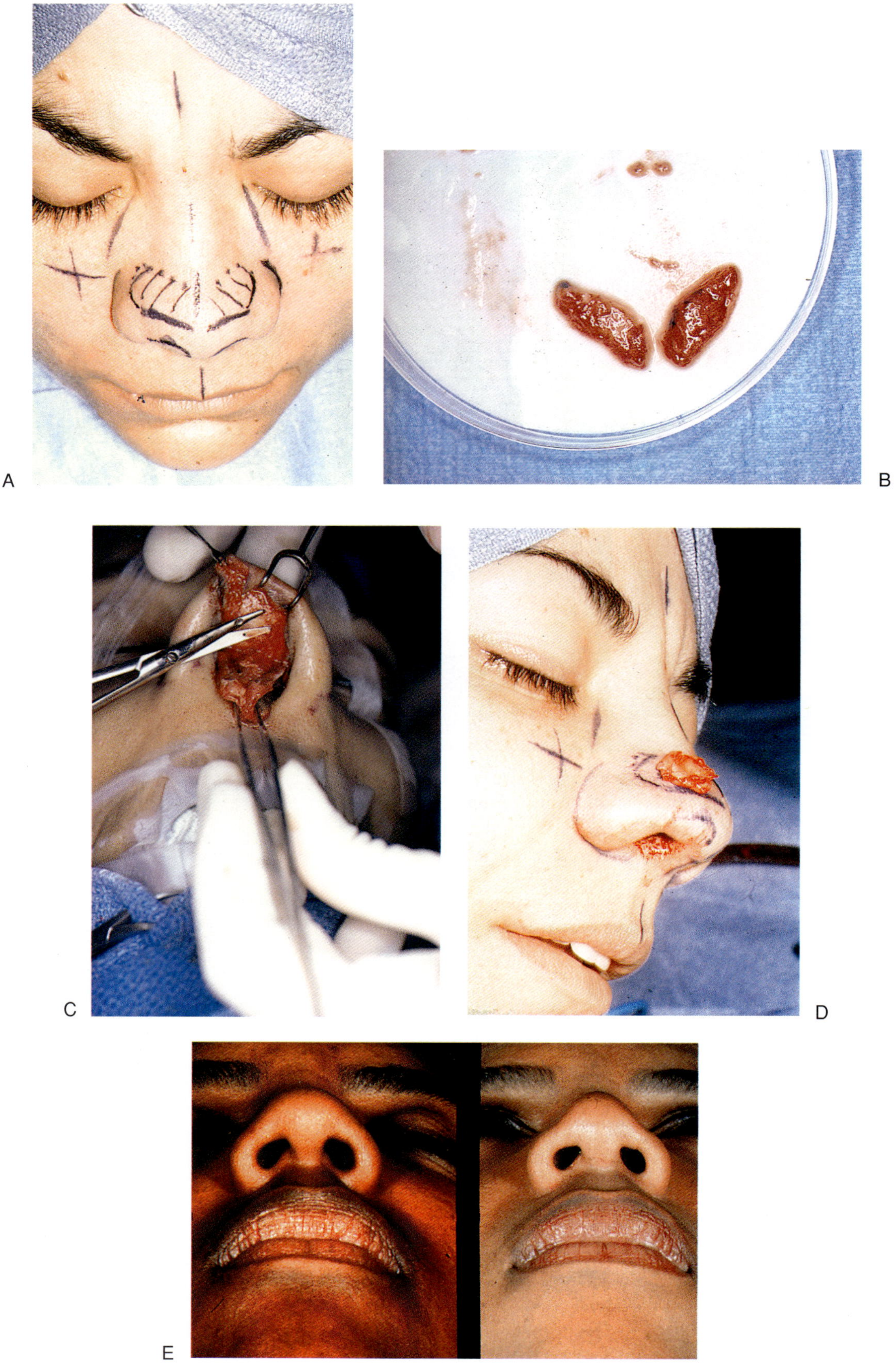

A B C D E

Figure 5. A–E: Tip defatting, previously advocated, is ineffective in defining the tip and supratip in the presence of thick skin. Aggressive defatting contributes to prolonged edema and minimal improvement in tip definition as shown 18 months post-operatively (E). Only limited tip narrowing results from tip defatting. We advise that the surgeon trim only the fatty film overlying and between the lower lateral cartilages.

Figure 6. The endonasal approach. **A:** Infracartilaginous and transfixion incisions allow access to the medial and lateral crura and the septum. **B–C:** For full mobilization of the alar cartilages, the two incisions may be interconnected. **D:** Cephalic rim resection must include the bulbous portion of the tip. Conservative resection is ideal, especially in males. **E–F:** A strut is then affixed to the septum for proximal stability and tip lengthening. **G–H:** Intercrural fixation provides anterior fixation and softens crural diastasis and tip redefinition.

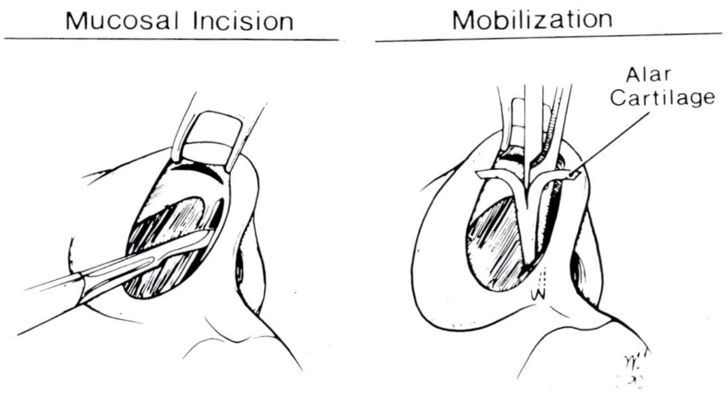

A, B

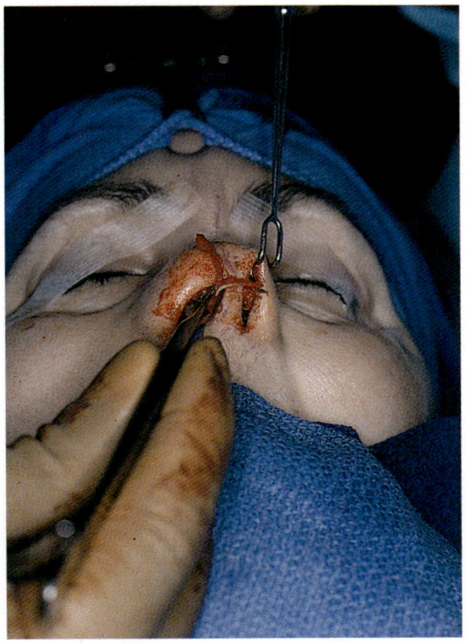

C

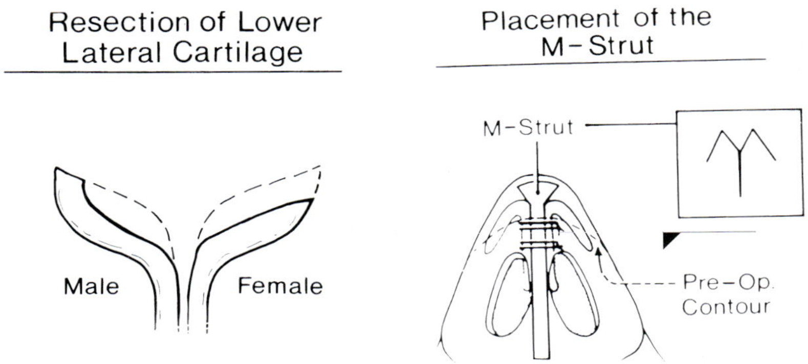

D, E

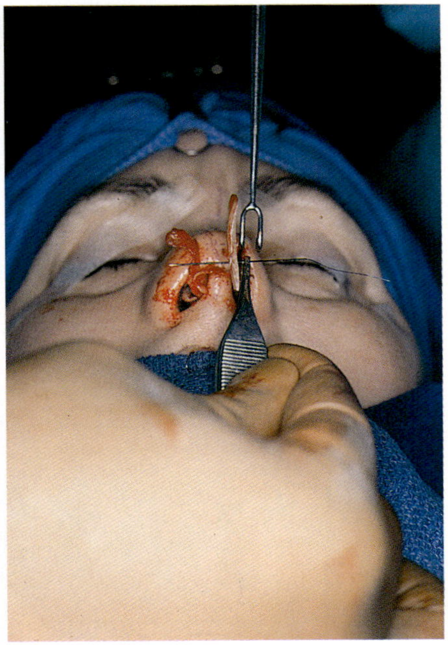

F

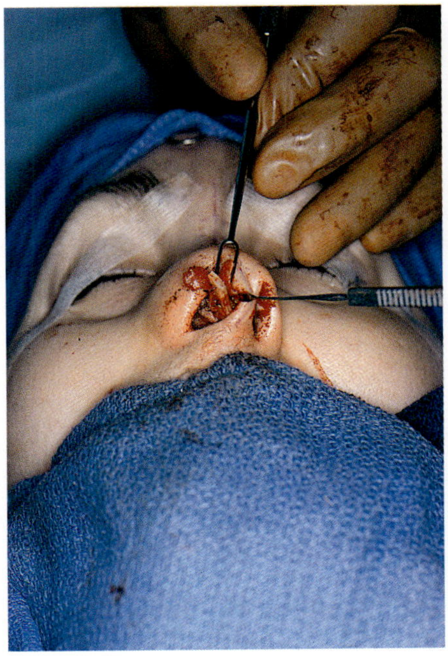

G

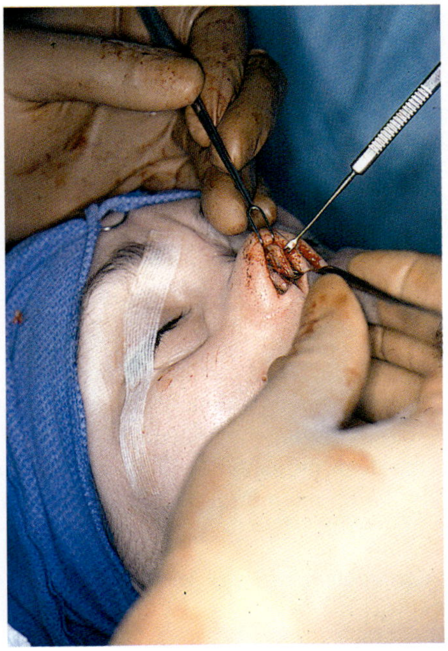

H

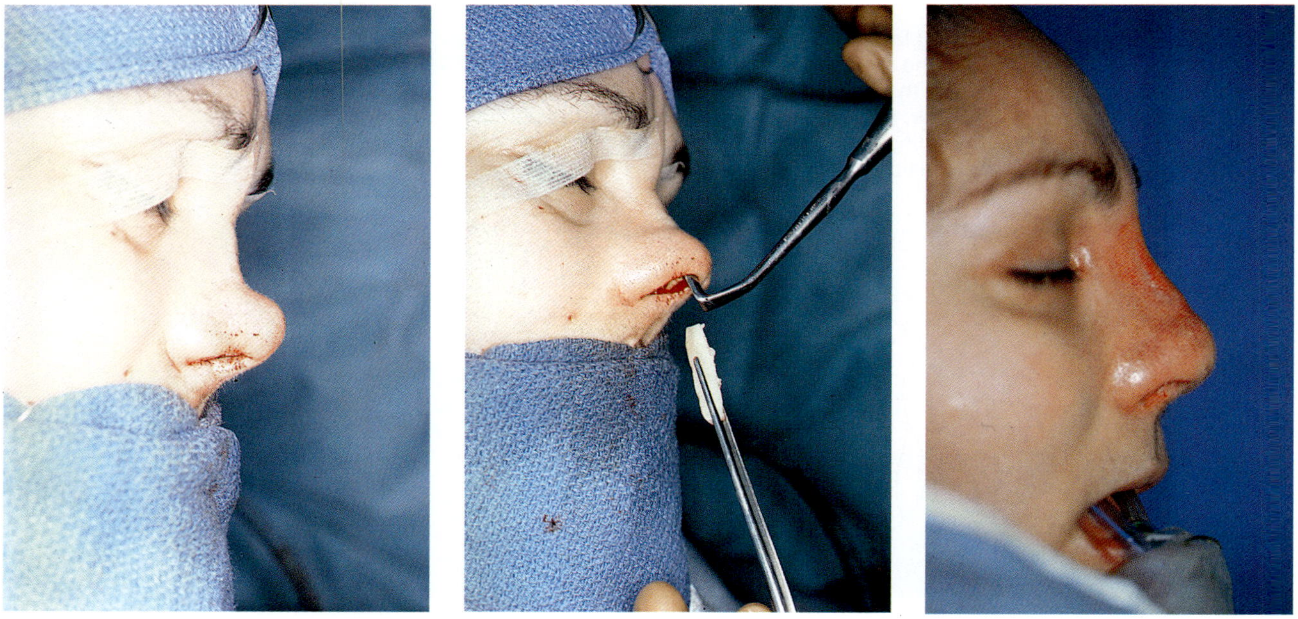

I, J K

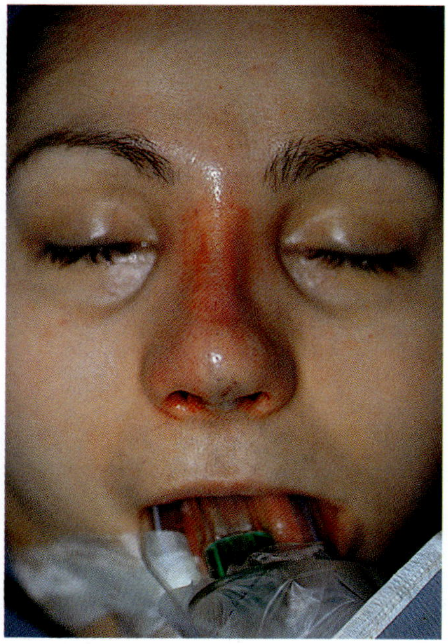

L

Figure 6 *(continued).* **I–K:** Dorsal augmentation is most appropriate for the saddle nose configuration. **L:** In the occasional patient, 30–35 mm × 3–5 mm thick long strips of septal cartilage can be used to improve dorsal contours.

and ability of the septal cartilage to support the tip and dorsum are defined. For the septal cartilage to be deemed adequate for one or multilayered dorsal strips, a septal tip strut must be 35–40 mm for the dorsum and 22–30 mm for the septal-to-tip strut. The strut is placed on either side of the septum with its vertical dimension shaped to 4–6 mm. Tip contouring is left until after intercrural positioning has been assessed.

Tip Enhancement with the M-Strut

Optimal tip positioning is assessed by trial-and-error rotation of the intercrural strut (Fig. 6E–H). Its position creates an M configuration that is formed by the genu and the strut, thus leading to the description of this design as an M-strut. Once two mattress sutures with 4-0

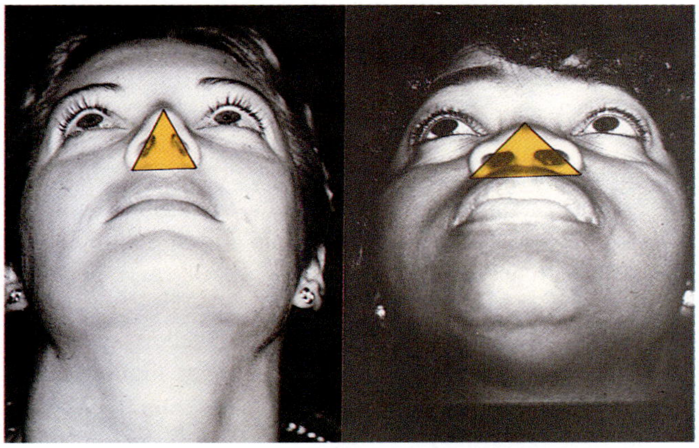

Figure 7. Alar flaring is defined as the amount of alar rim that extends lateral to the alar attachment to the cheek. The patient on the left exhibits very little if any flaring in sharp comparison with the model on the right. (From Matory WE, *Plastic Reconstructive Surgery*, Little Brown & Co.)

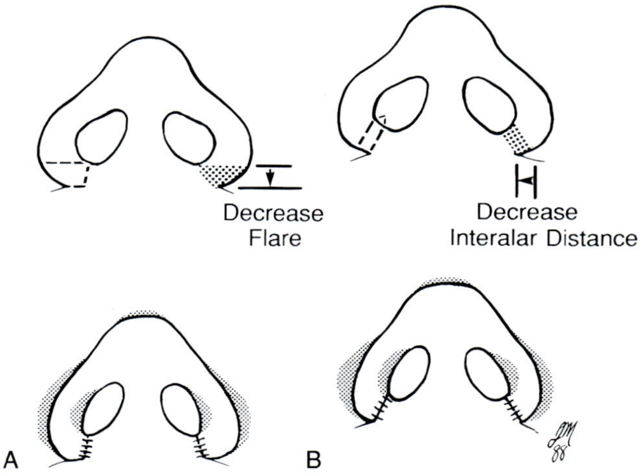

Figure 8. Flare reduction **(A)** can be achieved only with a vertical resection of the ala. Interalar reduction is minimally achieved with alar base resection (Weir) **(B)**.

polypropylene on a straight needle are positioned to secure the M complex, the actual height and length are determined by the strut's position with the septum. A Keefe needle can be used to temporarily affix septal and intercrural position. The strut length relative to the genu is marked and an additional millimeter of anterior height is advanced to encounter subsequent gravitational forces. Two mattress sutures are placed to secure the graft to the septum. If the septal graft is particularly thick, it can be split for a length of ~5–7 mm so that it can flank the septum. Two 4-0 mattress sutures are placed with a straight Keith needle. The septal support of this graft significantly minimizes late tip drooping that is promoted by the heavy nasal tip. Additional grafts may be placed inferior or parallel to the medial crura as described by Sheen, Hoefflin, and Gunter. Thick skin often compromises detail that may be achieved with onlay grafts.

By supporting the medial footplates, additional tip support and advancement can be achieved in addition to increased visibility of onlay grafts. Mattress sutures are used to approximate the medical footplate diastasis. Approximation to the septum can be adjusted to optimize tip height.

Alar Rim Sculpturing

In addressing the alar rim, it is crucial that one understand two distinct concepts: those of alar width and flaring. The aesthetic ideal in the Caucasian is such that the triangle formed by the tip and the alar attachments to the cheek is a nearly equilateral triangle, with the anterior height being slightly greater than the base (Fig. 7). The interalar distance in the African American often exceeds that of the tip height, particularly due to the presence of a shortened columella. That portion of the alar rim that extends lateral to the alar attachment to the cheek is considered flaring, as opposed to the wider interalar distance, which contributes to the breadth of the nose. Resections of the alar rim that decrease vertical height of the alar will diminish flaring (Fig. 8A). Resections that diminish transverse width of the alar rim will have a modest effect on interalar distance (Fig. 8B).

ADDRESSING FLARING

Let us spend a few moments outlining different strategies to address flaring. Alar base resections as defined by Weir allow a reduction in alar excess, but there are several limitations. One is a difficulty in determining the amount of alar rim to resect (Fig. 9). Second, asymmetries pre-operatively and therefore post-operatively are quite common (Fig. 10). Third, over-reduction leads to alar rim and tip deformities along with an unnatural appearance of the nose (Fig. 11).

Alar Base Resection

Photographs should be studied pre-operatively to identify asymmetries. The amount of alar to resect is determined (Fig. 12) by assessing the point *a* where the resection would lead to a straight-line alar rim. In that there are no straight lines in nature, adding 2 mm to the point that would straighten the alar rim will achieve a nice, natural, gentle curve. This approach also minimizes asymmetry.

It is important to preserve a 1-mm strip of alar rim attached to the base/cheek so that appropriate dermal and epidermal approximation can be completed. Improper alignment may result in unattractive or hypertrophic scars (Fig. 13). It is my personal feeling that the potential problems associated with alar base resection far outweigh the benefits achieved.

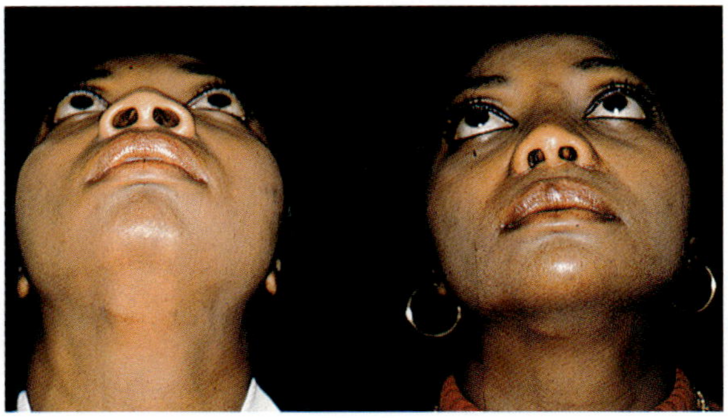

Figure 9. Alar base resection (Weir) was performed on this 32-year-old woman complaining of excessive flaring. (Courtesy of Matory WE and Falces E, *Plastic and Reconstructive Surgery*, Little Brown & Co.)

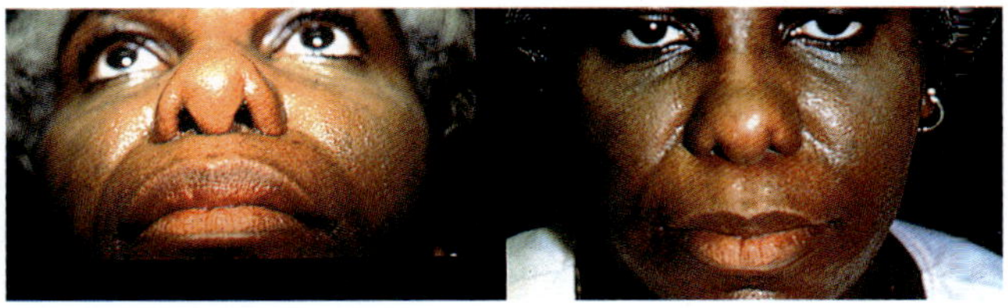

Figure 11. Over-resection of the alar base leads to tell-tale deformities that are irreparable. (Courtesy of Matory WE and Falces E, *Plastic and Reconstructive Surgery*, Little Brown & Co.)

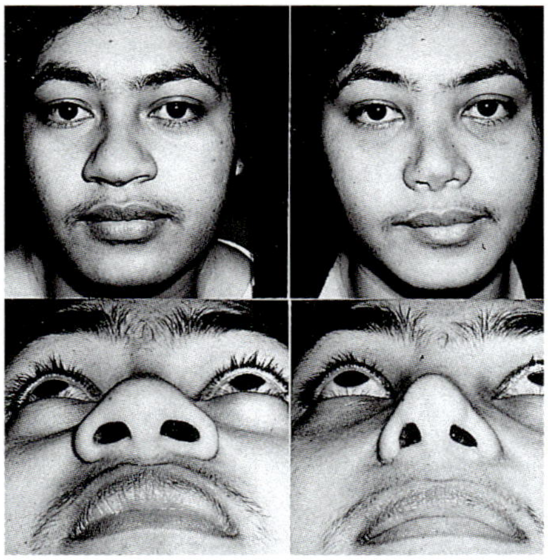

Figure 10. If pre-operative asymmetries are not identified, they will persist or magnify after surgery. (Courtesy of Matory WE and Falces E, *Plastic and Reconstructive Surgery*, Little Brown & Co.)

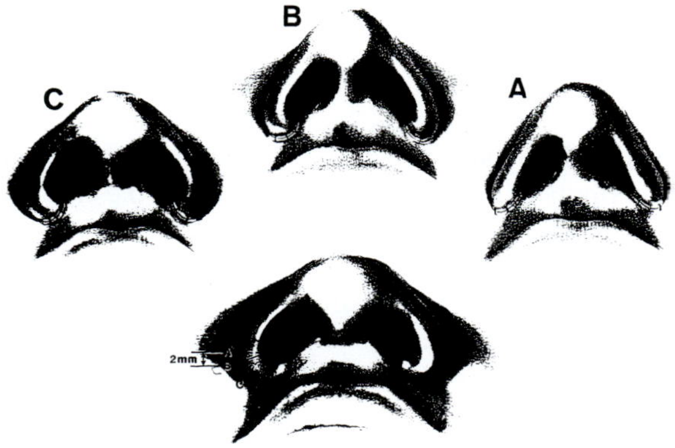

Figure 12. Determining the ideal amount of alar base resection. By discerning the resection that would straighten the alar **(A)** and adding 2 mm, a gentle natural curve is achieved **(B)**. Undersection leaves persistent flare **(C)**. (Courtesy of Matory WE and Falces E, *Plastic and Reconstructive Surgery*, Little Brown & Co.)

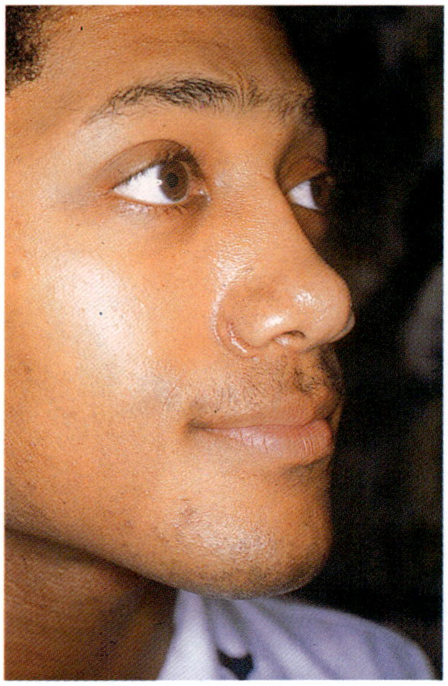

A

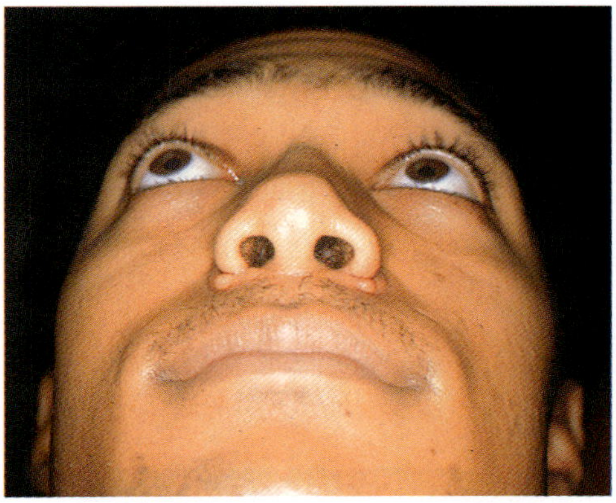

B

Figure 13. A–B: Hypertrophic or keloid scarring is rare, but this risk can be avoided by not using alar base incisions or by preserving a 1-mm strip of alar rim along the alar base. (Courtesy of Patrick McManamin, M.D.)

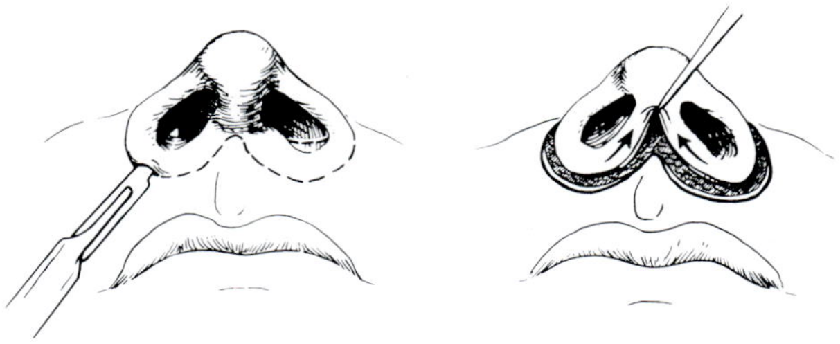

A

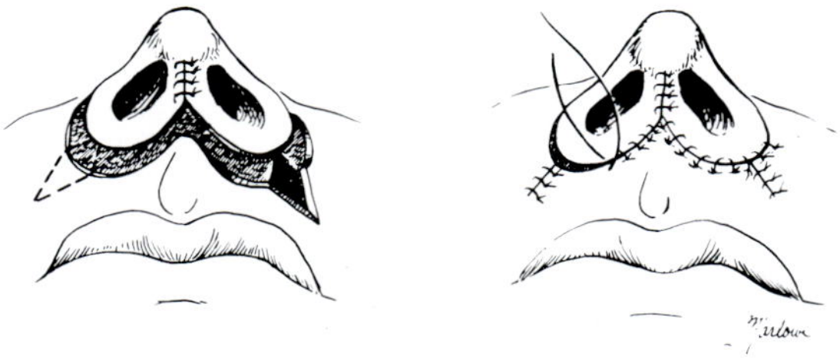

B

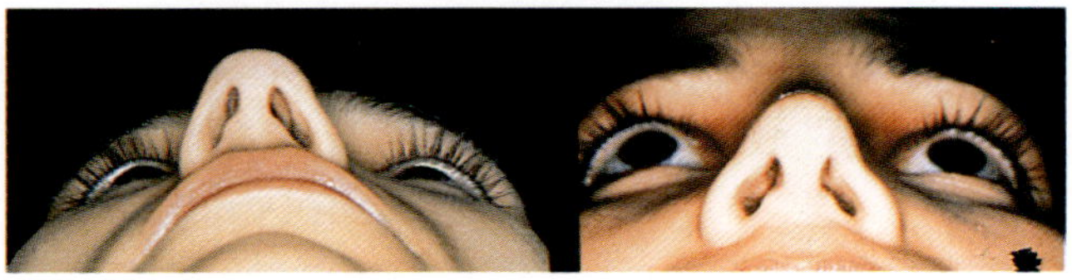

C

Figure 14. Alar sill advancement can be used to achieve modest flare reduction. The alar sill and base are mobilized **(A)** and rotated medially **(B–C)**. Excess along the nasolabial fold is resection. (Courtesy of Matory WE and Falces E, *Plastic and Reconstructive Surgery*, Little Brown & Co.)

Alar Sill Advancement

Alar sill advancement techniques as described by deAvelar allow reduction of flaring and interalar width simultaneously (Fig. 14). The alar base and lateral rim are fully mobilized and centralized with resultant advancement of the columella in a V-Y fashion. A small wedge is resected from the nasolabial fold to eliminate dog ears. This technique is most effective in the patient with mild to moderate flaring and/or minimally widened interalar width. The technique is rather extensive and potentially problematic with regard to potential scarring and likely worsening of edema.

Preferred Technique for Flare Reduction

The technique that I prefer to use for reduction of alar flaring is tip enhancement with or without a vertical resection of the alar rim (Fig. 15). The broad and flared ala is significantly

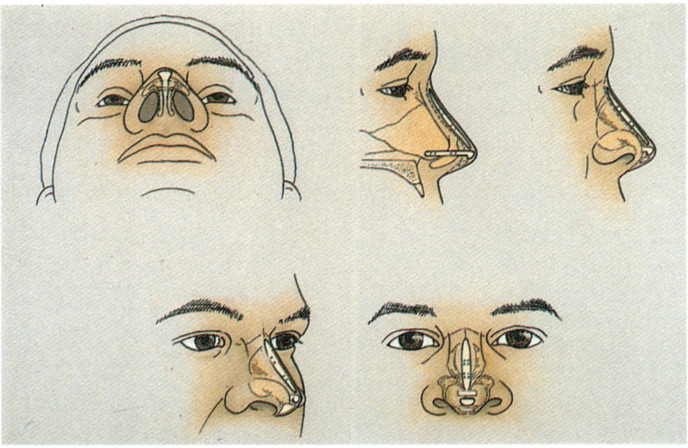

Figure 15. Ideal management of increased alar width utilizes tip lengthening along with height enhancement. By raising the tip, alar rim excess is lessened, routinely eliminating the need for alar base resection.

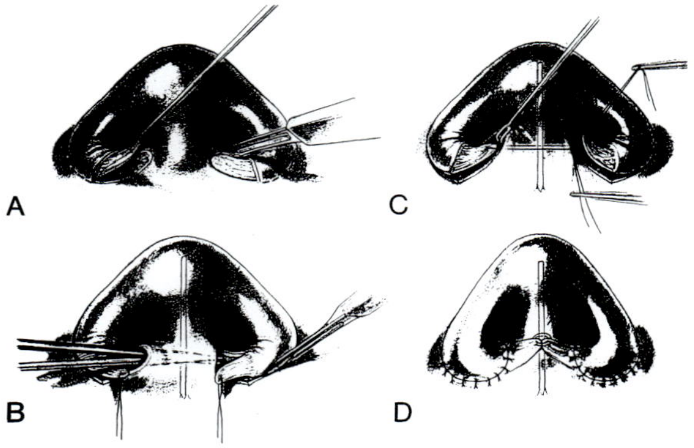

Figure 16. **(A–D)**: Interalar reduction is best addressed by deepithelializing the alar sill along with medial rotation and fixation to the septum. Asymmetry of the alar rim can be adjusted as needed.

A

B

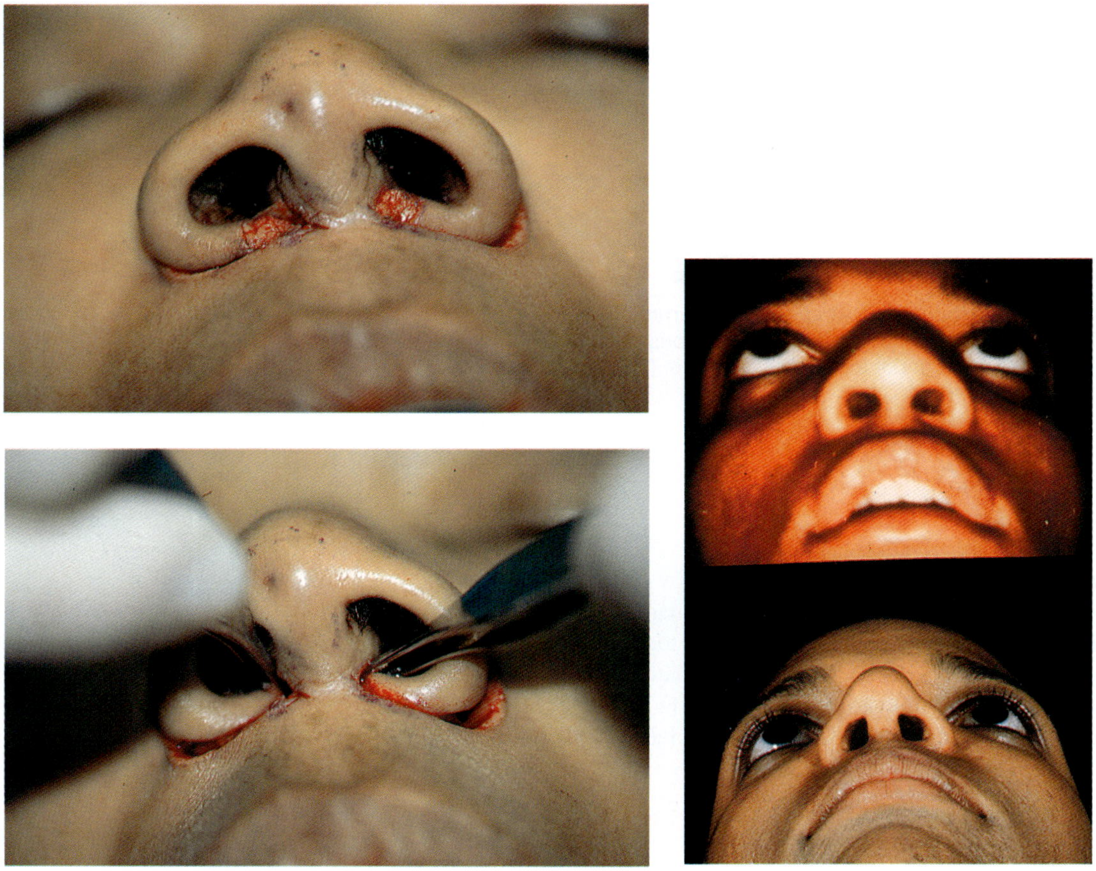

C

Figure 17. Reduction of the interalar distance can be accomplished with mattress sutures that fixate the alar sill to the septum. Once the sill is mobilized **(A)** and deepithelialized **(B)**, suture fixation effectively narrows interalar distance **(C)**.

improved by enhancing tip position. Central advancement of the tip decreases the amount of alar flaring and improves the relative dimensions of the tip versus the width of the basal triangle. When ideal tip height is achieved with the M-strut, the degree of alar flaring as well as the perceived pre-operative interalar width are significantly diminished.

Use of grafts inferior to the genu is not adequate to give long-term support to the often thick nasal tip in the African American. With time, tips with unfixated graft support tend to drop and thus are not advised.

Adjustments in Interalar Width

The interalar cinch procedure as described by Millard is most effective in reducing interalar width. The alar sill advancement of deAvelar can be used as well, with noted limitations of excessive swelling and scarring.

A closed or open approach can be used. When a mildly increased alar width is noted, cinching of sutures can be made, grasping the deep fibrofatty tissue within the alar base on each side. The 4-0 Keith needle is passed through the septum, along a medial rotation of the alar base. Separate sutures can also be used on each side, particularly if there is a notable degree of asymmetry. Small stab incisions can be used for ligation and/or burying the knot.

Wide interalar distances are best addressed with alar sill skin resection, medial advancement, and septal fixation. A 15 scalpel is used to incise along the alar base attachment to the cheek and beneath the nostril sill (Fig. 16). Medial attachment of the alar sill at the footplates is released, thus fully mobilizing the lateral and basal nose (Fig. 17). The medial attachments are advanced to determine the ideal amount of rotation. This point is marked for deepithelialization. A 4-0 Proline suture on a Keith needle is used to approximate the deepithelialized dermis to the septum. One suture is used to capture both medial segments and the septum (cinched and tied).

While we have found this technique to be effective in many patients, I now feel that it is necessary in only a few (Fig. 18). If appropriate tip enhancement is completed, the need for

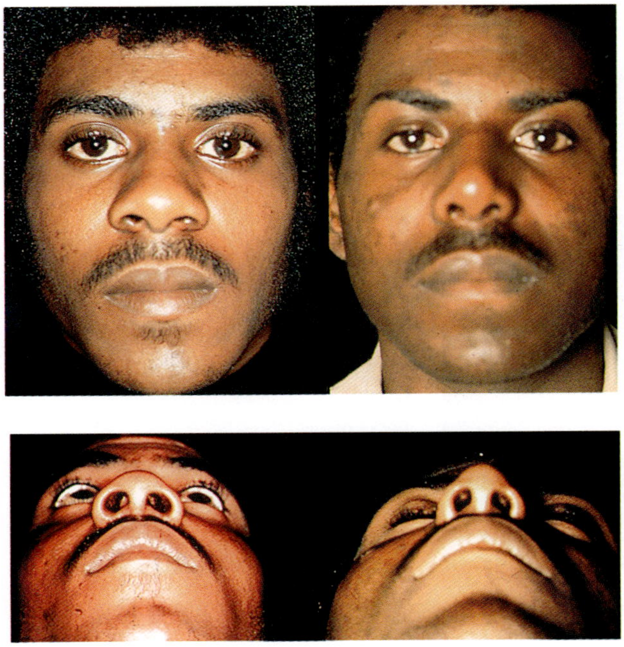

Figure 18. Tip enhancement along with alar base resection and interalar reduction *(top)* achieved the outcome 7 years later *(bottom)*. (Courtesy of Matory WE and Falces E, *Plastic and Reconstructive Surgery*, Little Brown & Co.)

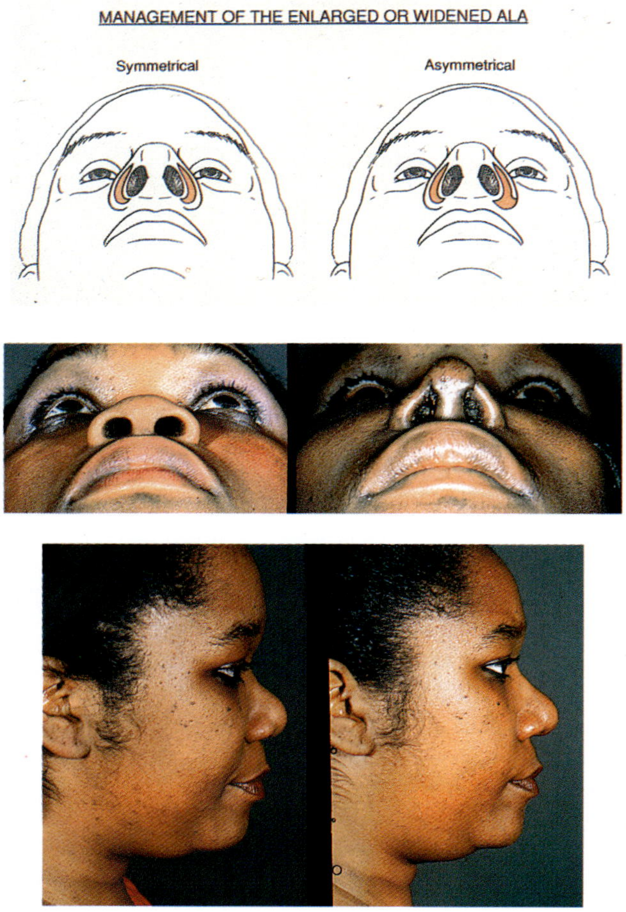

Figure 19. Following tip enhancement *(top)*, excess alar rim width can be reduced by resecting a vertical ellipse of skin and subcutaneous tissue. Tip enhancement without alar resection *(middle and bottom)* is illustrated in this woman with a blunt bifid tip. Alar rim thickness and/or asymmetrical length can be addressed by resecting skin and dermis from the rim. Alar rim scars heal with minimal visibility.

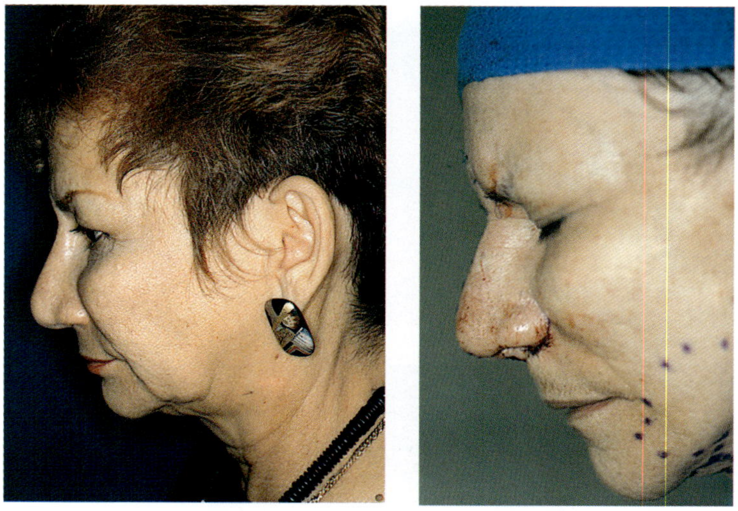

Figure 20. In my experience, grafts that are placed in soft tissues are unable to support thick skin for extended periods, ultimately resulting in a dividing tip.

alar base resection or for interalar width reduction is minimized or eliminated. Following tip enhancement, any excess alar rim width is most easily and naturally adjusted by excising a vertical elliptical strip of skin and subcutaneous tissue (Fig. 19). A simple running cutaneous 5-0 Proline approximates epithelial edges with minimal scar visibility (Fig. 17C). Adjustments can be made for asymmetry as needed.

Some authors (e.g., Hoefflin and Gunter) advocate cartilage grafts placed in subcutaneous tissue to yield tip support. This technique can be very effective but short lived in my experience. The nearness of tip skin overwhelms soft tissue and sometimes cartilaginous support, resulting in loss of tip height (Fig. 20).

In summary, alar adjustments to flaring and interalar width are best made by tip enhancement with or without vertical alar rim resection (Fig. 21). The latter achieves an improved relationship of the dorsum and nasal tip and typically diminishes the relative breadth of the basal triangle. When possible, one should avoid alar base resection or interalar reduction techniques to minimize scarring, asymmetry, and unnatural outcomes (Fig. 22). The thickened alar rim can be addressed with a vertical skin resection along with the removal of a wedge of underlying fibrous tissue. If asymmetry of the length of the alar exists, a transverse resection can be added, leaving medial and lateral skin intact. The resultant closures are natural, without deformities that are commonly noted after Weir resection.

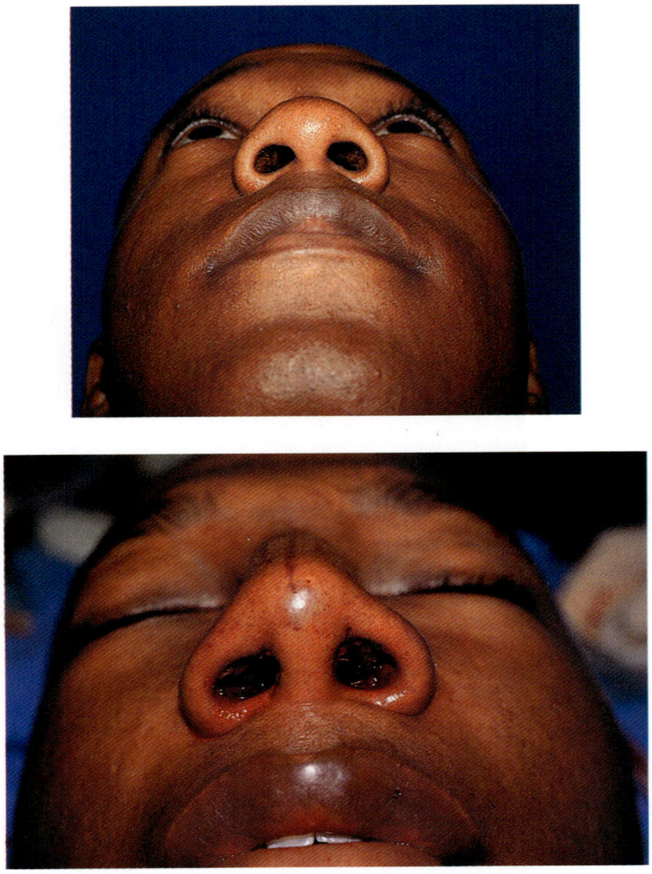

Figure 21. Tip enhancement nicely softens flaring in the male. Males are particularly disfigured by an unnatural alar base resection.

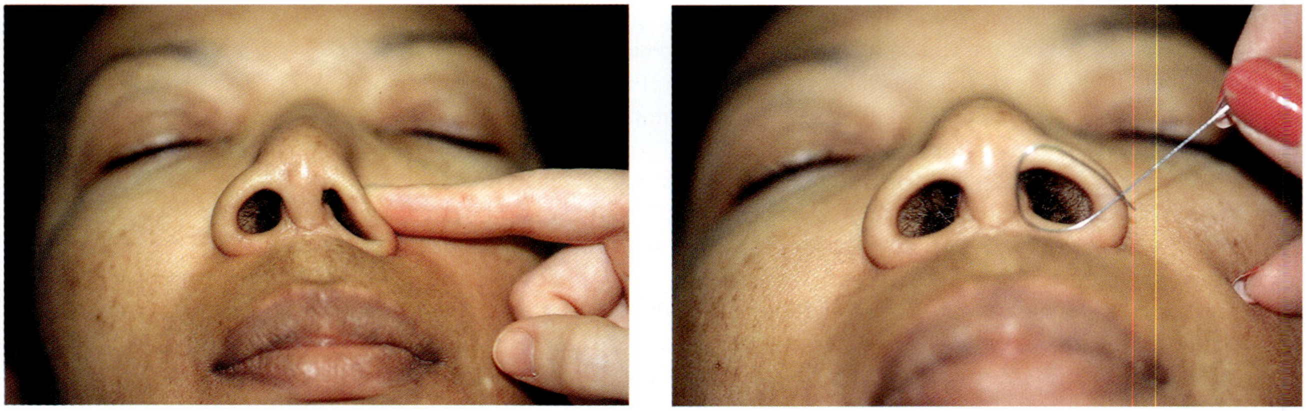

Figure 22. Prior to all alar base surgery, one must evaluate potential damaging effects on airway and symmetry. A nose template is made of one nostril and is flipped to assess the opposite side.

DORSAL AUGMENTATION

Alloplastic and autogenous grafts are frequently necessary to supplement the depressed nasal bridge commonly seen in the African American. L-shaped grafts used in the distant past have been notoriously problematic, particularly with frequent deviation or extrusion (Fig. 23).

Alloplastic Grafts

The alloplastic of choice in my practice is polytetrafluoroethylene (PTFE). Polytetrafluoroethylene is easily carved and, when implanted, is well tolerated by human tissues. As demonstrated by extensive burn experience, exposures routinely heal with topical dressings and implant removal is rarely necessary. At the present time, this is the ideal option for dorsal augmentation for my practice (Fig. 24).

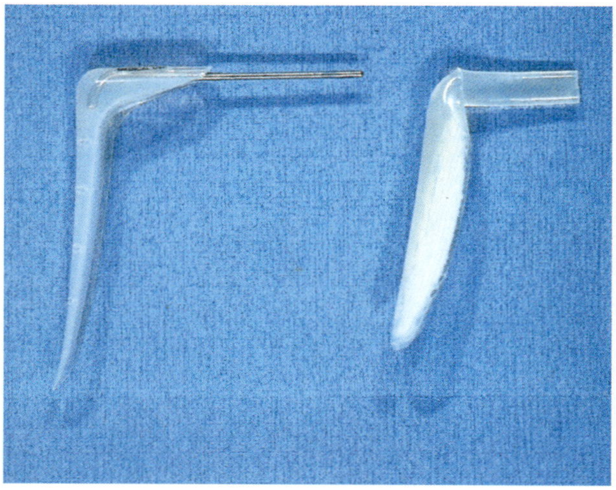

A

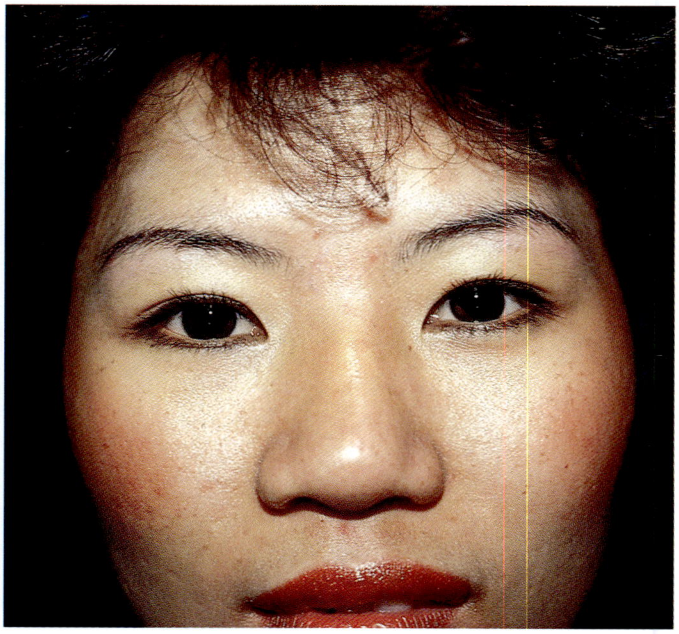

B

Figure 23. Dorsal augmentation. L-shaped struts do not correlate anatomically **(A)** and are prone to displacement **(B)**.

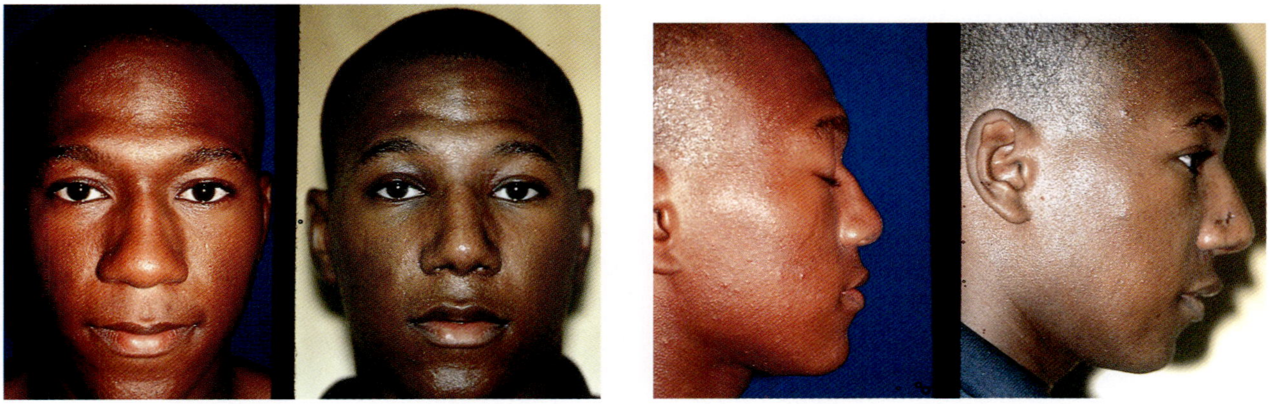

Figure 24. In my experience, among alloplastic implants, a custom-contoured polytetrafluoroethylene implant yields the most consistent and aesthetic results as noted 2 years after augmentation and tip enhancement.

Autologous Grafts

A number of autologous graft options have been utilized, with each having limitations. Conchal cartilage, even when crushed or with the utilization of a relatively straight segment of ear cartilage, has a strong tendency to curl and is frequently not long enough for the 28- to 32-mm deficits in the African American dorsum. As an example, conchal cartilage was used by a very talented rhinoplasty surgeon from another institution (Fig. 25) and has resulted in a graft of inadequate length and curling dorsal irregularity.

Septal cartilage can be effective, but its use is frequently limited because of the smaller size and thickness of septal cartilage in the African American. In general, the septal cartilage is somewhat foreshortened (20–25 mm) and thin (1–2 mm) (Fig. 26). Ethmoid bone can be used along with the cartilage, but somewhat problematically with regard to bony fixation. Only one layer of dorsal graft can typically be harvested. The need for dorsal augmentation frequently requires two or three layers of septal graft. Patch grafting or supplementation with cephalic alar trim may be necessary.

Temporal fascia is a reasonable alternative, particularly in association with a forehead lift or facelift procedure. The fascia is tubularized, and all free ends are secured so that the graft is not spread when placed within the dorsal pocket (Fig. 27). Results are shown 18 months after dorsal augmentation using temporal fascia (Fig. 28). Temporal fascia can resorb within the first 3–6 months, as noted in this patient 5 months after dorsal augmentation using temporal fascia (Fig. 29).

Rib cartilage graft was used most commonly during the initial phases of my practice. Incisions are typically made along the medial inframammary crease and measure 4–5 cm in length (Fig. 30A). The straightest portion of the rib is selected, and minimal carving should be performed to minimize resultant warping. With a 40-mm length, three separate grafts are harvested: two dorsal grafts and an M-strut that has a comma-shaped or triangular segment for the nasal tip (Fig. 30B). These techniques have been used with and without perichondrial stripping, and most frequently the cartilage maintains its midline position (Figs. 31–34). However, it is not unusual to see some short- or long-term warping and/or resorption, necessitating subsequent dorsal graft replacement.

The extra dorsal graft can also be used to replace an intraoperative fracture of the M-strut or dorsal graft. Excess cartilage can be replaced in the donor site, or it can be banked in the temporal scalp for easy retrieval. It can also be used for dorsal tip grafts. Tip grafts under thickened tip and supratip skin may lose definition, but in the medium-thickness or thin-skinned patient, tip grafts can be very effective.

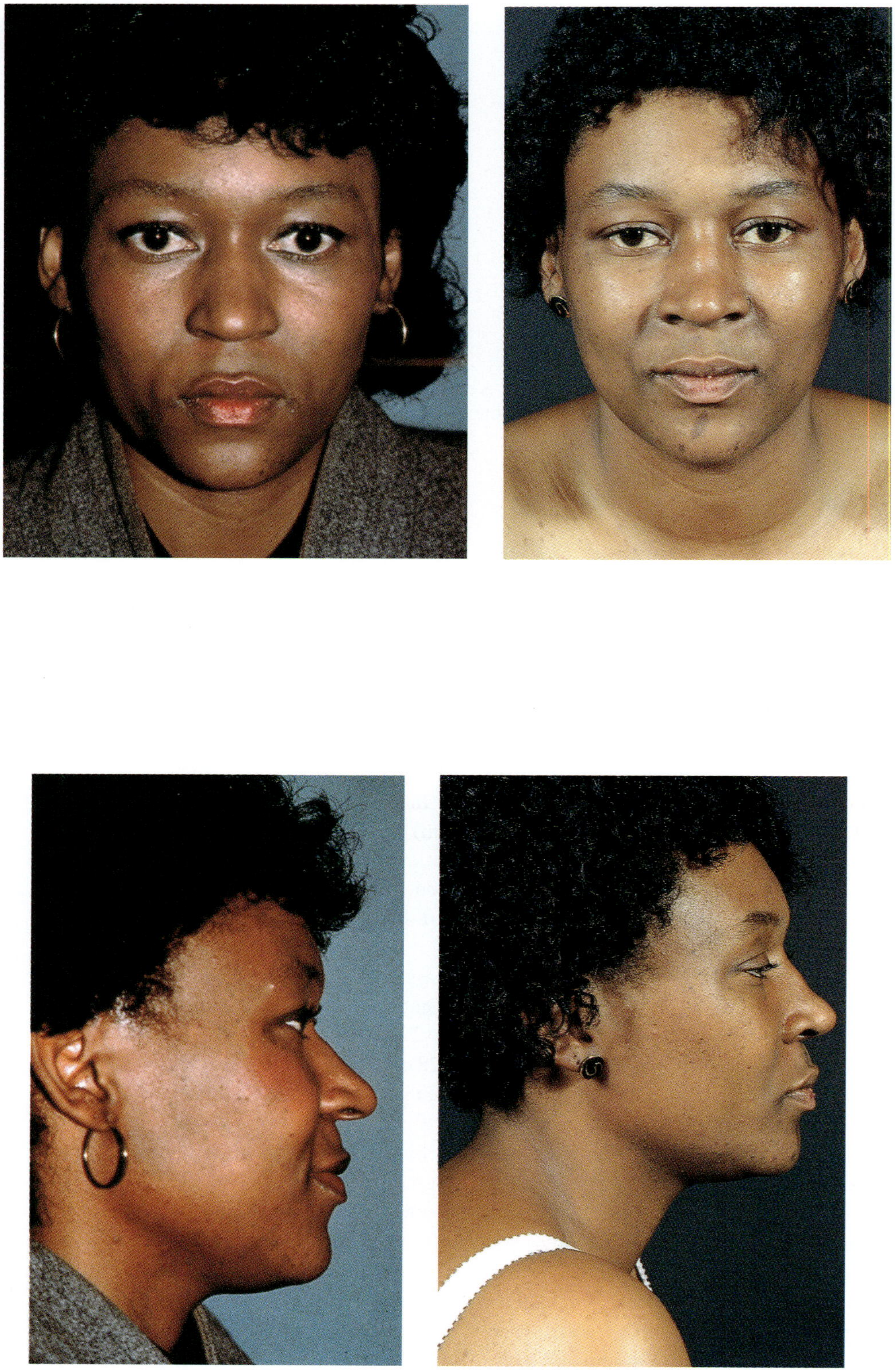

Figure 25. Conchal cartilage grafts, as used by another surgeon in this patient, provide inadequate length and straightness to yield optimal long-term results (25 above l/r, 25 below l/r).

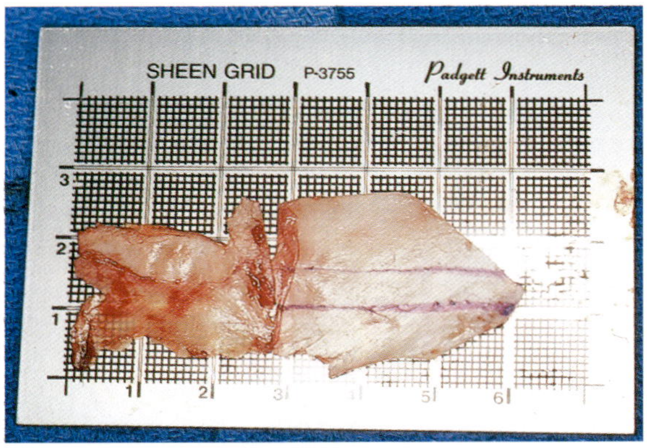

Figure 26. Septal cartilage is usually inadequate in meeting the dorsal length requirements of 30–35 mm × 4–5 mm.

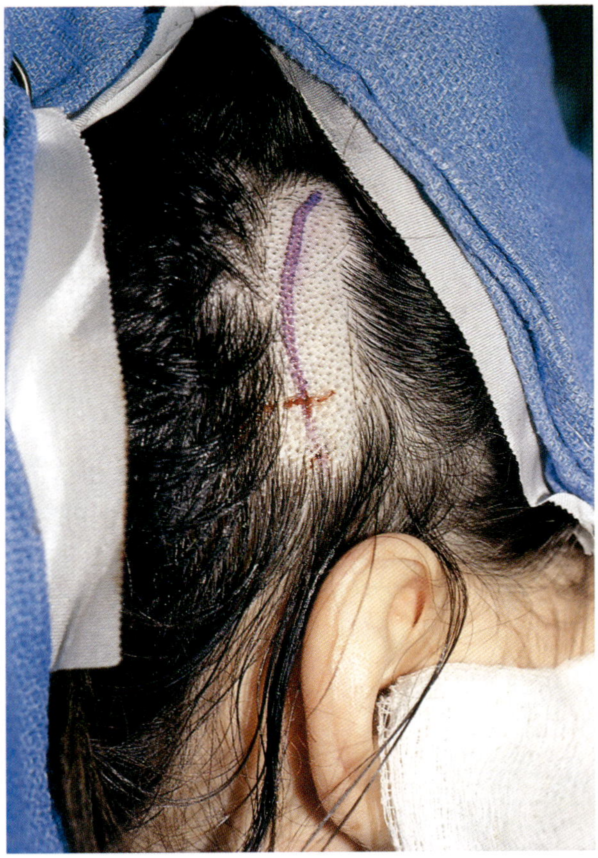

A

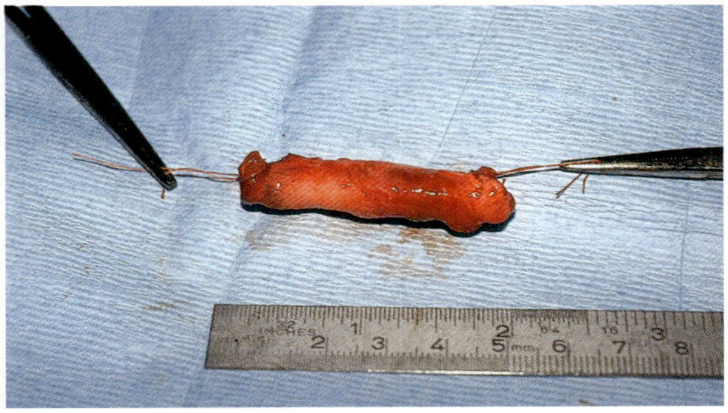

B

Figure 27. Temporal fascia can be easily harvested with minimal donor deformity **(A)**. By tubularizing the fascia height, width and handling are optimized **(B)**.

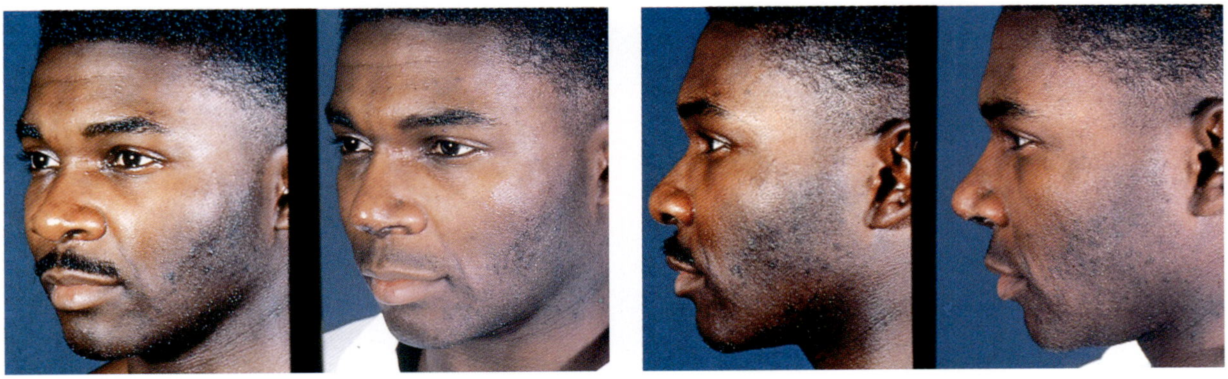

Figure 28. The results are shown in this 25-year-old man 18 months after dorsal augmentation with temporal fascia (28 l/r).

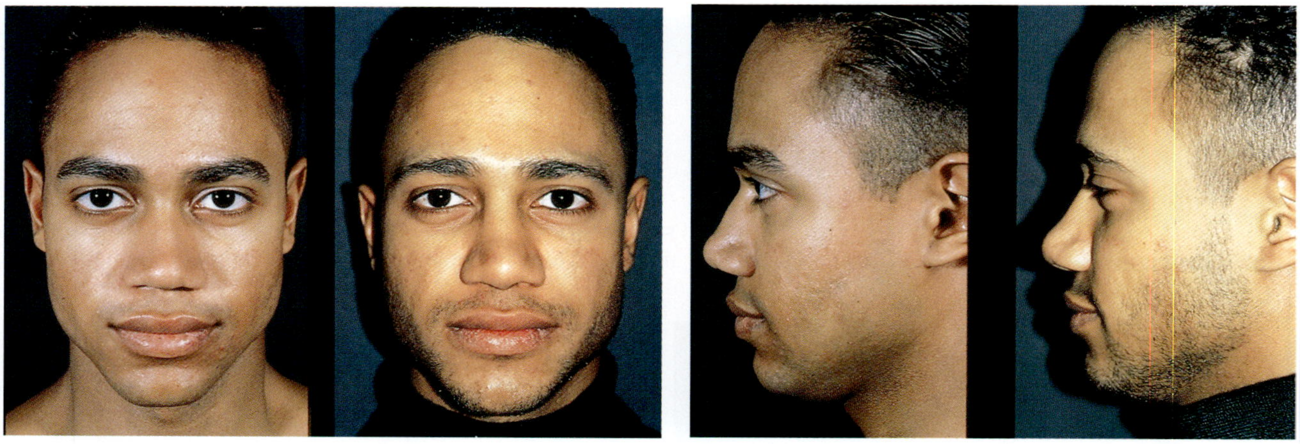

Figure 29. Occasionally temporal fascia absorbs, as noted in this 24-year-old man 5 months post-operatively (29 l/r).

Figure 30. Rib cartilage has been the most frequently used autologous graft source in my practice. Use of the costal margin **(A)** provides the straightest possible graft. With minimal carving, a dorsal and strut graft and a back-up can be harvested **(B)**. Excess can be banked at the donor site or scalp if desired.

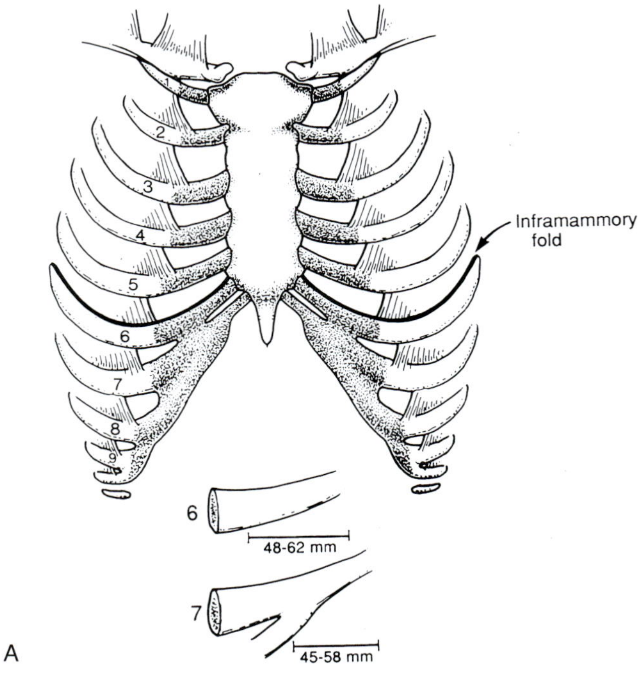

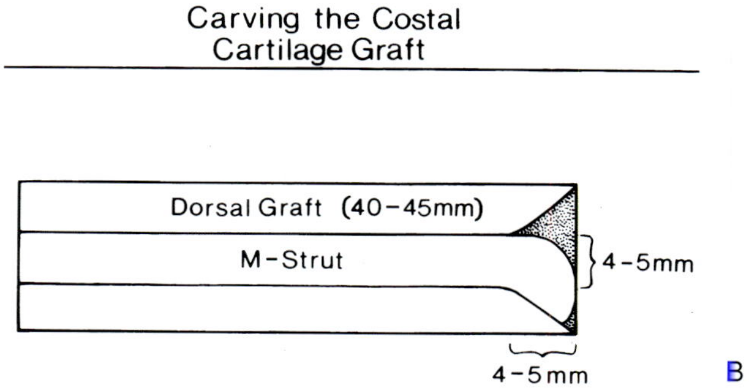

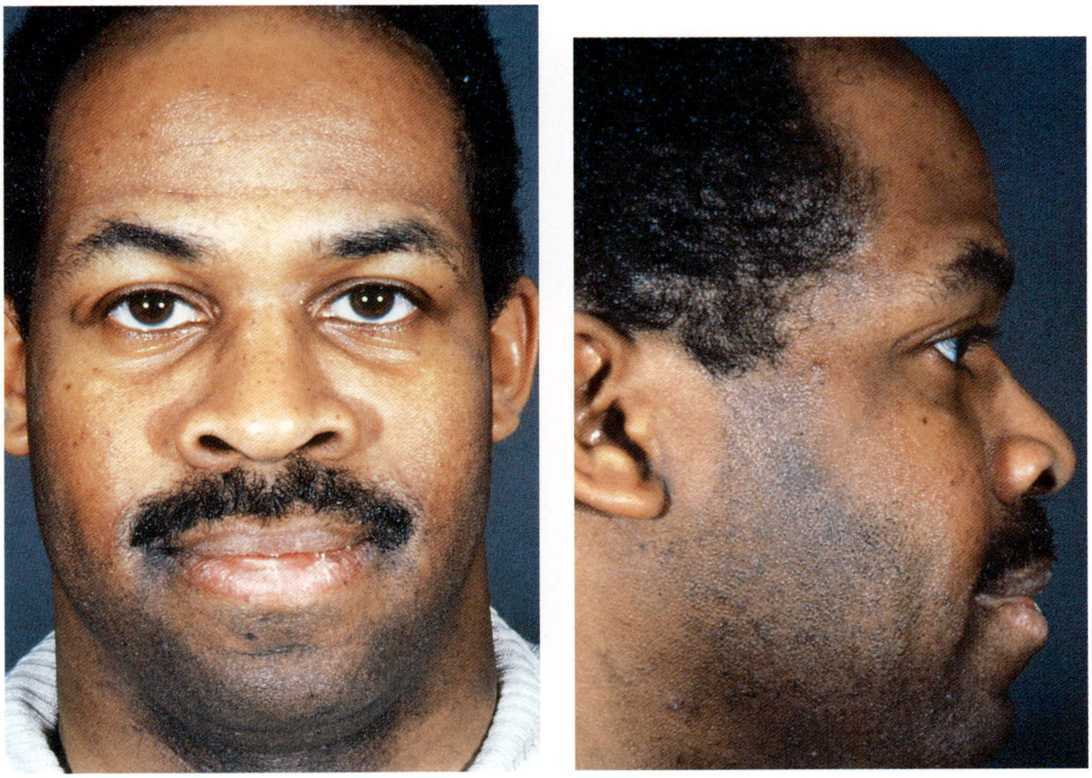

Figure 31. This 34-year-old male presented with concerns about lack of tip definition and alar flaring. Note the dorsal and nostril asymmetry, along with malar hypoplasia and microgenia.

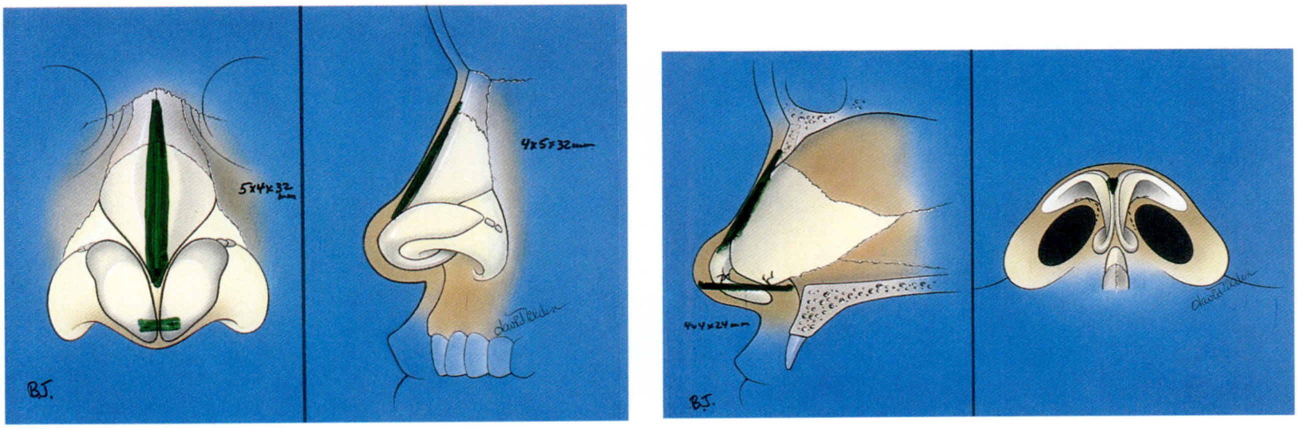

Figure 32. An M-strut is utilized to provide tip support concomitant with dorsal augmentation using a 4 × 36–mm contoured rib graft for the dorsum. A 4 × 3–mm onlay graft is placed to complement the columella.

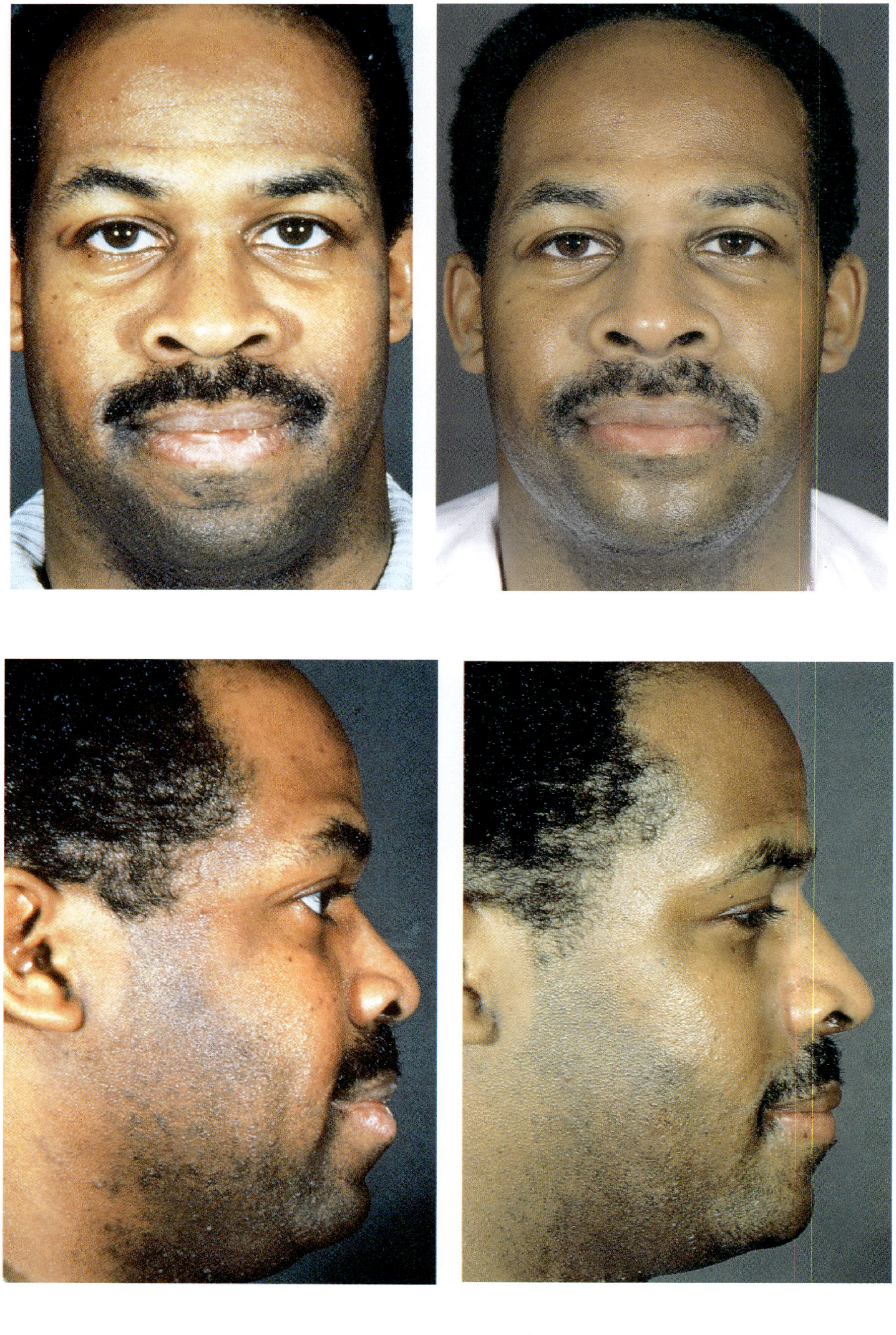

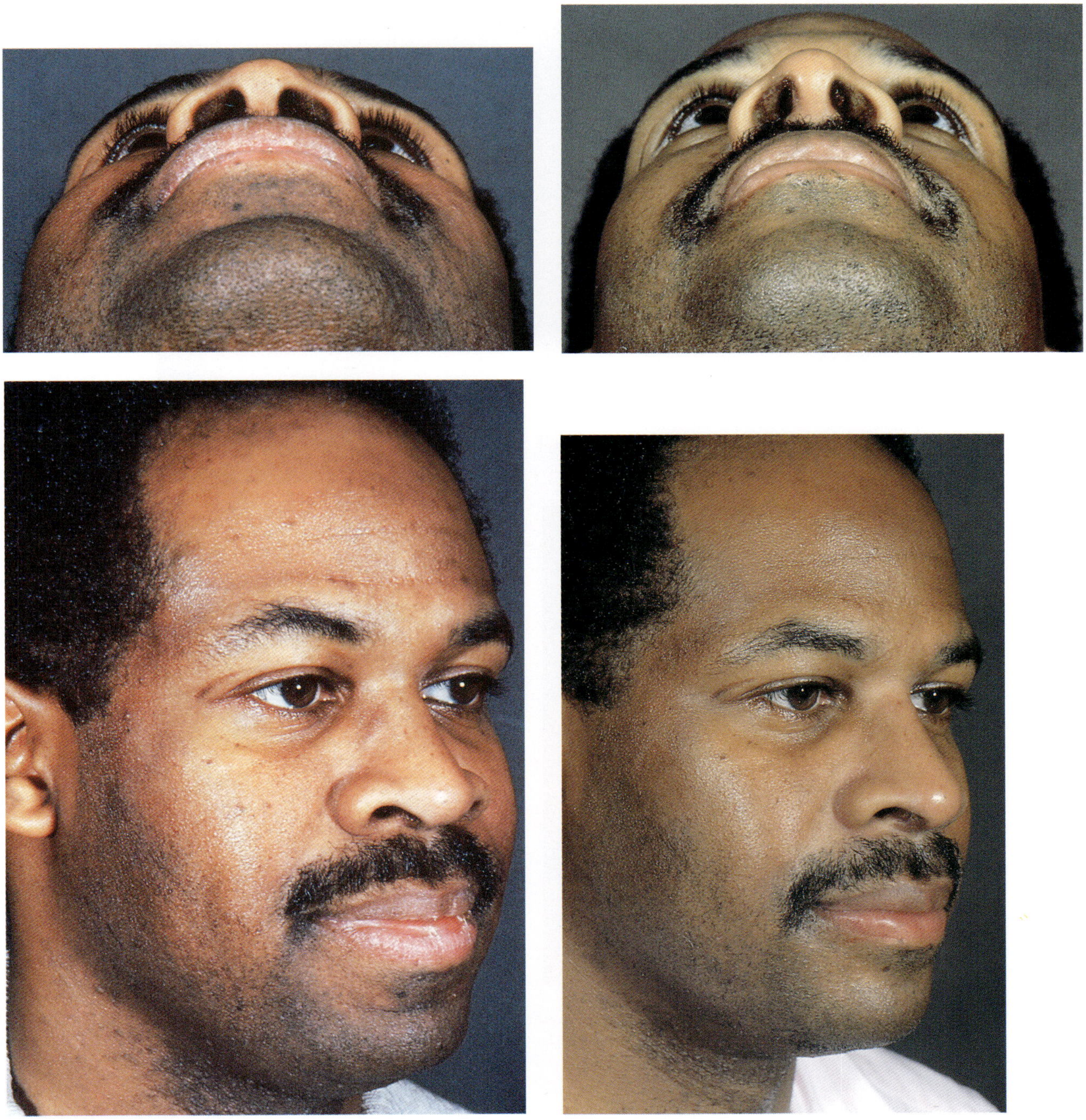

Figure 33. Pre- and post-operative views are shown 26 months after dorsal augmentation with rib cartilage, an M-strut, alar rim reduction, and alloplastic chin augmentation.

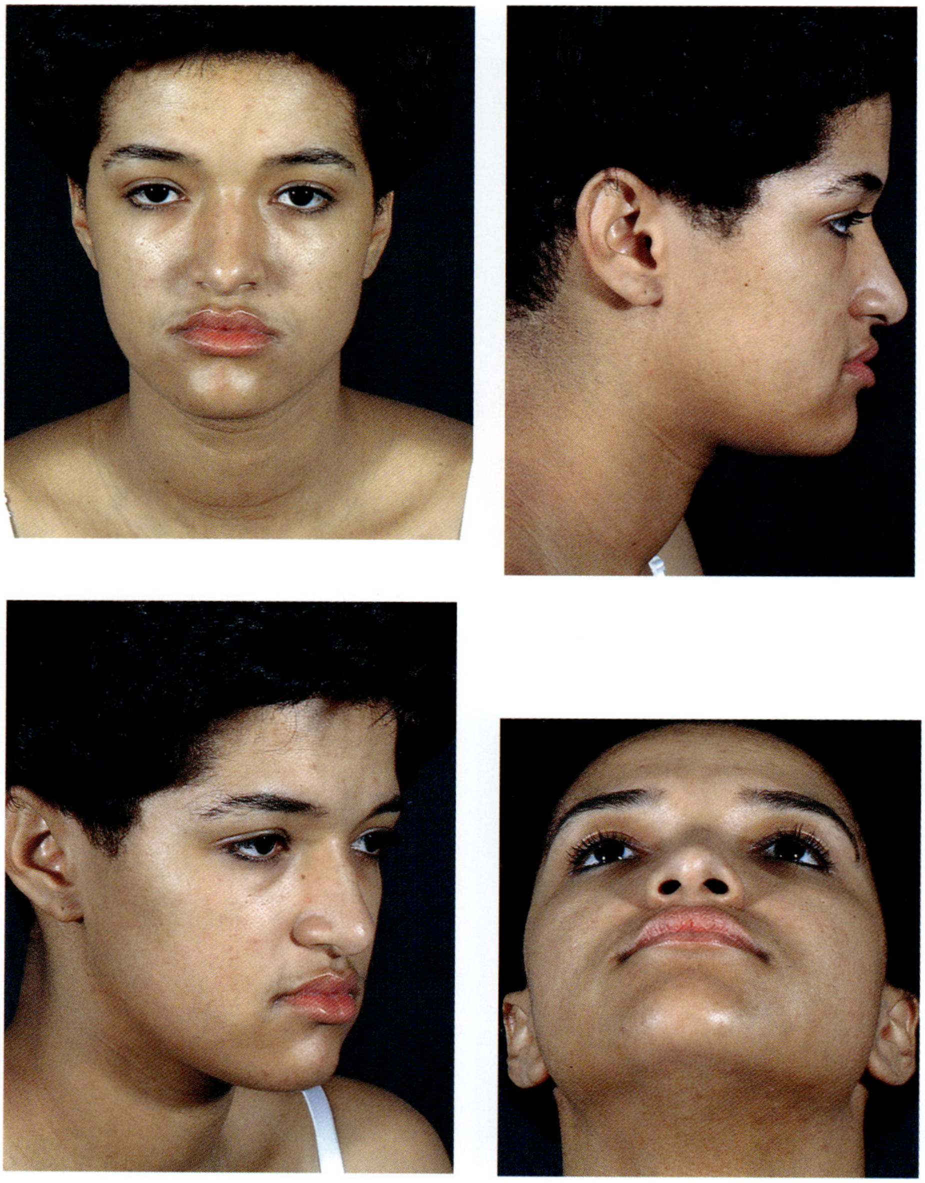

Figure 34. A–D: This 30-year-old woman presented with a diving nasal tip with mild tip stasis. Tip height was blunted, resulting in rounded nostrils.

Suture fixation of the dorsal cartilage graft can be used to minimize the tendency for warping. Two points of fixation are appropriate: to the septum distally and to the mid upper lateral canthage proximally. An open approach is routinely necessary to fixate the cartilage.

THE OPEN RHINOPLASTY

Based on the experience of the surgeon, the key indications for open rhinoplasty are extensive tip manipulation and/or pre-operative asymmetry and/or convoluted septal manipulations. The patient demonstrates a diving tip with a wide nasal bridge and pyramid along with a poorly defined tip. Tip augmentation was performed with an M-strut secured to the septum along with dorsal augmentation using rib cartilage graft, lateral infracture, as well as malar and chin augmentation with autologous fat.

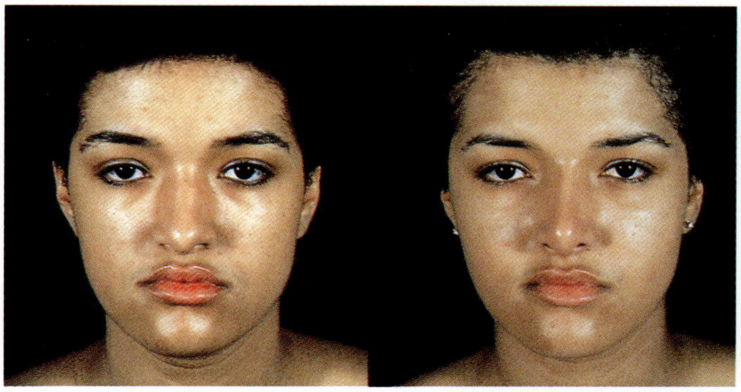
E

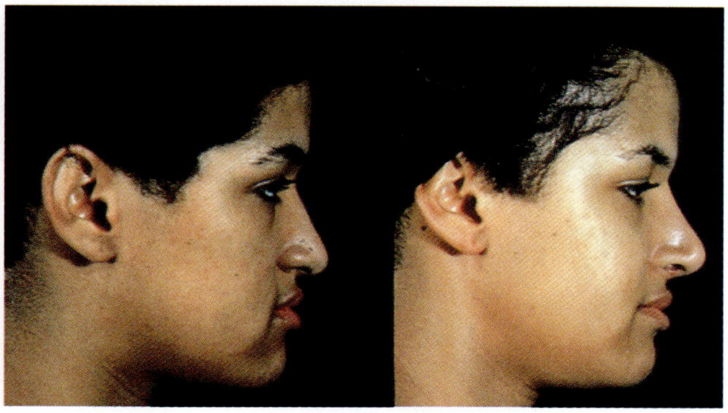
F

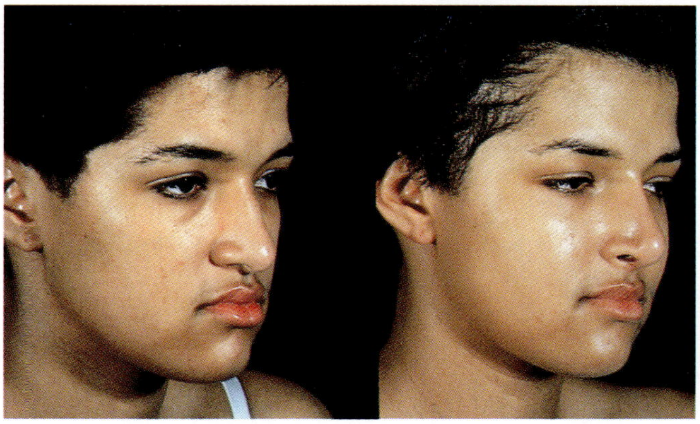
G

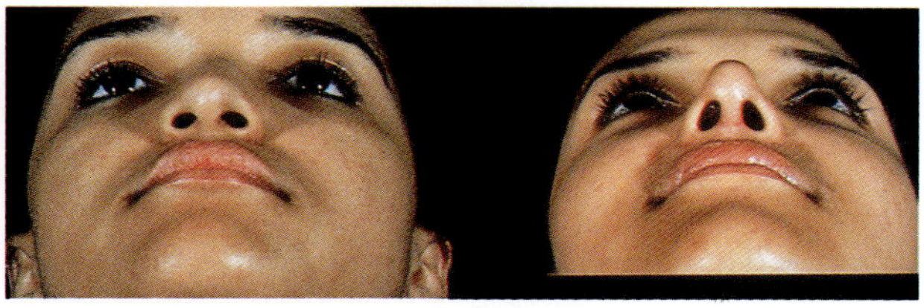
H

Figure 34 *continued.* **E–H:** With elevation of the tip by using an M-strut, dorsal height necessitated a small dorsal graft measuring 32 × 4 × 3 mm. Increased tip height is noted in the basal view.

Given experience with >1,000 open and closed rhinoplasties in the African American, I feel that closed rhinoplasty with a delivery technique is less traumatic, less devascularizing, and less likely to promote subdermal and dermal scarring. On the other hand, the open technique is more precise and allows better fixation and correction/prevention of dorsal asymmetries.

THE THICK-SKINNED NOSE

The thickness of African American skin, particularly in the supratip and tip areas and the alar rim, presents the most significant challenges to the rhinoplasty surgeon (Fig. 35).

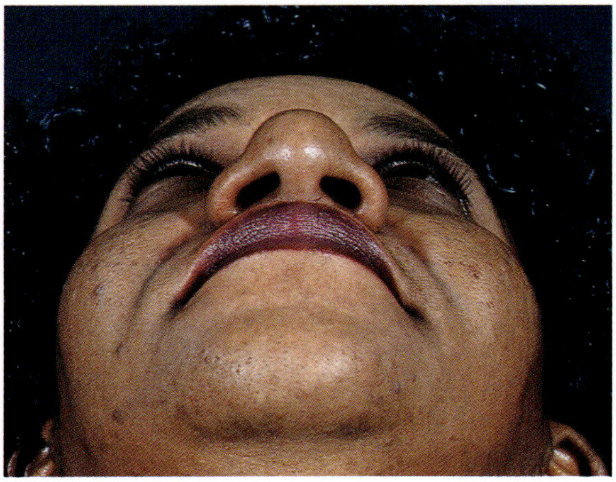

Figure 35. The thick-skinned nose represents a major challenge for every rhinoplasty surgeon. In the African American, tip thickness is maximal in the supratip and tip areas, ranging from 2 to 5 or 6 mm as in the depicted nose. Skin thickness defies tip contouring, unless the skin thickness is lessened.

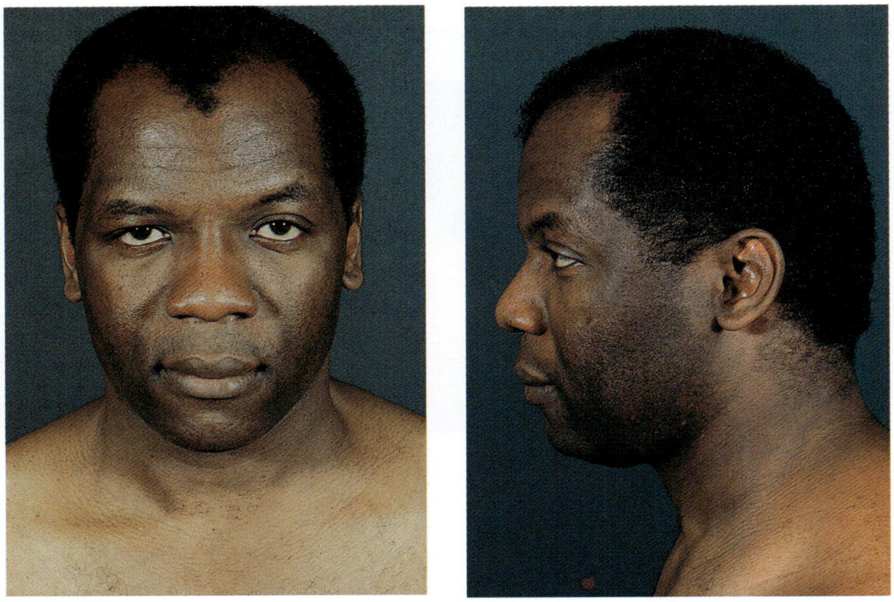

A, B

Figure 36. A–B: This 40-year-old man demonstrated 3 mm of dorsal skin with 4-mm thickness of the tip. He was concerned about the lack of tip definition, which is primarily secondary to skin thickness. **C–E:** The surgical plan was outlined as trimming of the dorsal irregularity of bone and cartilage, a 4-mm resection of the cephalad lower lateral cartilage, and wedge resection of the asymmetrical alar rim. An M-strut and dorsal rib cartilage graft (34 × 4 × 3 mm) is used to stretch the thickened skin envelope. Tip skin was put on stretch, decreasing relative tip thickness and improving tip definition. **F–G:** The definition of tip and dorsal skin were enhanced by putting the skin on stretch. Malar augmentation along with suction lipectomy of the nasal labial fold and submental area were performed along with chin augmentation.

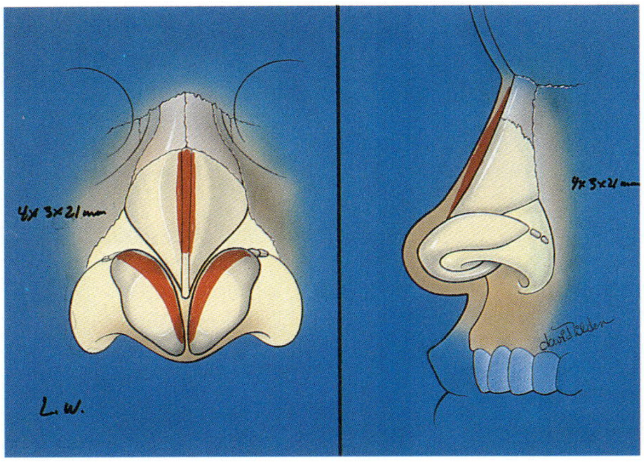

C

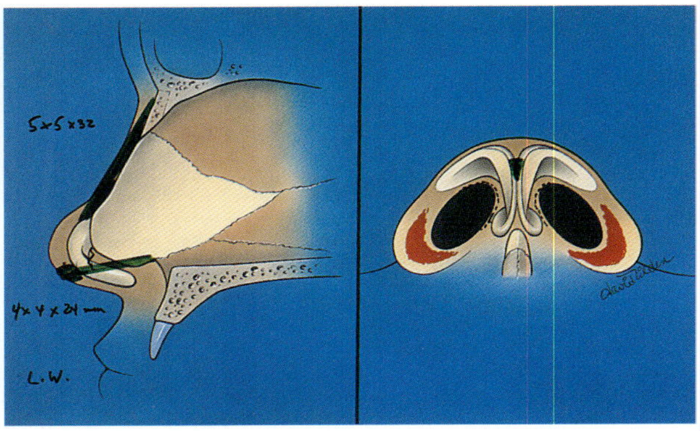

D

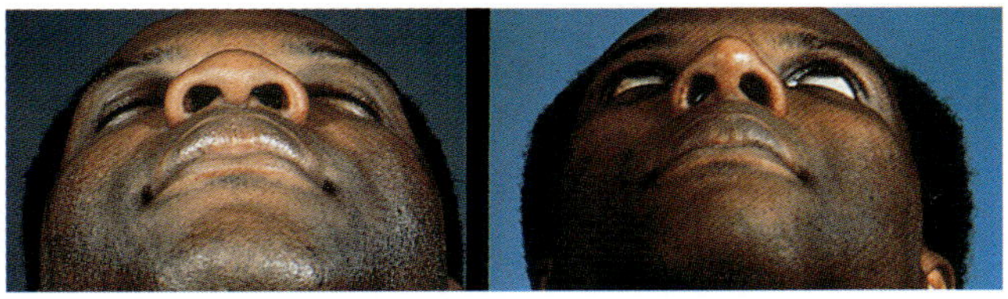

E

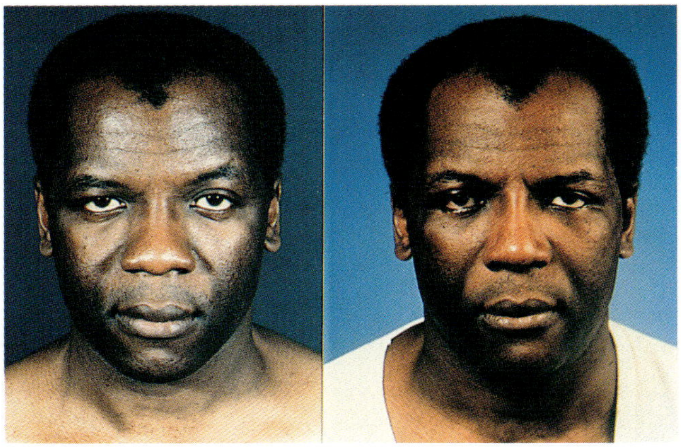

F

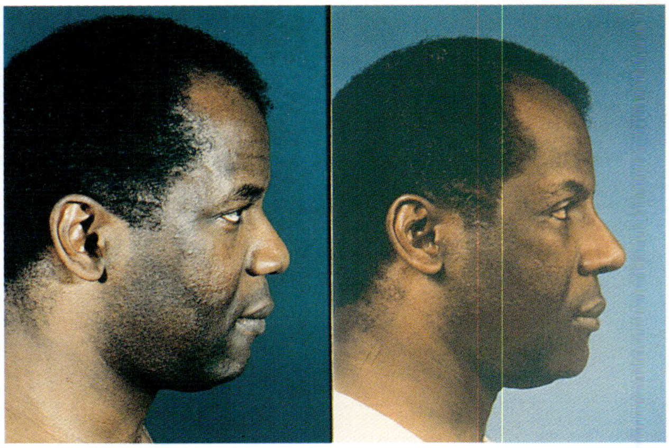

G

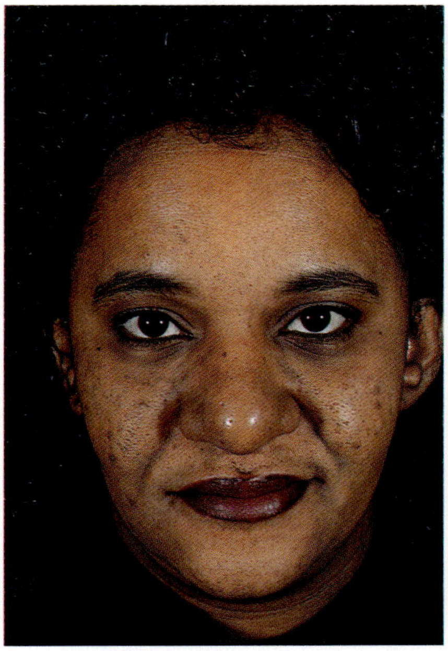
A

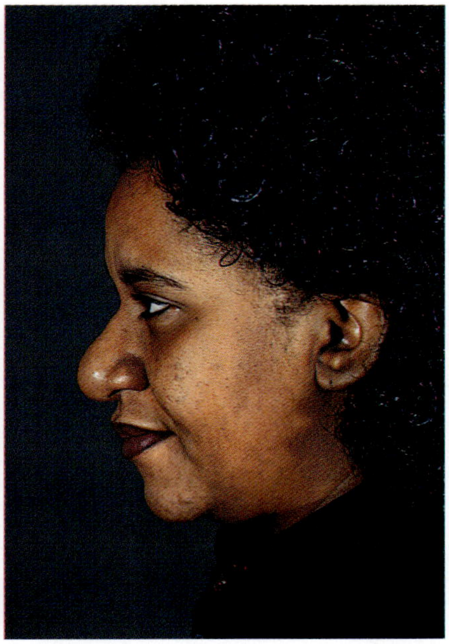
B

Figure 37. A–B: This 48-year-old woman had been chided for most of her life because of a large, bulbous, elongated tip. The most predominant observation on examination was the skin thickness measuring 5 mm along the tip and alar rim. **C–D:** Surgical plan includes smoothing the dorsal bone and cartilage and a 4-mm cephalad resection of the lower lateral cartilage. An open approach was used to resect a portion of the columella. Dorsal irregularities were hidden by the skin thickness. **E–F:** A columellar incision was used along with placement of an M-strut fixated proximally to the septum along with medial rotation of the lower lateral cartilages. A mattress suture was utilized for fixation. Resection of the alar rim and columella excesses were outlined and completed.

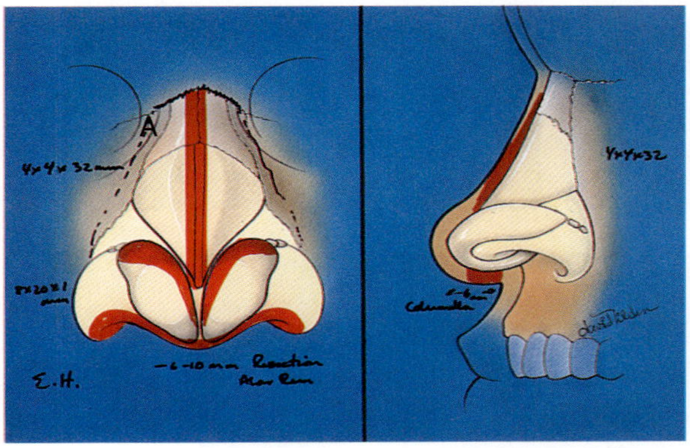
C

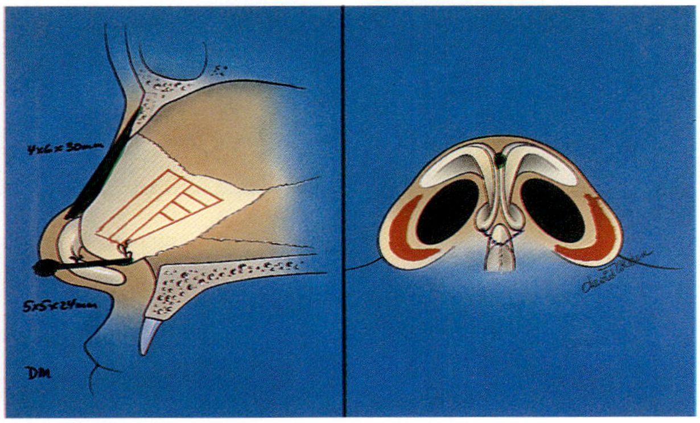
D

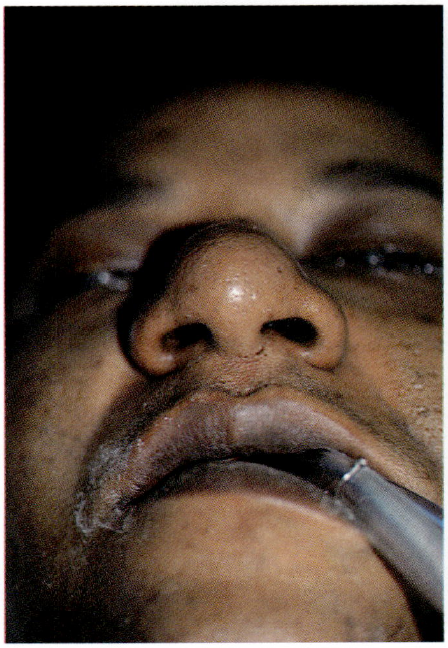
E

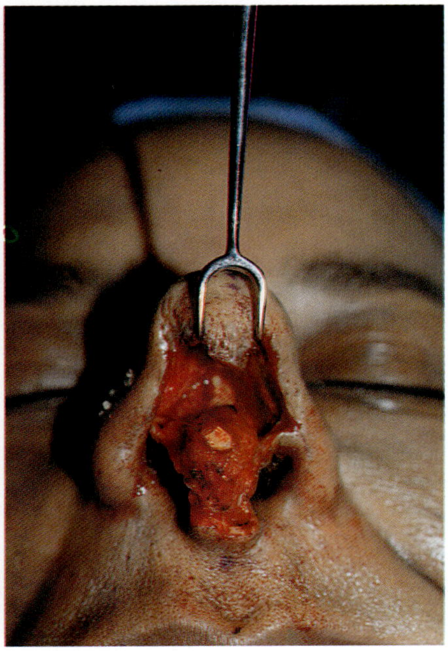
F

Figure 37 *continued.* **G:** A 34 × 4 × 5–mm cartilaginous rib graft was used to redefine dorsal skin. The cephalad rotation of the tip was noted with a resultant decrease in tip skin thickness. **H–M:** The patient is shown 18 months following rhinoplasty. There is some buckling of the dorsal cartilaginous graft. The tip is softened with improved definition.

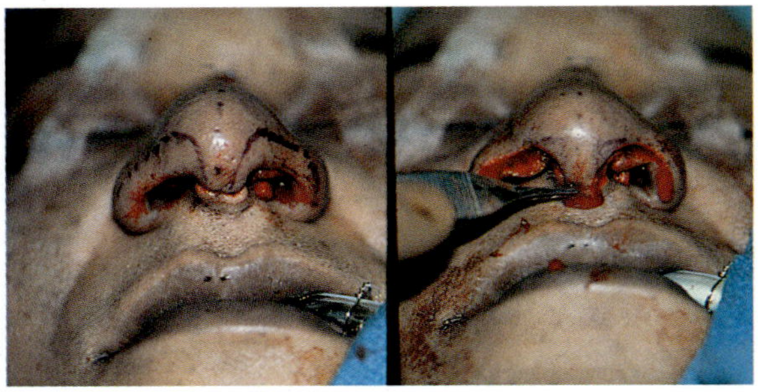

G

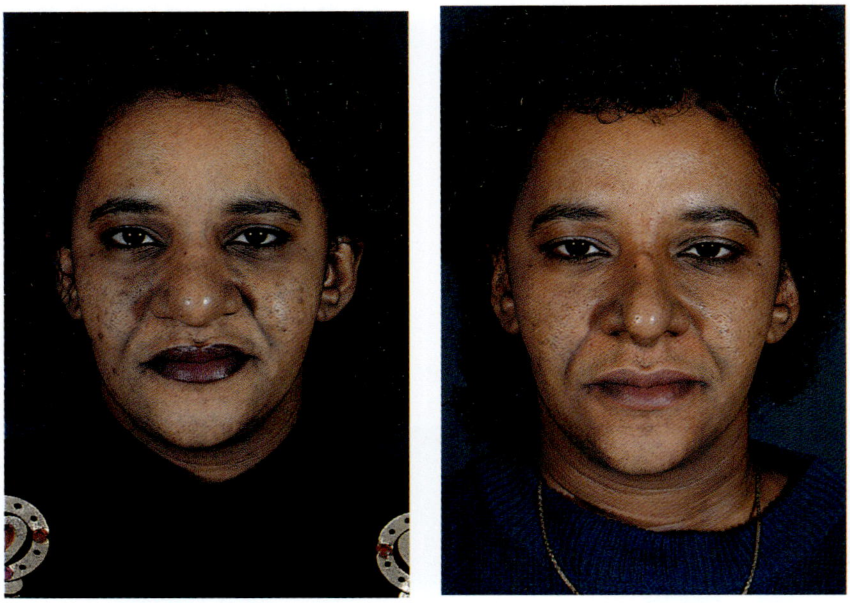

H, I

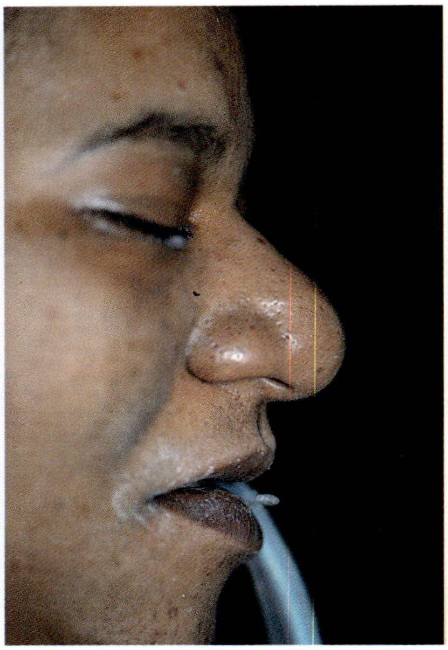

J

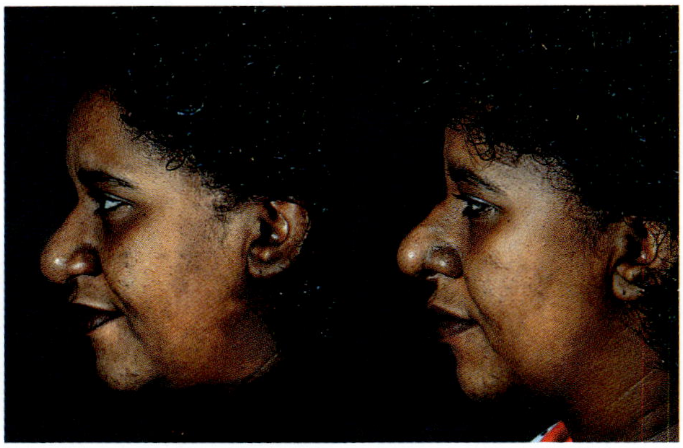

L

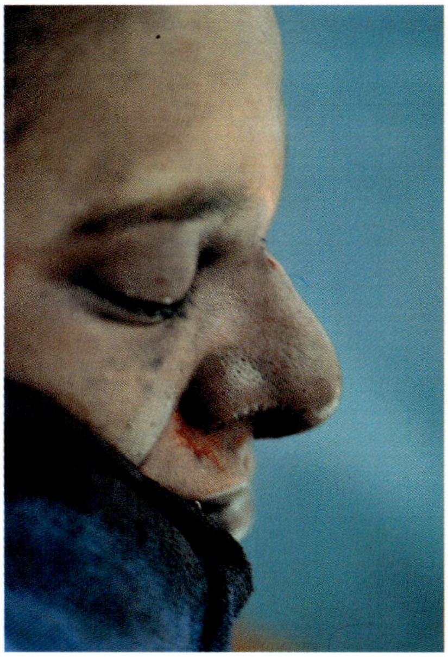

K

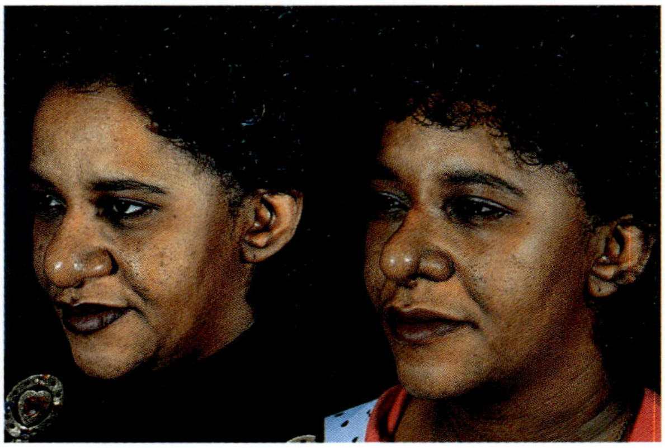

M

Figure 38. **A:** This 27-year-old woman had undergone 14 prior procedures for cleft lip and nasal deformities. **B–C:** There was considerable thickness of the dorsal and tip skin along with displacement of a previously positioned dorsal graft. **D–F:** Upon reviewing surgical options with the patient, we pointed out the problem of skin thickness diminishing the likelihood of achieving desired tip definition. Additionally, extensive scarring throughout the nose would complicate significant undermining. A direct excision of excess dorsal skin was opted for. **G–H:** The septum was mobilized and straightened using cartilaginous scoring and mattress fixation sutures. Closure was completed, approximating the deep dermis with Vicryl followed by a running cutaneous suture.

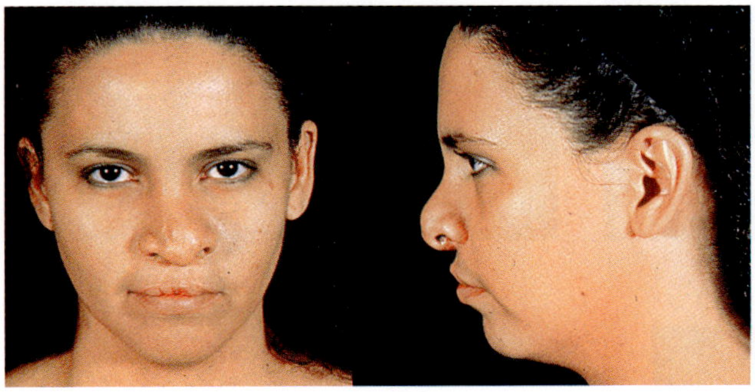

A

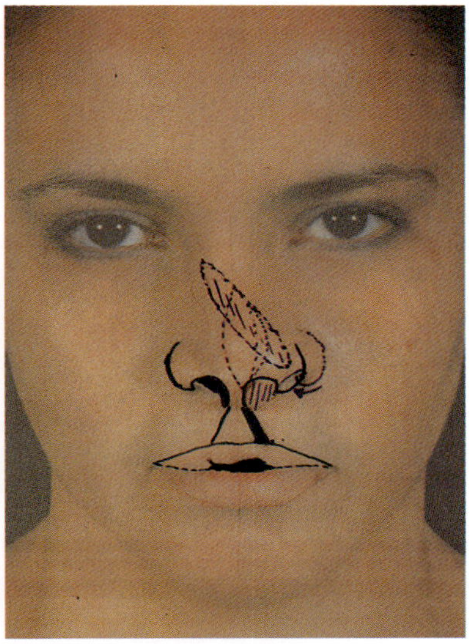

B

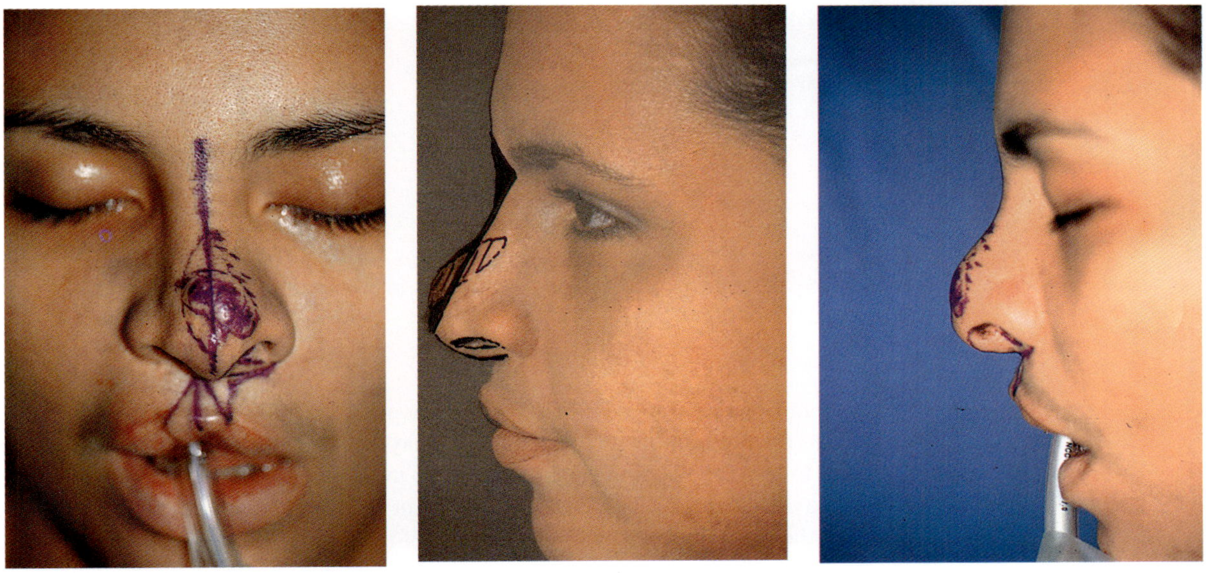

C, D

E

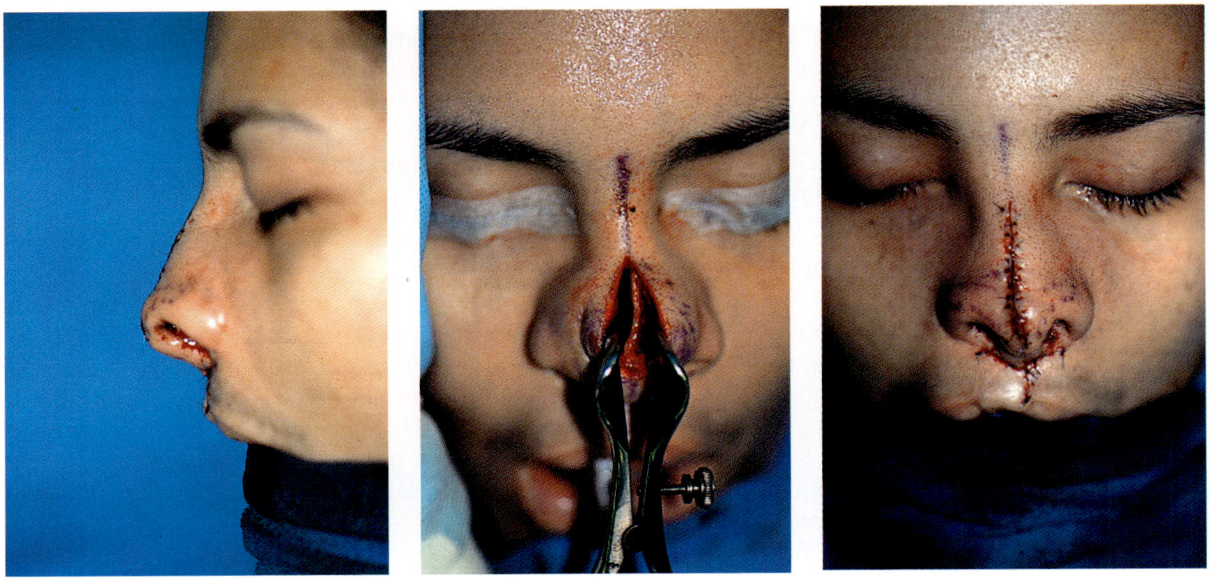

F, G

H

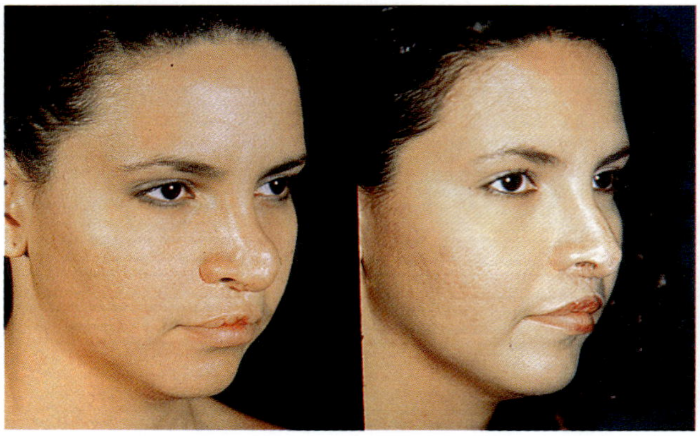

I

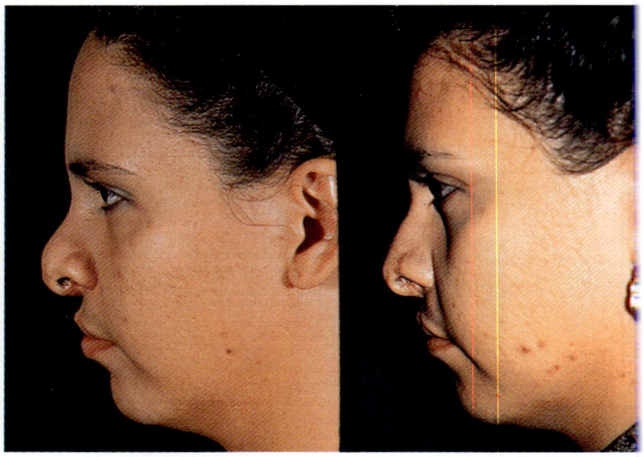

J

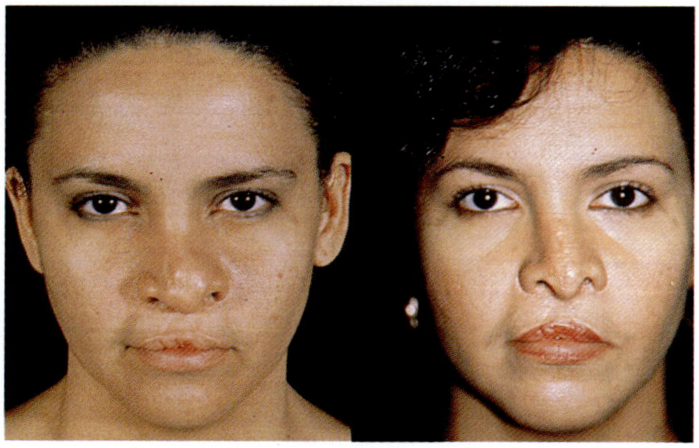

K

Figure 38 *(continued).* **I–K:** Post-operative results are outlined 24 months following the procedure.

Commonly noted thicknesses in these areas may vary from 0.5 to 2–3 mm. The thick-skinned tip, not infrequently encountered, may be 4–6 mm in thickness. The basic problem seems to be a foreshortened nose that results in an accumulation of skin in the supratip and tip areas. This effect, along with a concomitant shortened columella, leads to a severe blunting of the nasal tip and a marked flattening of the basal triangle. The lower lateral cartilage tends to be weak, relative to the tip thickness, and with aging, there are additional drooping and blunting of the nasal tip due to decreasing tip support.

Ideal management of the thick-skinned nose is best achieved by lengthening the nose spreading out of the thick skin of the nasal tip, providing firm tip support with proximal fixation to a rigid structure, i.e., the septum, along with columella lengthening (Figs. 36 and 37). A V-shaped incision at the columella base can be advanced as a Y to yield additional columellar length. Dorsal resection and alar rim skin resection can also be utilized to lessen excess rim and tip skin (Fig. 38).

SUBOPTIMAL RESULTS

Cartilage warping with the rib cartilage graft is perhaps the most common problem that we face during our initial rhinoplasty experience. The patient illustrated in Fig. 39 shows the intra-operative outcome immediately following dorsal augmentation and tip refinement utilizing the techniques described above. Three months later, the degree of warping is noted. Subsequent replacement of the dorsal rib graft with Proplast is demonstrated at the 6-month period. Rib donor sites routinely heal well but are not infrequently accompanied by hyperpigmentation (Fig. 40).

The full, broad-faced patient is best addressed by lengthening the nasal tip rather than

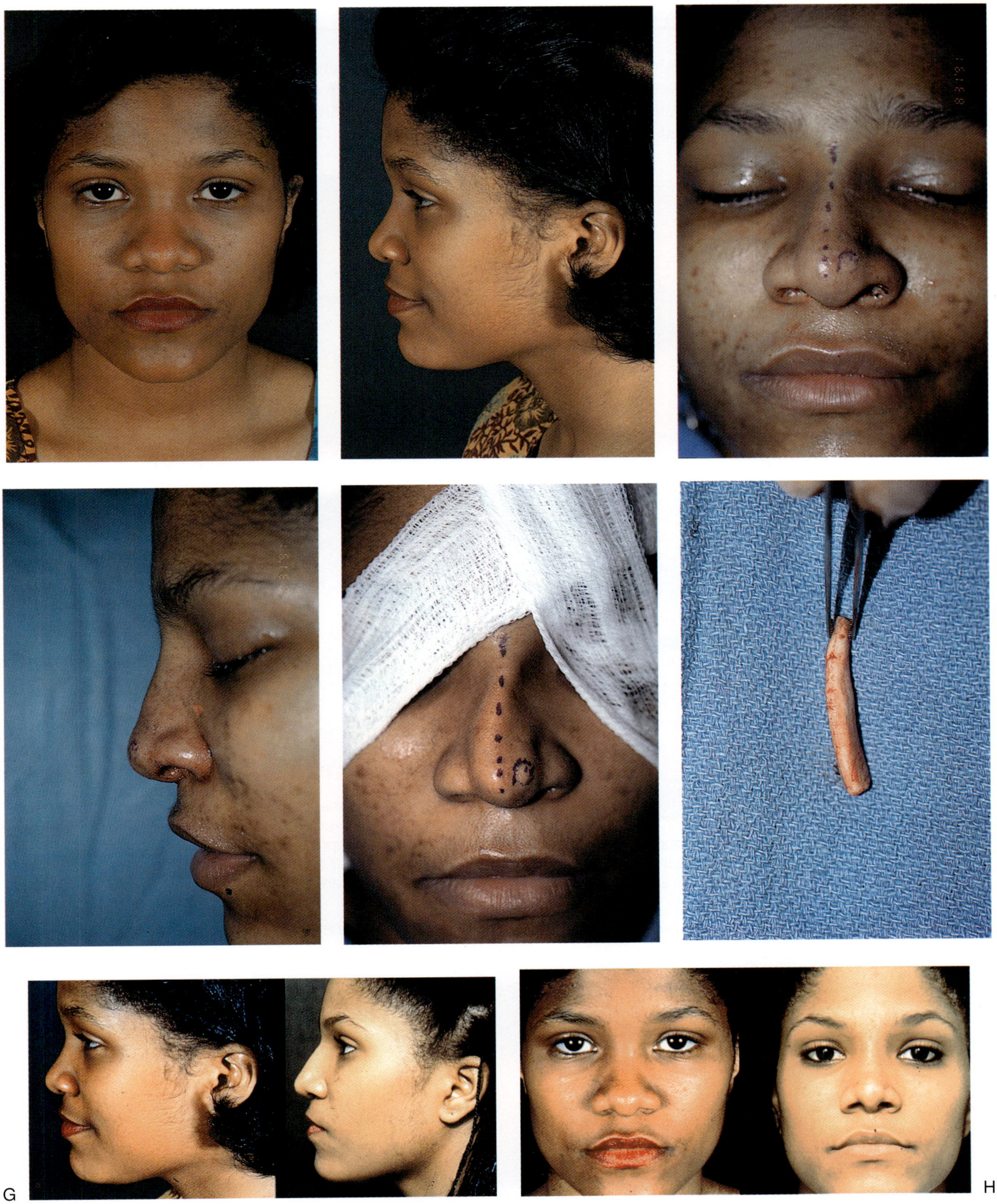

A, B C D, E F G H

Figure 39. A–B: This 19-year-old female model presented with concerns about enhanced tip definition. **C–D:** She is shown intraoperatively following a closed approach with placement of a dorsal rib cartilaginous graft measuring 32 × 5 × 5 mm. **E–F:** Alar cartilage diastasis was softened by using an M-strut, and 6 months later the patient presented with warped dorsal rib cartilage. **G–H:** After removal of dorsal rib cartilage graft and placement of a dorsal alloplastic proplast graft. (Courtesy of Matory and Falces.)

foreshortening. The alar rim should not be shortened with even incisions because the length is necessary to accommodate tip lengthening. Over-resection of the alar rim and excessive foreshortening lead to altered nasal facial proportions, resulting in perceptions of facial or racial incongruity (Figs. 41 and 42).

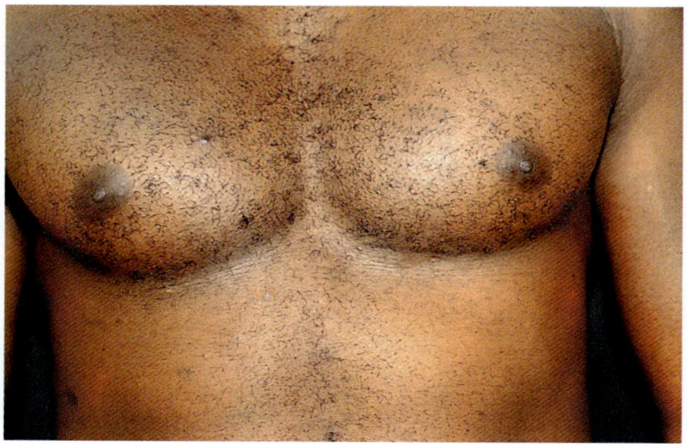

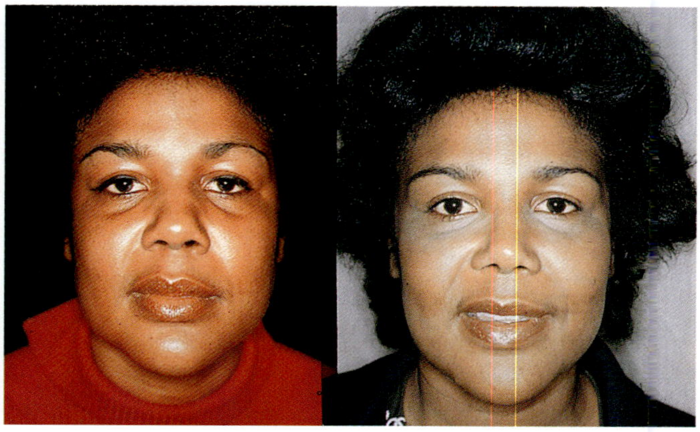

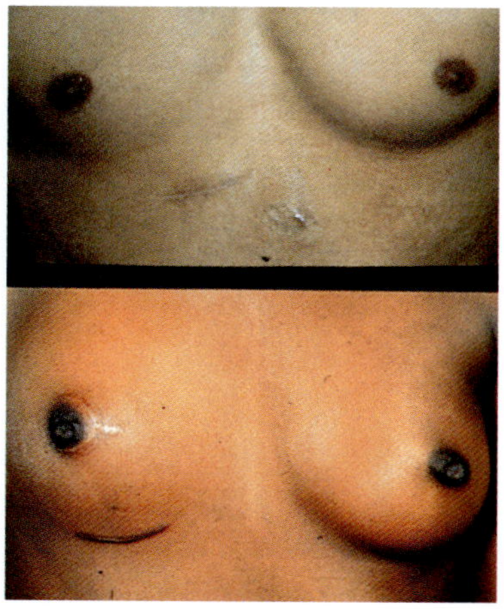

Figure 40. Rib cartilage grafts are optimally placed along the inframammary fold. Running dermal polypropylene is left in for 2–3 weeks to optimize subsequent healing.

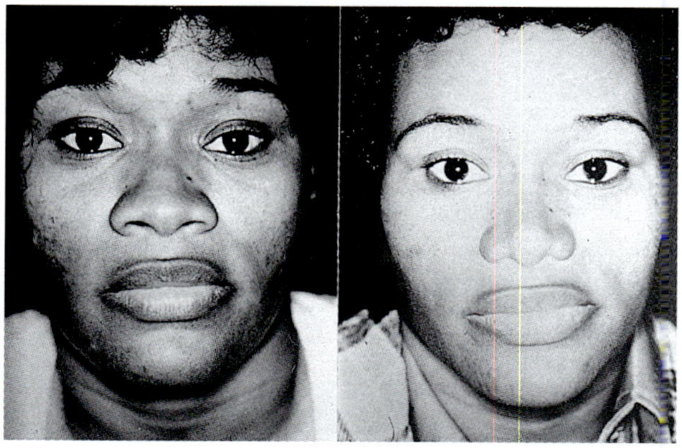

Figure 41. The patients shown were very satisfied following rhinoplasty. However, on review, the results demonstrate an overaggressive approach to rhinoplasty, yielding unnatural distortions. It is far better to be conservative in one's approach to the African American nose.

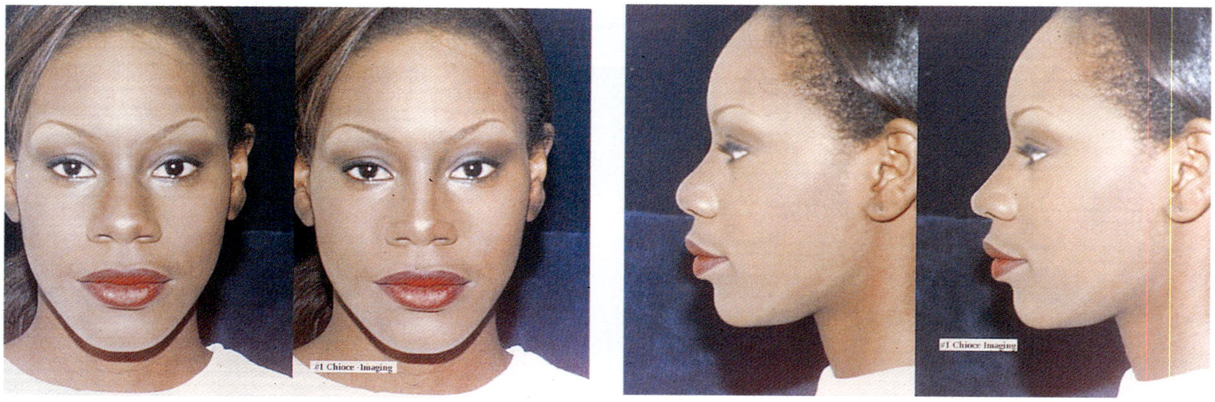

Figure 42. Video imaging is a particularly helpful method of avoiding unsatisfactory results. A surgical plan commensurate with the patient's desires is more easily accomplished. Lateral infracture, dorsal augmentation from radix to tip that lengthens the nose and lowers the tip-defining point, and M-strut augmentation of the tip and columella achieved satisfactory enhancement for this patient.

SECTION VII

The Asian Patient

Ethnic Considerations in Facial Aesthetic Surgery, edited by W. Earle Matory, Jr.
Lippincott–Raven Publishers, Philadelphia © 1998.

18

The Asian Patient

Editor's Commentary

W. Earle Matory, Jr.

ASIAN VERSUS ORIENTAL: WHAT IS APPROPRIATE?

Oriental is a geographic term that encompasses a host of non-Occidental peoples including Indians, Pakistanis, and Russians. Asian is a more inclusive term describing those of Han ancestry including ethnically similar groups, i.e., Japanese, Chinese, Korean, and southeast Asian. To refer to Asians as Oriental is comparable with defining ethnicity in the United States by using the term "American." America comprises a profoundly diverse ethnic make-up.

As we view three attractive Asian faces in Fig. 1, note distinctive differences in facial morphology. Han characteristics span a wide variety of ethnic groups varying from northern and southern Chinese to northern and southern Korean, to Japanese, to Thai, to south Indonesia, to Polynesian and Philippine. With this broad mix of ethnic backgrounds, aesthetic features vary considerably. We observed some common characteristics in our analysis of attractive models. A broad, prominent forehead with non-ptotic brows allows the orbit to have a bright-eyed appearance. The malar prominence should be full with a phi relationship with the vertex–menton. The nose may vary in length, but the attractive alar width al-al is almost always equal to en-ex. Alar width has a phi relationship with intercanthal width en-en and with the width of the mouth the intercommissural distance. A prominent jawline with absence of chin recession is a key characteristic of attractiveness in the Asian. Malar width is most attractive when the zyg-zyg is phi with the length of the head, vertex–menton. In viewing the model on the left, the malar eminence is particularly

W. E. Matory, Jr.: A New You Plastic Surgery Medical Group, Irvine, California 92714

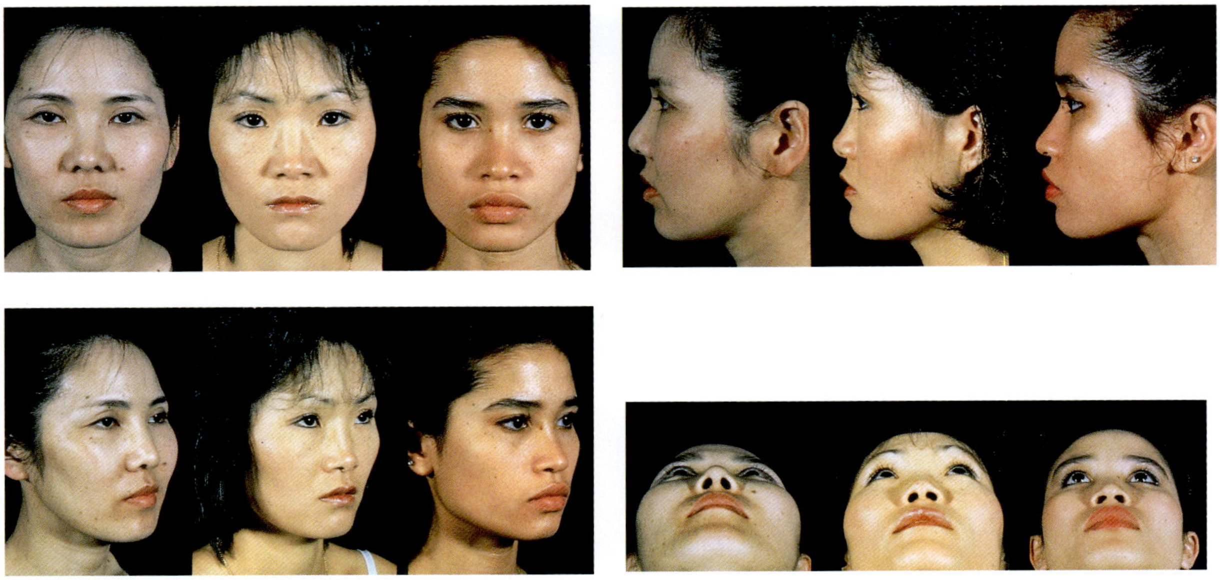

Figure 1. The exotic attractiveness of the Asian is demonstrated in facial features from Mainland China, Vietnam, and Tahiti. With each appealing face, there are many characteristics that are similar and a number that are distinctive. The prominent forehead, rounded malar eminence, and pleasant jawline are consistent in the attractive Asian woman. The bright, open eye tends to be more receptive and therefore more appealing. The malar eminence (zyg-zyg) has a phi relationship with the vertex–menton distance. The trichion–menton has a phi relationship with both the temp-temp and the gon-gon, with the latter dimensions formulating an oval-shaped face. There is extra fullness in the lower malar and proximal mandibular areas, which contribute to a roundness of the Asian face.

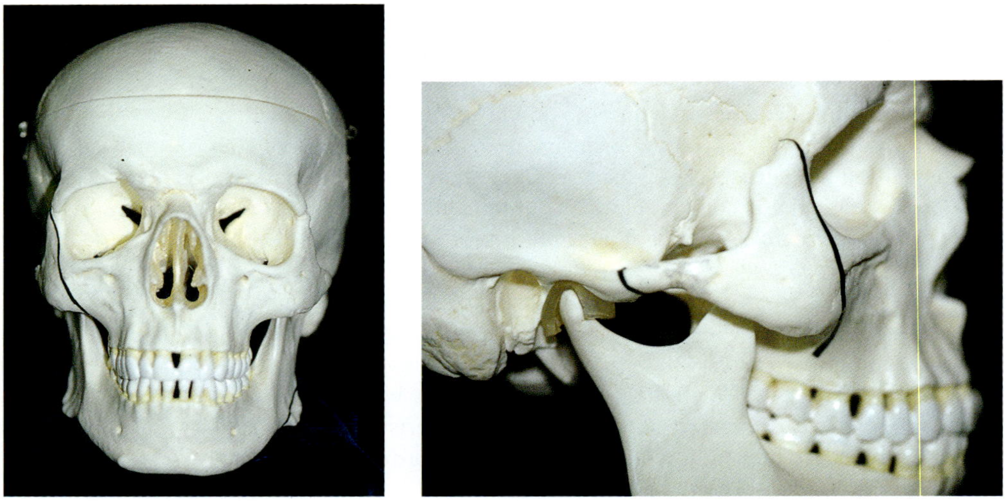

Figure 2. When malar fullness exceeds the phi relationship, an excessively rounded appearance is noted. Asymmetrical malar bones are best addressed by performing ostectomies through a coronal incision as outlined.

broad, giving a more rounded facies. Excessive malar prominence is a common concern for many Asian patients and in some cultures denotes negative social connotations.

EXCESSIVE MALAR PROMINENCE

A full malar prominence can be addressed through a coronal incision, which yields full exposure of the malar bones. Malar contouring can be performed through a limited incision, using a guarded burr, or conversely, if significant asymmetry exists, coronal exposure along with osteotomies can be performed to allow back table zygomatic contouring (Fig. 2). Once osteotomies have been completed, the degree of asymmetry is noted and burring can be performed to optimize malar symmetry (Fig. 3). Interosseous wiring is then be used to stabilize the malar bones (Fig. 4). Pre- and post-malar reduction is noted radiographically and photographically in Fig. 5. The same patient presented for osteoplastic rhinoplasty because of a lack of tip definition and a broad nasal pyramid (Fig. 6). The surgical plan is

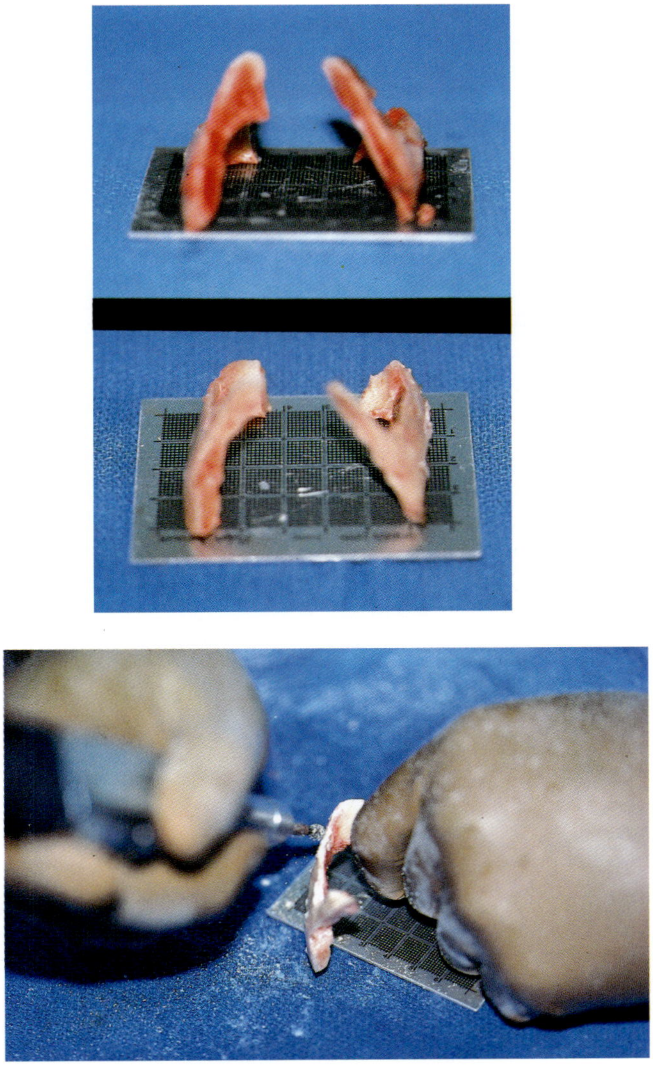

Figure 3. Upon completion of osteotomies, improved contouring and symmetry can be achieved on the back table. The lower diagram illustrates final contouring.

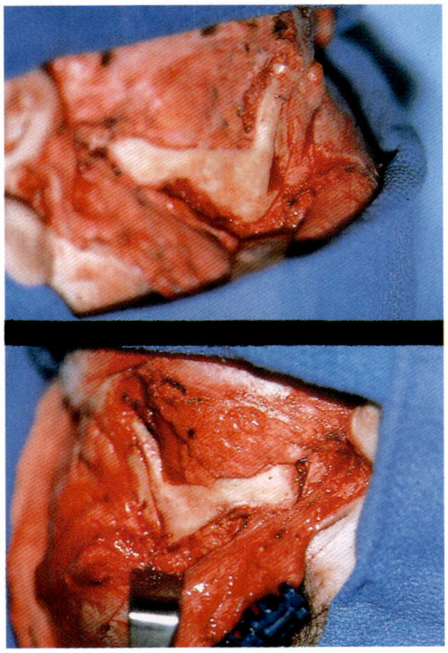

Figure 4. Interosseous plates and wires can be used to reposition and fix the malar bones.

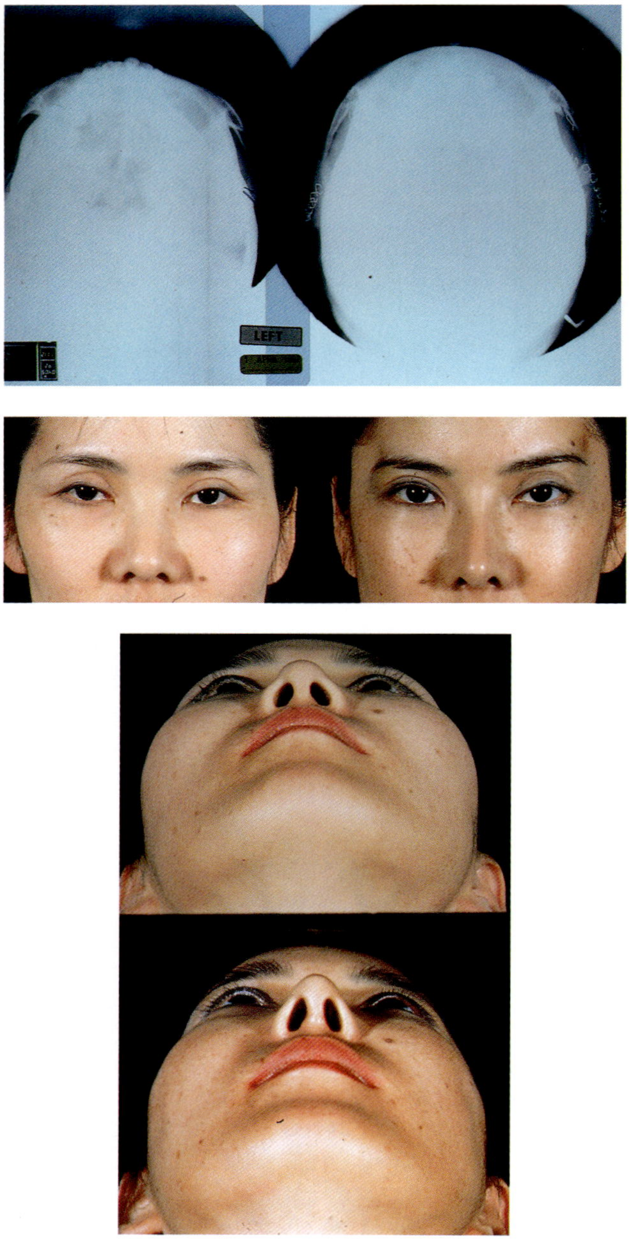

Figure 5. Results are shown radiographically and photographically 2 years following malar reduction.

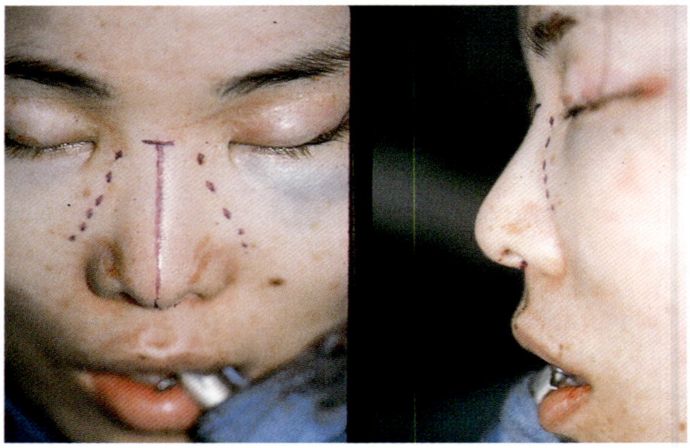

Figure 6. The same patient in Figs. 2–5 underwent nasal contouring to address a lack of dorsal and tip definition.

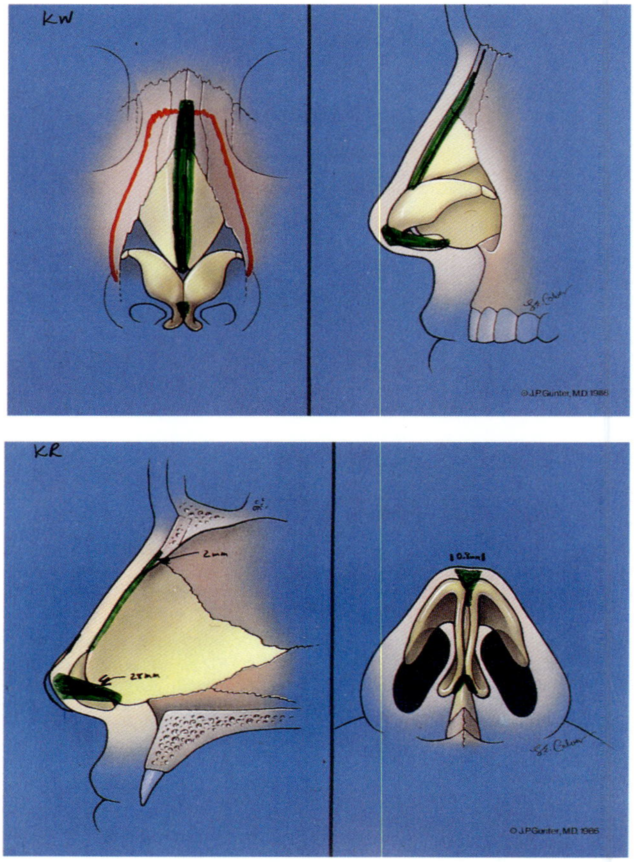

Figure 7. The surgical plan is outlined. This included lateral osteotomies, dorsal contouring, followed by a 30 × 4 × 2–mm dorsal graft. A septal graft was also utilized for the M-strut, which was fixated proximally to the septum and dissolute to the genu.

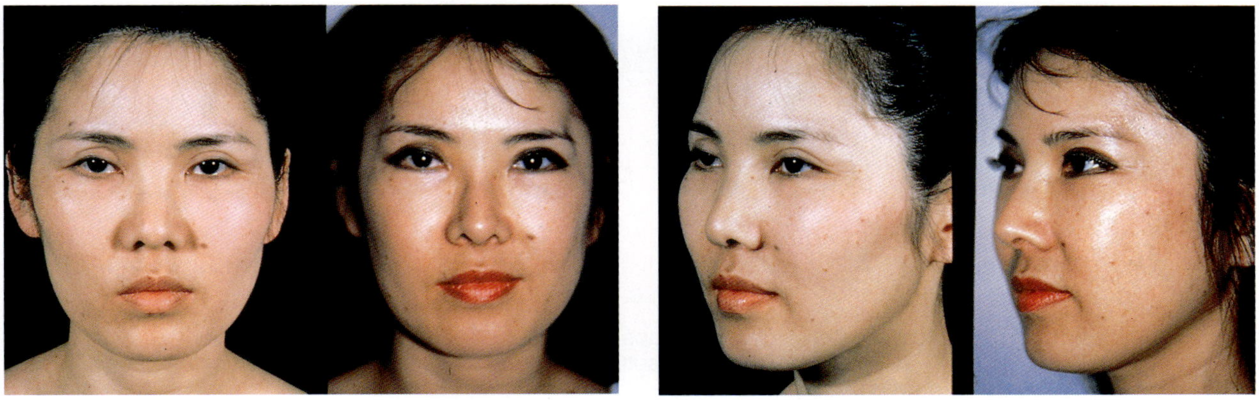

Figure 8. Photographs illustrate results in this 34-year-old Korean two years following transcoronal malar reduction and augmentation rhinoplasty using costal cartilage.

outlined (Fig. 7) for a lateral infracture and tip enhancement with an M-strut and dorsal augmentation with a 4 × 30–mm septal graft, one layer in thickness. Septal cartilage was used for the M-strut. Results are shown 2 years following malar reduction and the described rhinoplasty (Fig. 8).

EYELIDS

Conservatism in the placement of the supratarsal fold is crucial. Ideally the supratarsal fold should be placed no higher than the superior border of the tarsus. Given a patient's input, it is preferable to leave epicanthal folds intact. By adhering to these principles, a natural attractive improvement can be achieved (Figs. 9–11).

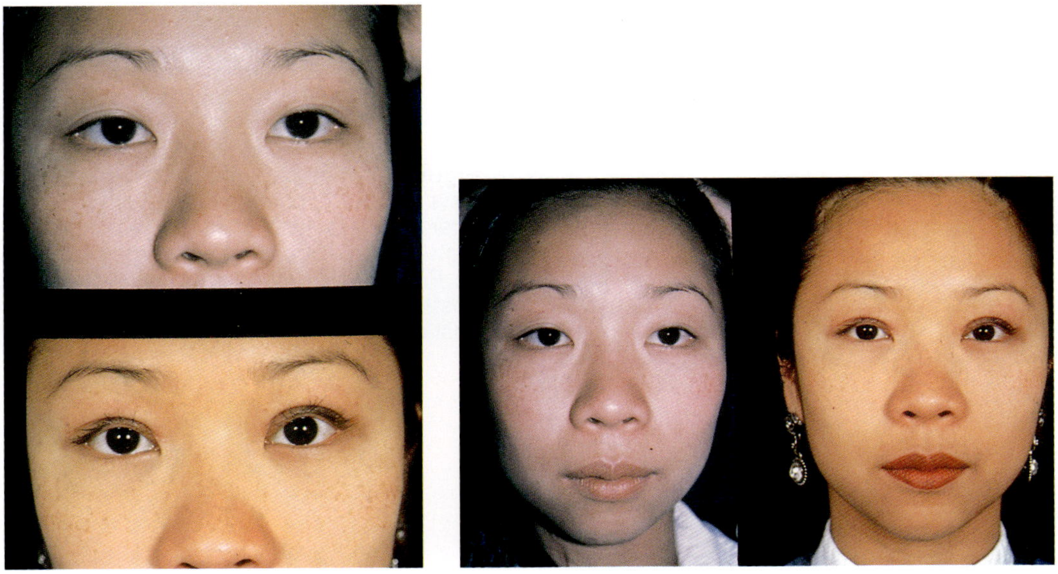

Figure 9. We encourage conservative management of the Asian eyelid. Preferable placement of the supratarsal fold is at the superior pole of the tarsus. Epicanthal folds, when preserved, yield a much more natural and ethnically compatible outcome.

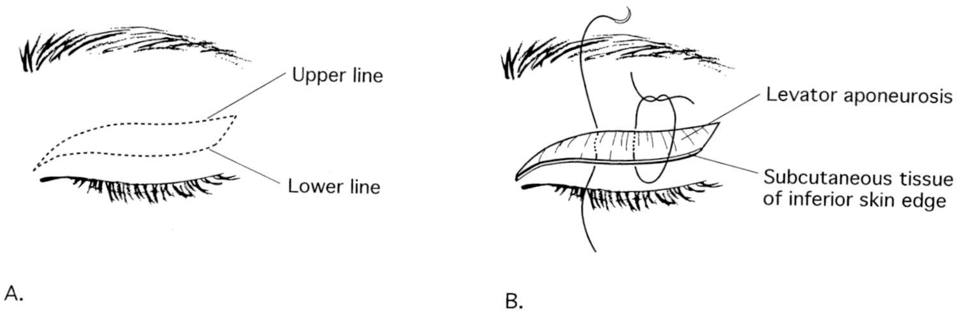

Figure 10. **A:** Design for a parallel or nasally tapered crease including the upper and lower lines of incision. **B:** The editor prefers to use a suture that courses from the dermis to superior tarsal border to dermis. This yields a deep permanent supratarsal fold.

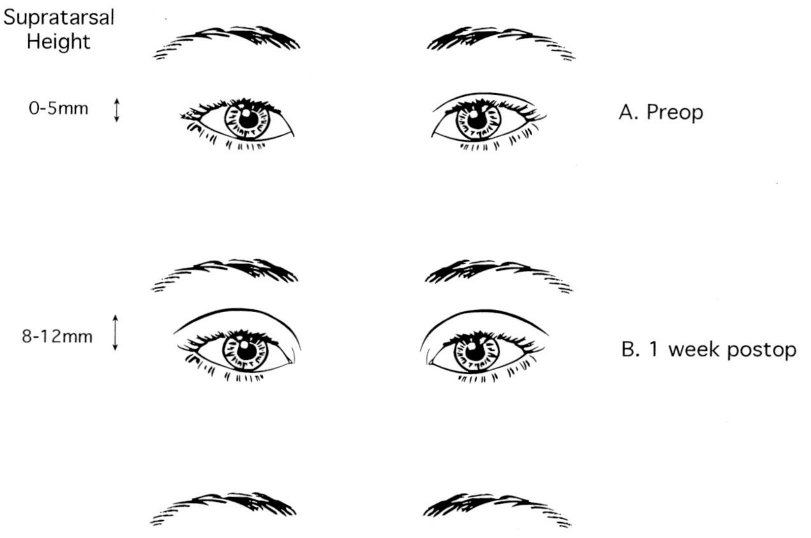

Figure 11. The patient should be prepared for a number of changes that typically occur after blepharoplasty, including a temporarily high appearance of the supratarsal fold. **A:** Pre-operative appearance. **B:** One-week post-operative appearance. **C:** Eight-week post-operative appearance.

Ethnic Considerations in Facial Aesthetic Surgery, edited by W. Earle Matory, Jr.
Lippincott–Raven Publishers, Philadelphia © 1998.

19

The Asian Patient

Leonard Gray, Edmond A. Zingaro,
and Edward Falces

The Ideal has many names, and beauty is but one of them.
— W. Somerset Maugham

Nearly half of the entire world population is of Asian descent. The history of Asia is as old and as rich as that of all humanity. Centuries of cultural growth have been accompanied by an expanding population. The number of Asians living in the United States, according to the 1990 U.S. Census, has increased 89% from 3.8 million to 7.2 million within the last decade. Within California, there has been such a massive immigration that it is estimated that Asians will make up over 50% of the state's population by the year 2000. In the San Francisco Bay Area alone, there are 294,000 Filipino and Pacific Islanders and 625,000 Orientals.

CULTURAL CONSIDERATIONS

As the Asian population has increased, so has the number of Asian Americans undergoing facial aesthetic surgery. Old myths and taboos from the East that were contrary to cosmetic surgery have given way to an acceptance of what can be achieved with today's plastic surgical techniques. There has been a growing appreciation of the personal aesthetic and psychological benefits of cosmetic surgery.

Contrary to what many believe, most Asians seeking plastic surgery do not want to have their features "Westernized." Rather, there are certain aesthetic improvements that are sought to achieve an enhanced but still identifiably ethnic appearance.

L. Gray, E. A. Zingaro, and E. Falces: San Francisco, California 94109

FACIAL CHARACTERISTICS

In general, Asian skin is more pigmented than that of the Caucasians and as such is less susceptible to the ravages of sun exposure in addition to being less likely to undergo the downward pull of gravity. The number of Asians requesting rhytidectomy is much less than that in fair-skinned populations. In our practices, the techniques used for face and brow lift in this segment of the population are not unique. In this chapter we will discuss the areas of facial aesthetic surgery that are distinctive in the Asian population: namely, blepharoplasty and rhinoplasty.

Creation of the upper eyelid crease and nasal enhancement are the most common cosmetic procedures performed in Asian countries and are probably the most common reason for Asian Americans to visit their plastic surgeon in the U.S.A. The surgeon must have a strong appreciation for Asian concepts of aesthetic balance and genuine beauty as well as a thorough understanding of what constitutes realistic expectations. In general, Asians are conservative, seeking modest and gradual change rather than dramatic transitions that alter ethnic character. Expectations are high and anticipated outcomes are not always clear in the patient's mind. There are inherent obstacles to achieving full patient understanding of preoperative details. The surgeon is advised to expand counseling efforts to overcome these omnipresent cultural, linguistic, and perceptual barriers.

EYELID SURGERY

Asian blepharoplasty dates back to the late nineteenth century, when Mikamo described the closed technique to create an eyelid crease. Mauro in 1928 described the first open technique for blepharoplasty in the Asian eyelid. In 1950 Ohashi introduced a cauterization technique to create the supratarsal fold (3). Sayoc, in 1954, presented a technique that would popularize the operation for creation of the supratarsal fold (3). He included a supratarsal incision, orbicularis muscle slip excision, resection of excess supralevator fat, and lower skin flap dermal attachment to the levator insertion. In 1960, Fernandez improved our understanding of the aesthetic quality of the results obtainable with the open technique. This method of creating lidfolds has become the standard by which others are measured. Most recently, Flowers has popularized the anchor blepharoplasty, a technique designed to make the fold neat, crisp, and youthful in Caucasians.

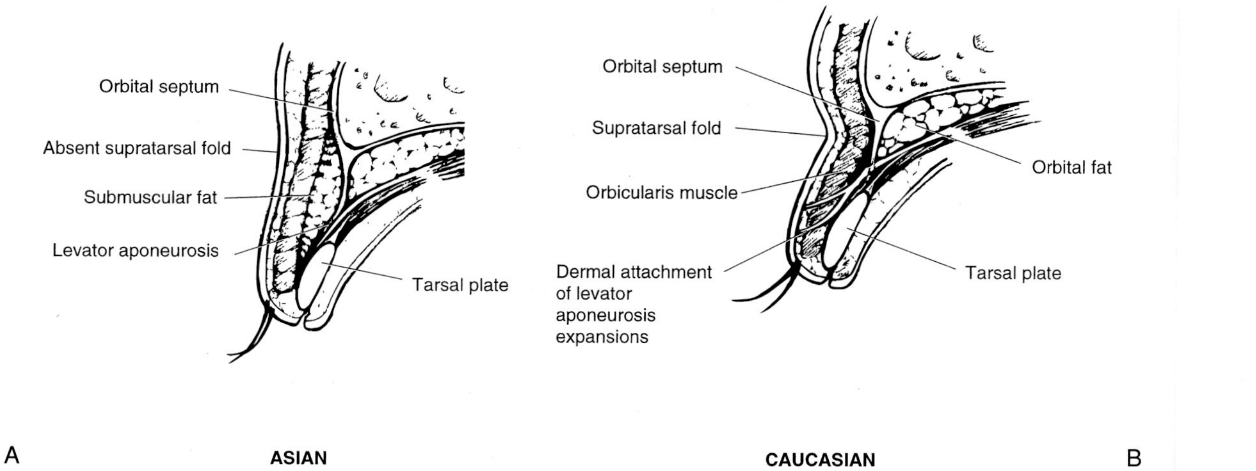

Figure 1. Anatomy of typical Asian eyelid. Note the absence of levator aponeurosis extensions to dermis **(A)** in comparison with the typical anatomy of the Caucasian eyelid **(B)**.

Anatomic Considerations

The unique anatomy of the Asian eyelid demands thorough study and detailed pre-operative evaluation (Fig. 1). The Asian perception of beauty thus incorporates a graceful eyelid crease that brightens the patient's appearance, with smooth but adherent pretarsal skin and soft mobile supratarsal skin.

Within the Oriental ethnic classification, there are many distinctive features that exist based on individual as well as ethnic contributions. The Chinese, Japanese, Korean, Malaysian, Filipino, Polynesian, and a multitude of other Asiatic subgroups each present us with individual, cultural, and anatomic variations that must be analyzed prior to surgical intervention. Approximately 50% of the Asian population inherits supratarsal folds. As a result, the upper lid appears less full and the eyelash curves upward. Lack of attachment of the levator to the tarsus medially allows the orbital septum and the underlying junction to lie between the skin and conjunctiva (Fig. 1A). This bulge creates an epicanthal fold that is sometimes exaggerated by an extra layer of preseptal fat. With 40% of individuals lacking epicanthal folds, absence of folds is sometimes deemed as a desirable.

Mild to moderate degrees of ptosis that hide the upper limbus are common. Absences of upper lid ptosis with the presentation of a brighter-eyed look has always been an admired trait in the Orient. The Asian perception of beauty thus incorporates a graceful eyelid crease that brightens the patient's appearance, with smooth but adherent pretarsal skin and soft mobile supratarsal skin.

In general, the Asian orbit is smaller with a tarsal height of 3–5 vs. 7–10 mm in the Caucasian. As a result the septum courses more distally, allowing the underlying fatty compartments to yield a fuller/puffier supraorbital prominence.

Operative Technique

The upper lid is everted to identify and measure the tarsal height. Creation of the lid crease along the superior edge of the tarsus will yield the optimal eyelid and facial balance. On the other hand, many patients seek a more subtle change, with a lower crease fold. A select few opt for a higher, more dramatic crease. Alternative positioning of the crease must be discussed, with the surgeon noting the more natural options. The decision, however, is based on the patient's educated wishes, not on the leanings or perceptions of the surgeon.

Upper lid skin redundancy is assessed. Conservatism is key. If the patient desires, a limited skin resection is outlined, incorporating the excess skin contributing to the epicanthal fold.

The creation of visible signs of cosmetic surgery may result in significant peer disapproval for the patient and medicolegal ramifications for the surgeon. The epicanthal fold, if present, should be left untouched, unless adjustments are specifically requested. Scars that result from attempted resection of the epicanthal fold are less appealing than the ethnically attractive and natural epicanthal fold.

A skin/muscle flap superficial to the tarsus is then elevated to the level of the ciliary margin, and redundant pretarsal fat is excised (Fig. 2). The orbital septum cephalad to the conjoined union with the levator aponeurosis is incised, and excess fat is teased out with the aid of a cotton swab and amputated with the cautery. Conservative resection will avoid a sunken superior lid, a tell-tale sign of surgery. One can always return to remove more fat. A resultant cadaveric appearance, devastating for any patient, is especially so for the Asian. A 2-mm strip of orbicularis muscle is removed from the previously elevated skin/muscle flap (Fig. 3). Several 6-0 non-absorbable buried sutures are used to approximate dermis and orbital septum to the superior border of the tarsus, and the caudal levator aponeurosis skin is approximated with a continuous subcuticular suture with 6-0 polypropylene. Cool compresses are placed on the eyes and the head of the bed is elevated 30° for 48 h. The polypropylene suture is removed at 5 days.

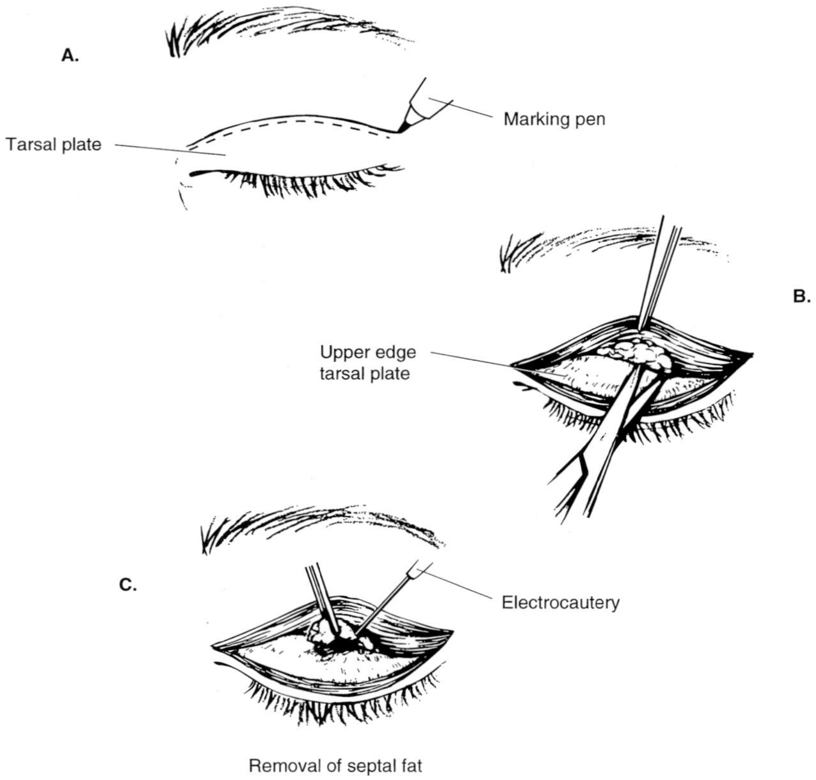

Figure 2. Removal of preseptal fat.

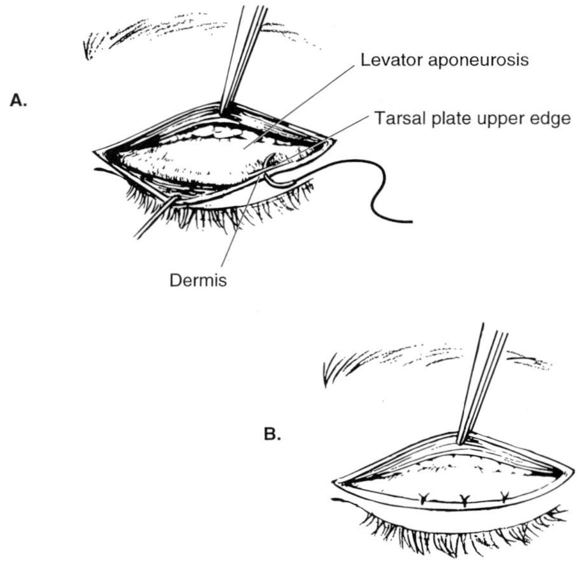

Figure 3. Dermis of inferior wound edge is sutured to the superior edge of the tarsal plate.

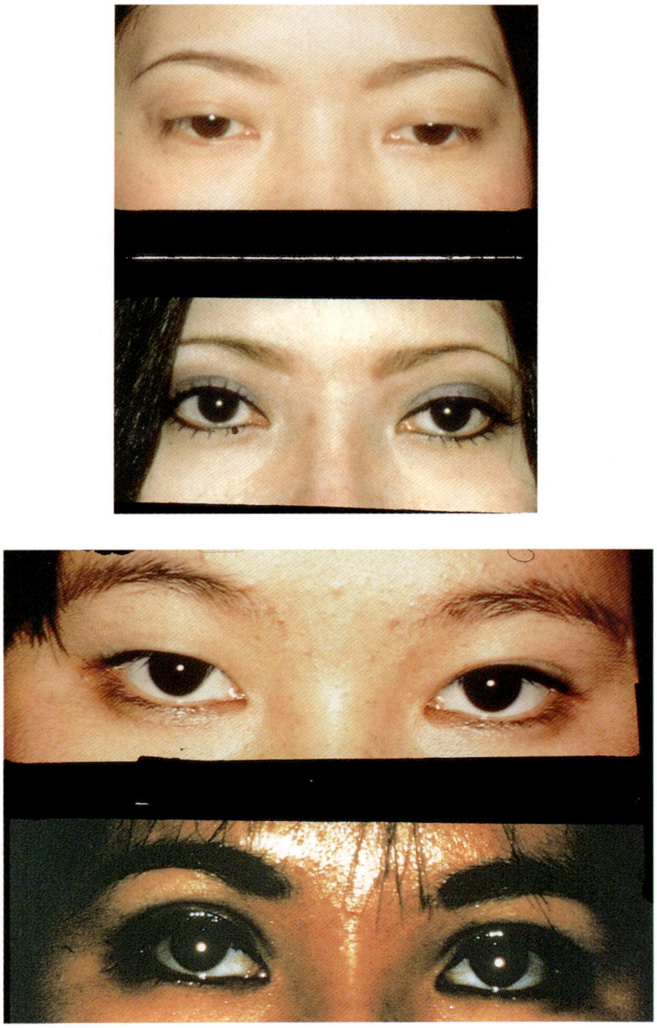

Figure 4. Pre- and post-operative appearance following blepharoplasty.

Redundant skin of the lower lid is less common in Asian subgroups. The transconjunctival approach is ideal in that there are no visible scars. In addition, the potential complication of lower lid ectropion is greatly reduced.

Thus, the goals of blepharoplasty in the Asian include smooth, graceful upper lids with dynamic, crisp fold contoured to the curvature of the globe and at a level that is consistent with that patient's wishes (Fig. 4).

RHINOPLASTY

The goal in Asian rhinoplasty is to proportion the nose to complement the graceful curvature, symmetry, and attractiveness of the Asian face. While a high, narrow dorsum with a sharply sculpted tip is an appealing result in those of European ancestry, this is rarely desirable and to some degree incompatible with the Asian face. Beauty requires a smooth, harmonious, and coordinated blend of facial features. A nose that is fuller and shorter than that desired in the Caucasian may better complement the broad and short Asian face.

Asian noses are short with a broad, somewhat amorphous tip. Excess fat is present at the level of the dome and also overlies the upper and lower lateral cartilages. The skin is thick.

Nostrils are rounded with a slight horizontal orientation. The soft triangles are often blunted or not visible. Lower lateral crura are usually small, thin, and weak. A low placement of the genu further contributes to tip broadness and flaring of the alar base. The columella is wide with some degree of retraction and associated with an acute nasolabial angle. A short, broad bony dorsum forms a widened, sometimes flattened nasal pyramid.

Operative Technique

A number of techniques have been used to refine the features of the Asian nose. Alloplastic materials both porous and solid, such as silicone elastomer, have been advocated by some. While results using alloplastic materials can be very favorable, the incidence of infection, extrusion, and displacement is more common than with autologous implantation. These complications are problematic for any patient. In the Asian the resultant permanent disfigurement may magnify negative peer pressure and might inspire litigation. We prefer autogenous materials whenever possible.

Our technique, that of crural advancement, better defines the nasal tip and changes the shape and orientation of the nostrils. In addition, tip projection is improved and the soft triangle is highlighted. The broad, low nasal dorsum may be augmented and wide nostril flaring is reduced (Fig. 5).

Following general anesthesia or local sedation and infiltration with xylocaine 1% with 1 : 200,000 epinephrine, a transverse columellar incision is made and extended as a rim incision. Skin is elevated up over the dome, revealing tip and supratip fat. Defatting is performed over the entire lower lateral cartilages and inbetween the medial crura. Of note, the vestibular skin on the mucosal side of the alar cartilages is left intact. The medial and lateral crura are then sutured to each other and advanced from the base past the genu using buried sutures of 5-0 clear nylon. This process of closing the intercrural distance continues

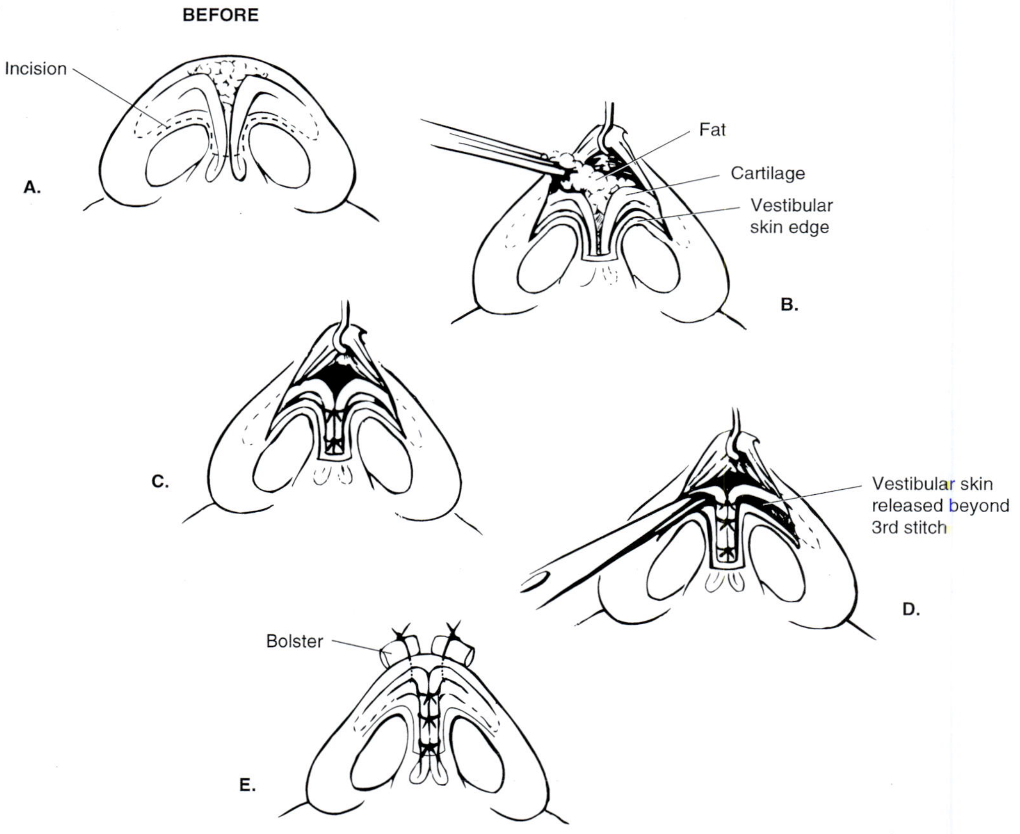

Figure 5. Tip augmentation and reduction of nasal flaring.

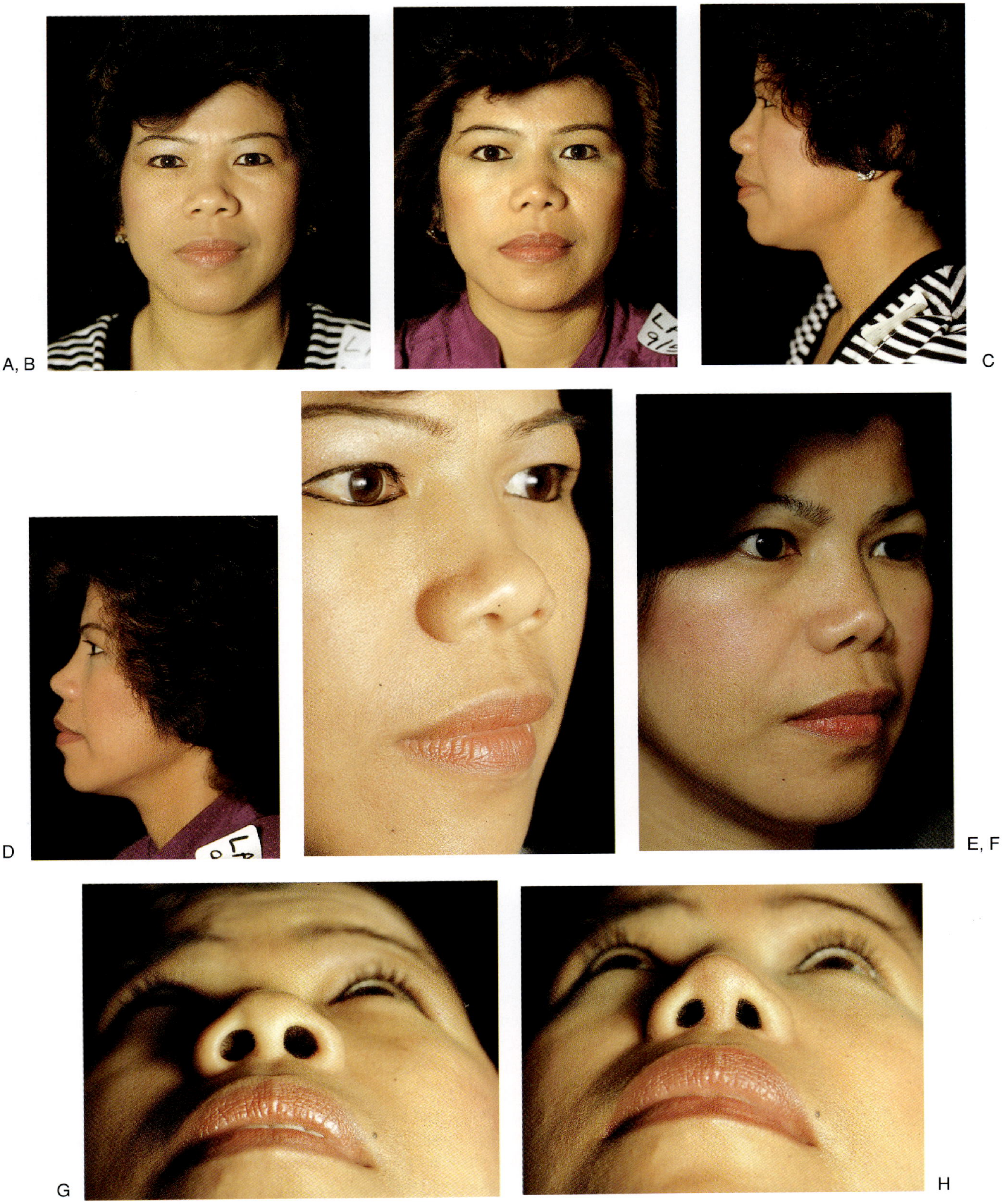

Figure 6. Pre-operative **(A, C, E, and G)** and post-operative **(B, D, F, and H)** appearance after placement of a dorsal implant, tip defatting, crural advancement, and alar wedge excisions. Note the vertical midcolumellar incision used. No cartilage grafts or struts were used.

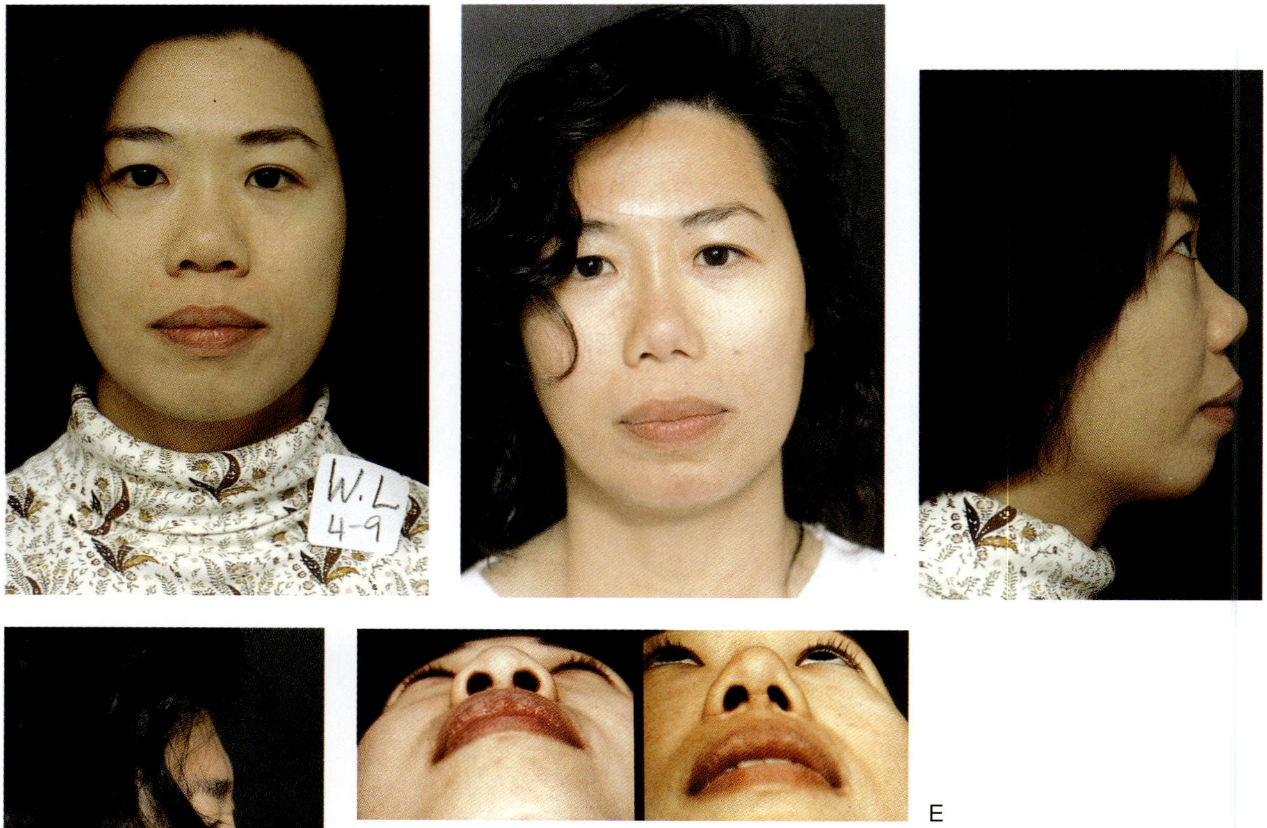

A, B C E

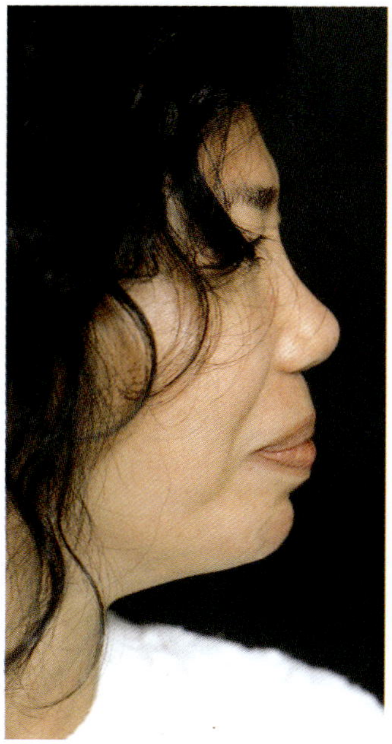

D

Figure 7. Pre-operative **(A, C, left half of E)** and post-operative **(B, D, right half of E)** appearance after placement of a dorsal implant, tip defatting, crural advancement, and alar wedge excisions.

until the desired cartilage projection is achieved. Usually three to four sutures are needed, some of which may extend cephalad and/or lateral to the genu. With intact vestibular skin, this process changes the nostril from a round shape to a more vertical one. The vestibular skin lateral to the new genu may then be released, allowing the skin to redrape and thus permitting the new more appealing soft triangle to reform. The cephalic portion of the lower lateral cartilages is trimmed symmetrically as needed.

If the bony dorsum is wide or with ridges, contouring is accomplished by rasping. Subsequent augmentation corrects the low, flat appearance of the dorsum. Septal cartilage is the preferred alternative when available. Conchal cartilage, rib cartilage, or bone from the iliac crest, ulna, tibia, cranium, or rib may also be used. We use a technique described by Gunter, where an elliptical piece of septal cartilage is scored and then fractured. This piece, which is now in an "inverted U-frame shape," is then placed over the dorsum.

Transcutaneous bolster sutures are placed and maintain the genu at maximal projection. Columellar skin is closed with 6-0 nylon and nasal mucosa with 5-0 chromic. Should the nostrils still be deemed flared or widened, alar wedge excision is performed, along with undermining of the ala (Fig. 6).

The resultant orientation of the tip and dorsum is directed toward achieving a natural but enhanced appearance that is in harmony with the ethnic characteristics of the Asian face (Fig. 7).

RECOMMENDED READING

Baek SM. Oriental blepharoplasty—single stitch non incision technique. *Plast Reconstr Surg* 1989;83:236.

Fernandez LR. Double eyelid operation in the Oriental in Hawaii. *Plast Reconstr Surg* 1960;25:257.

Flowers RS. Blepharoplasty and periorbital aesthetic surgery. *Clin Plast Surg* 1993;20:2.

Gunter JP. Advanced concepts in rhinoplasty. Course 2-452, ASPRS National Meeting, New Orleans, LA, 1993.

Mikamo M. Plastic operation of the eyelid. *Chingai Iji Shinpo Tokyo* 1896;17:396.

Sayoc BT. Surgery of the Oriental eyelid. *Clin Plast Surg* 1974;1:157.

Song IC. Surgical management of the Asian eyelid and nose. Course 1-306, ASPRS National Meeting, New Orleans, LA, 1993.

Ethnic Considerations in Facial Aesthetic Surgery, edited by W. Earle Matory, Jr.
Lippincott–Raven Publishers, Philadelphia © 1998.

20

Facial Surgery in the Asian Patient

John A. McCurdy, Jr.

Her eyes, her lips, her cheeks, her shapes, her features
Seem to be drawn by love's own hand; by love
Himself in love.
— Dryden

While the physical characteristics of Asians show substantial individual variation, certain distinct facial features do necessitate formulation of unique surgical approaches for aesthetic modification. The most notable of these anatomic characteristics for which surgical manipulation is commonly requested are the following:

1. The upper eyelid, characterized by an absent or poorly defined superior palpebral fold, abundant periorbital (and frequently suborbicularis) fat, and an epicanthal fold of varying configuration and size.
2. A nose with poor lobular definition and deficient anterior projection of both pyramid and lobule. Additionally, the lobular columella is often retracted and the alar base may be somewhat widened.
3. Hypoplasia of the midface manifested by maxillary retrusion associated with an anterior inclination of the maxillary incisors.

Skin texture and pigmentation exhibit substantial individual variation. In general, those Asians originating from more southerly latitudes show darker pigmentation. Approximately 75% of central Asians (i.e., Northern Chinese, Koreans, Japanese) have lightly colored, somewhat milky skin pigmentation. The yellowish tint of Asian skin is largely a consequence of the number and distribution of melanin granules rather than variations in the skin lipoproteins.

Regardless of the extent of skin pigmentation, Asians generally demonstrate a thicker dermis than equivalently pigmented Caucasians. This greater collagen density is mani-

J. A. McCurdy, Jr.: Department of Surgery, University of Hawaii, John A. Burns School of Medicine, Honolulu, Hawaii 96813 fested in a tendency toward a more vigorous fibroplastic response during wound healing, which results in hypertrophic scarring and prolonged redness during scar maturation, in an incidence worthy of note even in lightly pigmented Asians. Clinically, hypertrophic scarring is most common in the epicanthal region and the post-auricular (and occasionally temporal) incisions for rhytidectomy. For unknown reasons, hypertrophic scarring rarely if ever occurs on the lower eyelids or following alar base excision. In spite of the fact that hypertrophic scarring is common in the noted areas, frank keloid formation is rare, occurring most commonly in the ear lobule after piercing.

Increased dermal thickness may account for a substantially lower incidence of fine facial rhytides in both darker and fair Asians as compared with Caucasians of equivalent age. Asian skin tends to respond to sun exposure with an accelerated development of pigmented dermatoses (lentiges, actinic keratoses, seborrheic keratoses, etc.) as compared with Caucasian skin. Skin malignancies, however, of all types are markedly less common in Asians than in Caucasians.

CULTURAL CONSIDERATIONS

An understanding of cultural differences among Asian nationalities is perhaps of equal importance in achieving optimal surgical results as is thorough comprehension of anatomic factors. Effective communication between patient and surgeon is of utmost importance in pre-operative planning as well as in management decisions during the post-operative healing period. Appreciation of cultural and personality characteristics facilitates precise interpersonal communication. Miscommunication predicated on failure to understand such differences is all too often the basis for inappropriate surgical decisions and manipulations (initial and/or corrective).

In spite of the significant influence of the Western world on the East, the tremendous differences between Western and Eastern cultures soon becomes obvious to Westerners who associate with native Asians. Although these differences are less defined in the generations descended from the immigrant populations, certain powerful cultural influences often persist, and these may exert significant effects on attitudes concerning (or behavioral reactions following) cosmetic surgery. As stressed above, a basic appreciation of these cultural factors is of great assistance in providing insight into the psychological make-up of the diverse Asian nationalities and will enable the surgeon to communicate more effectively with, and respond more appropriately to, the concerns and desires of Asian patients.

One of the basic foundations of Asian philosophy is a strong belief in fate, destiny, and the importance of luck, both good and bad, in daily affairs. Many Asians have strong beliefs in certain maxims, proverbs, and superstitions and apply these beliefs and superstitions to important situations encountered in their daily lives.

Asian cultures also place great significance on physiognomy—the relationship of physical traits are characteristics to behavior and personality—as well as to prospects for success in business, friendship, marriage, and other human relationships.

Most Asians exhibit great respect for higher education and those in positions of authority. This degree of respect may result in a deference to surgeons that may impair effective communication. Questioning the physician is considered to be a sign of disrespect, and thus patients may be reluctant to request clarification of matters that they do not completely understand.

Asian patients frequently feel that their surgeon will automatically know (and do) what is best. An unsatisfactory result, however, frequently fragments this patient/physician bond, unleashing emotions and behavioral forces that could have been attenuated by effective pre-operative communication.

IMPORTANCE OF BEAUTY

Physical beauty is often particularly important to Asian women, as there is a general cultural belief that if a woman does not remain attractive to her husband, he has every right to wander in search of other sources of affection. Before the advent of cosmetic surgery, a fatalistic attitude toward appearance was predominant, a stance that to a large extent—at least in more urbanized areas—has been supplanted by a strong desire to undergo surgery for improvement in appearance. Submission to cosmetic surgery, however, often results in subconscious feelings of guilt and in some cases may complicate the healing period. A major source of such guilt is a strong attachment to family and the belief that it is disrespectful to one's parents to alter physical characteristics that were "given" to an individual by parents. A belief in the importance of beauty and its relationship to personal success has, to a large extent, overwhelmed this cultural tradition.

Alternatively, guilt over having undergone cosmetic surgery may result in withdrawal ("hiding") from family and friends. Such self-imposed isolation robs the patient of much needed emotional support during the critical post-operative period that may contribute to obsessive and/or delusional concerns. The surgeon must be cognizant of these potential disruptive forces during the early post-operative healing period and firmly resist request for inappropriate revision procedures. One prominent Vietnamese surgeon admonishes his patients in printed material, "Please do not look in the mirror for you will surely be disappointed!"

The Asian appreciation for harmony and symmetry, the basic elements of beauty, as well as an eye for detail are manifested in the precision of their craftsmanship. However, this appreciation for perfection may translate into an anxiety about post-operative asymmetry and other appearances during the healing period, requiring considerable patience and understanding on the part of the surgeon. Asian patients often solicit the opinions of family and friends about their appearance during the early post-operative period and are very susceptible to unflattering comments during this stage. This is a common source of early post-operative unhappiness and dissatisfaction, and the surgeon must firmly resist requests for inappropriate revision procedures during this time.

NATIONAL CHARACTERISTICS

While many of the basic cultural nuances discussed are common to all Asian cultures, each ethnic group shares certain common behavioral and personality traits and attitudes that, while not universal, tend to characterize and distinguish members of these nationalities.

The concept of "national identity" is certainly familiar to Westerners. The British, for instance, are being characterized as polite but formal, having a "stiff upper lip," and Germans are stereotyped as stern, diligent, and perfectionistic. In the United States, the characteristics of citizens from different regions provide a basis for such stereotyping. Texans, for example, are characterized as friendly and relaxed with a tendency toward exaggeration, while New Yorkers are often thought of as impatient, blunt, and sarcastic.

In the same manner, Asian nationalities recognize certain typical characteristics among themselves and stereotype various nationalities according to commonly observed traits. Whenever I lecture on surgery in Asian patients, without exception, one of the most common questions asked is, "I just can't seem to get through to my Asian patients. How do you communicate with them effectively?" An understanding and appreciation of ethnic differences and stereotypical traits of the many Asian nationalities may be helpful in this endeavor. The following discussion is based solely on my experiences formulated during 20 years of practice and numerous discussions with ethnic Asians about the differing traits and personality characteristics of various nationalities.

Japanese

The Japanese are often described as exceedingly polite, respectful, and patient. These characteristics are favorable to successful cosmetic surgery, particularly in terms of psychological and emotional adaptability. Japanese patients generally understand the concept that improvement, not perfection, is the goal of cosmetic surgery. They rarely complain during post-operative recovery, consistent with their tendency to avoid direct personal confrontation. If revision procedures are indicated, the Japanese patient is frequently apologetic, expressing concern that somehow her/his lack of attention following initial surgery may have contributed to the post-operative result. If a surgical result is suboptimal, the surgeon should not hesitate to initiate a frank discussion of the problem as occasionally a Japanese patient would rather consult another surgeon rather than risk offending the original surgeon by complaining about an unsatisfactory result. Similarly, if unhappy with advice or treatment recommended by a surgeon, the Japanese patient will often simply seek another opinion rather than complain or ask questions.

Korean

In contrast to Japanese attitudes, Koreans are often perfectionistic, assertive, and intolerant of minor defects and asymmetries. The typical Korean patient is rarely reluctant to express concerns and dissatisfaction, often in an aggressive or overbearing manner. S/he is more likely to be impatient during the post-operative healing period. Koreans are honest and hard working, but because bargaining is an integral component of Korean culture, they may use expressions of dissatisfaction as a lever to extract concessions (i.e., fee discounts) on surgical procedures for themselves or friends.

Perhaps the best approach in dealing with any unrealistic requests or temperamental behavior of Korean patients is one of firmness and honesty as these attributes are respected in Korean culture. Koreans are very responsive to the honest feelings and concerns of others. Most importantly, surgeons should not allow themselves to be intimidated into performing inappropriate or unnecessary surgery (particularly revision surgery) on this patient population.

Vietnamese

Vietnamese people tend to be exceedingly polite, respectful, and self-effacing. These characteristics persist as long as events proceed according to their hopes and expectations. Vietnamese, in my experience, tend to mistrust authority—perhaps as a result of the exploitations suffered during their French colonial history. They may become withdrawn, sullen, and even hostile if the post-operative period does not proceed according to their expectations. The suspicion of authority may lead Vietnamese patients to be unconvinced by the surgeon's attempts to explain imperfect results or why the healing process may be proceeding more slowly than anticipated. It is not unusual for a dissatisfied Vietnamese patient to tell the surgeon that s/he is satisfied with the surgical result while complaining mercilessly to friends (and other surgeons consulted) about the result and the ineptness of the surgeon.

Honest and open discussion is the most effective method of interacting. The surgeon should never attempt to deny or "smooth over" concerns that arise, however trivial they may seem. Maintaining effective rapport requires (a) responsiveness to the questions and insecurities that present and (b) employment of a "do something" approach to perceived or real concerns. For example, assist tincture of time by recommending local massage or by the application of topical treatments like 1% hydrocortisone cream. Sensitivity to patient concerns and the TLC that should accompany post-operative care with all patients can be particularly important in this patient population.

Chinese

It is difficult to characterize the attitudes and reactions of Chinese patients to cosmetic surgery as the behavioral characteristics of this diverse group (many distinct "subnationalities") are so varied. Many patients are withdrawn, fatalistic, and reluctant to express emotions, making communications between patient and surgeon difficult and sometimes frustrating. Others may be impatient, emotionally labile, irascible, and inclined to indulge in face-saving behavior, occasionally involving petty dishonesty. Some may be highly suspicious of authority, which can impede frank and open discussion.

Chinese have extremely strong ties to the family and often harbor unconscious feelings of guilt and shame in altering facial features. In general, however, Chinese patients show a realistic attitude toward the benefits and limitations of cosmetic surgery. They respond rationally to open and honest discussion.

Filipinos

The culture of the Philippines values politeness, honesty, and respect for the physician, rivaling that of the Japanese. These traits make patients of Philippine ancestry excellent candidates for cosmetic surgery. Filipinos faithfully follow post-operative instructions and are generally patient in awaiting the final post-operative outcome. They are understanding if convalescence is prolonged or minor complications arise. Few patients are more genuine and effusive in their expression of appreciation for a good result. The surgeon, however, must not take these desirable attributes for granted, for if the patient's confidence and trust are abused, emotional lability and volatile confrontation may result.

Thais

Thailand is called the "land of smiles" as its people are known for their relaxed and trusting attitudes. Thais are generally very patient, responsive to explanations regarding the healing process, and tolerant of minor imperfections and asymmetries.

INTERACTING WITH THE ASIAN PATIENT

As a group, Asian patients tend to be reserved and self-effacing, necessitating open, somewhat probing discussions to extract pertinent information and form realistic expectations, both before and after surgery. The surgeon should (a) encourage the patient to communicate any fears, worries, or disappointments honestly and (b) be, likewise, frank and straightforward when discussing expectations, realistic results, and possible complications.

BLEPHAROPLASTY IN THE ASIAN EYELID

General Considerations

Surgical modification of the upper eyelid has become increasingly popular in Asia since World War II and, at the present time, is the most commonly performed aesthetic operation in the Far East. While surgery of the Asian eyelid is similar to blepharoplasty in other ethnic groups, important anatomical and technical differences do exist, and the surgeon must be familiar with these variations to maximize aesthetic results.

As a group, approximately 50% of Asians exhibit a "single eyelid," so-called because, in the absence of a superior palpebral fold, the lid hangs like a curtain from the supraorbital ridge. Creation of a palpebral sulcus divides the lid into well defined pretarsal and palpebral segments, producing the "double eyelid" desired by many Asian women as well as an increasing number of men.

The incidence of the single eyelid, of course, is higher in Asian populations that have remained homogeneous (i.e., Japanese, Northern Koreans), while a double eyelids are more common in heterogeneous populations (i.e., Vietnamese, South Koreans, Southeast Asians, and Filipinos). Most Asians with natural double eyelids, however, exhibit a small fold accompanied by abundant periorbital and submuscular fat as well as excess skin with considerable pretarsal laxity.

It would be erroneous to assume that the popularity of the double eyelid operation is related solely to Western influence. Asian cultures have long regarded the bright-eyed look associated with the double eyelid as an aesthetically desirable feature. Many Oriental women produce double eyelids by using various tapes and glues to encourage adherence of the pretarsal portions of the upper lid skin, resulting in a palpebral fold. As such rituals are time consuming and temporary, surgery is frequently requested after reaching the age of 15 or 16.

Because many Asian cultures regard the double eyelid as an aesthetically desirable facial feature, it is important for the surgeon to understand that a request for surgical modification of the single eyelid is not necessarily a request for Westernization of the lid. Many patients, particularly those who have been born in North America, simply desire a small double eyelid while maintaining ethnic character.

Westernization of the eyelid, on the other hand, requires reduction of the characteristic puffiness of the Asian lid by removing excess skin and fat and, in many cases, modification of an epicanthal fold. In general, recent immigrants to Western countries request creation of a large eyelid (i.e., higher palpebral fold), while individuals born or raised in Western society usually request a more "natural" lid with preservation of their ethnicity.

Anatomic Considerations

The commonly accepted anatomic explanation of the differences between single and double eyelid is as follows: In the Caucasian eye, filaments of the levator expansion penetrate the orbital septum and orbicularis muscle and attach to the overlying dermis, creating a superior palpebral fold when the eye is opened. In the Asian lid, the levator aponeurosis does not penetrate the orbital septum of the orbicularis muscle but terminates on the superior margin of the tarsus.

Recent studies, however, suggest that the anatomic basis for formation of the superior palpebral fold is somewhat more complex. Rather than attaching directly to the dermis, filaments of the levator aponeurosis appear to extend inferiorly into the pretarsal portion of the lid, interdigitating with fibrous septa coursing from the tarsus (penetrating the pretarsal orbicularis) to the pretarsal skin, thus producing adherence between the pretarsal skin, orbicularis muscle, and tarsus. The actual mechanism of lid fold creation appears to relate to this adhesion of pretarsal skin, orbicularis, and tarsus. The preseptal skin, in contrast, is non-adherent to the preseptal muscle and thus is relatively mobile. As the levator contracts, the mobile preseptal skin folds over the relatively rigid pretarsal lid (skin, orbicularis, and tarsus) that is elevated as a unit, thus forming the fold. This concept is consistent with the fact that in eyelids without a well defined palpebral fold, the pretarsal skin is redundant because it lacks attachments to the pretarsal muscle and tarsus. Surgical procedures that create a superior palpebral fold achieve this goal by virtue of the fact that the process of supratarsal fixation effectively produces an adhesion between the pretarsal skin and the lid-opening mechanism, thus allowing its elevation as a single unit on levator contraction. This modified understanding of the anatomic basis for the lid fold has clinical implications in double eyelid surgery because a more stable adhesion in the pretarsal lid and tightening of the pretarsal skin can be achieved by undermining the pretarsal skin several millimeters prior to placement of fixation sutures.

Furthermore, the lack of adherence between pretarsal skin, orbicularis, and tarsus allows a wedge of periorbital fat (bounded anteriorly by the levator aponeurosis and posteriorly by the orbital septum) to descend inferiorly, anterior to the tarsal plate, producing the characteristic "puffiness" of the pretarsal lid. An abundant layer of suborbicularis fat is often present in the Asian lid, contributing to fullness in the pretarsal area. Interestingly, the location of the palpebral fold in all ethnicities appears to coincide with the point of fusion between levator aponeurosis and orbital septum, the descending wedge of fat bounded by these structures acting as a barrier preventing adherence of pretarsal skin, orbicularis, and tarsus. Clinically, this barrier of fat must be surgically excised inferior to the point at which the palpebral fold is created to create permanent adhesion of pretarsal tissue layers. Failure to adequately remove this tissue is frequently the cause of "falling out" of the surgically created fold and occurs most commonly in the lateral aspect of the eyelid.

Pre-Operative Considerations

The major goal of blepharoplasty in the Asian upper lid is creation or enhancement of a crisp, well defined palpebral fold. Because of the many possible variations in achieving this goal (i.e., the level of the palpebral fold, the depth of the palpebral sulcus, as well as the appearance of the epicanthal region that can be controlled by variations in surgical technique), careful pre-operative evaluation and counseling of each prospective patient are mandatory in planning this operation. Many patients desire only the creation of a palpebral fold and wish to retain the other characteristics of the Asian eyelid. Others, however, prefer more radical Westernization that requires modification of the epicanthal fold as well as reduction of lid puffiness by removal of redundant skin and fat.

Several methods assist the surgeon and patient in selecting the type of eyelid transformation desired. In my practice, patients are advised that three basic decisions are necessary: (a) the size of the "new" eyelid, (b) the shape of the "new" eyelid, and (c) the disposition of the epicanthal fold.

For planning purposes, double eyelids are arbitrarily divided into small, medium, and large sizes, depending upon the amount of visible pretarsal skin and the depth of the palpebral sulcus. Likewise, eyelids are classified as either round or oval in shape.

In discussing the epicanthal region, differences between the so-called "inside" and "outside" folds are demonstrated with pre- and post-operative photographs, enabling a more rational discussion of possible variations (Fig. 1).

Patients are then shown pre- and post-operative photographs illustrating the various sizes and shapes of eyelids (Fig. 2). In many patients, it is possible to demonstrate the approximate size and shape of the lid (while the patient is looking into a mirror) by manipulating the eyelid skin with a bent paper clip or forceps.

Some patients bring pictures of magazine models to their consultations, and, while it must be stressed to the patient that a surgeon cannot construct an eyelid to the patient's exact specifications, examining these pictures in conjunction with pre- and post-operative photographs allows the surgeon to determine the general size and shape of eyelid that each individual desires.

Anesthesia

The operation is performed under local anesthesia (0.5 bupivacaine or 1% lidocaine with epinephrine 1:50,000) with intravenous sedation. The vast majority of cases are performed as outpatient procedures in an office surgical facility. As frequent opening and closing of the eyes during surgery are helpful in evaluating symmetry, general anesthesia is not

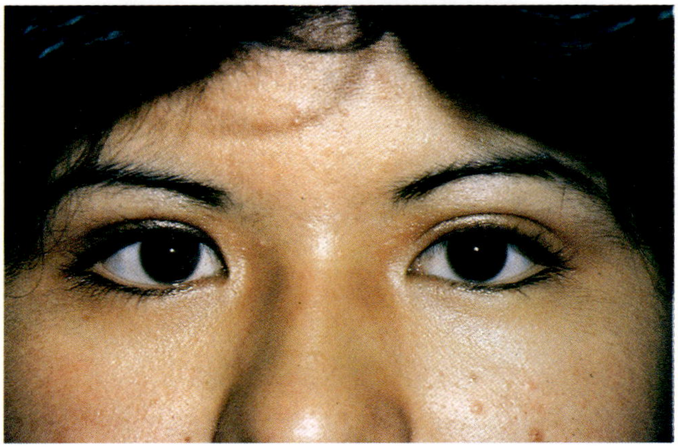

Figure 1. The left eye exhibits an outside fold, while the right eye exhibits an inside fold, maintaining the epicanthus.

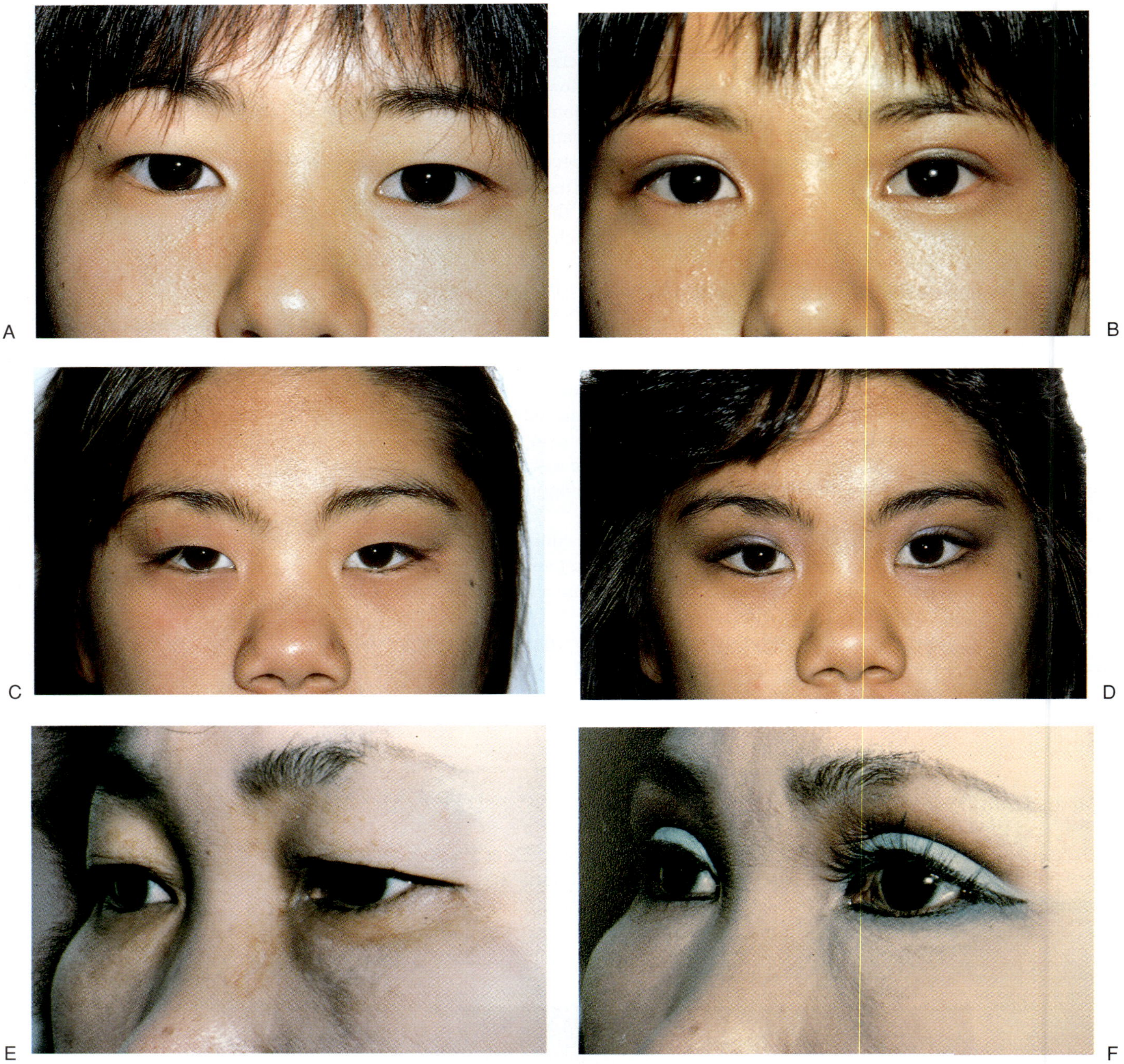

Figure 2. A–B: Pre- and post-operative photographs showing surgical creation of a small double eyelid with an inside fold. **C–D:** Surgical creation of double eyelid that is oval in configuration with an inside fold. **E–F:** Pre- and post-operative photographs showing surgical creation of a large double eyelid with an outside fold.

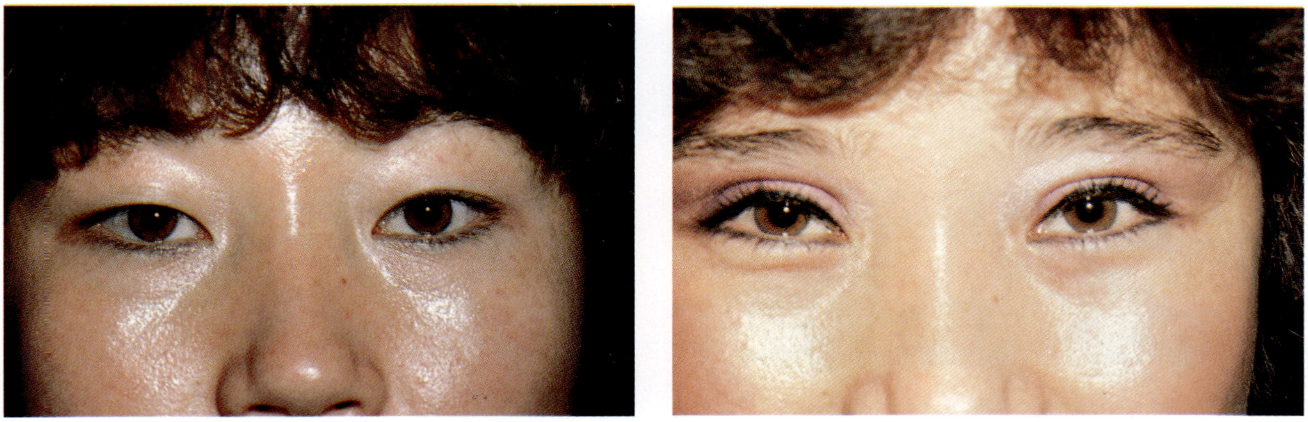

G H

Figure 2 (*continued*). **G–H:** Pre- and post-operative photographs showing surgical creation of a medium-sized double eyelid with a compromise fold.

recommended. For the same reason, the level of sedation during surgery should be light. Diazepam and midazolam are best avoided as both agents frequently interfere with lid opening.

Operative Procedure

The key to success in upper lid blepharoplasty in Asian patients is to perform each step (from pre-operative making to final suturing) with the goal of achieving eyelid symmetry. Proper pre-operative markings are of the utmost importance and are determined by the size (small, medium, large) and shape (round, oval) of the desired eyelid transformation. The most important factor in determining the level of the superior palpebral fold is the distance from the ciliary margin at which the inferior lid incision is drawn, ranging from 6 to 10 mm. For creation of a small double eyelid, the incision is placed 6–7 mm above the ciliary margin, while in patients desiring a medium-sized lid, the incision is placed 8 mm above the ciliary margin. For a large eyelid, the incision is marked 9–10 mm above the ciliary margin. While tensing pretarsal skin to the point of lash eversion, an initial mark is placed at the desired height at the level of the lateral limbus following which the entire inferior incision is drawn. To create an eyelid with an oval shape, the incision is configured so that it is ~2 mm more inferior when it reaches the medial canthus while remaining at approximately the same level at the lateral canthus as in the center of the lid. The incision is then extended slightly superiorly and laterally so that it will fall in a periorbital line. If a round eyelid shape is desired, the lateral aspect of the incision is drawn so that it is ~2 mm more inferior at the level of the lateral canthus than at the level of the lateral limbus. Individual desires regarding management of the epicanthal region determine the location of the lid inci-

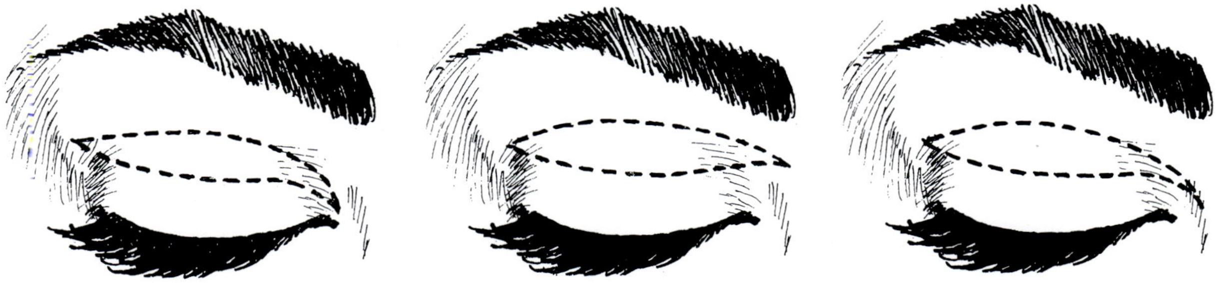

A B, C

Figure 3. Incisions used for the creation of an inside fold **(A)**, an outside fold **(B)**, and a fold terminating on the origin of a small epicanthus **(C)**.

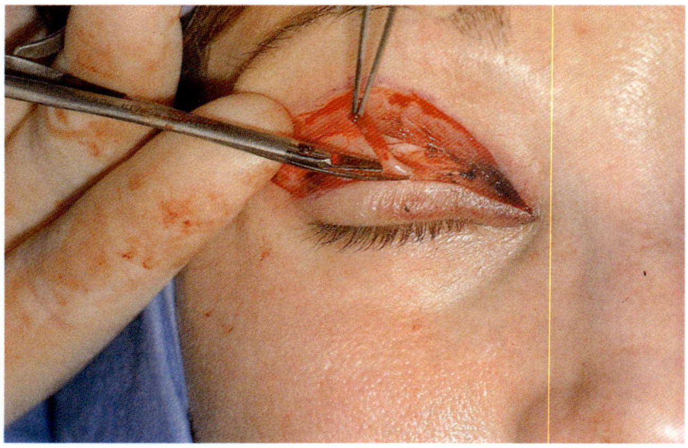

Figure 4. Excision of a 2- to 3-mm strip of muscle beneath the skin at the level of the inferior skin incision.

sion in this area. If an inside fold (i.e., no epicanthal modification) is requested, the incision is drawn lateral to the existing epicanthus (Fig. 3A). If a outside fold (epicanthal effacement) is desired, the incision terminates medial to the epicanthal web (Fig. 3B and C). The level of the superior incision, which determines the amount of skin to be excised, is determined by pinching the skin with forceps and asking the patient to open and close the eyes as in a standard blepharoplasty procedure. The average amount of skin excised is 3–10 mm, depending upon the age of the patient and the type of eyelid desired. It is important to individualize the amount of skin removed according to the size of eyelid requested, as this factor is important in determining the amount of pretarsal "show." For the patient who desires a small double eyelid, only 2–3 mm of skin is excised. For creation of a medium-sized lid, half of the maximal amount of skin that can be removed (as determined by forceps pinching) is actually removed; i.e., if 12 mm of skin could be maximally removed, the incision is placed 6 mm above the level of the inferior skin incision. If a large, Westernized

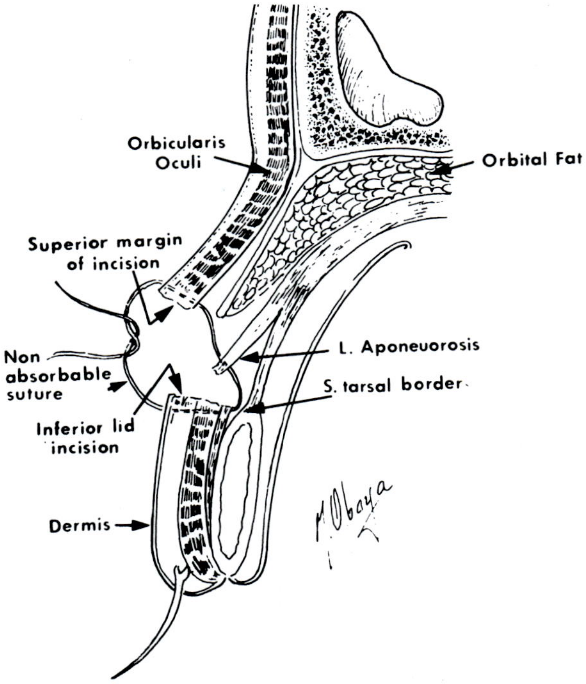

Figure 5. Placement of an external fixation suture (6-0 nylon).

lid is desired, 2–3 mm less than the maximum amount of skin that could be removed as determined by forceps pinching is actually excised. The superior incision is marked so that it courses parallel to the previously marked inferior incision, joining it at the medial and lateral canthal areas.

Following infiltration of local anesthetic, skin and subcutaneous tissues are excised exposing the orbicularis muscle. A 3- to 5-mm strip of orbicularis is excised above the tarsal plate. The orbital septum is then incised, exposing periorbital fat. If a deep "Western" palpebral sulcus is desired, removal of all visible fat in the central and lateral compartments is performed so that the levator expansion is completely cleared. Removal of medial fat, however, is more conservative, as creation of a deep hollow in the medial aspect of the lid does not produce the aesthetically desirable effect that often results from sculpturing this area in the Occidental eye. Excessive fat removal medially also predisposes to hypertrophic scarring as more tension is placed on the skin closure. Little or no fat in any compartment is excised if a small double lid is desired; in such cases the fat is carefully separated so that the levator expansion can be identified.

Prior to placement of fixation sutures, a 2- to 3-mm strip of muscle is removed from beneath the skin at the level of the inferior skin incision (Fig. 4). This maneuver effectively undermines the skin 2–3 mm, providing a wider base of adhesion for formation of the palpebral fold, and allows tightening of pretarsal skin during fixation.

Fixation sutures of 5-0 nylon are then placed, incorporating the skin edge of the inferior incision, the levator aponeurosis, and the superior skin incision (Fig. 5). Buried "internal" fixation sutures of permanent or absorbable suture incorporating only the inferior skin edge and levator may be substituted for the "external" fixation suture, but including the upper skin edge in the fixation enhances interoperative determination of symmetry as the extent of "hooding" contributed by the suprafold tissues is more easily determined. Three fixation sutures are utilized: laterally at a point approximately one-half the distance between the lateral canthus and lateral limbus, centrally at the midpupillary level, and medially at the level of the medial limbus. The lateral fixation suture is placed initially, followed by the middle and medial sutures. Assessment of symmetry is enhanced if the sutures are placed sequentially in the right and left eyelids; i.e., the lateral fixation suture is placed in the right eyelid following which lateral fixation suture placement is performed in the left lid. With the eyes open, symmetry is assessed by inspection and direct measurement following which the middle fixation sutures are placed, etc. One or two additional medial fixation sutures are often placed in the medial aspect of the lid to efface the epicanthal fold if desired. On occasion, more advanced techniques of epicanthoplasty are necessary. The entire incision is then approximated with a running suture of 6-0 plain gut. Fixation sutures are removed in 7 days.

Post-Operative Course

The early post-blepharoplasty period is characterized by marked edema of the pretarsal portion of the lid as well as by variable degrees of blepharoptosis. The extent and duration of this ptosis are directly related to the level of fixation as well as the amount of skin and fat excised, being more significant if a larger lid is created. Blepharoptosis is generally not objectionable following removal of the fixation sutures on the 7th post-operative day but may occasionally cause persistent concern because of resultant asymmetry. Slowly resolving asymmetric ptosis is often related to hematoma or edema of Müller's muscle. Occasionally, residual pretarsal edema may be detectable for up to 6 months but is usually satisfactorily camouflaged by cosmetics following suture removal.

Complications of Blepharoplasty

Perhaps the most common source of dissatisfaction in Asian patients undergoing upper lid blepharoplasty is post-operative asymmetry of the lid folds. This deformity occasionally occurs even in the hands of the most experienced surgeon.

Post-operative asymmetry is more likely to occur when lid or brow asymmetry exists pre-operatively, and each prospective candidate for upper lid blepharoplasty must be carefully evaluated in this regard. Minimal ptosis also predisposes to post-operative asymmetry. If asymmetry exists, it must be carefully pointed out to the patient, explaining that exact post-operative symmetry will be more difficult to achieve. Pre-operative asymmetry, of course, must be carefully documented in the medical record as well as by pre-operative photographs.

Strict adherence to certain technical points minimizes development of post-operative asymmetry:

1. The pre-operative markings on the upper eyelid must be performed while the skin is stretched cephalically. The skin is tensed until the eyelashes begin to evert, a checkpoint that will facilitate symmetrical placement of the pre-operative marks bilaterally.
2. After completing the markings, they are rechecked using a ruler prior to infiltration of anesthetic. On rechecking the incisions, it will be surprising how often a millimeter of asymmetry is discovered, allowing appropriate correction before beginning the operation.
3. After placing the initial fixation suture (usually at the lateral-most fixation point), a corresponding fixation suture is placed in the opposite lid, following which the height of both sutures above the ciliary margin is carefully measured. In placing this initial as well as subsequent fixation sutures, the pretarsal skin is stretched to the point where the eyelashes begin to evert, a visual check also utilized in pre-operative marking as described above. If a difference of even 1 millimeter is noticed on measuring the height of the initial fixation sutures, it should be corrected at this time. Following placement of subsequent fixation sutures, a similar measurement is performed.
4. Avoid excessive sedation during the operative procedure as it may interfere with voluntary lid opening, making it more difficult to assess the effect of fixation of the pretarsal skin.

Use of an external fixation suture that incorporates both upper and lower skin incisions facilitates intraoperative assessment of the palpebral fold as the contribution of the upper skin segment to the final eyelid size and shape can be visually assessed during actual construction of the fold as described above.

Slight asymmetry in the early post-operative period is very common because of differential swelling of the eyelids as well as the slight degree of ptosis that may temporarily follow fixation procedures. Although many patients are concerned about this asymmetry, the surgeon should carefully explain this problem and firmly refuse to consider revision until edema has resolved. Occasionally more marked lid asymmetry due to obvious failure of one or more fixation sutures deserves earlier correction, repair easily being accomplished by replacement of the failed sutures.

MANAGEMENT OF THE EPICANTHUS

Although ~90% of Asians exhibit an epicanthus, the size of the fold, although varying widely among individuals, is usually relatively small, and thus aesthetically successful effacement only rarely requires complex procedures advocated for management of this condition in the Caucasian. A major reason for the relative ease in managing the Asian epicanthal fold is that, in contrast to epicanthus encountered in Caucasians in which a vertical shortage of skin is problematic, the epicanthal fold in the Asian lid is usually associated with skin redundancy of the entire upper lid. This can be demonstrated by medial displacement of the skin with a cotton-tipped applicator. Successful effacement of the fold can be conceptualized as an advancement procedure. The goal of this advancement, in addition to removal of the fold itself, is to elongate the entire palpebral fold in a medial direction. Further benefits of this maneuver are the production of an enlarged eye and eyelid and a narrowing of the nasal bridge, a wide bridge being a concern of many individuals with prominent epicanthal folds.

Determining the Approach to the Epicanthal Fold

In many patients, no specific intervention in the epicanthal area is necessary. This group includes those who desire an inside fold as well as other patients with a small, almost rudimentary epicanthus in whom the surgical approach used to create the palpebral fold results in sufficient medial advancement of the epicanthus to achieve effacement.

The major advantage, of course, in minimizing surgery in the medial canthal region is the reduced risk of hypertrophic scarring. This region exhibits a biologic predisposition to hypertrophic scar formation, and thus even the most meticulously performed procedure in this area may be complicated by an aesthetically unpleasant scar.

In keeping with the known propensity for scar formation in the medial canthal area, it is best to encourage patients who are either unaware of their epicanthal folds or uncertain if they really desire modification of this region to defer epicanthaplasty at the time of primary surgery. I counsel such patients that epicanthal modification can be performed as a secondary procedure.

Epicanthaplasty, if desired or indicated, is usually performed in conjunction with upper lid blepharoplasty. One of three approaches is used to efface the epicanthus, depending upon the size of the fold requiring modification. Each procedure is based on the general principle that effacement can be successfully accomplished by medial advancement of the existing fold.

Advancement of a small fold is performed in conjunction with the incisions used for creation of the palpebral fold. These incisions are carried medially and inferiorly to the level of the lacrimal caruncle. The pretarsal skin in the area of the epicanthus is undermined to within 1–2 mm of the ciliary margin. Underlying soft tissue, including orbicularis muscle, is excised. The skin is then advanced medially and secured by placing one or two external fixation sutures (Fig. 6). If a small "dog ear" develops, it is excised in the direction of the skin fold, occasionally extending onto the medial aspect of the lower eyelid.

If additional advancement is required, a "half Z-plasty" is utilized (Fig. 7). The epicanthal fold is incised near the medial terminus of the palpebral wound, creating a triangular flap that is undermined and advanced nasally into the triangular defect previously created. The resulting dog ear is trimmed in the direction of the skin lines as described above.

Effacement of a larger epicanthus may require a greater medial advancement than is possible with Z-plasty techniques. Such a fold often terminates on the medial aspect of the lower lid, necessitating modification in this area as well. An excellent aesthetic result is generally achieved by a W-plasty advancement procedure:

1. The desired position of the inner canthus is marked (this is a point ~2 mm medial to the desired position of the inner canthus) following which two V-shaped flaps, forming a W, are outlined, the triangular flaps having their bases on the segments of the epicanthus located on the upper and lower lids (Fig. 8).
2. The outlined W is incised and the triangular flaps undermined toward the inner canthus.

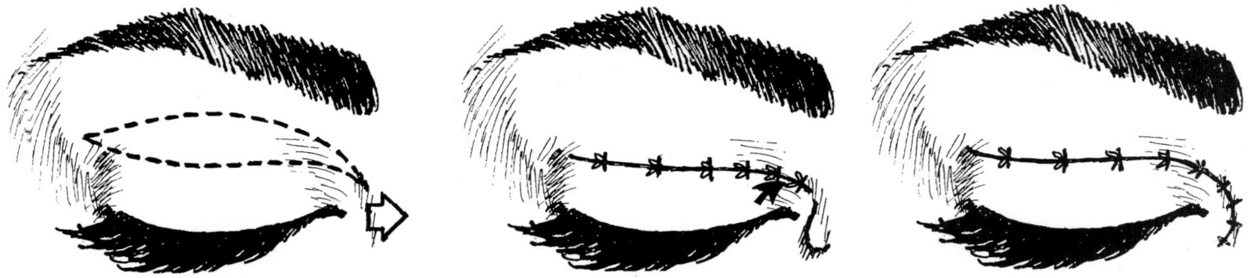

Figure 6. Effacement of a small epicanthus by medial fixation sutures combined with excision of a small dog ear.

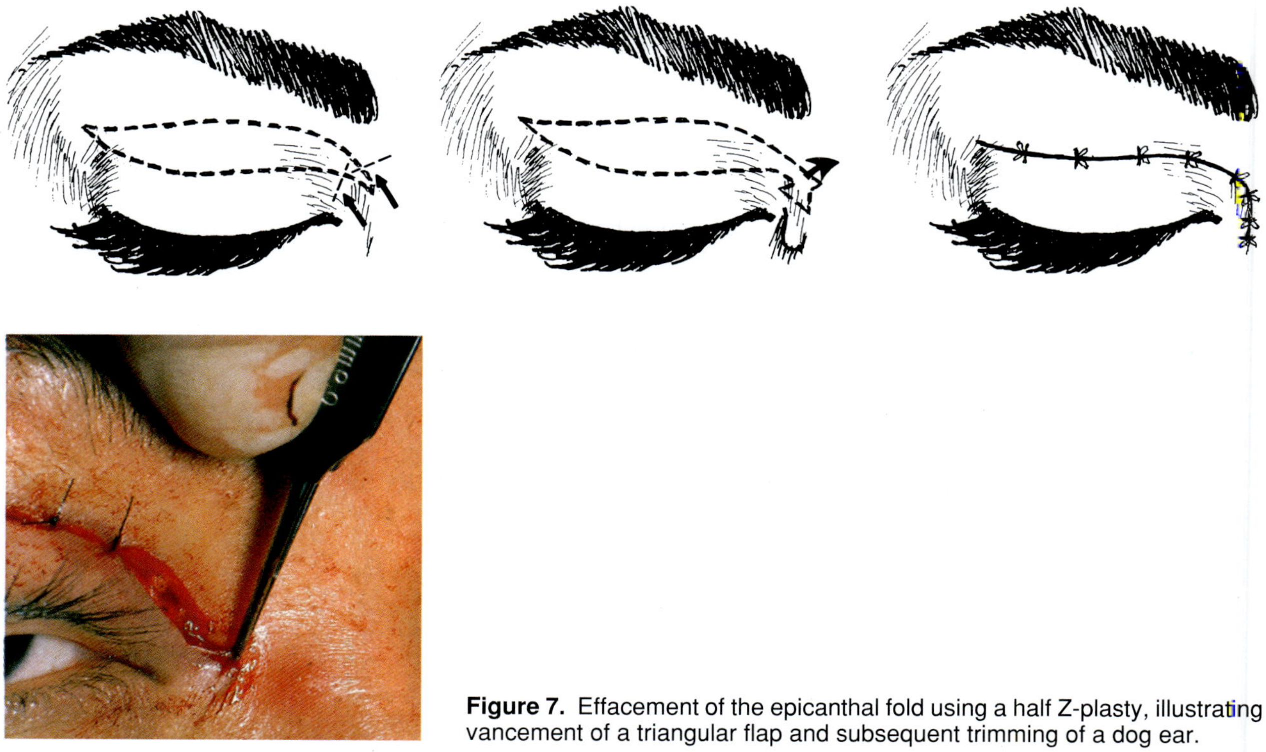

Figure 7. Effacement of the epicanthal fold using a half Z-plasty, illustrating advancement of a triangular flap and subsequent trimming of a dog ear.

3. The skin medial to the apex of the W is incised linearly toward the inner canthus, allowing advancement of the epicanthal fold medially.

4. The position of the new inner canthus is established by suturing the skin at the terminus of the above incision to the apex of the W (6-0 nylon) as illustrated in Fig. 7.

5. The undermined triangular flaps are then advanced medially, trimmed to fit precisely into the W, and sutured into place (6-0 nylon).

6. Sutures are removed in 5–7 days.

Complications of Epicanthaplasty

As previously stressed, even the most meticulously performed epicanthaplasty is often complicated by development of hypertrophic scar regardless of the technique utilized. One of the keys to success, then, is to anticipate this problem and aggressively treat incipient scarring with topical and, if necessary, intralesional steroids.

Asymmetry is another potential complication of epicanthaplasty. The surgeon should al-

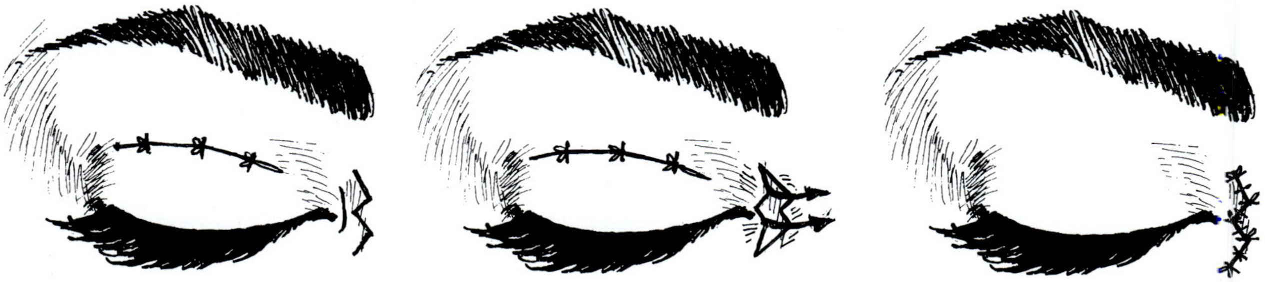

Figure 8. Epicanthaplasty with the W-plasty advancement procedure.

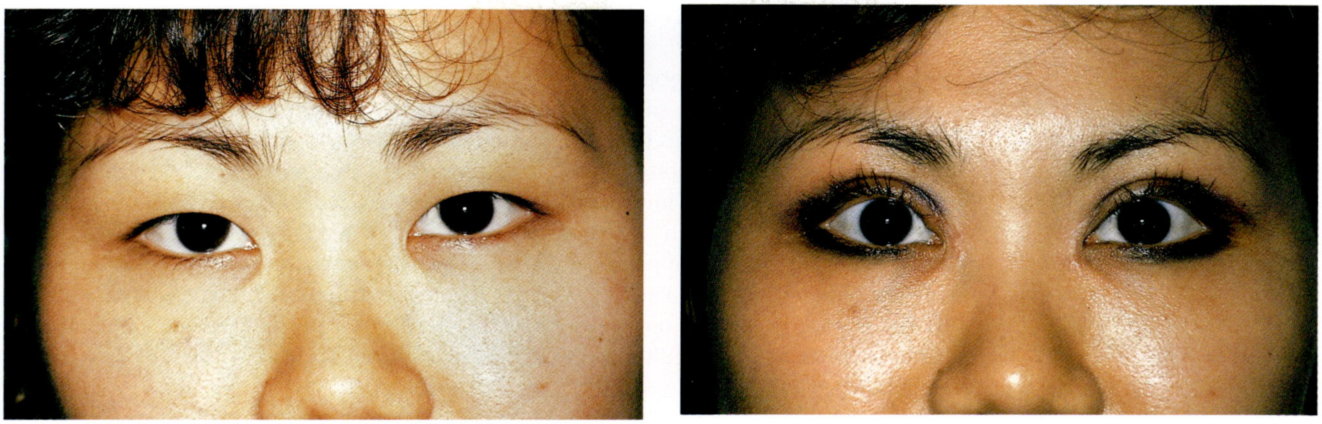

Figure 9. Effacement of an epicanthal fold using the W-plasty advancement procedure.

ways inform patients about asymmetry that exists pre-operatively in the eyelids, epicanthal region, and palpebral fissures as they most often will persist or become more apparent post-operatively. Patients must understand that differences in post-operative edema between the two eyelids frequently translate into post-operative asymmetry and that judgment regarding final symmetry may be unreliable for 6 months or more post-operatively.

Pre-operative counseling must stress proposed management of the epicanthal fold, and if a patient is uncertain as to whether modification of the fold is desired, epicanthaplasty may be best performed as a secondary procedure. Once the epicanthal fold is removed, it can never be reconstructed. It is helpful to inform patients that in general effacement of the epicanthus produces a more Westernized appearance while preservation or only slight modification of the fold preserves Asian characteristics.

In addition to improving facial balance by elongating "small eyes," epicanthaplasty improves the appearance of the nose, as the nasal bridge may appear excessively wide when the lateral dimension of the eyes is decreased by a large epicanthal fold (Fig. 9).

LOWER LID BLEPHAROPLASTY

As in the upper eyelid, the Asian lower lid characteristically exhibits a considerable volume of periorbital fat that frequently produces a "puffy" appearance even at an early age. In many patients, considerable fat is present in the pretarsal plane (superficial to the orbital septum), accentuating fullness.

Although a wide spectrum exists, Asian skin is generally thicker than Caucasian skin and deeply etched rhytides extending laterally (i.e., laugh lines or crow's feet) occur less frequently. Eccrine syringomas occur on the lower eyelid skin in some individuals, and such patients must understand that these blemishes will not be eliminated by blepharoplasty. Pigmented lesions (seborrheic keratoses, lentiges, etc.) are also common on the lower lid.

Frequently hypertrophy of the orbicularis muscle is present. Such patients must be counseled regarding the differences between puffiness caused by fat protrusion and orbicularis hypertrophy, as well as the aesthetic and technical limitations of partial muscle resection.

The puffiness of the Asian lower lid may tempt the surgeon to recommend a transconjunctival approach. Most Asian patients, however, are firmly convinced that "too much skin" is a component of their problem, and thus dissatisfaction often follows with an operation that does not remove skin. This observation coupled with the fact that transconjunctival blepharoplasty does not allow modification of orbicularis hypertrophy makes the skin/muscle flap approach the procedure of choice for all but the very young patient with no concern about skin excess or men whose only concern is "bags" resulting from fat protrusion.

AUGMENTATION RHINOPLASTY

The goal of aesthetic rhinoplasty in the Asian nose is similar to that in Occidental rhinoplasty: creation of a strong, smooth dorsum exhibiting a prominent origin at the nasion but not competing with the tip as the leading point of the nasal profile. A delicate, well defined lobule with definite columellar "show" and an oblique anteroposterior orientation of the nares constitute an equally important but seldom emphasized goal.

The characteristic anatomy of the Asian nose requires that the surgeon plan an augmentation procedure rather than reduction rhinoplasty. Augmentation rhinoplasty is requested with increasing frequency in areas with large Asian populations. While it might be assumed that the popularity of this operation reflects a desire for "Westernization," it should be noted that in many Asian cultures, the high, narrow nasal bridge is an aesthetically desirable feature.

Historically, many materials have been employed to augment the Asian nose. At the present time, Western surgeons prefer autogenous material, while in the East, use of silicone implants predominates. Many Western surgeons preach against the use of alloplastic nasal implants, apparently ignoring the fact that the long-term results using this material in the Asian nose have been excellent. The incidence of infection, displacement, and/or extrusion is substantially lower than would be expected on the basis of experience in augmentation of the non-Asian nose with solid implants. The reasons for this tolerance are unknown but may perhaps be related to greater thickness of skin and subcutaneous tissue. Complications, as is the case with other cosmetic procedures, are most commonly due to technical error rather than an inherent problem with the operation itself. While the basic principle that autogenous material, when available, is preferable to alloplastic implants is certainly valid, many Asian patients are unhappy with the results of nasal augmentation using autogenous cartilage and bone as satisfactory sculpturing of the lobule is often not achieved. Techniques of tip rhinoplasty that are highly successful in the Caucasian nose are frequently unsatisfactory in the Asian because the attenuated lower lateral cartilages are not strong enough to accentuate tip projection and support and the lobular skin and subcutaneous tissue is too thick to reflect sculpturing of the delicate cartilage. Thus, if tip projection is to be enhanced, the surgeon must reinforce or buttress lobular cartilage with cartilage grafts.

Asian craftsmanship, renowned throughout the world, is characterized by a pragmatic concern for function coupled with a keen eye for beauty and symmetry and meticulous attention to detail. Augmentation rhinoplasty using silicone implants has been refined by conscientious, experienced, and well trained Asian surgeons, and any temptation to label such procedures as inherently dangerous or unreliable should be tempered with respect for the experience and accomplishments of our colleagues in the East. Evolution in the technology of silicone implants has continued as softer grades of silicone elastomer have be-

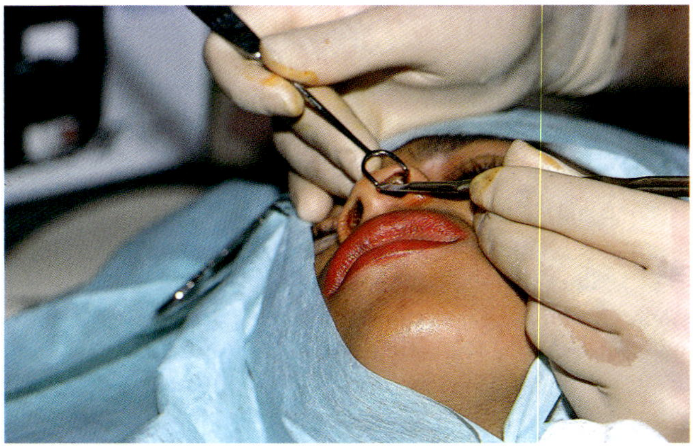

Figure 10. Marginal incision used for augmentation rhinoplasty.

come available for implant fabrication. Softer implants translate into increased flexibility, resulting in reduced tension at the implant/tissue interface.

Frustration over the dissatisfaction of Asian patients with the results of tipplasty using techniques that produced excellent results in the Caucasian nose led me to begin exploration of the possibilities of alloplastic implants. In some cases, only subtle augmentation of the dorsum is required, and in such cases autogenous cartilage is an excellent choice.

Mersaline mesh, Gortex, or homograft materials are alternatives to silicone implants in these patients. The decision to use autogenous or alloplastic material is individualized according to the desires of each patient with regard to the extent of lobular sculpturing and dorsal augmentation. Anatomic factors such as skin thickness and the configuration of the lower lateral cartilages assist in determining the type of procedure to be employed. Silicone implants are preferred in many patients who desire increased lobular definition and/or tip projection. Thin lobular skin constitutes a relative contraindication to the use of silicone implants. Given the current social and medicolegal environment, feelings of each individual patient regarding use of foreign materials must be considered.

Pre-Operative Considerations

It is of utmost importance that the candidate for augmentation rhinoplasty completely and carefully communicate the specifics of the nasal transformation that is desired. Many Asian patients assume that the surgeon knows best and will automatically construct a nose to their exact specifications. If communication between patient and surgeon is unclear or imprecise, disappointment may ensue regarding such matters as dorsal height, lobular configuration, and tip projection. The surgeon must determine whether the patient wants the tip to be narrow or relatively broad. Is the desired nasion wide or narrow? Does the patient wish the dorsal profile to be straight or slightly convex? Pre- and post-operative photographs of various augmentation rhinoplasty procedures are often helpful in this regard. It should be stressed to the patient, however, that a surgeon cannot promise to construct the nose to exact specifications.

The goals, limitations, and possible complications of surgery are thoroughly discussed. Language barriers and preconceived notions of the patient regarding the goals and limitations of the procedure should be recognized and addressed during pre-operative consultation.

Surgical Technique for Alloplastic Implants

Augmentation rhinoplasty is generally performed under local anesthesia in an office operating suite. An oral cephalosporin or its equivalent is initiated on the day prior to surgery and antibiotic prophylaxis continued for 3 days post-operatively.

1. Access to the dorsum and lobule is obtained via a marginal incision that extends into the columella (Fig. 10). Dissection of a precise midline pocket is facilitated by initiating the dissection via the columellar portion of the incision. The lower lateral cartilages are freed from the lobular skin but are not otherwise modified as the implant will rest on their anterior surfaces.
2. The silicone implant is not premeasured but is individually tailored at the time of surgery. This tailoring is accomplished by placing the implant into the dorsum, determining its effect, and then removing it for modification as indicated by the desires of the patient as well as the aesthetic sense of the surgeon.
3. A columellar strut is always utilized as it stabilizes the proximal portion of the implant in the midline, thus decreasing the incidence of wobbling and asymmetry. It is important to understand that the function of the columellar strut is not to thrust the tip anteriorly, and thus the strut does not extend to the nasal spine. Overzealous attempts to enhance tip support with a strut are ill conceived maneuvers that increase the incidence of implant extrusion.

4. The distal end of the dorsal implant terminates at a point halfway between the interbrow and intercanthal lines and should be sculptured to blend inconspicuously with the nasion so that it is not readily palpable. The nasofrontal angle should be preserved.

5. If the surgeon experiences difficulty freeing both lower lateral cartilages via a single marginal incision, a similar incision should be made on the opposite side to ensure symmetrical placement of the implant in the lobular area. The subcutaneous pocket should be of generous size. If resistance is encountered upon placing the implant, the pocket is too small and should be enlarged to prevent excessive tension on the nasal skin. If a small dorsal hump is present, it is easier to rasp the dorsum than to modify the implant to accommodate this hump.

6. Following satisfactory placement of the implant, the nasal alae are analyzed, and if necessary, an alar rim reduction procedure is performed.

7. Some patients may benefit from narrowing of the nasal pyramid achieved by lateral osteotomy.

Implant Configuration

The nasal implant that I recommend for routine use differs from other commercially available implants primarily in its columellar aspect (Fig. 11). The columellar strut has two functions: (a) stabilization of the proximal segment of the implant in the midline thus resisting displacement and subsequent malposition; (b) sculpturing the columella, i.e., displacement of the characteristically retracted columella inferiorly, thus increasing its "show." If hard elastomer is utilized for the columellar strut, it can be relatively short and thin as the firm material is resistant to deformation by columellar tension. The fibrous capsule that naturally forms around the implant often exerts a rotational force on the implant, resulting in lateral displacement of the strut with resultant perforation at the vestibular aspect of the columella, i.e., the incision (the most common sight of implant extrusion). These rotational forces are less likely to be transmitted to a columellar strut fabricated from a soft elastomer because of the flexibility at the lobular/columellar junction of the implant. However, this flexibility will result in superior deformation of the strut (by columellar tension) unless the strut has sufficient breadth to allow it to be wedged between the caudal septal cartilage and columellar skin. During surgery, the flared columellar strut is carefully trimmed so that it is wedged between the skin and caudal septum at the most anterior point that allows aesthetically sufficient inferior displacement of the columella (producing columellar show).

The inferior inclination (angulation) of the columellar strut with respect to the dorsal component assists in achieving this goal. (Other commercially available nasal implants are constructed so that the columellar strut projects at a 90° angle from the dorsal component.)

Following final trimming, the columellar strut never extends posteriorly for a distance >75% of the length of the columella. Allowing the strut to contact the nasal spine results in a "tent pole" effect—an invitation to disaster in the form of implant extrusion secondary to pressure necrosis of the lobular skin. Always remember that the function of the columellar strut is not to project the lobule in a tent pole fashion. Lobular projection is

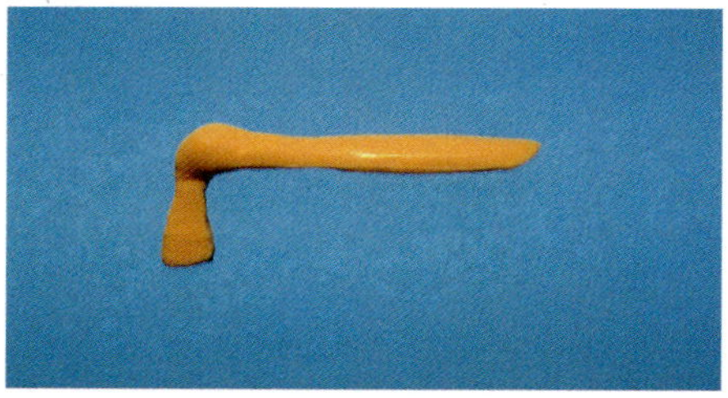

Figure 11. Design of a silicone nasal implant. Note flared columellar strut.

achieved by the sheer volume of the rounded, slightly elevated (i.e., mound) lobular component, similar to the cantilever effect of bone grafts utilized for total nasal reconstruction.

Because of complaints that clear silicone implants may be visible through the nasal skin under bright indoor lighting, the implant should be a neutral color (i.e., beige). Like other commercially available implants, soft elastomer is used for its fabrication.

Complications

Asymmetry as a consequence of improper placement of the implant or subsequent displacement of its distal aspect is the most common complication of augmentation rhinoplasty in the Asian nose. In the early post-operative period, apparent asymmetry may merely be the result of edema. Slight asymmetry is often successfully managed by instructing the patient in manipulation of the distal aspect of the implant. If noticeable asymmetry persists, however, correction can only be effected by removal and replacement of the implant.

Infection requires immediate removal of the implant. Antibiotic therapy is initiated and continued according to the results of culture and sensitivity studies. The infection resolves rapidly, following which subsequent augmentation can be performed. Although many surgeons recommend deferring revision surgery for 6–12 weeks, if thinned, stretched skin in the lobular region is not supported within 2 weeks of implant removal, contraction will commence, resulting in a surface dimple that is difficult to efface. Support of the thinned skin is best achieved with autogenous cartilage.

Delayed extrusion is the most worrisome complication of augmentation rhinoplasty in the Asian nose. The incidence of this complication is extremely low and is generally a consequence of technical error. Perhaps the most common reason for delayed extrusion is excessive tension in the lobular region secondary to ill conceived attempts to enhance tip projection with a columellar strut. The surgeon must be conservative in attempts to increase tip projection and explain the reasons for this conservatism to each patient. The incidence of delayed extrusion is also reduced by ensuring that the implant does not fit too snugly in the dorsum, thus reducing skin tension in this area. Extrusion is also reduced by the presence of a columellar strut as this reduces wobbling of the implant.

Impending extrusion is suggested by progressive thinning of the lobular skin. If recognized at an early stage, salvage of the implant can often be achieved by prompt removal. The implant is sculptured to a smaller size, a dermal or temporalis fascia (or crushed cartilage) graft sutured over the lobular component, and the implant replaced into the existing nasal pocket.

The major goals of rhinoplasty in the Asian nose include augmentation of the nasal dorsum in conjunction with refinement of the lobule. Although various materials may be used to achieve these goals, individually sculptured solid silicone implants are presently the most commonly used prostheses. Some surgeons currently advocate the use of cartilage grafts to enhance tip projection while continuing the use of silicone implants for dorsal augmentation. Although I remain firmly convinced of the advantages of silicone implants because of their proven efficacy and reliability (as well as for their cost/benefit ratio), I applaud the efforts of those surgeons exploring the more successful use of autogenous materials in the Asian nose. Although recent reports suggest that long-term survival of cartilaginous grafts of the onlay type in the nose is excellent, consider that the fate of columellar struts subject to stresses of a different magnitude may well be different. Is it significant that proponents of such grafts recommend "overcorrection"?

The surgeon should be conservative in selection of implant size, remembering that subtle enhancement often produces substantial aesthetic benefit. Conservatism is of utmost importance in attempts to enhance tip projection as excessive tension on the lobular skin is a prime factor in delayed extrusion of alloplastic implants. Infection is a secondary cause of implant extrusion and abscesses most commonly develop in the columellar region, but can occur over any portion of the implant.

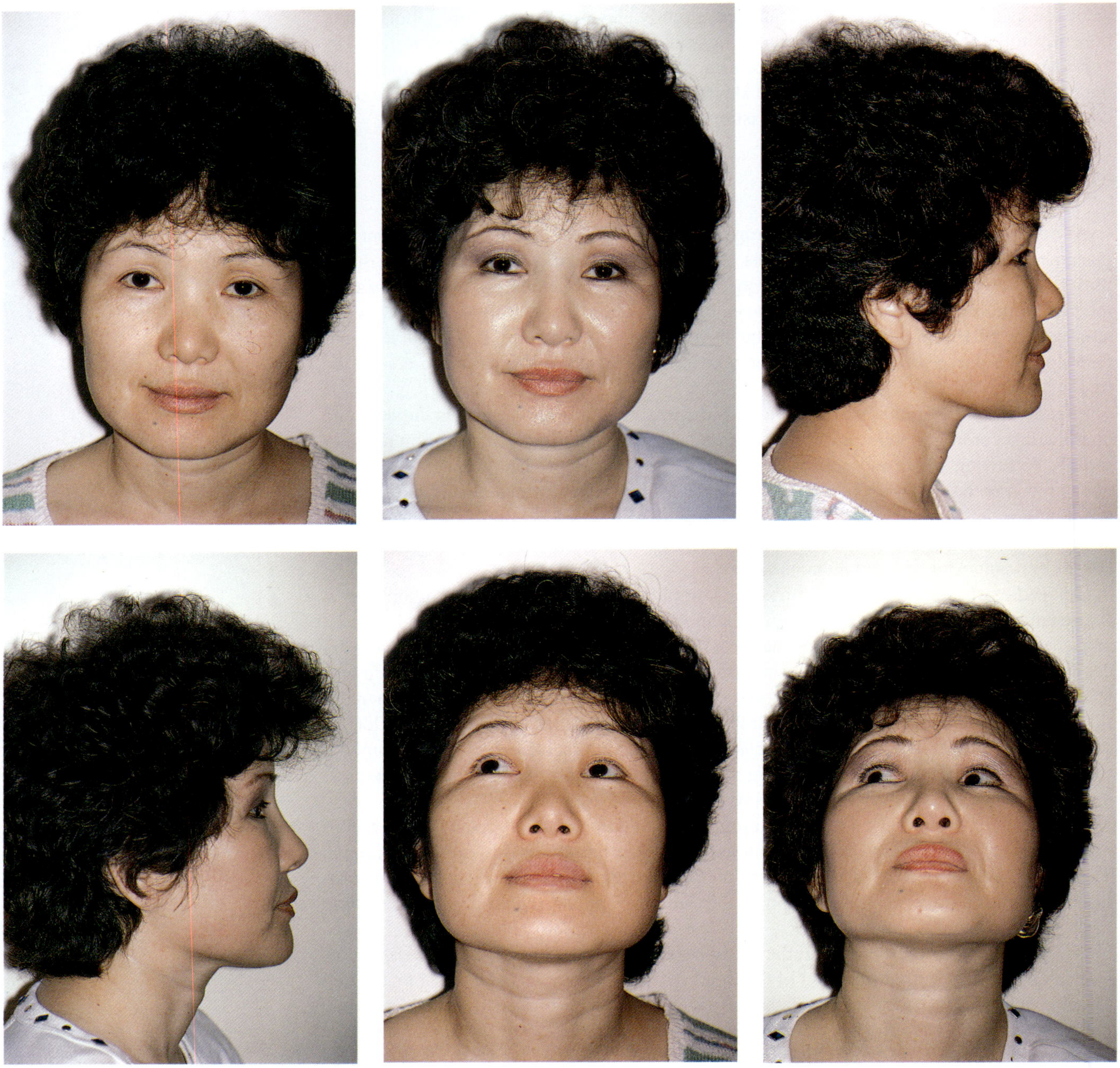

Figure 12. Pre- and post-operative photographs demonstrating the results of augmentation rhinoplasty using a silicone implant.

Successful aesthetic rhinoplasty in the Asian nose requires knowledge of anatomic variables, appreciation of nasal aesthetics and social and cultural concerns, thorough preoperative evaluation and patient counseling, along with careful attention to detail.

Careful and considered use of silicone implants in augmentation rhinoplasty offers plastic surgeons an opportunity to utilize their aesthetic senses to the fullest extent, enabling them to produce dramatic changes in nasal appearance (Fig. 12). When such surgery is properly planned and executed, the incidence of complication is low. Complications following augmentation rhinoplasty with alloplastic implants are frequently the result of technical errors and are not due to inherent deficiencies in the operation per se. A thorough un-

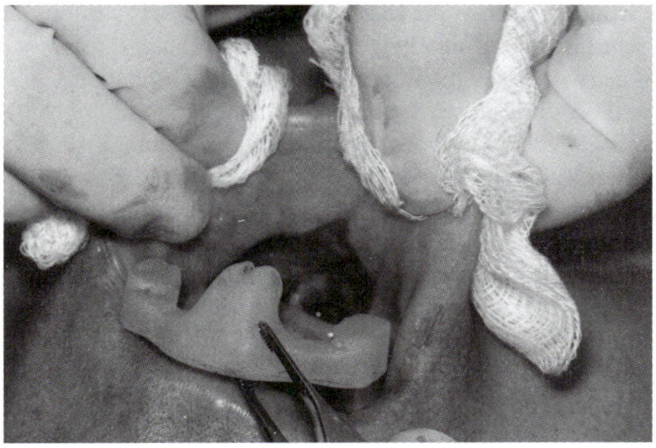

Figure 13. Preformed silicone premaxillary implant (Guinta design) placed via a sublabial approach.

derstanding of the basic principles and important safeguards when using such materials in the nose is essential for successful surgery.

MAXILLARY IMPLANTS

Bimaxillary protrusion resulting in a relatively depressed midfacial region is a relatively common characteristic of the central Asian face, often being accentuated by an anterior inclination of the maxillary incisors. With increasing age, this midfacial configuration tends to be associated with deepening of the nasolabial folds.

Although correction of this facial disproportion is an aesthetically rewarding procedure, the number of patients who are willing to undergo this relatively simple corrective operation is amazingly small.

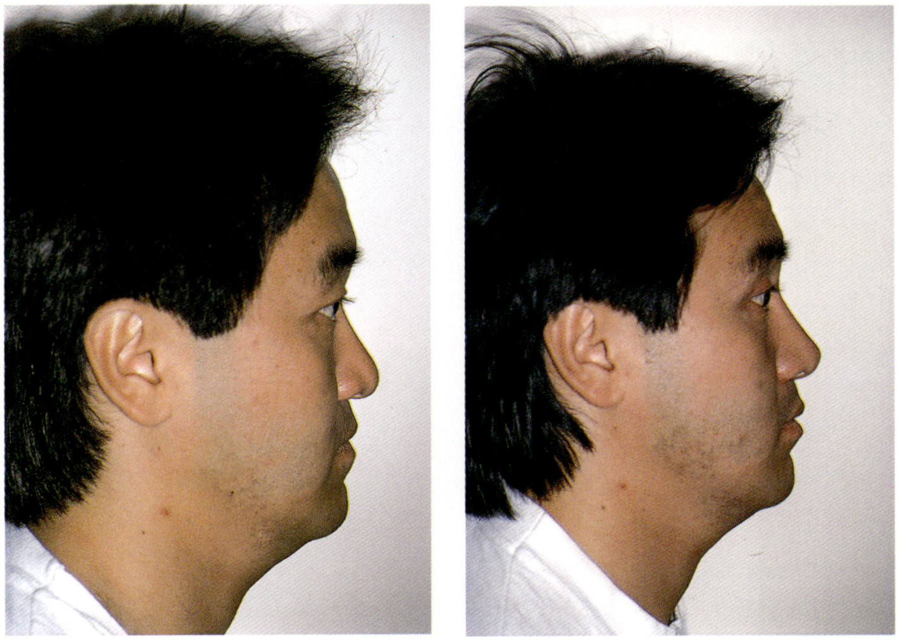

Figure 14. Pre- and post-operative photographs illustrating the results of maxillary augmentation using a silicone implant.

Correction of midfacial retrusion can be effected by using either silicone or Mersaline mesh implants. Mesh implants can be placed via an intranasal approach for correction of small degrees of retrusion, but the intraoral approach affords better visualization for correction of larger "deformities."

Either implant is placed in a supraperiosteal plane via a sublabial incision transecting the frenulum. When mesh implants are utilized, the lateral aspect of augmentation extends beneath the origin of the nasolabial fold.

Preformed silicone premaxillary implants (Guinta design) are available in two sizes. Regardless of the size selected, these implants usually require further sculpturing to fit individual facial anatomy (Figs. 13 and 14).

RECOMMENDED READING

Boo-chai K. Plastic construction of the superior palpebral fold. *Plast Reconstr Surg* 1963;31:74–78.
Boo-chai K. Sculpturing the nasal tip and lobule region. *Clin Facial Plast Surg* 1996;4:103–116.
Cheu MT, Lu SY. Secondary blepharoplasty for Oriental eyelid. *Facial Plast Surg Clin* 1996;4:49–54.
Fernandez LR. Double eyelid operation in the Oriental in Hawaii. *Plast Reconstr Surg* 1960;25:257–264.
Flowers RS. The art of eyelid and orbital aesthetics: multiracial considerations. *Clin Plast Surg* 1987;14:703–721.
Giunta SX. Premaxillary augmentation in Asian rhinoplasty. *Facial Plast Clin* 1996;4:93–102.
Hin LC. Oriental blepharoplasty—a critical review of technique and potential hazards. *Ann Plast Surg* 1981;7:362–374.
Hin LC. Unfavorable results in Oriental blepharoplasty. *Ann Plast Surg* 1985;14:523–534.
Hiraga Y. Complications of augmentation rhinoplasty in the Japanese. *Ann Plast Surg* 1980;4:495–499.
McCurdy JA Jr. *Cosmetic surgery of the Asian face*. New York: Thieme, 1990.
McCurdy JA Jr. Management of the epicanthal fold. *Facial Plast Surg Clin* 1996;4:25–33.
McCurdy JA Jr. Lower lid blepharoplasty. *Facial Plast Surg Clin* 1996;4:41–47.
McCurdy JA Jr. Augmentation rhinoplasty: implant selection and design. *Facial Plast Surg Clin* 1996;4:87–92.
Yang HH, Peterson RL. Asian blepharoplasty: suture technique. *Facial Plast Surg Clin* 1996;4:35–40.

Ethnic Considerations in Facial Aesthetic Surgery, edited by W. Earle Matory, Jr.
Lippincott–Raven Publishers, Philadelphia

21

The Filipino and Polynesian Patients

Marco Rizzo

A difference in degree may eventually become a difference in kind.
— Immanuel Kant

The Filipino and Polynesian ethnic group can be considered to be among the most exotic-looking people in the world. Certain geographic and migratory trends of early history explain some of the distinctive physical characteristics within these groups and assist in defining an origin of ancestry that can become enhanced by way of aesthetic surgery.

Being active island inhabitants, their physical features are favorable to a tropical climate as their dark skin and thick hair easily reveal.

The Filipino group consists of >7,000 islands. These islands became a colony of Spain in the early 1500s through the efforts of Ferdinand Magellan. Surprisingly, however, with as much Spanish influence as still exists in the Filipino culture, the Filipinos stem from the Malay race, which now occupies both Malaysia and Indonesia.

Early records of migratory trends suggest that groups from southeast Asia traveled into Indonesia and then to the Polynesian islands. Two routes were identified. There was a Micronesian route that extended from the Philippines to the Carolinas, branching out to the Marshall and Gilbert Islands, then into Polynesia and Hawaii. There was also the Melanesian route that goes through Indonesia through New Guinea, Fiji, and into the Polynesian islands of Samoa and Tonga, Tahiti, and the Marqueses, then into Hawaii, New Zealand, and Easter Island.

In favor of the Melanesian route, archeological findings of burials in the Hawaiian islands and study of cranial bones show a peculiar shape of the mandible that gives only two points of support on the body of the jaw instead of the usual three or four points in the Caucasian mandible. The two points might be unstable and tilted from chin to fold, creating a rocking, back-and-forth motion when placed on a flat surface, giving this characteristic the name of "rocker jaw." This is seldom found in European mandibles; however, it is especially typical of Maori and Moriori Polynesian people as well Australians and Melanesians.

M. Rizzo: Honolulu, Hawaii 96813

Although the Filipinos and Polynesians represent a small percentage of those undergoing surgery, these racial extractions can often be identified in Asians and Caucasians as a result of inter-racial breeding. Certain skin tones and hair textures are dominant characteristics of both ethnic groups.

ANATOMIC CHARACTERISTICS

With a usually long, yet slightly round face shape, the nose may have a medium to flat bridge with a moderately round to flat tip and wide nostrils. The shape of the eye demonstrates a trace of Asian ancestry as there is roundness of the upper eyelid and frequent slanting of the eyelid. Epicanthal folds are not uncommon in the Philippines. The jaw line is somewhat elongated but still produces a rounded face.

CULTURAL CONSIDERATIONS

Loyalty to the heritage and immediate family is a strong cultural bias among Polynesians and Filipinos. One's choice to modify facial features with aesthetic surgery may be perceived as an ethnic betrayal. These startling confirmations of cultural ethics were noted in an informal survey that was conducted among Polynesian and Filipino groups.

According to the survey, those with an Asian background seemed to be satisfied with facial and bodily features except for the nose. The interbreeding tends to predominately feature a wider, shallow bridge combined with the already round or flat tip. It was a common feeling that modifying the tip and creating a taller bridge would reinforce other inherent Polynesian characteristics. Another common concern was the weak chin, as it would exaggerate the roundedness of the face that some perceived as a mismatch with an often tall, athletic frame and thick, wavy hair.

Those with Caucasian admixture were less likely to change any facial feature, as the balance of rounded cheeks and elongated jawline was felt to appropriately complement full lips. In this population the hair texture is less curled and slightly wavy, which seems to coordinate with the longer forehead commonly seen in this admixture.

Thus, skin tone and hair texture are dominant indicators of Polynesian ancestry, thus allowing for the enhancement of existing exotic overtones. Many of the cultural issues described in the questionnaire identify some alternative surgical approaches that do not compromise ethnic self-perceptions.

Polynesians have interbred with a number of ethnic groups, primarily Asian and Caucasian. The Asian influence lightens the skin with a more olive tone, creates more of a slant in the upper eyelid, flattens the nasal bridge, and increases malar roundness. Polynesian features commonly represent combined characteristics of multiple nationalities.

Filipinos, on the other hand, have a smaller, more delicate frame, with thick, straight black hair that accentuates sharp cheekbones and a subtle roundness of the lower jaw and chin. The nose is usually narrow at the bridge, while gradually becoming wide and blunt at the tip. A "flat" nose seems to dominate the characteristics within an immediate family. The skin texture is smooth and frequently flawless with a rich, almost burgundy tone of brown.

In predominantly a Catholic country, the unwillingness to pursue modifications through aesthetic surgery stems from the desire to maintain the looks within the family or not wanting to be considered as vain or unappreciative of "what you were born with." Results from our survey showed that most of the men interviewed were content with their features, whereas almost 100% of the women wanted to change their nose to have a taller bridge and more refined tip. The chin was commonly mentioned as giving the overall look of "petiteness," being in good proportion to the slant of the eyes when smiling.

The Filipino with an Asian mixture is often concerned about the dominance of Asian features, frequently prompting a desire to enhance the Filipino genealogy by increasing the presence of the supratarsal fold. Facial width is broader with malar rounding, not infrequently accompanied by coarse, thick, straight hair. Skin is more acne-prone within this subgroup than noted in other Filipino admixtures.

Filipinos with Caucasian background note larger eyes and eyelids, lighter skin tone that achieves the burgundy hint when exposed to the sun, and a taller body frame with lighter shades of brown hair. The lips, however, may not be as full as those of their Filipino ancestors, and the refined shape of the sharp Filipino cheekbone may become overdramatized by a narrow jawline. Lip and mandibular augmentation are thus common requests.

The prominent but often recessed malar configuration exacerbates the nearly uniform short nasal length. The low frontonasal angle is often accompanied by frontal bossing, which further deepens and shadows the angle.

PRE-OPERATIVE EVALUATION

Filipinos, Polynesians, and Asians present a number of anatomic and aesthetic challenges. Hypertrophic sebaceous glands with acute and chronic acne further compromise the aesthetic outcome. Thus, chronic inflammation commonly accentuates scarring of any nasal incisions. The effect of any tip enhancement is minimized by prominent fibrofatty tissue and thick overlying skin. Pre-operative assessment must discern the amount of defatting that is indicated. More substantial dorsal and tip grafts may be required in light of the thick soft tissue envelope.

Cephalad rotation of the tip and a foreshortened columella contribute to visibly rounded nostrils. The columella may be hidden with overhanging ala and a high columella attachment to the nostril sill. Pre-operative recognition will direct the harvesting of several septal and/or conchal grafts.

The interalar distance is often widened and accompanied by moderate alar flare. Flaring is best addressed, in my hands, by wedge excision.

The surgeon, when faced with this multitude of challenging anatomic and aesthetic concerns, must evaluate and clearly understand the desires of the patient. After 20 years of experience in addressing the needs of Polynesian, Filipino, and Asian patients, it is clear to me that the surgeon's insight into the patient's goals is significantly enhanced by pre-operative video imaging. Once the aesthetic goal is discerned, the possibilities and impossibilities of achieving this goal are thoroughly discussed with the patient. One must note that changes that are dramatic or ethnically transforming may not prove to be satisfying to the patient's aesthetic taste or to the perceived self-image. The latter is particularly true for the older patient, in that social, psychological, and physical adaptability diminishes with age. Ethnic patients, in my view, are more demanding and require longer and more frequent consultations. The communication skills of the surgeon and his/her staff must be highly sophisticated and insightful to appropriately meet the needs of this patient population.

Assessment of Bone and Cartilage

I. A. Midline. The tip of the nose should be centered over the cupid bow. If deviation is present, identify the cause and correct with septal surgery or osteotomy.

B. The tip should have four defining points: the columellar/lobular junction, the dorsum/tip junction, and the two dome areas. A line connecting the dome areas should divide this into two equilateral triangles. The four defining points are not quite clear in the Asian due to flat domes and the fibrofatty tissue covering them.

C. The nasal tip projection is determined next. If the upper lip is in correct position, a vertical line is drawn between the alar/cheek junction. Sixty percent should lie anterior to the vertical line. Also useful is the ratio of the distance from the nasofrontal angle to the tip and the alar/cheek junction to the tip, which should be $\sim 0.6:1$. Here again, more projection is needed in the majority of cases, and this is obtained by all known methods of tip augmentation that we will be describing.

D. For tip rotation or nasolabial or columella/labial angle, I like 95–100° in females and 90–95° in males. Another common peculiarity of the Asian nose is the presence of an acute nasolabial angle, which is due to maxillary atrophy and is increased by alveolar projection. Maxillary or perinasal augmentation will improve this angle to an acceptable ratio.

II. A. Width of the alar base should approximate the intercanthal distance, which should also equal the width of an eye. The width of the nasal base, which is slightly wider in Asians, is compensated by the width of the intercanthal area, especially when the epicanthal fold is present. Many times both wedge excision of alar and W-plasty on epicanthal fold are indicated to improve the condition.

B. A line outlining the alar rims and the lowest portion of the columella should give a gentle gull wing appearance. It should hang just inferior to the alar rims. Here the gull wing appearance frequently is not present, the columella has a higher attachment, and correction is necessary, but not always successful.

C. On basal view, the nose should have the shape of an equilateral triangle. The lobular/columella ratio should be approximately one to two. The nostril should be a teardrop shape, with the long axis oriented medially. In the basal view, we see that the Asian nose does not have an equilateral triangle and the columella/lobule ratio is half-and-half. Also the position of the nostrils is different and difficult to correct.

III. A. Width of the body. Bony pyramid base should be slightly less than the alar width (three to four) or 80% of the ala. If higher, it should be narrowed at the time of osteotomy.

B. The deepest point of the nasofrontal angle should be at a level between the upper eyelashes and the supratarsal fold with the eyes in forward gaze. Consistently this point is found to be lower, and this gives the appearance of a short nose. It should be modified as necessary.

PERI-OPERATIVE DETAILS

Heavy sedation and local anesthesia are commonly used. I pre-medicate with intramuscular Demerol 100 mg and Vistaril 100 mg. Intravenous increments of valium, Versed, or fentamyl are given to achieve adequate sedation for the infiltration of Marcaine 0.25% and epinephrine 1:200,000. Nasal hair is trimmed. The skin and mucous membrane are prepped with Betadine solution.

During the procedure, intravenous cephalosporin is administered. Oral doses are continued for ~4–5 days.

After surgery, half-inch tape strips (Steri-strips) are used over skin adhesive (Mastisol) on the nose and ear. An aluminum splint is applied to the dorsum and taped for 7 days. Dental rolls are placed, in post-auricular sulcus, and taped with Steri-strips tightly.

SURGICAL TECHNIQUES

Rhinoplasty and blepharoplasty are the most common procedures that I perform on the Polynesian, Asian, and Filipino. This chapter will focus on rhinoplasty.

Rhinoplasty

The nasal lobule is supported by soft tissue and underlying elastic cartilage. The aesthetic goal should be to lengthen the nose and to enhance the tip, with preservation of a soft, flexible tip. The latter will tolerate the external forces exerted on the nose by the thick soft tissue envelope and will better tolerate minor trauma. To achieve this outcome, I use cartilage grafts for tip enhancement and elastomer silicone for the dorsum.

Tip Enhancement

An open approach through a transcolumellar incision with extension onto the mucous membrane optimizes exposure of the lower lateral cartilage. The cartilages are skeletonized, with the removal of fibrofatty tissue above and between the medial crura. The periosteal elevator is used to dissect onto the dorsum, beneath the periosteum when possible. A large pocket is made to ensure a comfortable and precise prosthetic fit. Attempting to avoid the skin or mucous membrane, the prosthesis is inserted. Two holes are made in the cephalad portion of the implant to promote tissue ingrowth. Implant immobilization is assisted by splinting for ~8 days. The inferior portion is fixed to the midline with a nonabsorbable 5-0 suture (Fig. 1).

To minimize shifting or lateralization, additional fixation can be used in the midportion of the prosthetic. I use an absorbable suture of 5-0 with a curve needle inserted percutaneously and just the nasal bones, taking in the bite, skin implant septum follow-through after the midline implant skin. Then the suture is delivered under the skin flap, where the knot is then placed. The nasal tip is then elevated with three conchal cartilage grafts, including intracrural graft and two shield grafts. The intracrural graft is taken from the septum (when available) or from the cavum of the concha cartilage of the ear. A graft 3–4 mm in width and 15–18 mm in length is harvested from the straightest portion of the cavum. If the curvature is excessive, I suture a similar-sized mirror image graft to straighten the curvature.

Shield graft no. 1 is shaped from the cavum portion of conchal cartilage, 10 mm × 7 mm in length, and is short, stubby, and strong. Shield graft no. 2 is retrieved from the cymba and is much more flexible, more rounded, and lighter. The latter is larger, measuring ~12–13 mm × 8–9 mm in the upper portion. This cephalad portion shapes the width of the nasal tip. It also gives flexibility and roundness and covers any irregularities that lie beneath it. The grafts are sutured to each other using 6-0 clear nylon in a laminated manner.

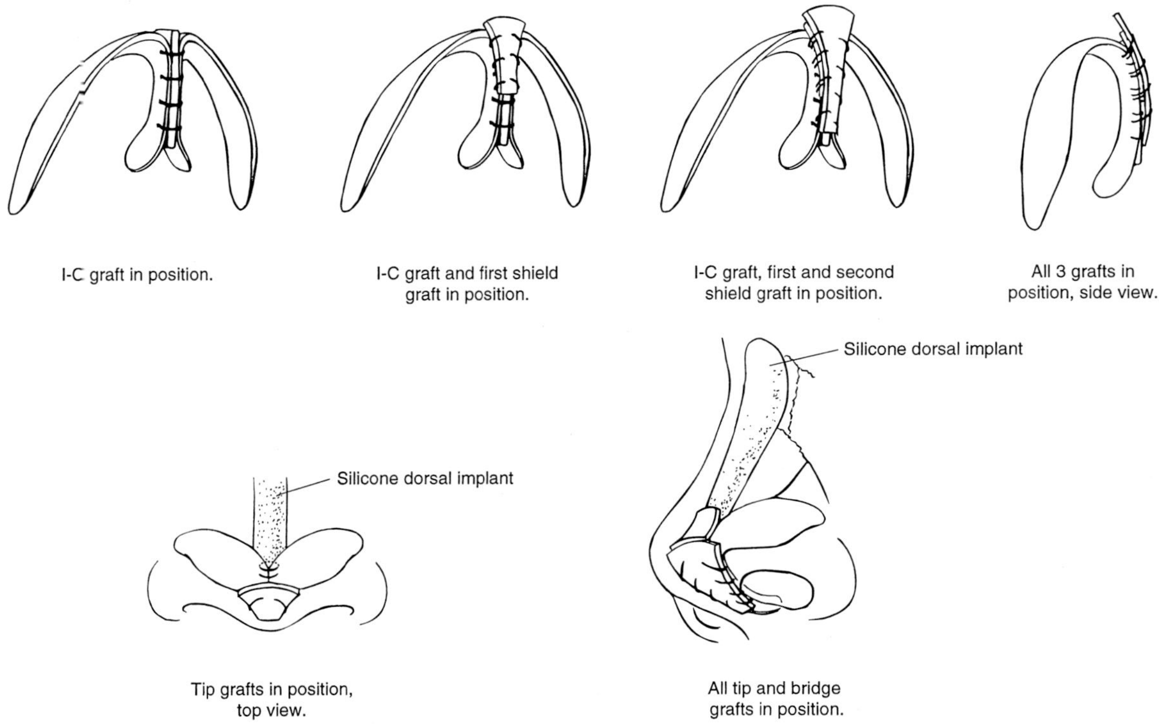

Figure 1. Tip graft sequence.

Autologous Grafting

Bone for Dorsal Augmentation

Bone is chosen over other materials for dorsal augmentation usually in severe saddle shape deformities most commonly seen in trauma. A lot of material is necessary to correct the problem. Its use has both advantages and disadvantages.

Donor sites include split calvarium, hip (bone) iliac crest, ulnar (non-dominant hand), and ribs. None of these is ideal.

Disadvantages include the following:

1. Most bone sources absorb or decrease in size over time. Iliac crest seems to be more predictable, with less absorption.
2. The need for general anesthesia.
3. The need for power tools for shaping and reduction.
4. Prolonged surgery.
5. Donor site pain (hip), scars, and complications (e.g., pneumothorax for ribs).

In summary, if pure bone graft is needed, the iliac crest seems to be the best source, and if cartilage is also needed for the tip, rib may be preferable.

Cartilage for Dorsal Augmentation

Following are some sources of cartilage for dorsal augmentation:

1. Rib is probably the most ideal but may be calcified in the older patient. A general anesthetic may be necessary. Warping may occur.

2. The septum in the Asian is routinely smaller in surface area and thinner than in the Caucasian. If septum is used, one must leave significant support to avoid dorsal collapse, at least 1.5 cm. Of note, the flattest noses that require the most cartilage for the tip and dorsum have the least amount available.

3. Ear is excellent for tip elevation, but it has irregular and uneven contours for dorsal elevation.

4. Radiated cartilage. Stay away from it. It is unpredictable, and complete reabsorption and/or warping are common.

Of the cartilaginous sources, rib is preferred because of the availability of adequate amounts, minimal absorption, adaptability to carving, and the small incision (3 cm). We like rib no. 7–8 or 9.

Tip Augmentation

Sources

Sources for tip augmentation include the following:

1. Ear is the most frequently used source.
2. Septum (prior surgery or trauma is a deterrent for its use).
3. Rib—as discussed earlier, not advisable if only tip cartilage is needed.

Technique

This procedure must be done with autogenous tissue, and cartilage is the most pliable and reliable of them all. There are two methods: floating and fixed augmentation.

The Floating Method. The floating method was used and described earlier by Peck with his umbrella graft and by Sheen with tip grafts. They are prone to change with time because of the weight and pressure of the overlying skin envelope. The soft tissue support mechanism is weak with a resultant loss of projection over time. These techniques are therefore less predictable than the fixed method.

The Fixed Method. This method was advocated by Gunther and Rohrick. Use a strong strut of cartilage, either septum or rib, and shape as in an inverted Y. The graft hugs the spine of the nose to avoid motion and lateralization. Suture fixation to the medial crus adds further stabilization and elevates the entire nasal tip from the base of the nose.

For the intercrural or columella grafts, use the foot of the medial crus as anchoring mechanism and all grafts are sutured to the medial crus to achieve tip elevation. Additional cartilage may be added to the tip to augment elevation and tip projection. The latter is my preferred approach.

Addressing the Skin Envelope

A prominent fibrofatty layer is defatted in the supratip and tip areas with blunt-tip small scissors. Care is taken to avoid injury to the subdermal vascular plexus. Thin skin and subcutaneous elements are supplemented with temporal fascia that may extend from radix to tip if necessary.

Dorsal Augmentation

I have found silicone to be the best material for dorsal augmentation, when utilized properly. Silicone is precise in shape and size, in addition to being reliable, economical, and well tolerated. The Asian, Filipino, and Polynesian are well aware of the benefits of silicone nasal implants and are quite comfortable with their use. Conversely, this population is often dramatically opposed to invasive surgery associated with autologous grafts. The occasional patient may reluctantly accept ear cartilage harvest.

The implant must be sterilized. After shaving or modification, or shortening, I routinely soak the prosthetic in Betadine solution prior to implantation. In placing the implant, one should avoid contact with skin or mucous membranes. Carving should be minimized, only involving small volume adjustments.

To meet our patients' needs, we utilize premolded implants by Implantech (Fig. 2). The highest point on the dorsum varies from 1.5 mm (extra small) to 5.5 mm (extra large). The prosthetic length of 4.5 cm approximates the distance from the frontal nasal to the supratip. This length usually requires shortening according to individual need, with nasal length ranging from 3.5 to 4.2 cm.

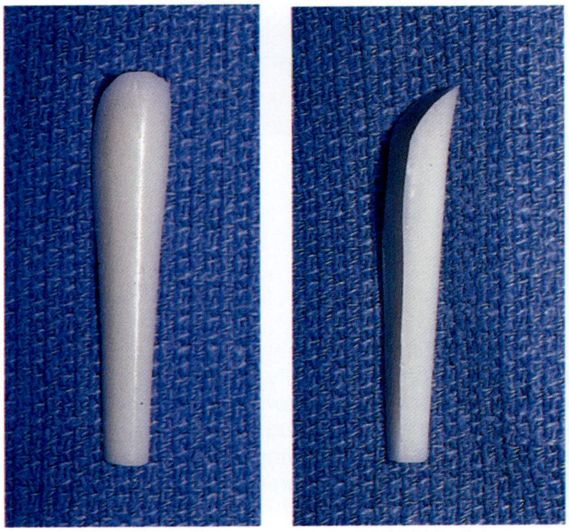

A, B

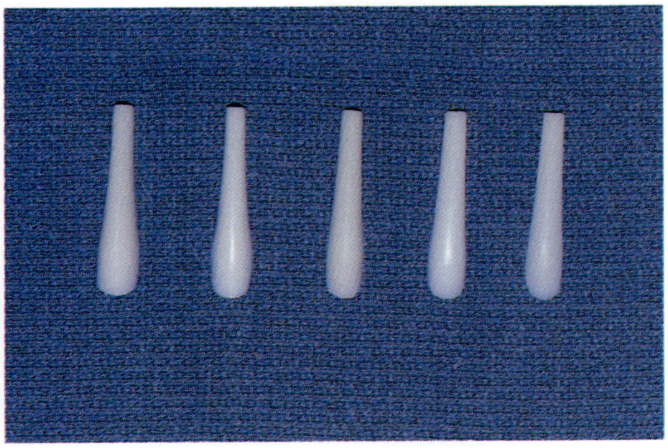

C

Figure 2. Implantech implants shown from top **(A)** and side **(B)** and in five different sizes **(C)**.

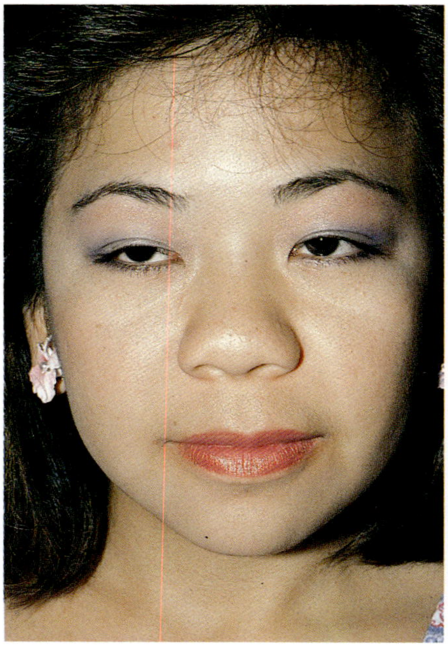
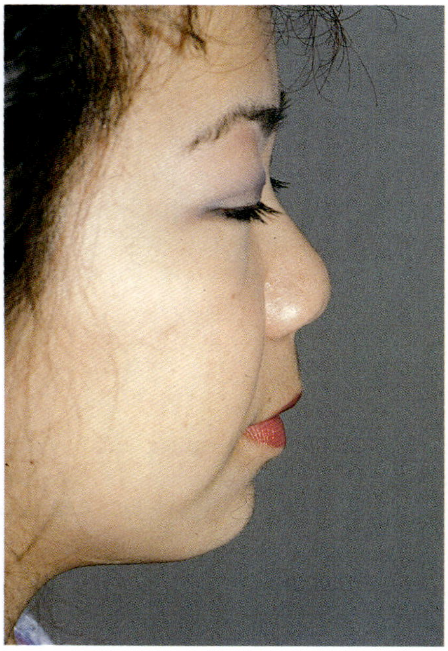

A, B

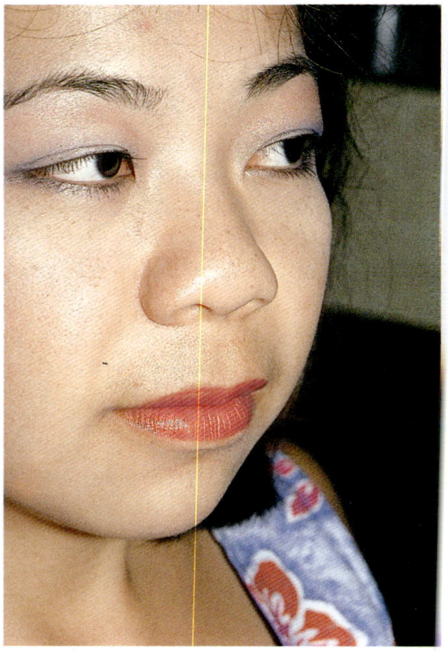

C

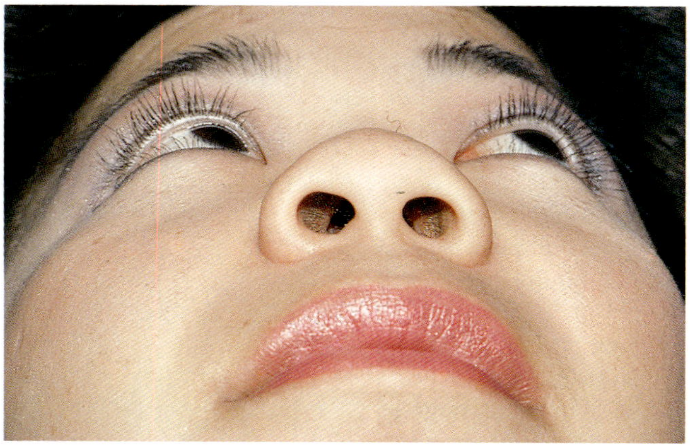

D

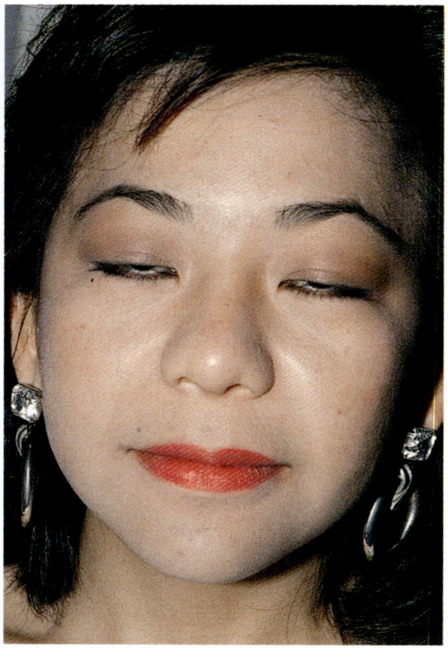

E

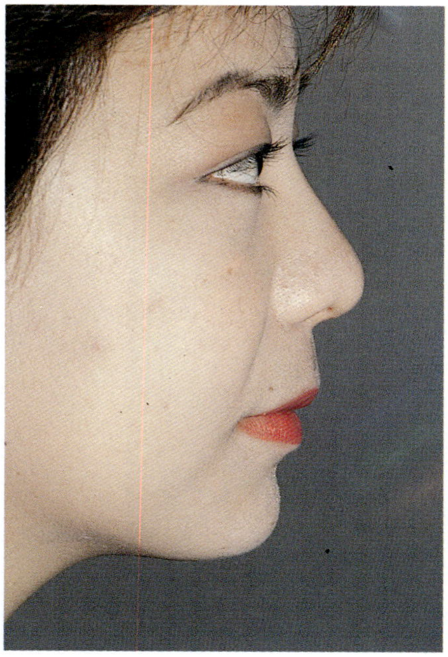

F

Figure 3. This patient presented for rhinoplasty and is shown pre-operatively **(A–D)** and post-operatively **(E–H)**. Planning of the operative procedures is also shown **(I–J)**. Lengthening of the nose, dorsal elevation, increased tip projection, decreased supratip projection, and narrowing of the alar base were acheived by augmentation with a premolded silicone prosthesis, small excision of the lateral crura bilaterally, and tip augmentation with conchal cartilage grafts and bilateral wedge excision. Chin augmentation with a premolded silicone prosthesis was also done.

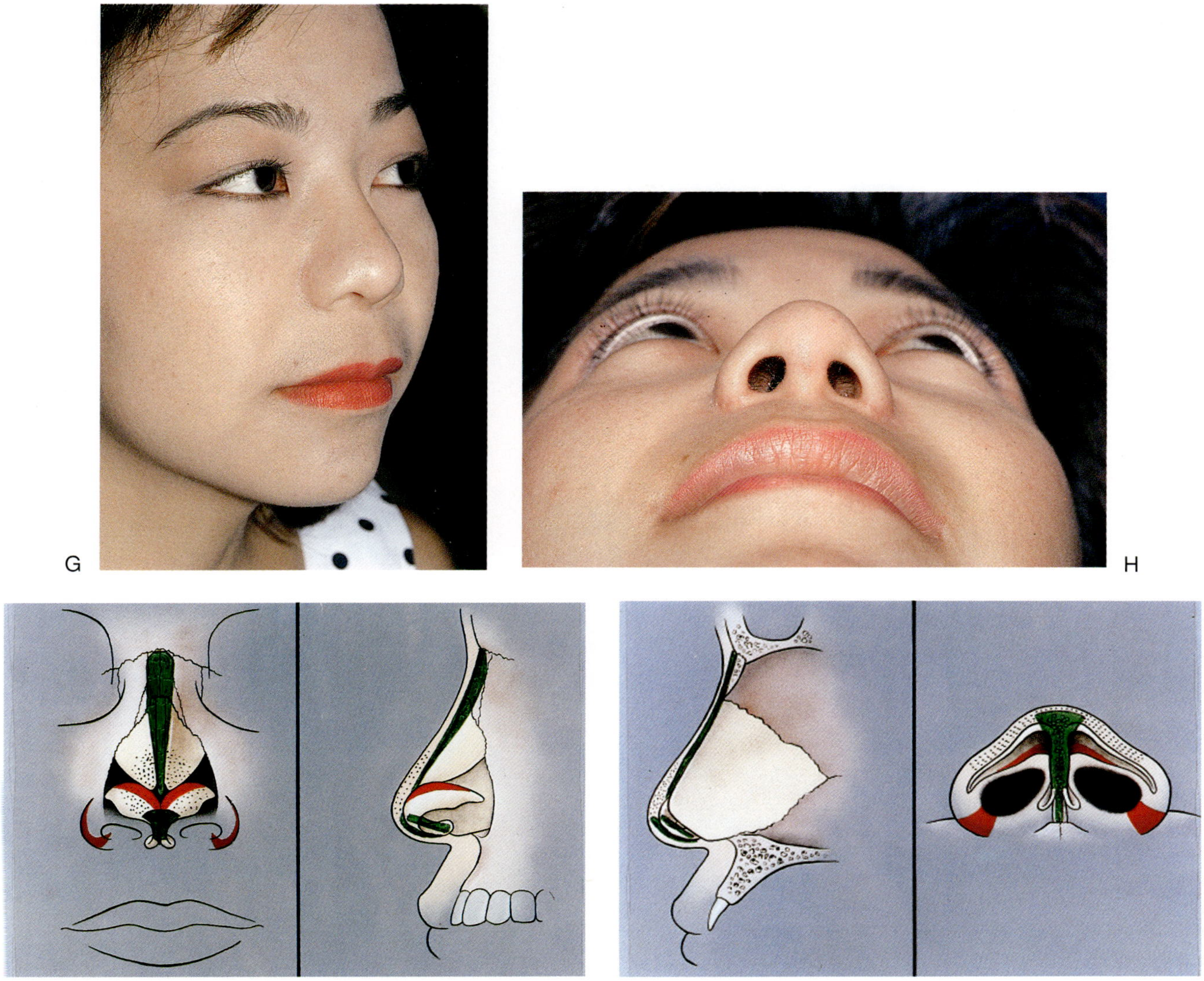

G H

I J

Figure 3 (*continued*).

The shape of the implant resembles the nasal bones and has two lateral wings in the upper dorsum only, which will hug the nasal bone (Fig. 2). They have two functions: The first is to increase the width bilaterally and gradually, and the second is to avoid lateralization of the upper portion. Two punctures, each 2 mm in diameter, are made on the side of the implant for tissue ingrowth. In the most cephalic portion of the prosthesis, there is a gentle elevation in the profile that will parallel nasofrontal contours. The inferior portion of the implant has a step-off that simulates the supratip break. Examples of these procedures are shown in Figs. 3 and 4.

Infection occurs infrequently, <0.5%, and mostly in the secondary rhinoplasty. Bacteriologic cultures yielded *Enterobacter aerogenes*, *Enterococcus*, and *Aerobacter* organisms. If infection develops, the implant need not be removed, but at least 3 weeks of Cipro should be given. If there is no response to this course of Cipro, the prosthesis then must be removed, preferably through an endonasal incision. The distal prosthetic is identified, the suture is cut, and the implant is removed. Only one absorbable suture is placed on the mucous membrane. The procedure is followed by 1 week of oral antibiotic treatment.

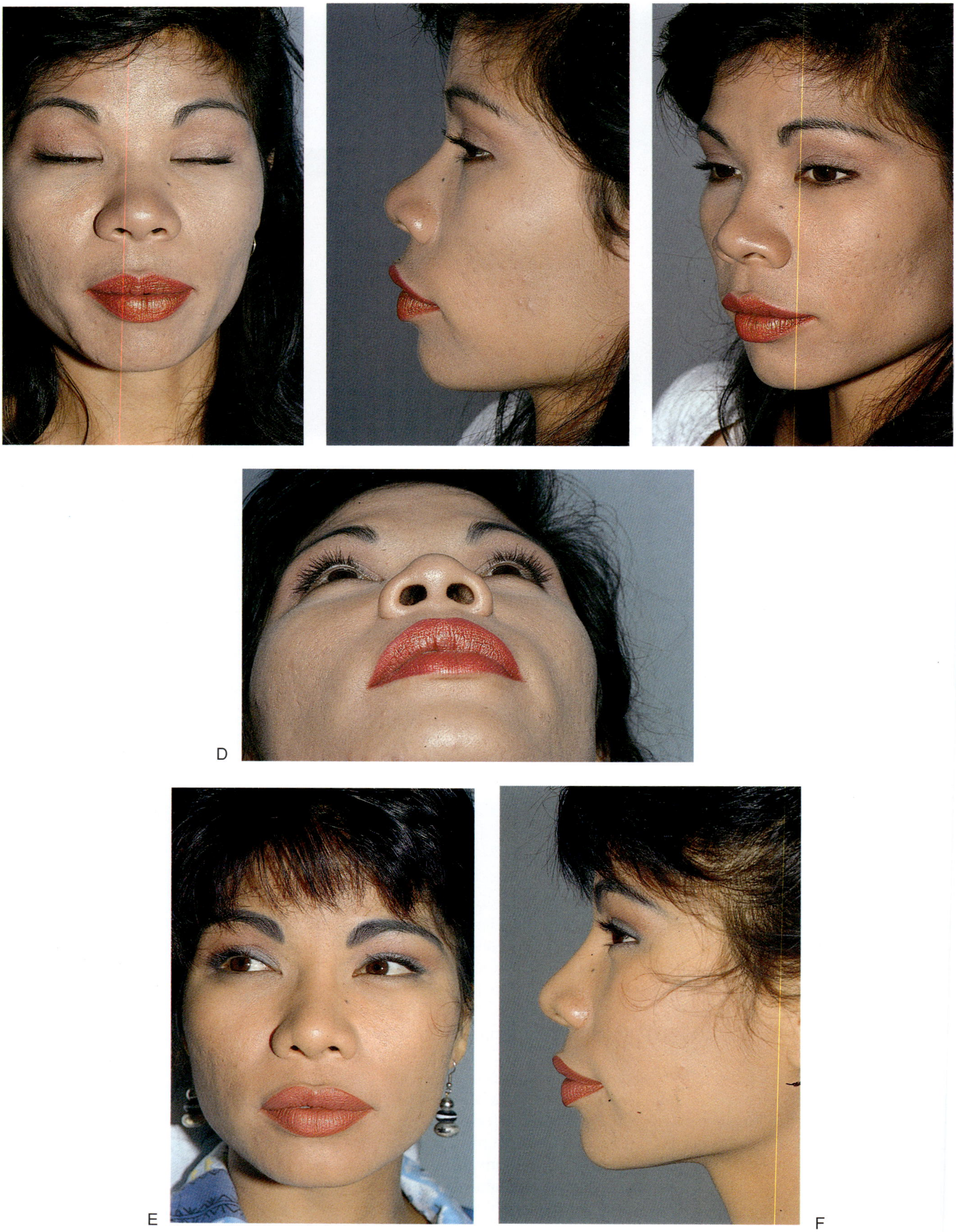

A, B C

D

E F

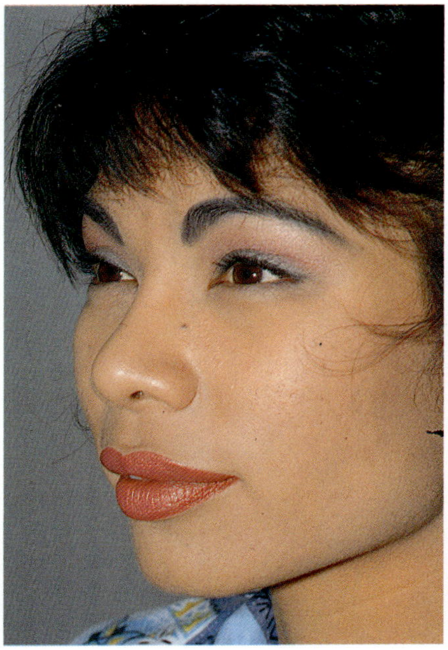

G

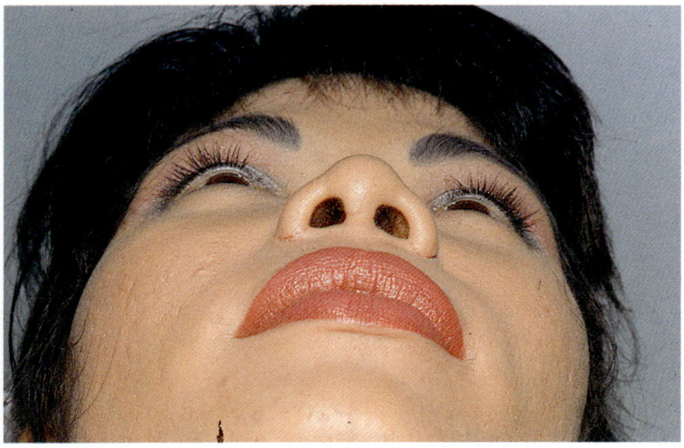

H

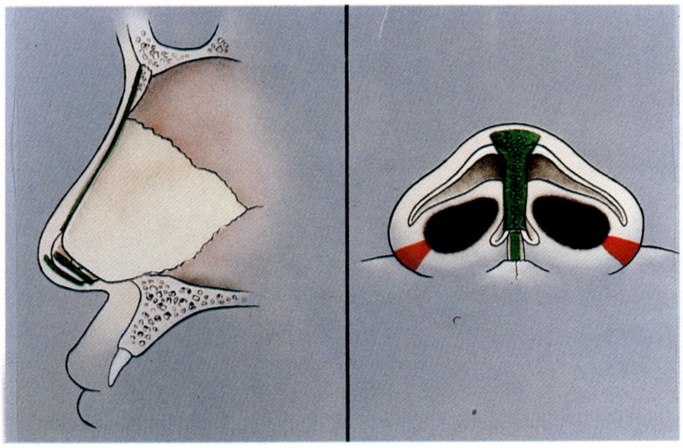

I

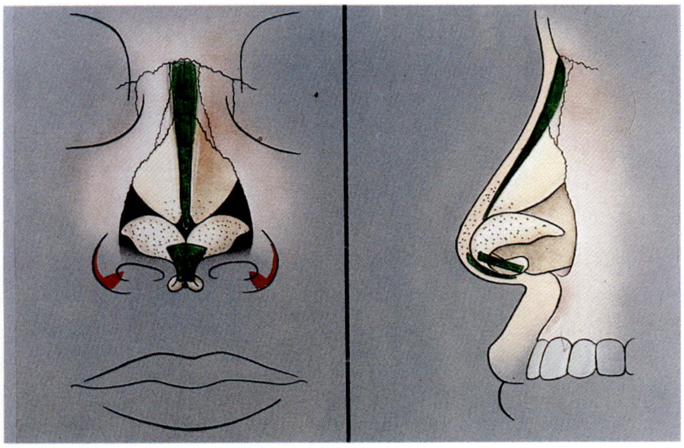

J

Figure 4. This patient presented for rhinoplasty and is shown pre-operatively **(A–D)** and post-operatively **(E–H)**. Planning of the operative procedures is also shown **(I–J)**. Lengthening of the nose, dorsal elevation, increased tip projection, and narrowing of the alar base were achieved with dorsal augmentation with a silicone prosthesis, tip augmentation with conchal cartilage grafts, and bilateral wedge excisions.

Secondary Rhinoplasty

During the early years of my practice, I saw a host of deformities following augmentation rhinoplasty. We photographed many but operated on few. The most frequent and the most severe deformities were seen with L-shaped implants. I recognized the basic problems but could not visualize the solutions. In addition, patients often refused implant removal even in the presence of malposition or suboptimal aesthetic improvement, similar behavior to that observed in breast implant patients. Open rhinoplasty uncovers the many anatomic disfigurements that result following the placement of L-shaped implant. We feel that all L-shaped implants should be removed sooner or later. External rhinoplasty allows surgical reconstruction in one stage.

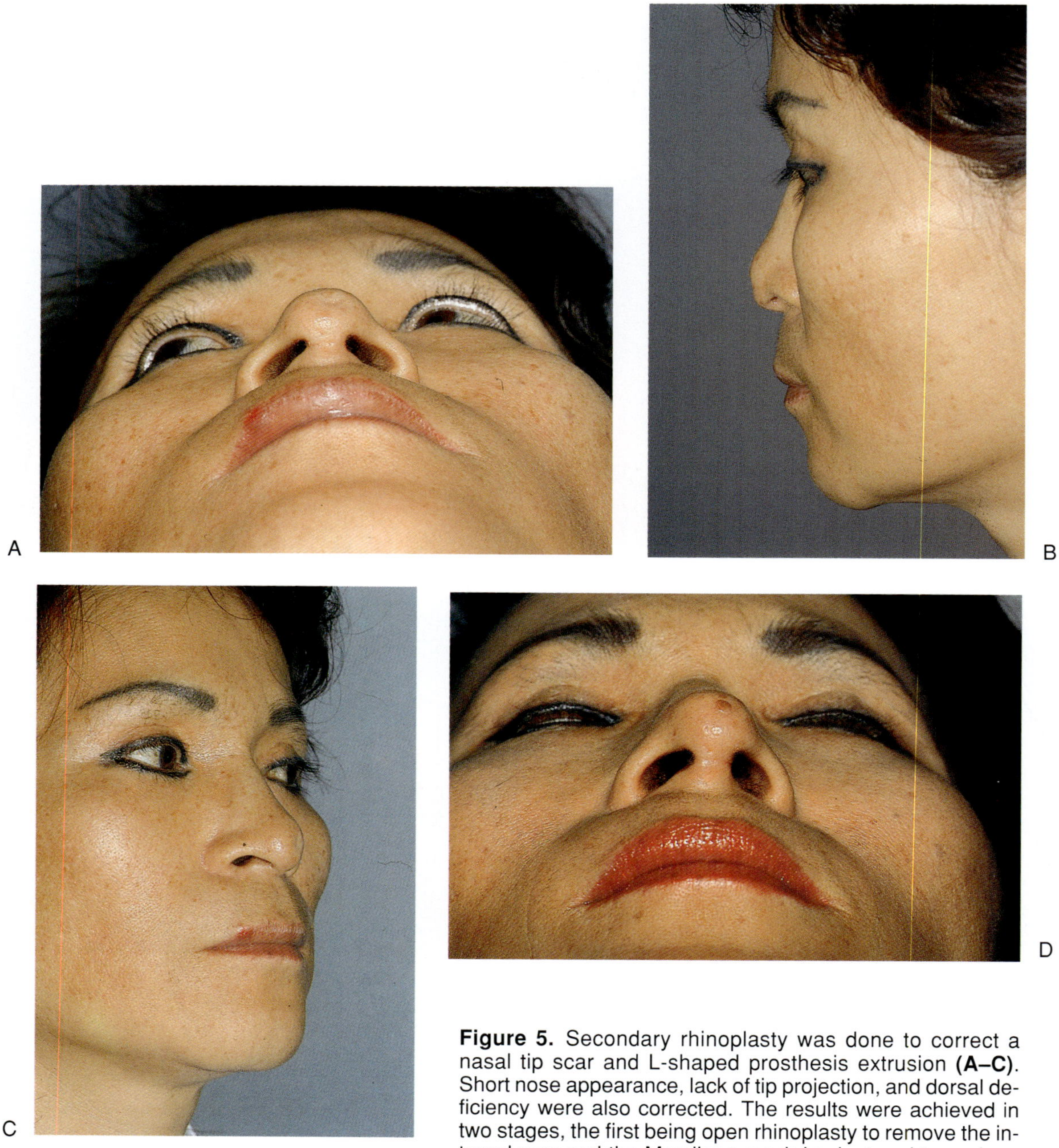

Figure 5. Secondary rhinoplasty was done to correct a nasal tip scar and L-shaped prosthesis extrusion **(A–C)**. Short nose appearance, lack of tip projection, and dorsal deficiency were also corrected. The results were achieved in two stages, the first being open rhinoplasty to remove the internal scar and the Mersilene mesh implant and to perform a tip graft using conchal cartilage. The second stage involved removal of skin scar with a 3.5-mm skin biopsy punch and placement of skin grafts from the forehead, which can be seen due to temporary hyperpigmentation in these early pre-operative photographs **(D–F)**. Planning of the operative procedures is also shown **(G–H)**.

E F

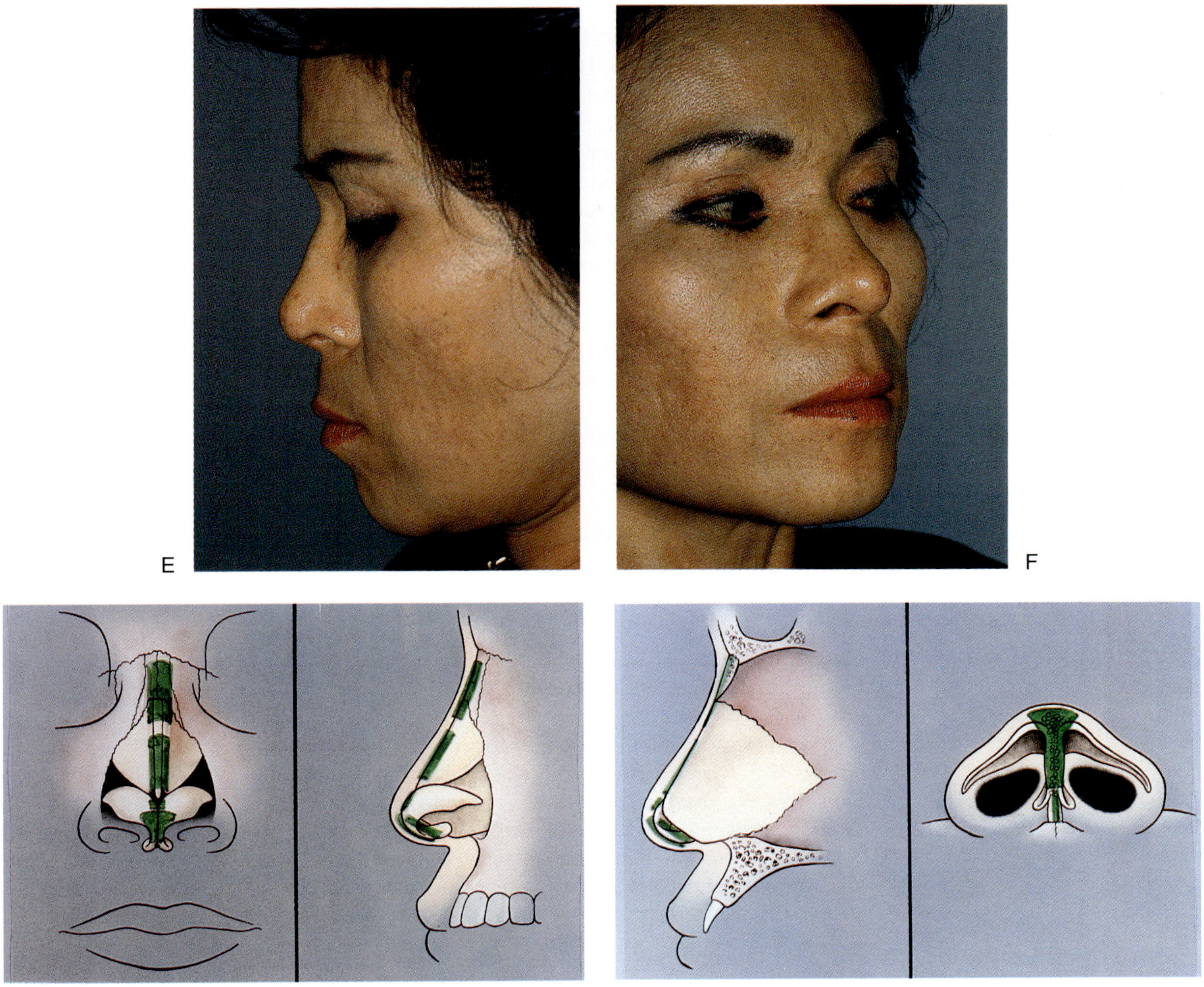

G H

Figure 5 (*continued*).

Deformities Following L-Shaped Implantation

Two anatomic deformities are common: that of the nasal dorsum and the nasal tip. The dorsum may be too large or irregular. Lateralization and distortion are not uncommon. Other deformities are more directly secondary to mechanical pressure, including a degree of redness, skin thinning, and impending or actual extrusion.

Tip distortions are due to compression of the lower lateral cartilages, resulting in tip widening and excessive projection or pointedness of the domes; inadequate tip projection may lead to nasal length/width disparity or impending or actual extrusion as exhibited by pain, pressure points, skin thinning, or infection.

Surgical Correction of the Sequelae of L-Shaped Implants

Patients must be advised of the potential sequelae that may occur as a result of implant removal. We routinely have been able to remove the implant and reconstruct the tip and dorsum in one stage through an open technique. Careful dissection of the lower lateral cartilage from the thin overlying skin is essential. Cartilage may be folded by pressure or scarred down and distorted. I use loop magnification and fine instruments to achieve a clear and atraumatic dissection. Upon removal of the implant, check the size and tenure of the capsule. If it seems too thick and visible, it may be removed with tender care. Removal of the posterior layer of the capsule is safer and is usually adequate.

Most problematic implants are located in the subcutaneous plane. Repositioning an autologous implant on a subperiosteal level, if possible, is preferable. If tip skin is thin, temporal fascia will camouflage underlying deformities. Reabsorption is far less with temporal fascia than with dermis or other soft tissue grafts.

In instances of actual extrusion, the residual scar is dealt with secondarily. Five to six months later, a small scar may be treated with full-thickness skin graft using a 3- to 5-mm punch graft. Forehead skin at the hairline as the donor site provides excellent color match. If necessary, a stuck-up graft is done for adequate thickness and deepithelializing the buried one; 7-0 nylon is used to stabilize the graft (Fig. 5).

This seems to be adequate treatment for small scars of the nasal tip. Larger scars may necessitate local flap reconstruction, e.g., a mucous membrane flap from the upper lip sulcus to nasal tip via columella or membranous septum tunnel.

PITFALLS AND COMPLICATIONS

We have experienced a number of potential untoward outcomes. The following discussion identifies frequently encountered obstacles to optimal results.

Suboptimal Placement of the Dorsal Implant

Improper positioning of the silicone implant is the leading contribution to commonly touted ill effects including infection, mobility, malposition, and redness. The cephalic portion of the prosthesis must be placed as deeply as possible to avoid a step-off from the forehead to the device. Pocket development and suture fixation must be perfectly contoured to prevent rocking motion that may raise the cephalic implant, resulting in a loss of definition of the nasofrontal angle. Lateral implant movement and rocker deformity along with visibility of implant edges occur when the implant is placed too superficially, i.e., in the subcutaneous plane. Skin circulation may thus be altered, often causing redness.

Persistent Dorsal Hump

Unrecognized or underestimated osteocartilaginous excess that is not addressed will allow a rocking/see-saw motion of the implant. If a suture is placed distally, cephalad rotation may show the implant edge. With the external approach, visualization of a smooth, straightened dorsum is a requisite to proper implant positioning.

Prosthetic Length

Inadequate prosthetic length results in a step-off deformity with visible implant edges noted at the nasofrontal angle or distally. An implant that extends distal to the septal angle may be visible or palpable or may ultimately erode.

Partial Augmentation of the Dorsum

Partial augmentation of the dorsum to fill an isolated radix or mid or distal height deficiency should be avoided. Even in the best of hands, segmental dorsal implants will be noticeable in photographs, especially those taken with dim lighting or inadequate exposure. Avoid or replace segmental dorsal prosthetics when possible.

Thin Skin

Thin skin that is noted preoperatively or that resulting from prior implantation results in visible nasal deformities. Visibility of irregularities or of implant edges can also be problematic. We suggest using temporal fascia to cover these defects. Varying thicknesses of fascia can be used to soften implant irregularities and to prevent prosthetic erosion.

Silicone Injections

Silicone injections have been commonly used in Asian and Polynesian populations. History or examination may not identify the presence of silicone injection. Minor amounts in the glabella or dorsum may result in chronic post-surgical edema along with dermal and subcutaneous irregularities. Autologous grafts are better tolerated in that they induce far less post-surgical inflammatory reaction.

In those noses, one concha and one septum is preferable particularly when strong supporting structures are necessary. A lot of those noses need to be elongated to look better. This is achieved by following surgical technique for a short nose advocated by Gunther and Gruber, plus an advancement of the lateral crus most of the time necessary by transecting the lateral crus 3–4 mm from this attachment and bringing it down or forward, then fixing it to the stump in a most caudal position (Fig. 6). Also the elevation of the nasal frontal angle with the prosthesis will help to elongate the nose. This procedure should not be done at the same time as the augmentation procedure, unless all autologous material is used.

So the sequence will be first the lengthening of the nose through a mucous membrane incision, then 9 months later the dorsal augmentation.

PREVENTING THE UNHAPPY PATIENT

Communicating the subtle changes that accompany cosmetic facial surgery in the Filipino, Polynesian, and Asian may be difficult. Often times, it may be more perplexing for the patient to translate his/her wishes. We have found computer imaging to be very helpful in finding the most successful road to patient satisfaction. Sophisticated features like calibration of implant size and measurement of facial angles allow the surgeon to facilitate the effective transfer of information. Imaging is particularly beneficial for the patient presenting for rhinoplasty who also needs adjunctive procedures like chin, malar, or maxillary aug-

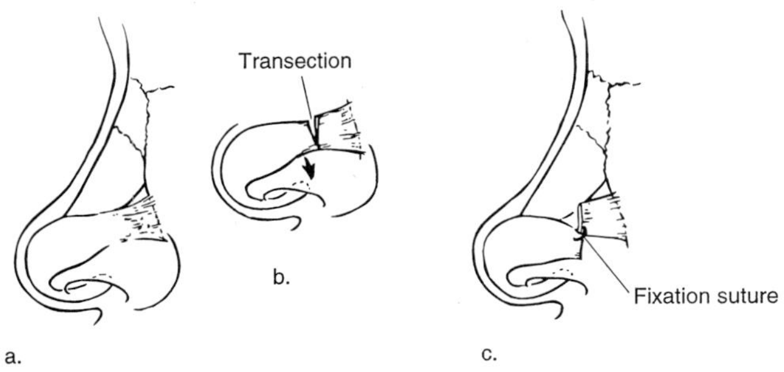

Lowering the lateral crus by transection.

(Releasing tension to allow lengthening. No change in rotation or nostril configuration,)

Figure 6. Lowering the lateral crura by transection.

mentation. A common source of dissatisfaction is too much or too little dorsal augmentation or nasal lengthening. Imaging is capable of translating the limitations of nasal lengthening or dorsal augmentation.

If you do not have access to computer imaging, a carved Silly Putty prosthesis and Mastisol over their noses is helpful. This can be adjusted to the patient's desire, then a photo taken for documentation. The Silly Putty would give you a good guide to follow for both the silicone implant shape and the measurements, but also for the graft. Silly Putty might not be as helpful in secondary work due to the present of an existing implant.

RECOMMENDED READING

Constantian M. The septal angle: a cardinal point in rhinoplasty. *Plast Reconstr Surg* 1990;85.
Ersek RA, Delerm AG. Processed irradiated bovine cartilage for nasal reconstruction. *Ann Plast Surg* 1988;20.
Juri J, Juri C. Secondary rhinoplasty. *Ann Plast Surg* 1987;18.
Juri J. Surgical treatment for secondary retracted nose. *Plast Reconstr Surg* 1990;86.
Megumi Y. Augmentation rhinoplasty with soft tissue and cartilage. *Aesthet Plast Surg* 1988;12:89–93.
Niranjan NS. An anatomical study of the facial artery. *Ann Plast Surg* 1988;21.
Park C, Lineaweaver W, Rumly T, Bunckle H. Arterial supply of the anterior ear. *Plast Reconstr Surg* 1992;90.
Parsa FD. Nasal augmentation with split calvarial grafts in orientals. *Plast Reconstr Surg* 1991;87.
Reich J. The application of dermis grafts in deformities of the nose. *Plast Reconstr Surg* 1983.
Straith R. Five long-term case reports (average 15 years) of saddlenose correction using cast Silastic implants. *Plast Reconstr Surg* 1991;88.

SECTION VIII

The Hispanic Patient

Ethnic Considerations in Facial Aesthetic Surgery, edited by W. Earle Matory, Jr.
Lippincott–Raven Publishers, Philadelphia © 1998.

22

The Hispanic Patient

Editor's Commentary

W. Earle Matory, Jr.

"Hispanic" defines a wide range of attractive facial features that may be broad or narrow or Castilian in nature. A sculpted nose, prominent cheeks, a defined chin and jawline, along with a long neck are consistent features in the attractive Hispanic (Fig. 1). The basal view may demonstrate a broad amorphous, an elongated, or a finely sculpted tip (Fig. 2).

CONTOURING OF THE FACE AND NECK

In my practice, tumescent suction-assisted lipectomy is the most commonly performed procedure on the Hispanic patient, with correction of facial aging and rhinoplasty close seconds. With the tumescent technique (Fig. 3), significant volumes of fat can be removed from the lower third of the face and submental area to achieve an improved facial shape, jaw, neck, and chin area.

Facial aging, malar sag usually associated with infra-orbital shadowing, jowl formation, and platysma banding are common findings in the Hispanic patient. Because of the strong propensity for post-auricular hypertrophic scarring, we prefer a mini-rhytidectomy as described in Chapter 12 (Fig. 4).

Permanent lash liner is a frequent request in the Hispanic American. We prefer black or very dark brown pigment in two to three layers to ensure the commonly desired heavy coloration. Perpendicular in a black passage of the dye is preferable. Not infrequently, these patients request highly stylized permanent lash liner. When possible, the surgeon should

W. E. Matory, Jr.: A New You Plastic Surgery Medical Group, Irvine, California 92714

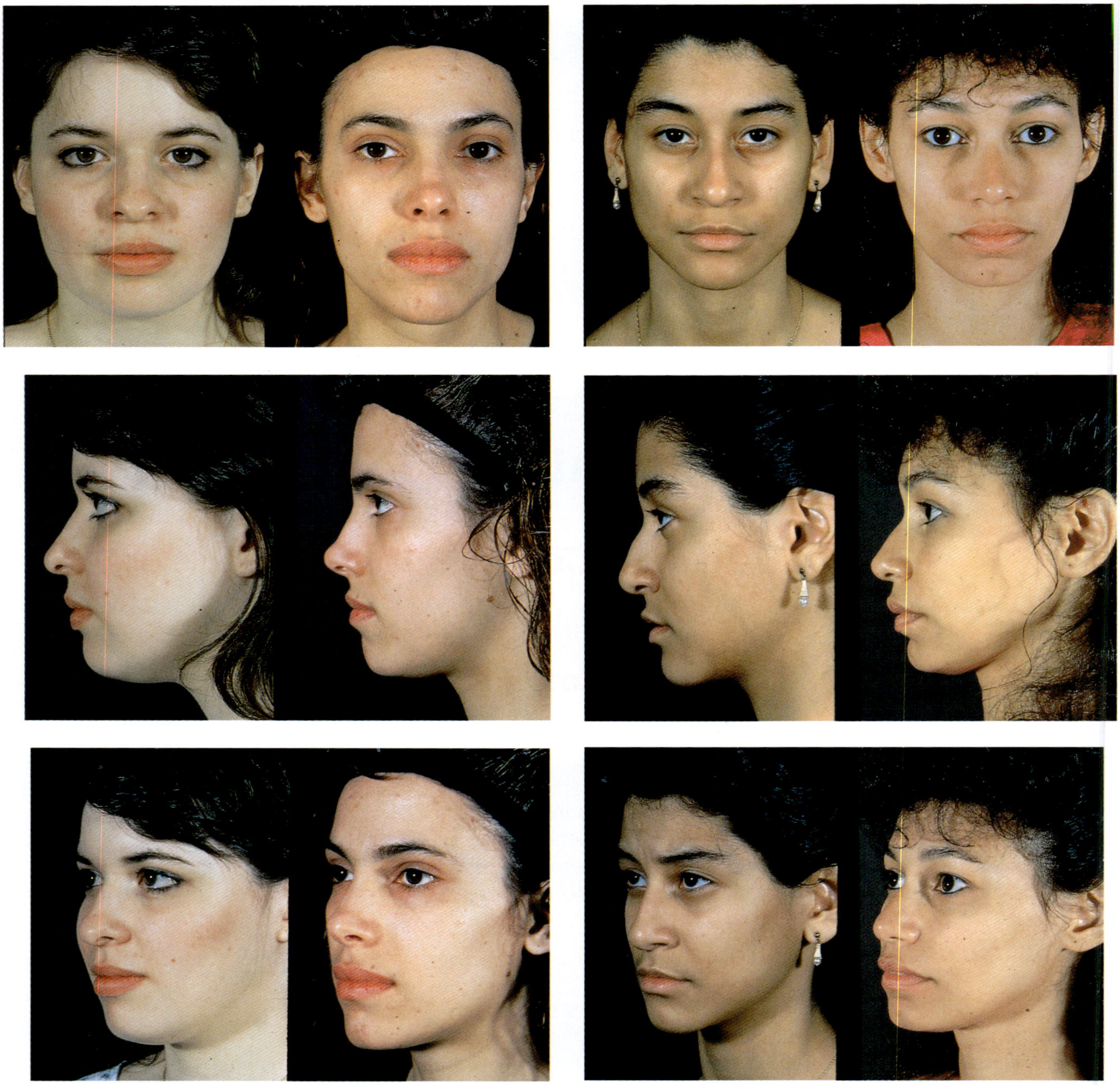

Figure 1. The Hispanic facies varies from highly sculpted and thin skinned; to the Castilian who features an elongated nose and facies and dorsal hump; to the broader facies that may or may not have significant African characteristics such as full lips and a broad amorphous tip with thick skin. Common features for the attractive facies include a high forehead, prominent malar eminences, a smooth, strong jawline, and a long neck.

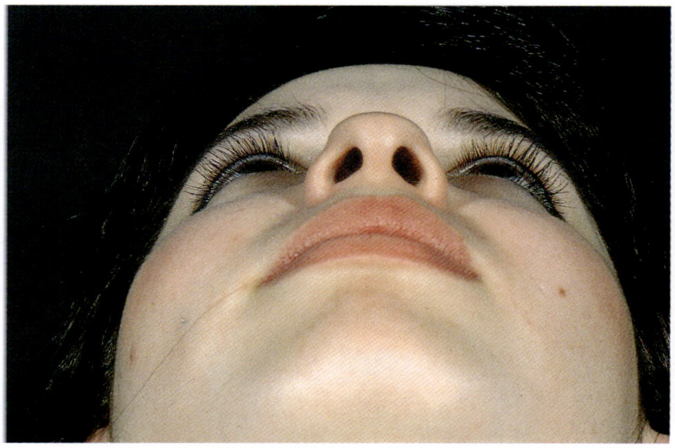
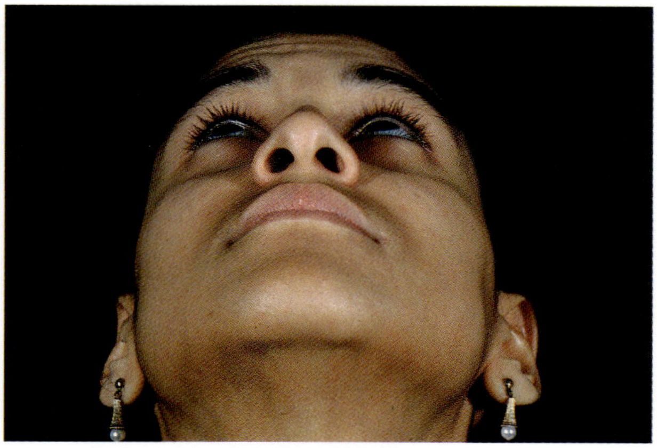
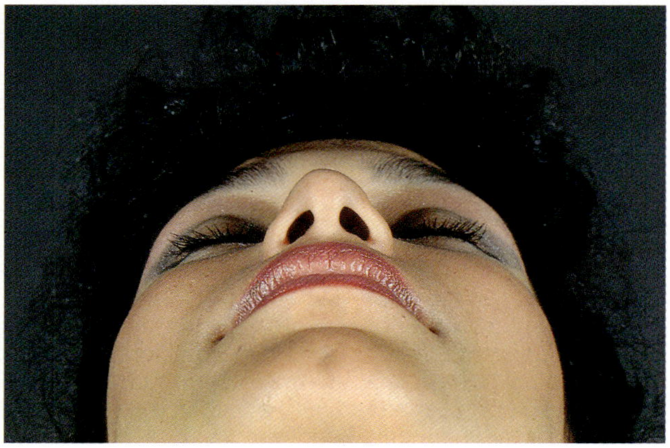

Figure 2. The basal view may demonstrate a variety of tip and alar width relationships.

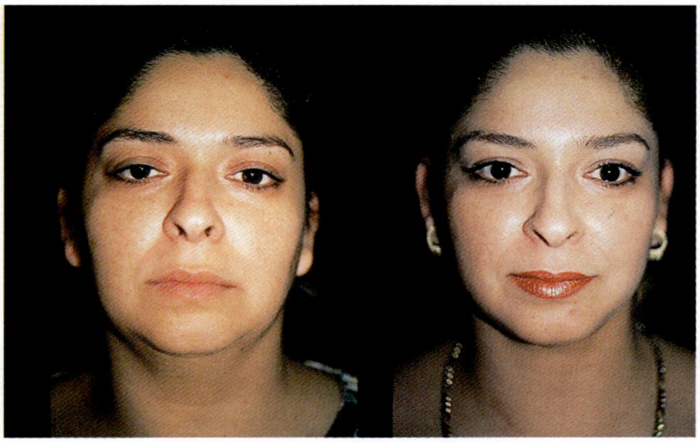
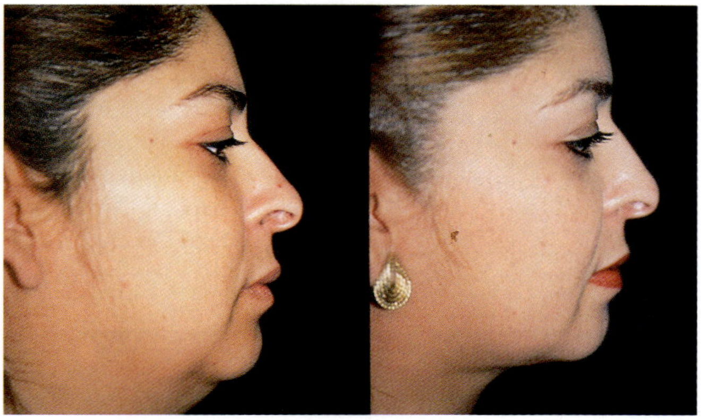
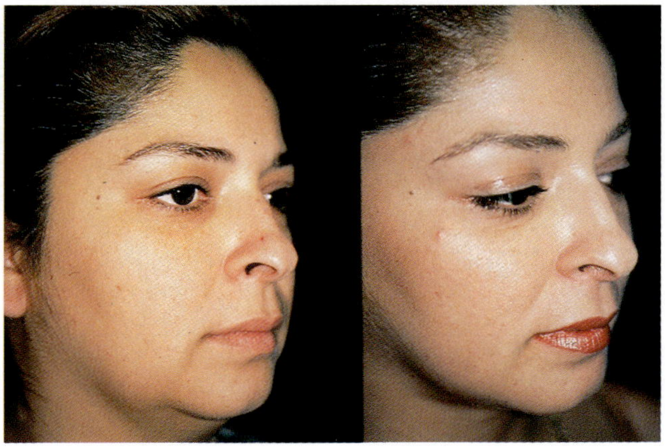

Figure 3. Results 1 year following tumescent liposuction of the lower face and neck, removing 25 cm^3 from each jaw and 50 cm^3 from the submental area.

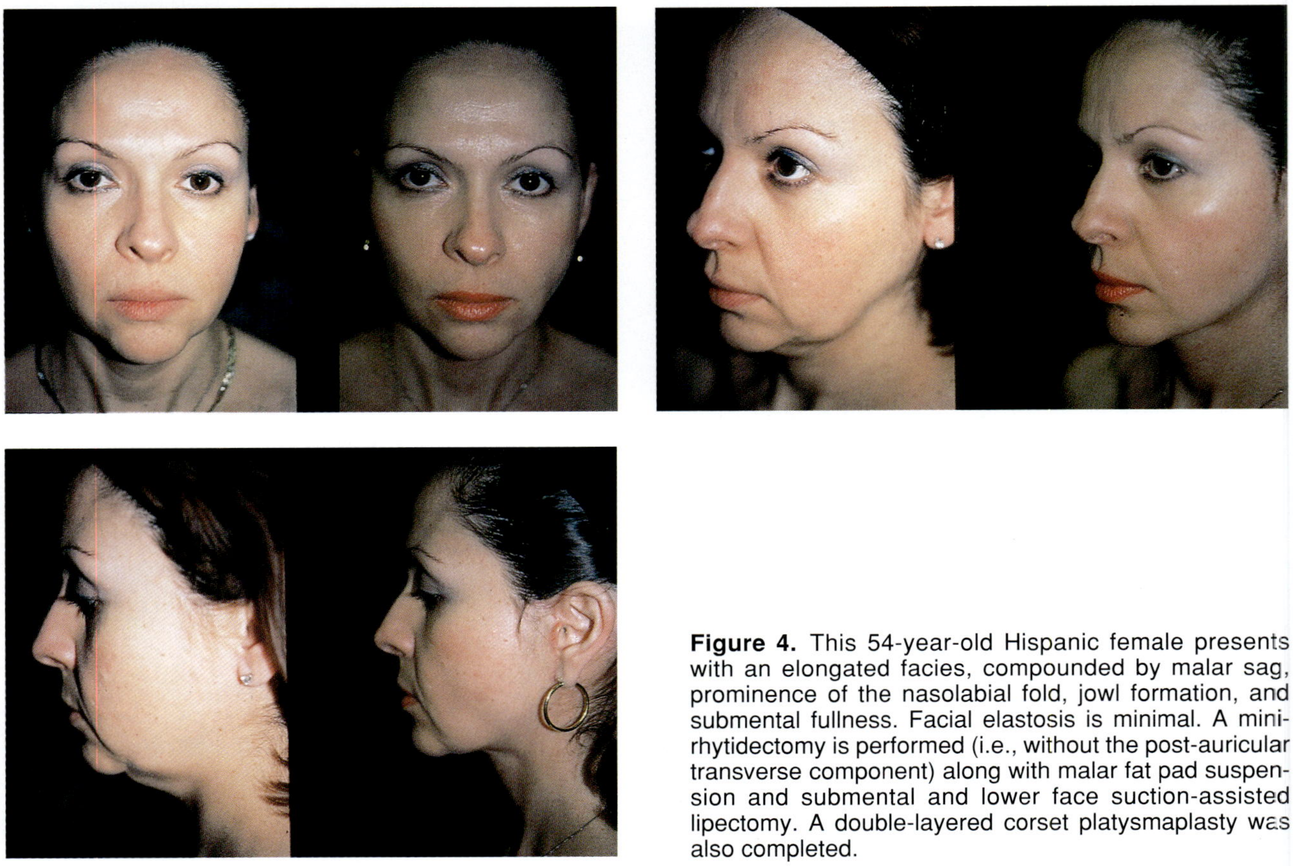

Figure 4. This 54-year-old Hispanic female presents with an elongated facies, compounded by malar sag, prominence of the nasolabial fold, jowl formation, and submental fullness. Facial elastosis is minimal. A mini-rhytidectomy is performed (i.e., without the post-auricular transverse component) along with malar fat pad suspension and submental and lower face suction-assisted lipectomy. A double-layered corset platysmaplasty was also completed.

lean toward a conservative style that can be adjusted by the patient's personal preferences (Fig. 5). This minimizes later complaints of dissatisfaction with certain styles.

Hispanic patients tend to be very grateful and often refer family members and friends. The medical practice should be directed to do all that is appropriate to encourage referrals. With Hispanic Americans representing the largest growing ethnic group, the surgeon can understand the importance of incorporating Hispanic staff members.

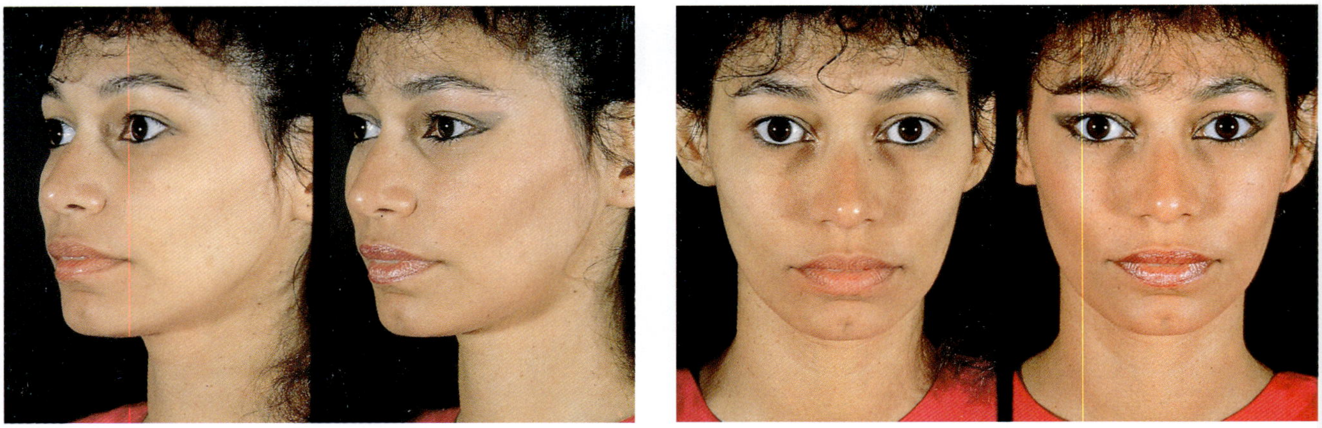

Figure 5. Permanent lash liner is best completed using black pigment. In spite of frequent requests for highly stylized application, the surgeon should lean toward a more conservative styling and allow personally customized adjustments to be applied as desired by the patient.

Ethnic Considerations in Facial Aesthetic Surgery, edited by W. Earle Matory, Jr.
Lippincott–Raven Publishers, Philadelphia © 1998.

23

Facial Surgery in the Hispano-American Patient

Oscar M. Ramírez

Experience is a series of errors seen retrospectively.
—Oscar M. Ramírez

CULTURAL CONSIDERATIONS

Hispanics living in North, Central, and South America, commonly called Hispanic Americans, represent a racial mixture between the European Spaniards and Native Americans. This admixture was particularly prominent in Central and South America, due to the religious, cultural, and economic effects of Spanish colonization (1). Forced African migration to the Americas added a third large component to the process of Mestizaje (2). During the last century, the migration of Asians and Central and Northern Europeans has further added to the Hispanic ethnic heritage.

Advances in communication via television, electronic media, satellite, cinema, airplanes, etc., promoting the "Occidental" look (Caucasian), have changed the concept of beauty throughout the world, particularly in Latin America. Influenced by intensive advertising, the Latin American Mestizo and particularly the Hispanic female looks to the Anglo–Saxon European model of beauty. Historically, there has been resistance among Mestizo males to change facial features through cosmetic surgery. This may be an expression of the strong self-esteem or "macho" character of the Mestizo male. In contrast, younger generations have different attitudes about cosmetic surgery. With increasing frequency in our practices, we see male patients requesting cosmetic surgery. This is particularly true for recent immigrants to the United States. The crucial factor in the rise of Mestizo patients seeking cosmetic surgery is the astonishing and spiraling number of Hispanic immigrants to the United States. Progressive increases in economic prosperity and the desire to be integrated more easily into the U.S. culture make cosmetic surgery appealing to many Hispanic Americans.

O. M. Ramírez: Lutherville, Maryland 21093

FACIAL CHARACTERISTICS

There is a wide variety in the facial structure and relationships of the eyes nose, lips, and teeth to the remainder of the face. These facial structures and relationships are consistent with the degree of racial mixture. The anatomical features of the face vary from the American Indian to the Caucasian. Inbetween these two extremes, the variations depend on the other inherited ethnic characteristics, for example, African or Asian. Frequently, patients will have a rich Indian–Negroid–Caucasian heritage with facial features blended from each of the racial components. This makes it particularly difficult to standardize a pattern of aesthetic abnormalities as well as specific general surgical procedures. Each case needs to be individually analyzed. Specific surgical planning must be tailored to each presenting complaint and to the aesthetic goals of the physician and more importantly the patient. However, important common denominators are noted: (a) Present cultural preference indicates that the model of beauty is the Caucasian Anglo–Saxon faces, (b) there is a higher degree of unrealistic expectation as compared with the Caucasian counterpart, and (c) Mestizo patients are extremely critical about the results obtained with surgical procedures.

In my practice, I see greater tolerance and a higher degree of satisfaction in the Caucasoid Mestizo as opposed to the more Indian-looking Mestizo. I believe that this is in part due to faulty analysis by the surgeon of the patient's facial characteristics as well as the high expectations that the patients have for minimal procedures to perform miraculous changes. A typical example is the patient who presents for rhinoplasty with a wide bizygomatic distance, bimaxillary protrusion, and very thick nasal skin. A standard rhinoplasty will not produce the desired outcome, often resulting in an operated and unnatural look, due to visible disproportions.

INDICATIONS

Aesthetic surgery on the Mestizo face is indicated when the patient defines realistic expectations of the desired outcome. Frequently, the unattractive craniofacial skeleton needs to be addressed. This can be dealt with, most often, utilizing limited facial skeletal surgery. If patients desire not to proceed with skeletal remodeling or minor osteotomies, then they have to understand the limitations of the surgical procedures that they are willing to undergo.

CONTRAINDICATIONS

Patients with unrealistic expectations should not undergo surgery. Patients who are looking for the perfect Caucasian model when the potential surgical changes are far from obtaining that model are likely to be unhappy irrespective of the outcome. The often thicker and coarser characteristics of facial skin may be problematic. The nasal skin envelope may be more difficult to redrape to the surgically altered osteocartilaginous framework. Thickened facial skin may also contour poorly following rhytidectomy. Secondary or touch-up operations as a result are more common. The patient must fully understand these eventualities. If the patient is not psychologically or financially prepared for the possibility of secondary procedures, surgery should not be performed. Hispanic Americans carry a higher risk of hypertrophic and hyper- or hypopigmented scars than the Caucasian counterpart. While this risk is not as high as in the Black population, potential scar deformities must be reviewed with and acknowledged by the patient.

PRE-OPERATIVE EVALUATION

During the initial consultation, I make an assessment of the facial characteristics. I identify and point out the craniofacial skeletal abnormalities and soft tissue disproportions to

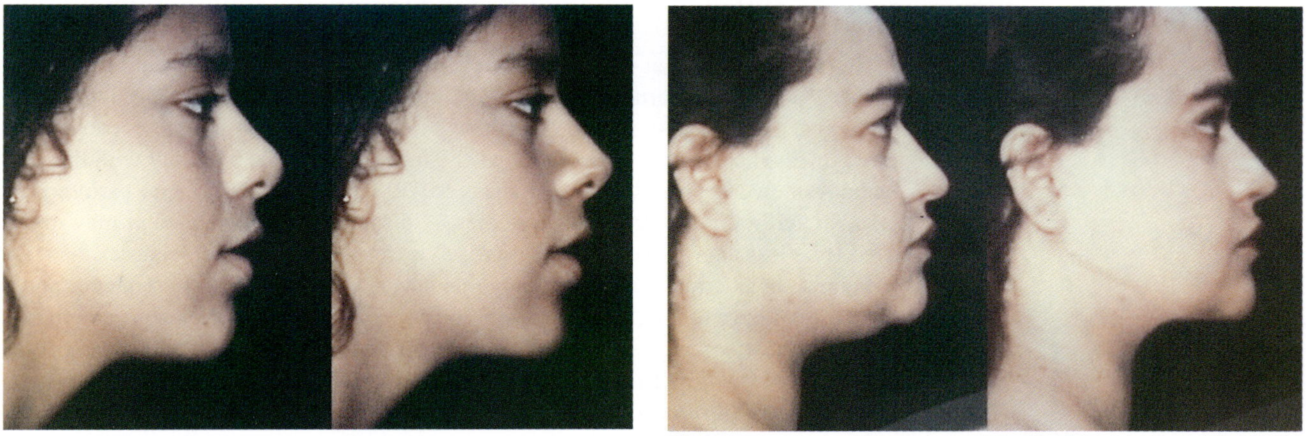

A B

Figure 1. A: Video imaging of a young female patient for rhinoplasty shown on the lateral view showing before and after the proposed changes. **B:** Video imaging of a middle-aged patient, proposing planned changes in the nose and the neck.

the patient. I try to discern the degree and type of ethnic contributions, particularly the Indian, African, or Caucasian phenotypes. One must discern the desires of the patient, in that the goals of the patient may not fit those of the surgeon or anatomic realities. The most common operation that the Hispanic American requests is rhinoplasty. Characteristic features of the Mestizo include a moderately broad nasal base, wide and short nasal bones, with a moderate nasal hump. Many of my patients have already undergone two or more operative procedures that have resulted in worsened nasal disproportions. In my practice, 70% present for secondary rhinoplasty in contrast to 30% for primary rhinoplasty. Patients coming for primary rhinoplasty, in addition to the features mentioned, commonly have very thick nasal skin, an acute nasolabial angle, and moderately wide nostrils. The incidence of microgenia is higher than in the Caucasian population, often requiring a sliding genioplasty and/or chin implant. It is important to point out that thick nasal skin limits the resultant definition of the nasal tip.

The incidence of bimaxillary protrusion is also higher than in the Caucasian population. For those individuals seeking correction of bimaxillary protrusion, I perform segmental bimaxillary surgery, followed in 3 months with an osteoplastic rhinoplasty. On occasion, combined procedures may be indicated. If there is a very low radix or prior septoplasty, I use rib cartilage to augment the nasal dorsum. Rib is also a good source for grafting the nasal tip. This will be reviewed in Operative Technique.

Video Imaging

During the pre-operative consultation, I use computer video imaging as a tool to promote realistic expectations on the part of the patient. Although there have been fears regarding false expectations that the computer can produce, in my practice, this has not been a significant problem to date. On the contrary, we have found video imaging to be a very useful technique for the patient to translate his/her expectations and for the surgeon to relay potential surgical results (Fig. 1). Other potential changes in the facial profile, particularly in reference to the lip/tooth relationship and the chin projection, can be translated to the patient. If I feel that the patient requires either a sliding genioplasty or a chin implant, I make the corresponding changes in the computer imaging and I discuss with the patient whether s/he wants to proceed with these changes. If not, I make specific emphasis in regards to the limitations that the rhinoplasty alone can give to the patient. If orthognathic surgery is anticipated, a cephalometric analysis and pre- and post-operative orthodontics are arranged.

PREVENTING THE UNHAPPY PATIENT

One must ensure that the patient's expectations are realistic. The entire face should be properly analyzed in terms of balance, symmetry, and quality of the skin. Based on the defined goals, the surgeon should determine whether the patient's requests can be achieved. The projected changes in one section of the face should be in harmony with the rest of the facial framework. If these planned changes will adversely affect facial harmony, the surgeon should rethink procedural strategies. A discussion with the patient may identify the need for a less aggressive surgical approach or sometimes other procedures.

Patient satisfaction in my patients seems to vary, dependent on the sequence and type of procedure. I have found that, going from the bottom to the top of the face, cervicoplasty and chin modifications with either a sliding genioplasty or a contour chin implant give a high degree of satisfaction. Likewise, orthognathic surgery to correct the bimaxillary protrusion has a high rate of satisfaction, as well as rhinoplasty, if properly performed.

Patient satisfaction in the Hispanic American is the greatest challenge in the peri-orbital area. Hispanic patients are very sensitive to changes in the eyelid slant. When the lateral canthal attachments are lower than the medial attachment, a slight modification of these attachments can significantly change the eye expression. Hispanic patients are very sensitive about "Orientalization" of their eye expression. Extreme caution should be taken when planning eyelid and peri-orbital surgery.

Conversely, fronto-orbital remodeling by reducing the fronto-orbital irregularities usually results in a high degree of satisfaction. Because of the tendency for thick scarring and thickening of the skin, especially around the nasal areas, the rhinoplasty should be approached with great care. The average Hispanic nose does not tolerate a classical reduction type of rhinoplasty. Likewise, excessive tendency to augmentation can make the nose protrude too much without optimizing nasal definition. Therefore, I prefer to balance between augmentation and reduction. By augmenting the areas that are deficient, particularly around the nasal bridge and increasing the projection of the nasal tip, and decreasing the nasal lobule and nostrils, aesthetic contours are achieved.

ETHNIC SPECIFICS

In spite of multiethnic contributions, there are a number of characteristics that are specific to the Hispanic Mestizo face. Classified as Euriprosopus by the anthropologists, the bizygomatic distance is increased in relation to the vertical dimension, giving the face a broad appearance (Fig. 2A). The length/width ratio (facial index) is <84 (3,4). The convexity angle is slightly higher than in the average Caucasian. The convexity angle in the Mexican adult, for example, is $+3{:}5$ (5) (Fig. 2B).

The convexity of the face is accentuated by the prognathic dental arches and by the slightly receding chin. The nasal index (relation length to width) is >85, making the nose broad in relation to the length. The dorsum is slightly convex with a small osteocartilaginous hump. The Castillian Hispanic, on the other hand, generally has a high nasal hump. The Mestizo has a wide nasal base and the nostrils are large and round with tendency toward the horizontal direction, particularly in the Negroid Mestizo. The columella is short with an acute nasolabial angle (70–80°). The angularity of the nasolabial area is decreased by the prominence of the dental arches in relation to the nasal spine and the downward prominence of the nasal tip. The lower third of the nose has a wide dome, with short medial crura that do not project into the columella.

Furthermore, the membranous septum is foreshortened and the columella is usually not seen below the alar rim on profile. The nasal skin is thick principally due to thickened subdermis along with generous subcutaneous fat covering the small osteocartilaginous framework, especially in the lower third of the nose. The common characteristics of the Mestizo face and nose are (a) convexity of the facial profile, (b) prognathic dental arches, (c) depressed piriformis area, (d) insufficient anterior projection of the nose, (e) small osteocar-

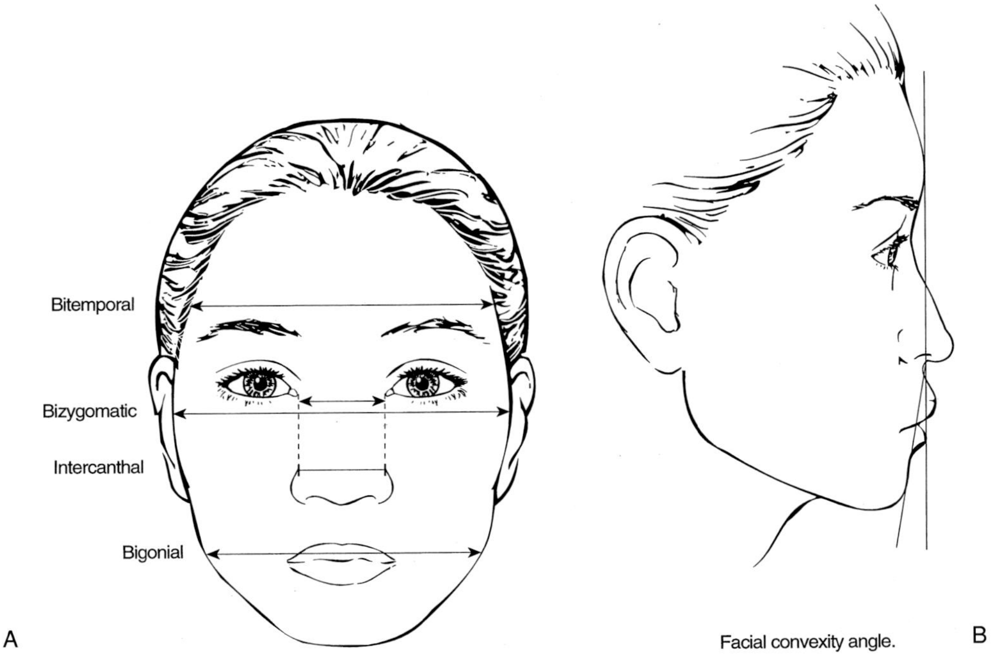

Figure 2. The Mestizo patient has an increased bizygomatic distance **(A)**, giving an appearance of broadness, and a higher convexity angle **(B)** than in the Caucasian.

tilaginous framework, (f) retracted columella and nasal spine, (g) acute nasolabial angle, (h) vertically long upper lip, (i) bulbous nasal tip, (j) thick skin, and (k) low bridge on the dorsum (6).

AGING

Facial skeletal characteristics include the lack of projection of the frontoglabellar area contributing to flatness of the forehead. The higher cheek projection is located more laterally than anteroposteriorly. The deep piriformis area accentuates the illusion of high cheekbones. Facial skin is generally thick with abundant sebaceous glands and increased subcutaneous deposits. There is a tendency toward sagging facial soft tissues at an earlier age. Brows tend to be implanted at a lower level with respect to the supra-orbital rim. Sagging of the cheeks and the nasolabial folds is common as is the early appearance of frowning of the mouth. Each of these factors combines to give the appearance of a sad look. Eyelids, particularly the uppers, tend to have an excess accumulation of fat deposits; the supratarsal fold is not well defined or is very low. Male pattern baldness, anecdotally, seems less common, and hair is usually straight, thick, and abundant.

To obtain facial balance of the nose and/or the facial skeletal structure, we prefer to augment rather than reduce. Because of the thick skin with a rich subcutaneous layer at almost every level in the face, it is more difficult to readapt these soft tissues to a smaller skeletal framework. For example, I prefer to treat a true mandibular prognathism with midface advancement rather than mandibular setback. As a result, the anterior nasal projection will increase and the likelihood of crowding soft tissues in the submental areas will be lessened.

DIAGNOSTIC AND THERAPEUTIC APPROACHES

A standard anteroposterior three-quarters view and lateral photographs are mandatory. Cephalometric analysis is performed when facial skeletal manipulation is anticipated. If an orthognathic surgery is planned, the occlusal anomalies are studied. Facial expansion versus reduction is carefully considered in every patient, with the optimal choice based on final aesthetic goals rather than absolute cephalometric analysis. Pre- and post-operative orthodontics are crucial.

If rhinoplasty is considered, a functional evaluation of the septum and the turbinates is made. Following reduction of the width of the nasal bones, turbinectomies minimize postoperative nasal obstruction.

OPERATIVE TECHNIQUE

Rhinoplasty

Nasal surgery is the most common aesthetic surgery that is requested by Hispanic Americans. The objectives of the operation have been well defined by Ortiz-Monasterio et al. (6):

1. Increase nasal protrusion.
2. Convert the dorsum to a straight or slightly concave.
3. Reduce width of alar bases.
4. Change shape of the nostrils.
5. Increase columellar strength.
6. Open the nasolabial angle.
7. Project columella below the alar rim.
8. Narrow the nasal tip.
9. Produce visual impression of thinner tip skin.
10. Modify the facial convexity.

Cartilage grafts are frequently needed to obtain the aesthetic goals with the recipient sites listed in order of frequency: nasolabial, tip, spreader, and dorsal grafts. The best and most readily accessible grafting material is the septum; however, following prior septal surgery, rib cartilage graft is an excellent alternative. In the very thick-skinned nose, ear cartilage graft is not strong enough to provide support. Ear cartilage may be used for filling contour irregularities.

The nasolabial columellar cartilage graft typically is a 1.5×0.75–cm triangle. Graft placement requires wide undermining with elevation of the depressor septi muscle of the bone. The graft is stabilized with transfixing 4-0 chromic catgut sutures. Cartilage applied to the dorsum of the nose usually extends from the nasoglabellar angle to the limits of the upper lateral cartilage. The dorsal graft should not be wider than 5 mm, and the borders of the graft are beveled. The nasal tip is reshaped using the available cartilage graft; however, most of the time, a small, tall, narrow shield graft is needed for refinement rather than for augmentation. If the nasal skin is too thick, wide undermining allows better redraping of the skin to the new shape. This is not recommended in heavy smokers who have a high probability for developing congestion, hyperpigmentation, and/or necrosis of the tip skin. I generally apply topically $\sim$5 mg of Kenalog around the tip and supratip areas at the end of the operative procedure to avoid the early formation of excessive scarring.

Nasal bone infracturing is done judiciously. If a dorsal cartilage graft yields the illusion of narrowing the dorsum, then I do not infracture. The short nasal bones in the Mestizo nose contribute to a tendency for nasal valve collapse. The spreader graft has been helpful as a preventative technical maneuver.

A wide nasal base that may not respond to nostril wedge resection is addressed with wide undermining at the subperiosteal plane, from the piriformis aperture to the midcheek level. This allows reduction of the interalar space with sutures applied to the base of the alae against the opposite member maneuvered through the transfixing incision and in some cases through the intra-oral approach. This maneuver also increases the nasolabial angle (Figs. 3 and 4).

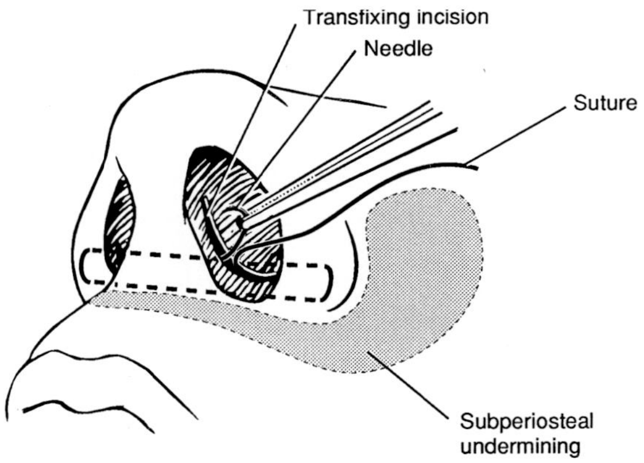

Figure 3. In many cases, particularly in patients with a strong African phenotype, wide subperiosteal undermining and the fixation sutures to the base of the alae are performed through the transfixing incision or the intra-oral approach.

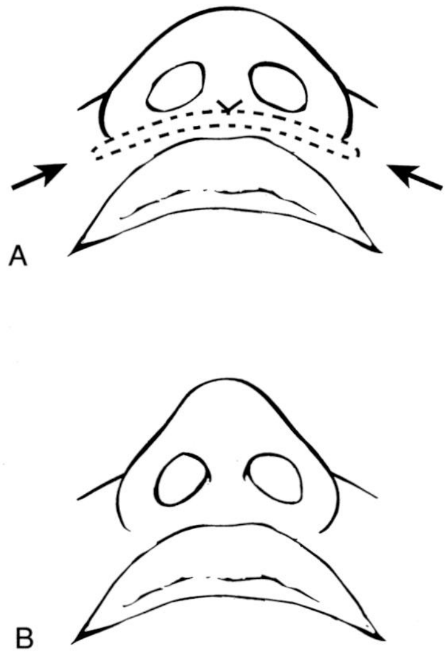

Figure 4. Schematic showing the location of the fixation sutures before suture tightening **(A)** and after **(B)**.

Orthognathic Surgery

Facial convexity is a common component of the Mestizo face, consistent with bimaxillary protrusion with associated microgenia largely along the central dental arch (premaxilla). This is probably an expression of the increased anteroposterior distance with a decrease in the transverse direction of the dental arch. Dental crowding allows for extraction of the first bicuspid. The anterior dental arches are repositioned (7–9). Pre- and post-operative orthodontics are needed to level and align the teeth. If a sliding genioplasty is required, this can be done simultaneously or in a delayed fashion. I prefer to delay the genioplasty to avoid potential fracture of the segment between the osteotomies.

Other Facial Aesthetic Procedures

Blepharoplasty

In many instances, brow ptosis is the reason for the redundant upper eyelid skin. With recent techniques for endoscopic brow lifting, this option is significantly more appealing to the Hispanic patient, especially the younger ones (10).

In patients that present with excess lower eyelid fat herniation, a word of caution is advised. The apparent herniation may be a manifestation of the lack of bony support of the anterior cheek. A small lower orbital rim implant and a sliding of the lower eyelid fat pads are the best options rather than a blepharolipectomy.

Facelift

Sagging of the soft tissues are more prevalent than wrinkling. The Mestizo patient usually has very thick skin resilient to stretching. I have encountered two problems with the Mestizo patient during facelifting. First, scars often become thicker than in the Caucasian. Second, there is a slightly higher tendency to stretch relaxation of the soft tissues. With the combination of subperiosteal facelift and a wide subcutaneous dissection, results following facelift surgery in the Mestizo are effective and long-lasting.

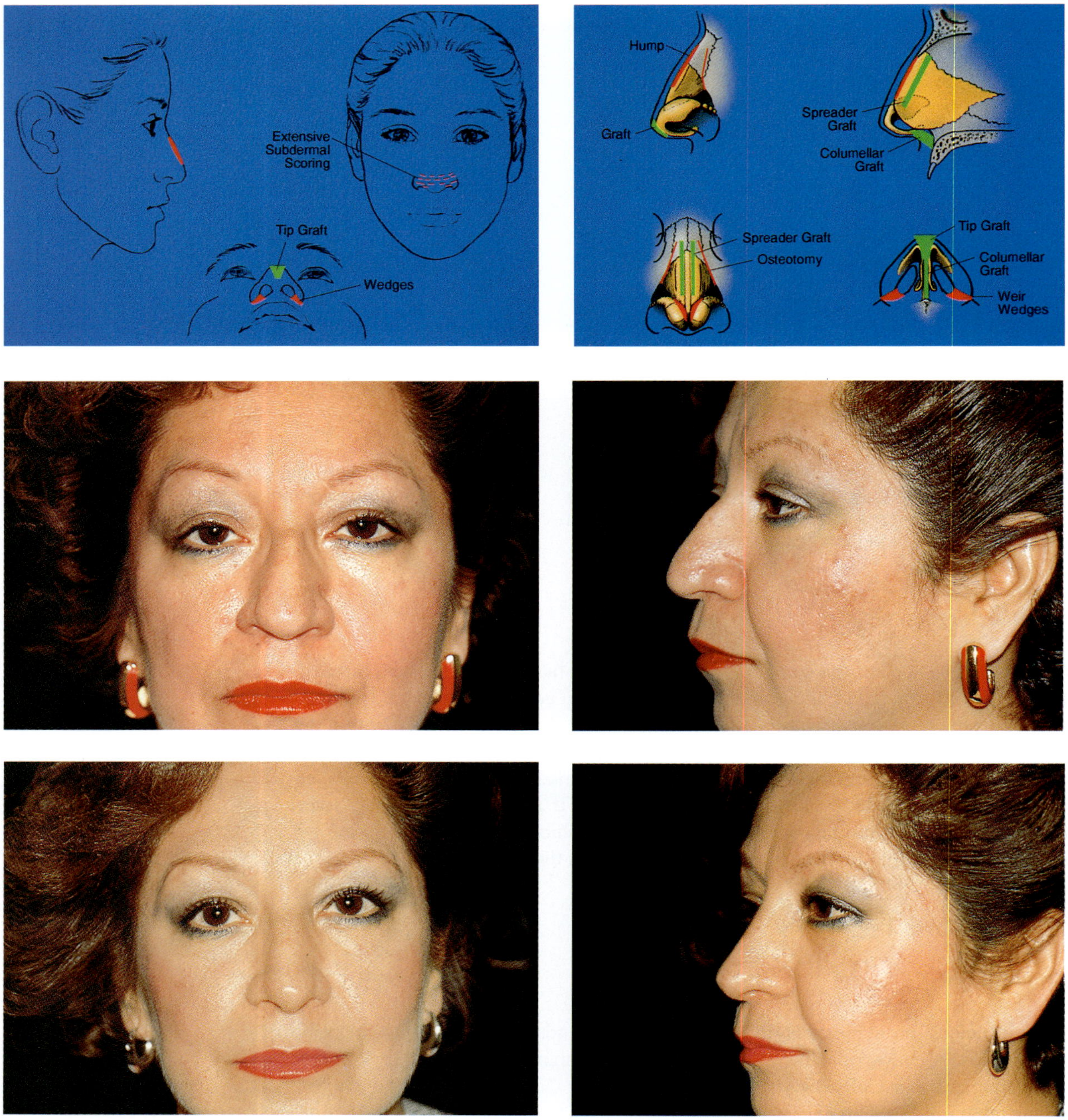

A B C D E F

Figure 5. **A:** Proposed areas of excision and augmentation on this patient's nose. **B:** Areas of bone and cartilage excision, nostril wedge excision, and the areas of support and augmentation with cartilage graft. **C:** Pre-operative appearance of a female patient with a strong Native American phenotype. She had a relatively large nasal hump and very thick nasal skin. **D:** The three-quarters view shows the small nasal hump, the acute nasolabial angle, and droopy tip. **E:** Reduction rhinoplasty provides an illusion of a straighter and smaller nose with better aesthetic lines. **F:** Note improvement of the nasal dorsum, nasal tip, and nasolabial angle.

Cheek Augmentation

This procedure is very rarely requested by the Hispanic patient because of relatively high cheekbones. However, many patients have a prominence of the cheeks that is more laterally oriented than in the anteroposterior direction. This should be analyzed and the corresponding aesthetic surgical decision made.

Suction Lipectomy

Because the Hispanic patient has considerable cheek fat, facial lipectomy is an effective technique for sculpting the soft tissues on the face. Bichat's fat pad excision is commonly performed.

Chemical Peeling

There is a greater tendency toward melasma as a result of pregnancy or of the use of oral contraceptives. However, trichloroacetic acid peeling (between 30 and 35%) is an acceptable adjuvant to correct facial hyperpigmentation commonly seen in the Hispanic face. On the other hand, phenol peeling is contraindicated in Hispanic patients because of the dark color of their skin.

COMPLICATIONS

Complication rates are related to the type of primary operative procedure. For rhinoplasty, the most common complications are nasal valve collapse, saddle nose deformity, disharmony of nasal proportions, and supratip deformity. The Hispanic patient has a higher tendency to develop hypo- or hyperpigmentation as well as hypertrophy of the scars. Following rhytidectomy, pre-operative facial asymmetries may become evident to the patient. A careful pre-operative analysis must identify and point out bony and soft tissue asymmetries to the patient before surgery.

CASE STUDIES

Case 1

Case 1 was a 50-year-old woman with a strong Indian phenotype. She presented with a large nasal hump and very thick nasal skin that was accentuated by the presence of acne rosacea. Rhinoplasty was carried out using the reduction rhinoplasty concept with defatting and thinning out of the skin at the subdermal plane, reduction of the nasal hump, increase of the nasolabial angle with columellar graft, nasal tip graft, and nasal wedge resections. Spreader grafts were also used to prevent collapse of the nasal valves (Fig. 5).

Case 2

Case 2 was a 38-year-old woman with a mixture of Hispanic, Negro, and Indian phenotypes. She had had a previous rhinoplasty with unsatisfactory results. Observe the lack of definition of the nasal tip and the low nasal bridge (see Fig. 6). There is an associated microgenia. The patient had a rhinoplasty with conservative osteotomies, nasal dorsum augmentation with septal cartilage graft, and a nasal tip graft. A small columellar graft was applied to increase the nasolabial angle. The ala was redefined using cartilage grafts, and the nostril wedges were resected. A small chin implant was also used.

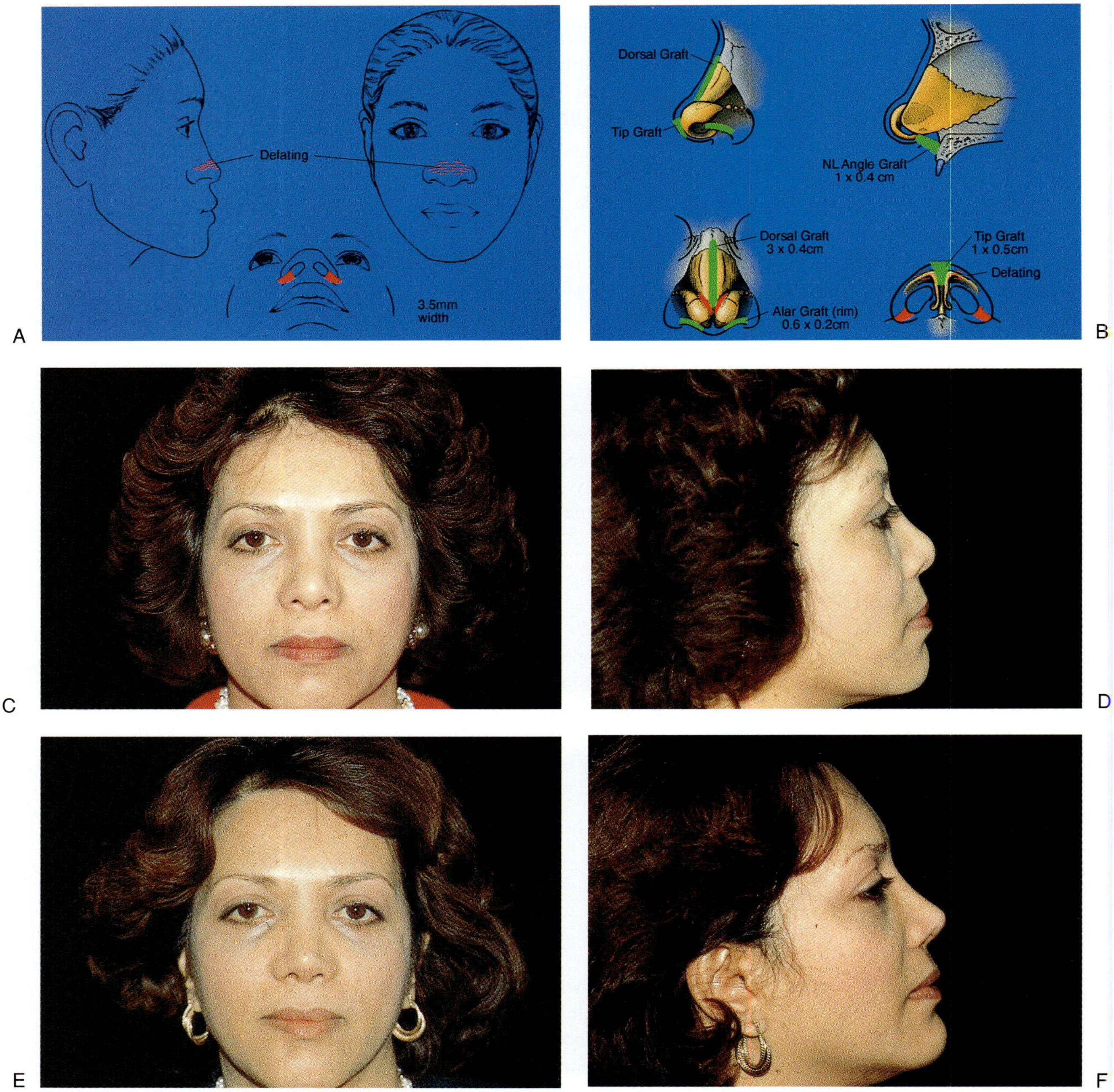

Figure 6. A–B: Schematic showing the planned areas of modification and the areas of excision, support, and augmentation. **C–D:** This 38-year-old patient had a broad mixture of racial phenotypes that included a broad nose with a flat tip and some break of the aesthetic lines at the midvault level. **E–F:** Improvement of the nasal aesthetic lines was achieved, along with thinning of the nose, correction of the mild collapse of the nasal valve, elevation of the dorsum, definition of the nasal tip, and a nasolabial angle of ~105°. Note also the shape and symmetry of the nostrils and the illusion of a short lip. A small chin implant was also done in this patient.

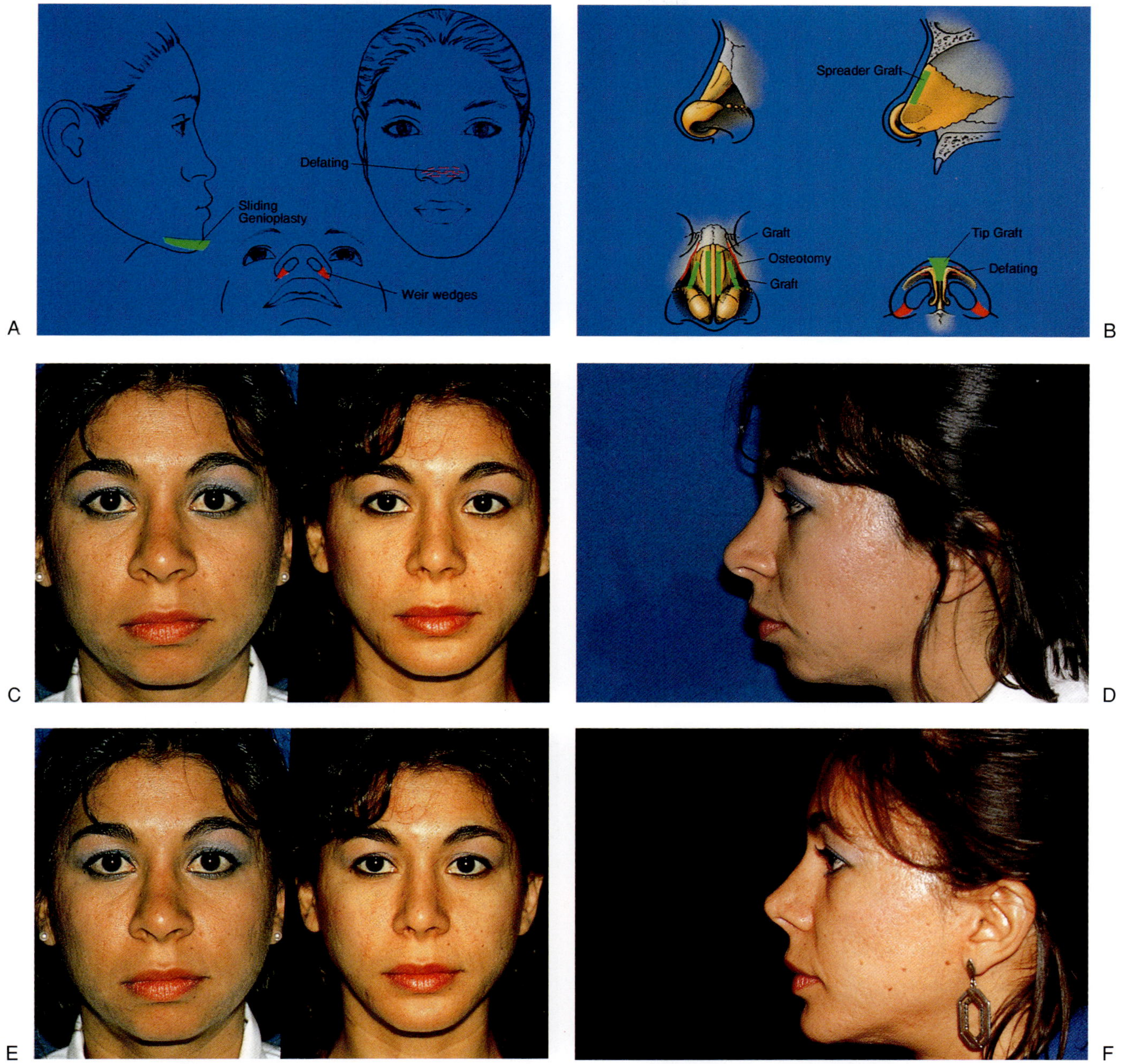

Figure 7. A–B: Schematic showing planned changes in the nose as well as planned sliding genioplasty. Note areas of augmentation and resection and the spreader graft and nasal supporting graft. **C–D:** Disproportion of the nose due to prior rhinoplasty. Observe the collapse of the nasal valve with disruption of the nasal aesthetic lines from brow to nasal tip. Nostrils are asymmetric and the nasal tip is wide and lacks definition. **E–F:** Post-operative photos show improvement of the nasal aesthetic lines with smooth flow from brow to nasal tip, which is now more defined. The columellar/alar relationships have improved and the nostrils are more symmetric. The sliding genioplasty results in less straining of the peri-oral muscles.

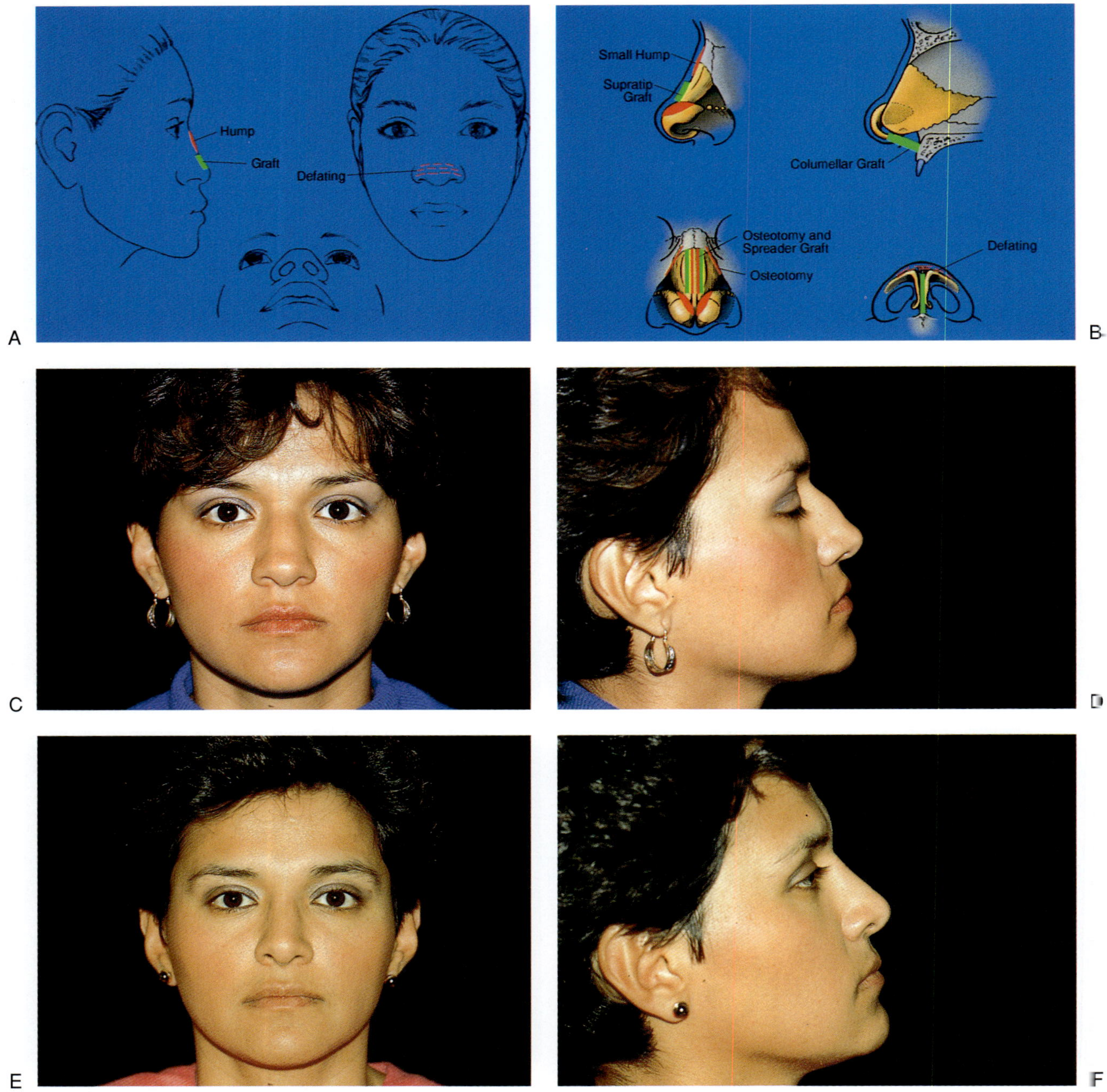

Figure 8. A–B: Schematic representation of planned changes on the patient's nose showing the areas of reduction and augmentation. **C–D:** This patient presented with a mixture of racial phenotypes including a broad nose and a wide bizygomatic distance. **E–F:** Postoperative photos show improvement of the aesthetic lines from the brow to the tip, with an illusion of a smaller and thinner nose, improved nasal dorsum, nasolabial angle, and alar/columellar relationship.

Case 3

Case 3 was a 35-year-old woman with Portuguese, Indian, and Negroid phenotypes. She had had two previous rhinoplasties. She presented with bilateral nasal valve collapse, a significant disproportion of the nasal components, and microgenia. The results follow a secondary rhinoplasty with defatting and thinning out of the fat and scar tissue, nasal os-

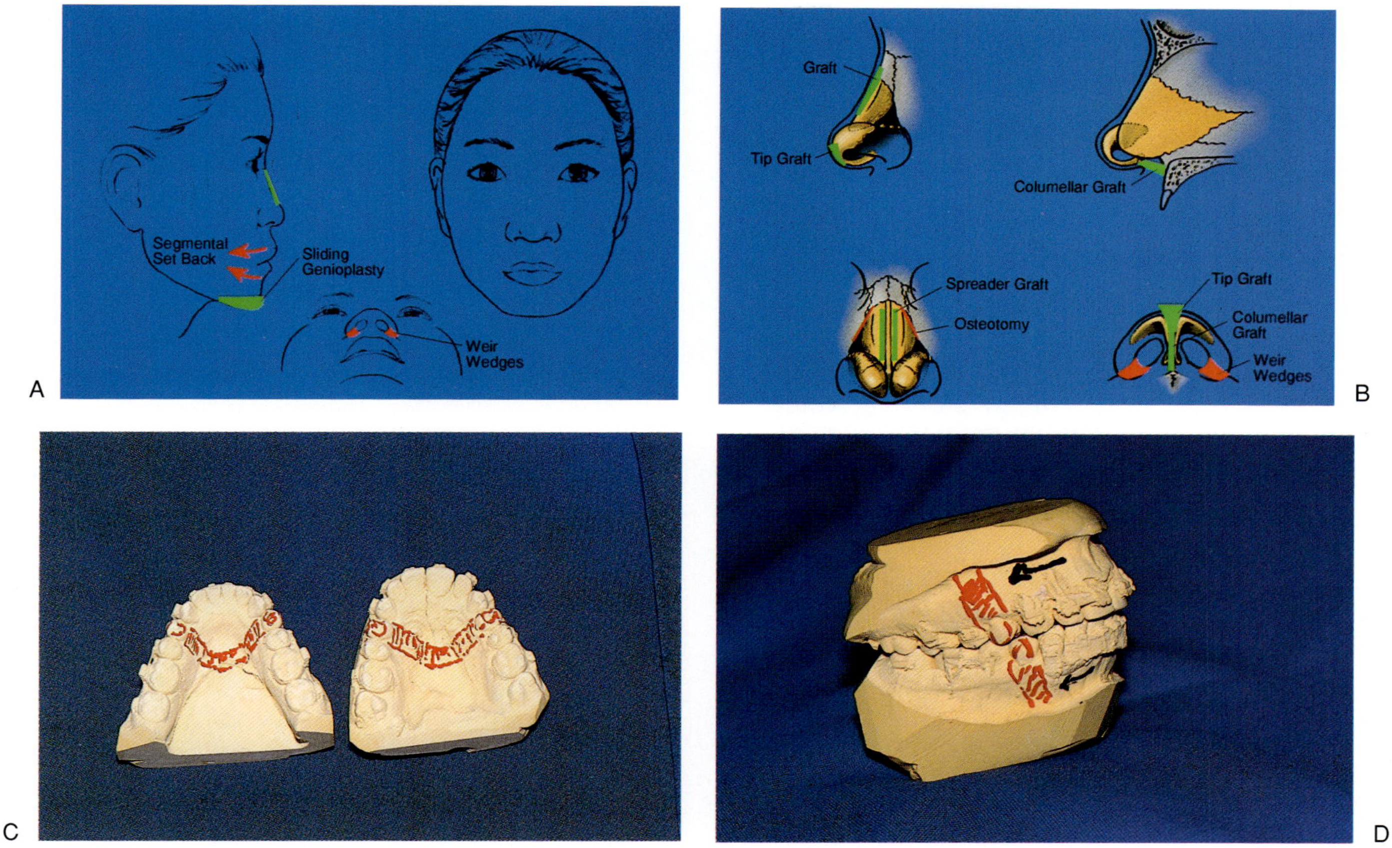

Figure 9. A–B: Schematic representation of planned areas of augmentation and reduction. Bimaxillary segmental osteotomy and sliding genioplasty are also planned. **C–D:** Dental model showing the planned areas of bone and teeth resection. Observe the increased anteroposterior dimension of the maxillary and mandibular segments. The lateral view shows the direction of the segmental osteotomy.

teotomies, spreader graft and a nasal valve-supporting graft, nasal tip graft, and nostril wedges. A sliding genioplasty was also performed (Fig. 7).

Case 4

Case 4 was a 30-year-old woman with Hispanic, Indian, and Negroid phenotypes. Observe the wide bizygomatic distance, the flat anterior cheek, nostrils with tendency to flaring, and wide nasal dorsum (Fig. 8). A reduction rhinoplasty utilized nasal osteotomies, hump removal, and nasal tip sculpting using her own alar cartilages. No tip cartilage graft was used in this case. However, a small supratip crest spreader graft and columellar graft were used.

Case 5

A prior rhinoplasty resulted in nasal valve collapse, asymmetry of the nasal proportions, and a wide nasal tip. Significant bimaxillary protrusion and microgenia were addressed initially with mandibular and maxillary segmental osteotomies with setback of the premaxillary segments after the resection of the first premolars. At the second stage, the patient had a secondary rhinoplasty with spreader graft, nasal osteotomies, dorsal, columellar and nasal

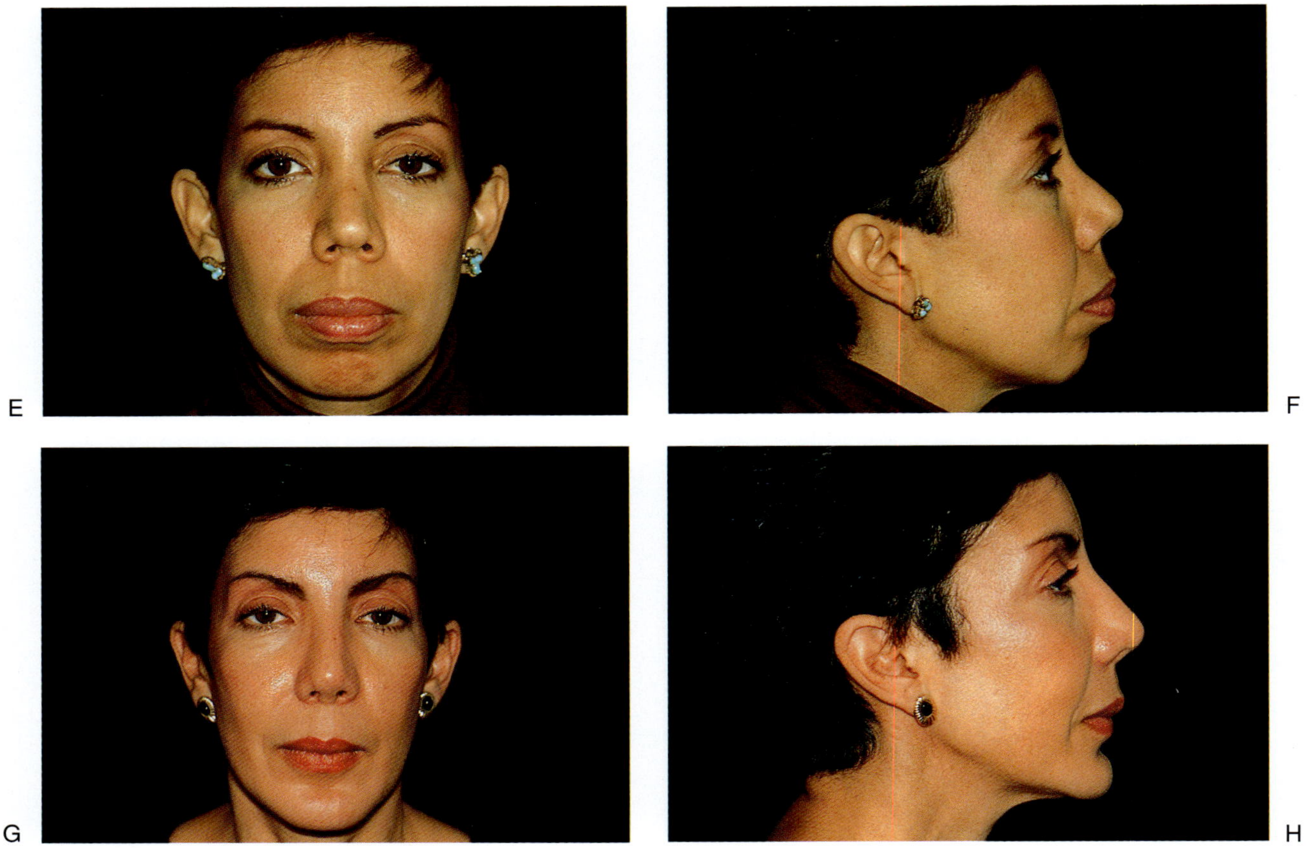

Figure 9 *(continued).* **E–F:** The patient had a significant nasal disproportion with an inverted V deformity on the dorsum, supratip deformity, columellar disproportion, and a slight depression at the keystone area. Bimaxillary protrusion, micrognia, and oral straining are also noticeable. **G–H:** Post-operative photos taken 9 years after surgery show the improvement of nasal aesthetic lines and nasal tip correction with a better columellar/alar relationship. Also observe the changes due to segmental maxillary and mandibular osteotomy and the sliding genioplasty.

tip grafts, nostril wedges, and concomitant sliding genioplasty. Results are shown 9 years after her secondary rhinoplasty and segmental bimaxillary surgery. The dental cast shows the increased anteroposterior distance of the dental arches and the bimaxillary protrusion. The planned segments of teeth and bone to be resected and the planned setback of the anterior segments (Fig. 9).

REFERENCES

1. Ramírez OM, Fuente del Campo. Hispanic and Mestizo male. In: Marchac C, Granick M, Solomon M, eds. *Male aesthetic surgery*. Boston: Butterworth-Heinmann, 1996.
2. Borah W, Cook SF. *El Mestizaje en la Historia de Iberoamerica*. Cultura, Mexico: Instituto Panamericano de Geografia e Historia, 1962.
3. Beals RH, Joijer H. *An introduction to anthropology*. New York: Macmillan, 1965.
4. Comas J. *Manual de Antropologia Fisica*. Universidad Nacional Autonoma de Mexico, 1965.
5. Ortiz-Monasterio F, Olmedo A, Trigos I, et al. Final results from the delayed treatment of patients with clefts of the lip and palate. *Scand J Plast Reconstr Surg* 1974;8:109.
6. Ortiz-Monasterio F, Olmedo A. Rhinoplasty of the Mestizo nose. *Clin Plast Surg* 1977;4:89.
7. Wassmund M. *Praktische Chirurgie des Mundes und der Kiefer*. Leipzy: Meusser, 1935.
8. Cupar I. Die Chiriurgische Behundeling der Form—un Stellungs—Veranderungen des Oberkiefer. *Ost Z Ostomat* 1954;51:565.
9. Kole H. Foreman des Offenen Bisses und ihre Chirugische Behanlung. *Dtsch Stomat* 1959;9:753.
10. Ramírez OM. Endoscopic techniques in facial rejuvenation. An overview. Part I. *Aesthet Plast Surg* 1994;18: 141.

SECTION IX

The Mediterranean Patient

Ethnic Considerations in Facial Aesthetic Surgery, edited by W. Earle Matory, Jr.
Lippincott–Raven Publishers, Philadelphia © 1998.

24

The Mediterranean Patient

Editor's Commentary

W. Earle Matory, Jr.

Some of the most attractive and exotic beauties of the world hail from the Mediterranean, for example, Sophia Loren and Angelina. In my experience, the most challenging and fulfilling operation is rhinoplasty. I prefer to identify the new tip-defining point, often necessitating cephalic rotation and some degree of nasal shortening in the elongated nose. Once this point is defined, the bony and cartilaginous humps can be rasped, burred, or resected (Figs. 1–3).

Because of pre-operative nasal deformities of significance, most patients from the Mediterranean are very thrilled and satisfied with the outcome even when minor irregularities persist.

W. E. Matory, Jr.: A New You Plastic Surgery Medical Group, Irvine, California 92714

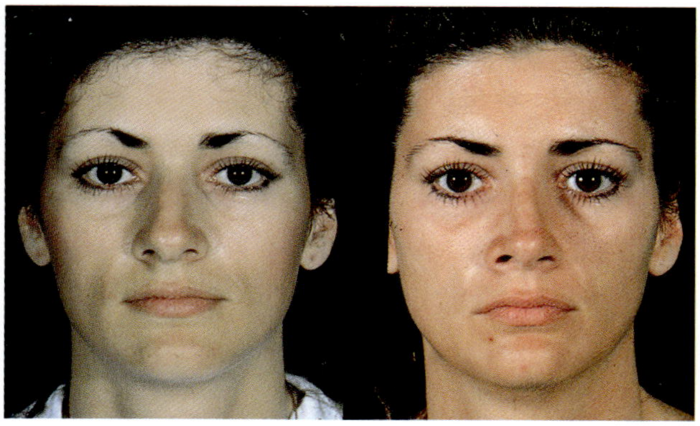

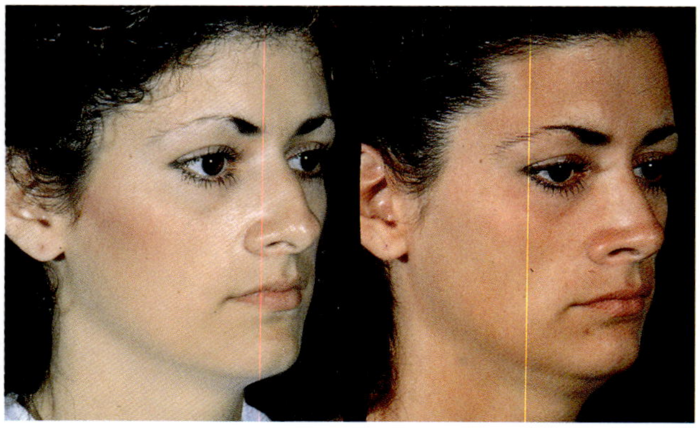

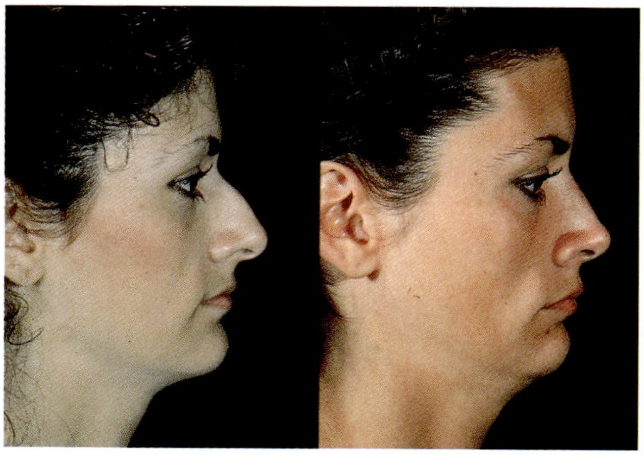

Figure 1. This 28-year-old woman presented with a bulbous bifid tip, a prominent/asymmetrical nasal bridge, and physiologic nasal valve collapse. Dorsal hump resection with the use of septal cartilage spreader grafts and cephalad resection of lower lateral cartilage were completed to achieve this outcome noted at 2 years.

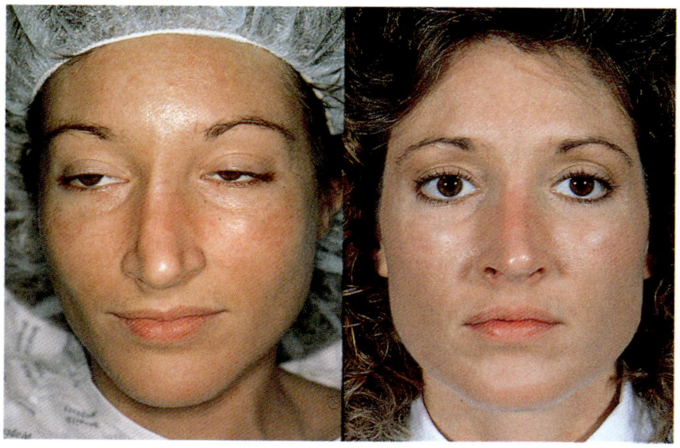

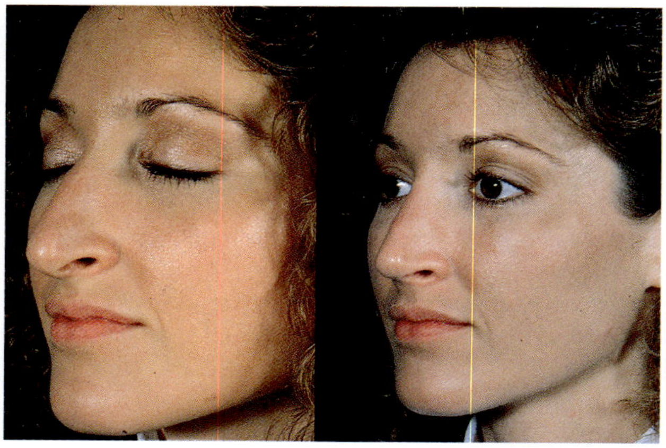

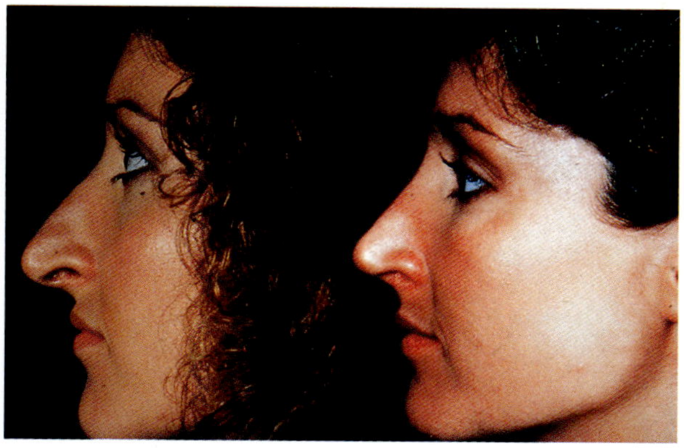

Figure 2. The elongated, deviated nasal dorsum and septum were addressed with cephalic rotation of the nasal tip, cephalic resection of the lower lateral cartilage, 2-mm dorsal osteocartilaginous resection from the dorsum, and the use of septal cartilage spreader grafts. Malar augmentation was completed with Proplast.

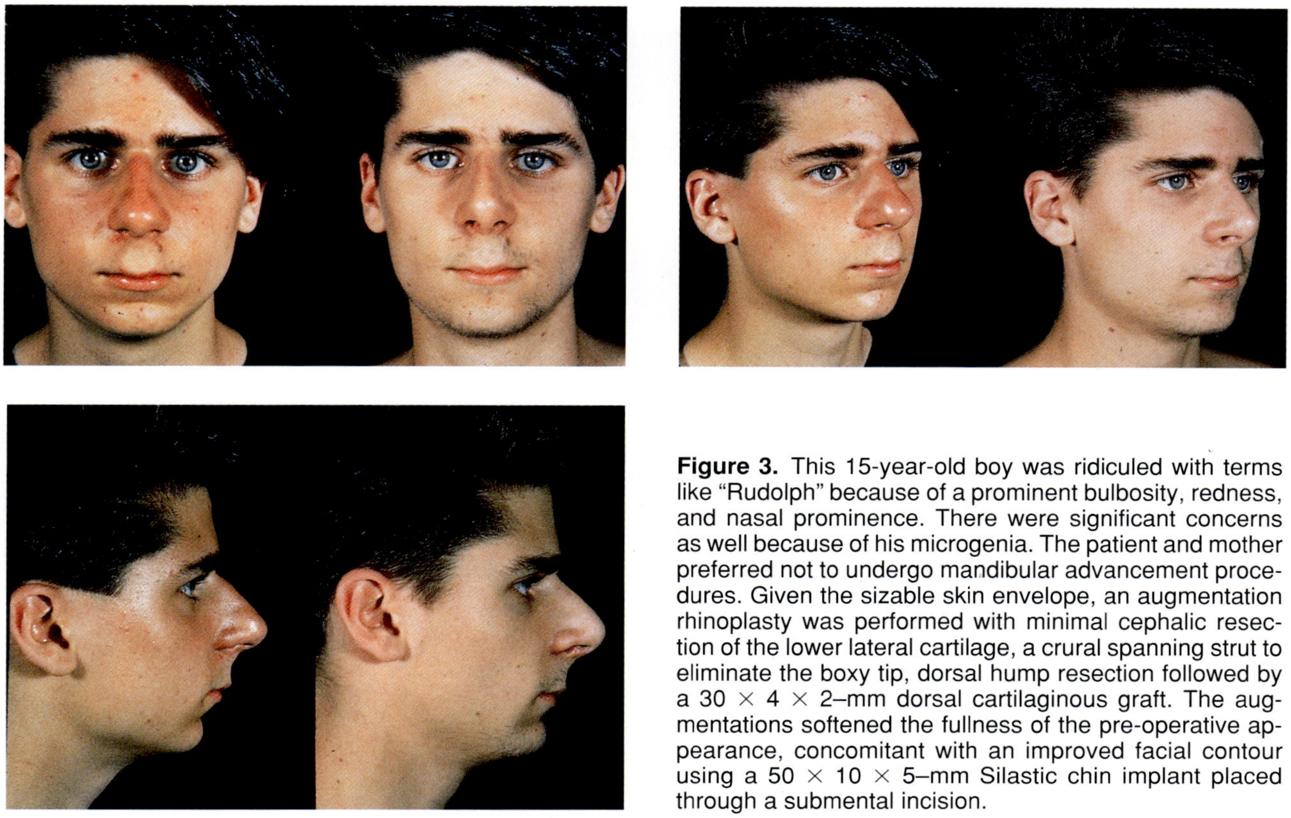

Figure 3. This 15-year-old boy was ridiculed with terms like "Rudolph" because of a prominent bulbosity, redness, and nasal prominence. There were significant concerns as well because of his microgenia. The patient and mother preferred not to undergo mandibular advancement procedures. Given the sizable skin envelope, an augmentation rhinoplasty was performed with minimal cephalic resection of the lower lateral cartilage, a crural spanning strut to eliminate the boxy tip, dorsal hump resection followed by a 30 × 4 × 2–mm dorsal cartilaginous graft. The augmentations softened the fullness of the pre-operative appearance, concomitant with an improved facial contour using a 50 × 10 × 5–mm Silastic chin implant placed through a submental incision.

Ethnic Considerations in Facial Aesthetic Surgery, edited by W. Earle Matory, Jr.
Lippincott–Raven Publishers, Philadelphia © 1998.

25

The Mediterranean Nose

Lorelle N. Michelson, George C. Peck, Jr., and George C. Peck

If the nose of Cleopatra had been shorter, the whole face of the earth would have been changed.
— Blaise Pascal

Proper projection of the nasal tip may be the most important factor in achieving correct nasal aesthetics. Many so-called "Mediterranean" noses lack not only good tip projection, but also have acute nasolabial angles, plunging tips, or foreshortened nasal tip pyramids (short columellae). Many Mediterranean people, in addition, have unusually thick, sebaceous skin. These tip problems along with thick skin are the two most important factors that render nasal surgery in the Mediterranean patient particularly difficult. We shall discuss our surgical techniques for achieving proper tip projection in this group of patients, with emphasis on those with plunging tips, short columellae, and thick skin. The indications for each technique and pre- and post-operative examples will also be depicted.

CULTURAL CONSIDERATIONS

Because of social–ethnic preferences in the choice of one's marital partner in America, many anthropologic truisms concerned with nasal types apply equally well whether they are referable to Europeans or to Americans of European ancestry. In the Mediterranean ethnic groups, typified by Italians, Spaniards, and Portuguese, the nasal shape is reputed to be either straight or convex in its profile. The retroussé dorsum is a rarity among Mediterraneans. In addition, the Mediterraneans are said to have nasal tips that are often "plunging" or inadequately projecting.

There may actually be marked differences in the alar cartilages in Europeans of German, Slavic, and Mediterranean backgrounds (Fig. 1). In Mediterranean noses, there may be a

L. N. Michelson, G. C. Peck, Jr., and G. C. Peck: The Peck Center, Clifton, New Jersey 07013

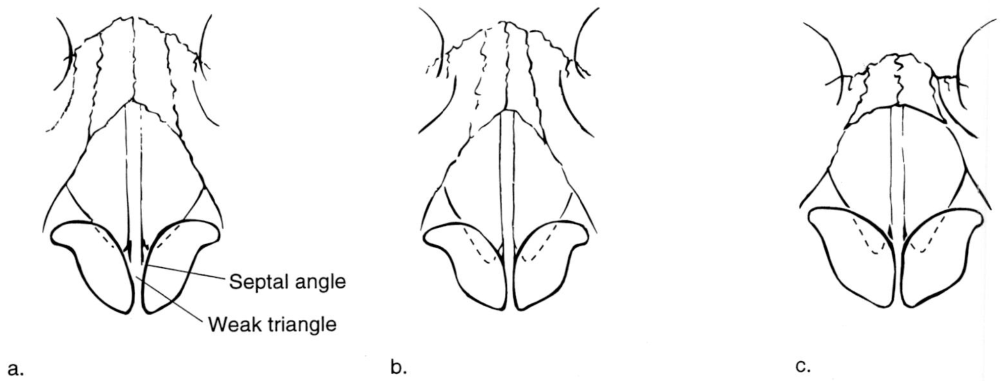

Figure 1. A: The Mediterranean nose. Lateral crura of the alar cartilages are said to be in vertical oblique position, with "weak triangle" between the lateral crura. **B:** The German nose. Lateral wings of the alae are wider than in the Mediterranean nose, accounting for less pronounced "weak triangle." **C:** The Slavic nose. Non-existent "weak triangle."

vertical oblique position of the lateral crura of the alar cartilages. This is reputed to be absent in most German or Slavic noses. It has been emphasized that a "weak triangle" exists between the medial margins of the lateral crura in the Mediterranean nose. There is also an aponeurosis covering this triangle (Fig. 1). Schmalix demonstrated, however, that the "German" nasal tip has a "weak triangle" that is just barely present since the lateral wings of the alae are wider and lie more oblique. Additionally, in the "Slavic" nose, the weak triangle is non-existent.

Regardless of ethnic background, the single most important factor in addressing any nose is ensuring proper nasal tip projection. Inasmuch as relative tip height is often foreshortened in the so-called "Mediterranean nose," ensuring proper tip height in the Mediterranean patient is even more difficult. Many Mediterraneans have thick skin as well, rendering refinement of the tip even harder to achieve. We will deal with our methods of producing proper tip projection, emphasizing those problems making this more difficult in the Mediterranean patient.

OPERATIVE TECHNIQUE

Tip Projection

In any primary rhinoplasty, sculpturing the lower lateral cartilages is the first step in ensuring proper tip projection (Table 1). If sculpturing alone does not achieve the desired projection, then one or more onlay grafts may be employed. If the onlays are not sufficient, then an umbrella graft is used. In some thick-skinned noses, a characteristic often present in Mediterraneans, an external shaving of the dorsal supratip area may also be performed. These procedures need not all be done at the same operation. If external shaving is performed, for example, this is often deferred until complete healing has occurred and the aesthetic lines have been established.

Lower Lateral Cartilage Sculpturing

Proper tip projection is always essential to good nasal aesthetics. The nasal tip should stand out from the straight line of the bridge by at least 2 mm. After drawing the approximate sculpturing line externally on the nasal skin, lower lateral cartilage sculpturing begins. The suction tip is placed intranasally in the dome area beneath the previously drawn sculpturing line (Fig. 2). An imprint is created by applying pressure with the finger against the tip of the suction cannula. This imprint then serves as a guide to mark the transcartilaginous or "sculpturing" incision.

Table 1. *Methods for achieving proper tip projection*

Lower lateral cartilage sculpturing
Onlay graft(s)
Umbrella graft
External shave

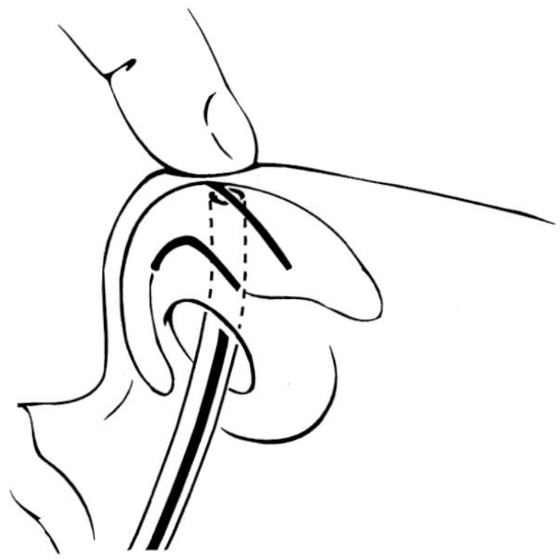

Figure 2. Suction tip placed intranasally in the dome area to create "imprint."

The incision is begun at the imprint and extended parallel to the alar rim. As the alar rim edge is everted with a double hook, the caudal border of the lower lateral cartilage is checked to be sure that sufficient width of cartilage is left in situ. Figure 3 diagrammatically shows the extent of the sculpturing incision.

A hemostat is then used to grasp the vestibular skin. By pulling downward, it is possible to expose the cephalad portion of the lower lateral cartilage and the contiguous fibroadipose tissue between the skin and the cartilage (Fig. 4). This exposed area represents the cartilage and fat that will be removed. The skin is then undermined from the fibroadipose tissue and cartilage beneath it (Fig. 5). This fibroadipose tissue must be removed with the segment of lower lateral cartilage to which it is attached. If this fibrofat is not removed, then unwanted supratip fullness can occur.

The vestibular skin is next held with a hemostat and separated from the intranasal side of the lower lateral cartilage with sharp dissecting scissors (Fig. 6). Figure 7 shows how the lower lateral cartilage is transected laterally and removed. The lateralmost portion of the lower lateral cartilage must be preserved when the cartilage is transected. Inadvertent removal of this "lateral tail" may eventuate in a pinched appearance in this area.

Sculpturing of the alar cartilage should produce a discrepancy in levels. If the "gull wing" sculpturing line has been properly placed, the resulting line imparts the desired aesthetic qualities to the nasal tip. The nasal tip thus has been modified by sculpturing but the continuity of the dome of the lower lateral cartilage has been preserved. The structural support of the nasal tip is left intact.

In contrast to this sculpturing procedure, and in techniques derived from Dr. Josef, shaping the nasal tip is based on removing portions of the lower lateral cartilage as well as tran-

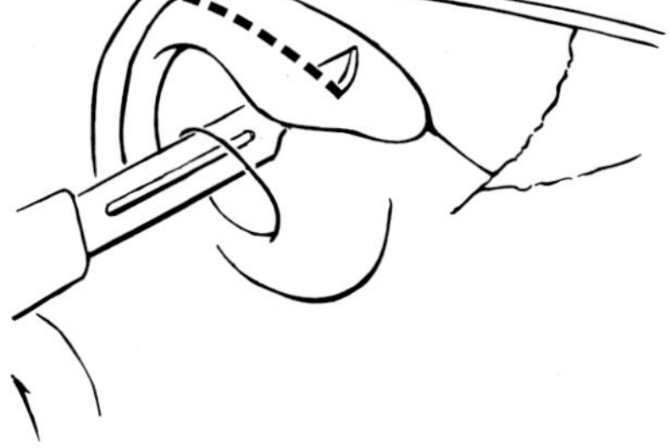

Figure 3. Extent of the sculpturing incision.

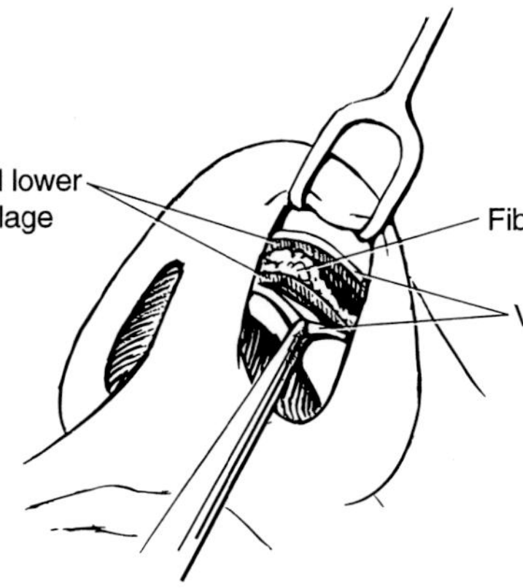

Figure 4. Cephalad portion of the lower lateral cartilage and its contiguous fibroadipose tissue, all of which need to be resected.

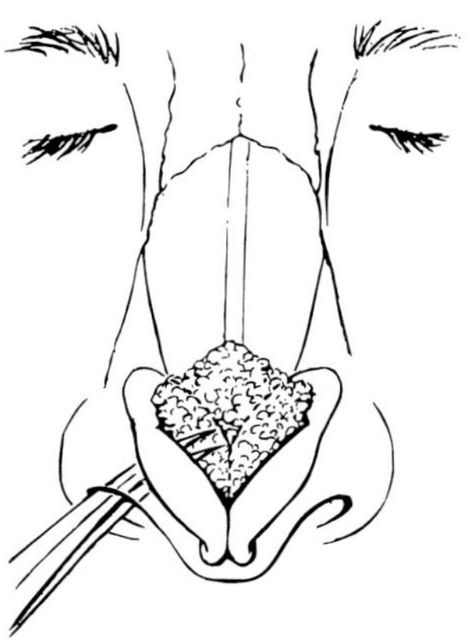

Figure 5. Undermining skin from fibroadipose tissue and cartilage beneath it.

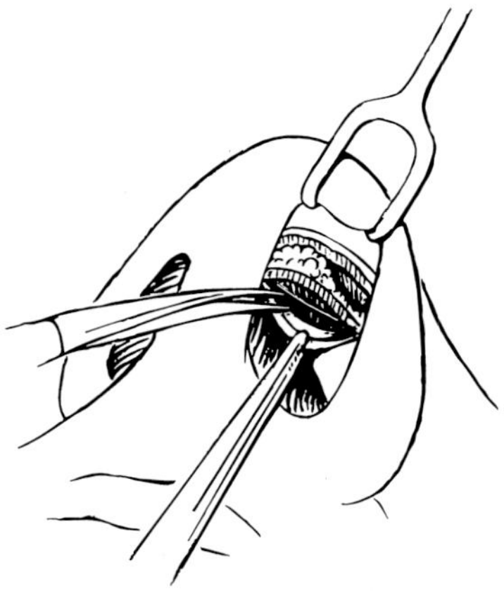

Figure 6. The vestibular skin is separated from the intranasal side of the lower lateral cartilage.

section of the domes. The problem inherent in any technique that transects the domes is that the union between the transected pieces is scar tissue, which does not have the rigidity of cartilage. In many cases, consequently, the dome transection results in kinking at the scar and in asymmetry of the tip. One of the transected ends of the crura may curl, in addition, producing sharp points in the skin.

After sculpturing the lower lateral cartilages, we perform a routine rhinoplasty. When indicated, this includes shortening and elevating the tip and lowering the bony and cartilaginous dorsum. If the tip still lacks projection, then we go on to an onlay or to an umbrella graft.

Onlay Graft

The onlay graft is an anatomical substitute for tip projection where that projection is most needed: at the highest portion of the alar domes. One should think of the onlay as merely an increase in thickness of the domes or as an "aesthetic contrivance" to produce the illusion of increased dome height. The beauty of the onlay is that it is shaped exactly like the domes and thus subtly augments them in those cases where their natural height is deficient.

A 4-mm infracartilaginous incision (Fig. 8) is made at the caudal border of the lower lateral cartilage near the junction of the dome with the lateral crus. A curved scissors creates a horizontal pocket of precise size above the domes (Fig. 9). The importance of being exactly horizontal above the domes is obvious, if one considers the onlay as merely a means

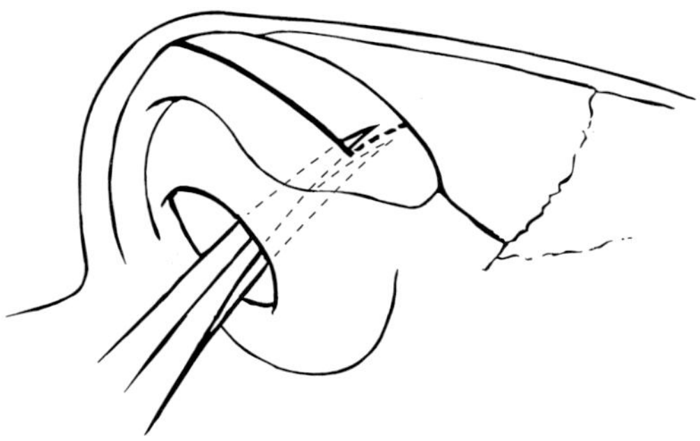

Figure 7. Lower lateral cartilage transected laterally with caution exercised to preserve the "lateral tail."

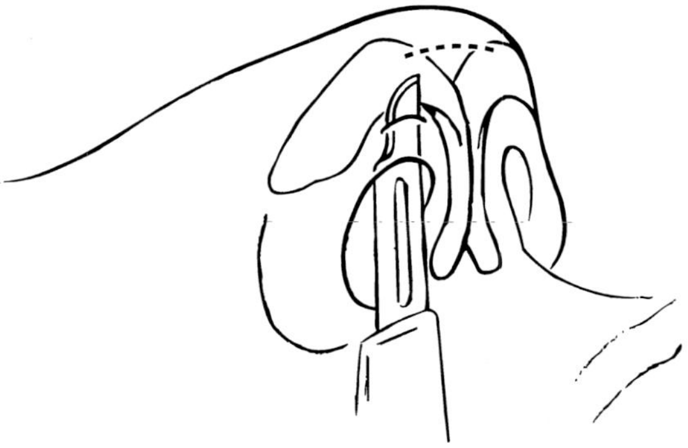

Figure 8. Infracartilaginous "stab" incision near junction of the dome with the lateral crus.

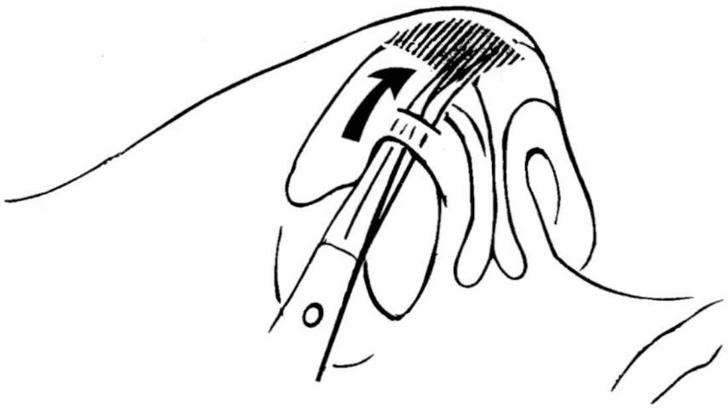

Figure 9. Horizontal pocket of precise size created above the domes.

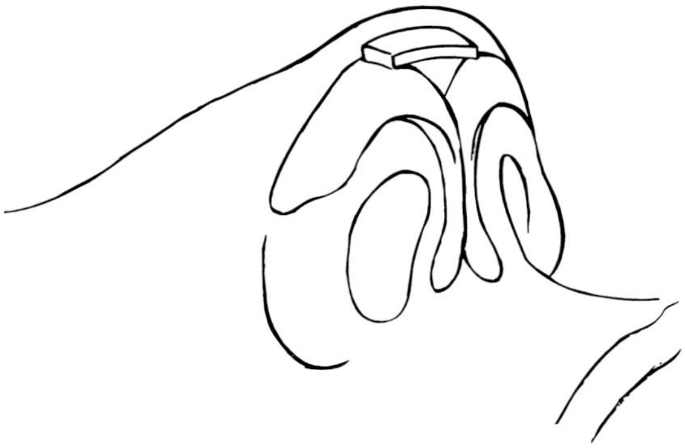

Figure 10. Since the onlay is a means of increasing dome thickness, the graft must be exactly horizontal above the domes.

of increasing dome thickness (Fig. 10). This is precisely where augmentation of tip projection is most aesthetic and is required.

The onlay of ~4 × 9 mm has a convexity resembling the nasal tip itself (Fig. 11). The edges may be shaved or softened, if necessary. For the thick-skinned nose, as is often the case in Mediterranean patients, a shorter graft provides better definition.

The graft should not be constricted within the pocket. Resorption does not occur, a fact that was amply documented by Peer. Several onlays may be used, and this is often necessary in the thick-skinned patient (Fig. 12). The grafts may be sutured together but are usually inserted individually, with the shortest onlay being closest to the skin or most superficial.

Since lower lateral cartilage is often available, this is the most often employed material for onlay grafts. Tip projection may frequently benefit from subtle augmentation with a double onlay of alar cartilage even when projection appears "correct" during the operation. In our experience, it has never been true that overaugmentation was performed. Rather, on the contrary, postoperatively, one wishes one had added more layers!

Onlay grafts of conchal cartilage may be used in those cases where the excised alar cartilage is insufficient. This is often true in secondary rhinoplasties, where the lower laterals have already been excised or where they are fragmented. To harvest conchal cartilage, an incision is made in the skin and then through the cartilage on the posterior aspect of the ear. Two or three onlays may be removed from contiguous conchal cartilage, leaving little residual donor site defect. One single layer of concha often proves to give adequate projection as opposed to alar cartilage where at least two layers are essential.

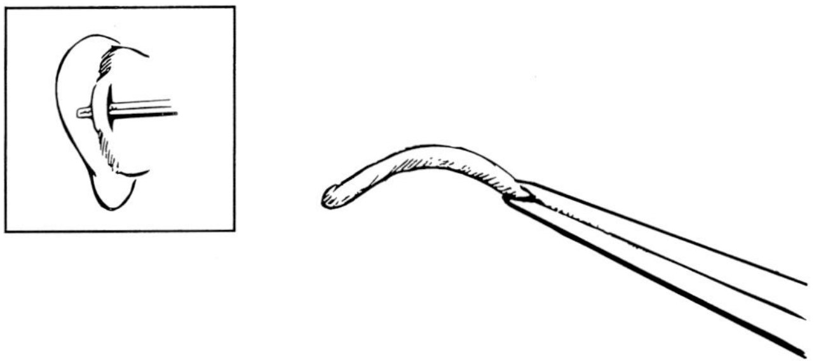

Figure 11. The onlay has a convexity resembling the nasal tip itself.

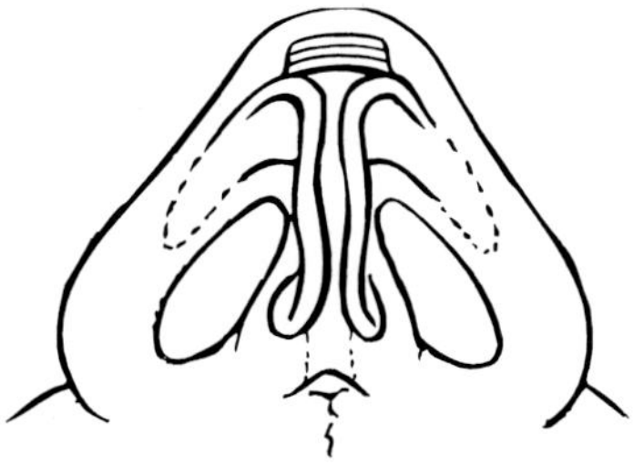

Figure 12. Several onlays may be necessary, particularly in thick-skinned patients, often the case in patients of Mediterranean extraction.

Table 2. *Indications for umbrella graft*

Loss of tip projection following rhinoplasty
Loss of tip projection after loss of septal support
Severe plunging tip
Thick skin tip
Amorphous tip
Congenital short nasal tip pyramid (short columella)

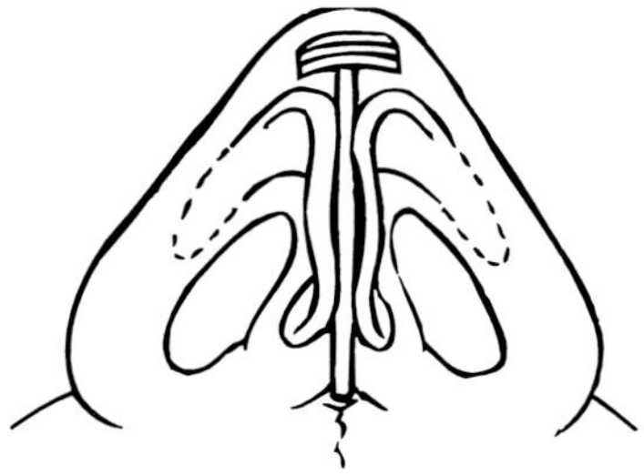

Figure 13. The "umbrella" consists of a strut plus onlay(s). The strut is placed between the medial crura in "sandwich" fashion.

Umbrella Graft

In cases where the onlay graft alone is insufficient, an umbrella graft is necessary. The indications for the umbrella graft are summarized in Table 2. Many of these indications are present in patients of Mediterranean descent.

The umbrella graft or "umbrella" consists of a strut plus one or several onlays (Fig. 13). The umbrella is one of the most useful techniques in the reconstruction of nasal tip projection. Like the simple onlay graft, the umbrella may be performed in both primary and secondary rhinoplasty. In his original description of this graft, the senior author referred to the "umbrella–sandwich technique," since the strut is placed between the medial crura in "sandwich" fashion.

The strut may be constructed from ear cartilage or from the septum, with concha being our first choice because of its elastic qualities and ease of insertion. The strut is "sandwiched" between the medial crura, such that one-third of the strut stands alone above the domes. The length of the strut is usually ~3 cm, but this length may vary according to patient requirement.

The strut alone under the skin could create a tip that is too sharp and pointed. For this reason, the superior tip of the strut is covered or "capped" by onlay graft(s). This combination produces the umbrella effect. It must be remembered that each of the components of the umbrella [strut plus onlay(s)] is in a separate pocket.

The strut is harvested from conchal cartilage in much the same way as described for the onlay graft. The straightest segment of cartilage available should be selected for the strut. The onlay may also be harvested from the concha or from lower lateral cartilage as already discussed. The fact that the strut may not be perfectly straight is not of concern. The

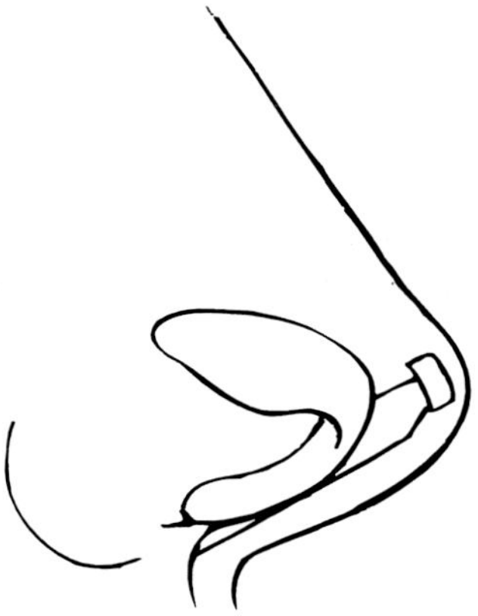

Figure 14. Lateral view of the relative positions of the strut and onlay.

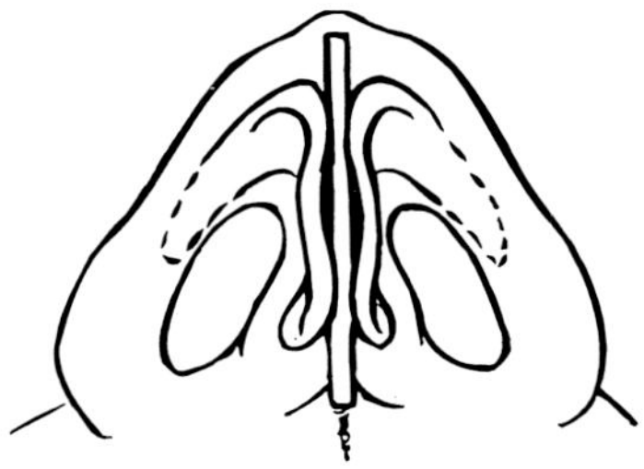

Figure 15. The strut must project 3 or 4 mm above the domes.

purpose of the strut is to give height and support to the nasal tip, and any irregularities in shape are usually camouflaged once the strut is inserted between the medial crura. Figure 14 illustrates the relative position of the strut and onlay as they will appear in the nasal tip.

An incision is made on the infracartilaginous side of the medial crus to place the strut. A vertical external columella incision may also be employed. A pocket is developed between the medial crura that extends from the nasal spine to the nasal tip. The strut is then inserted between the medial crura so that it projects 3 or 4 mm above the domes (Fig. 15).

An onlay graft is positioned horizontally over the domes as described in Onlay Graft once the strut is in place. The sandwiched strut is sutured in position between the crura by a transfixion suture. No sutures are required to close the stab incision used for placement of the onlay graft(s).

The patient in Fig. 16 is of Jewish ancestry. She is depicted two and a half years after three onlays of lower lateral cartilage were employed during rhinoplasty. Note the "plunging nasal tip" so characteristic of the Mediterranean patient.

The patient in Fig. 17 is of Jewish descent. She had had previous nasal surgery but was still unhappy about the lack of tip projection. She underwent an umbrella graft consisting of a strut (previously placed rib cartilage) and two onlays from ear cartilage. The procedure was performed 2.5 years prior to her post-operative photographs. Note the foreshortened columella characteristic of many Mediterranean patients (Fig. 17).

A

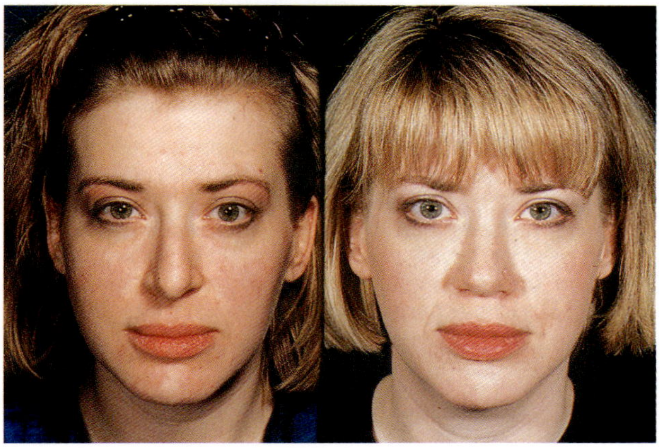

B

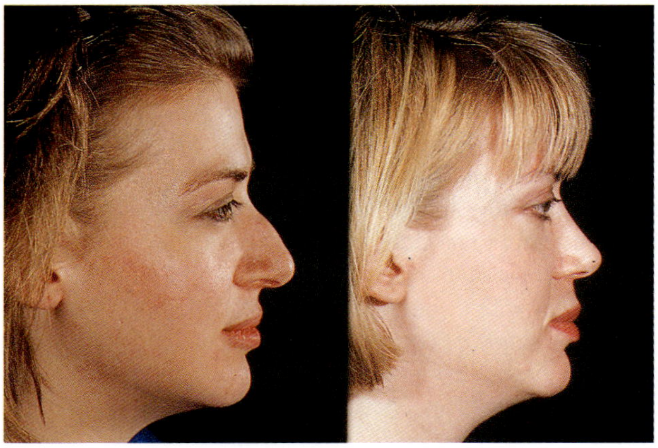

Figure 16. Patient of Jewish ancestry. Primary rhinoplasty employing three onlays of lower lateral cartilage. **A:** Pre- and post-operative front views. Reduction in nasal length is often necessary in patients of Mediterranean background. **B:** Pre- and post-operative profile views. The "plunging nasal tip" is often seen in Mediterranean patients.

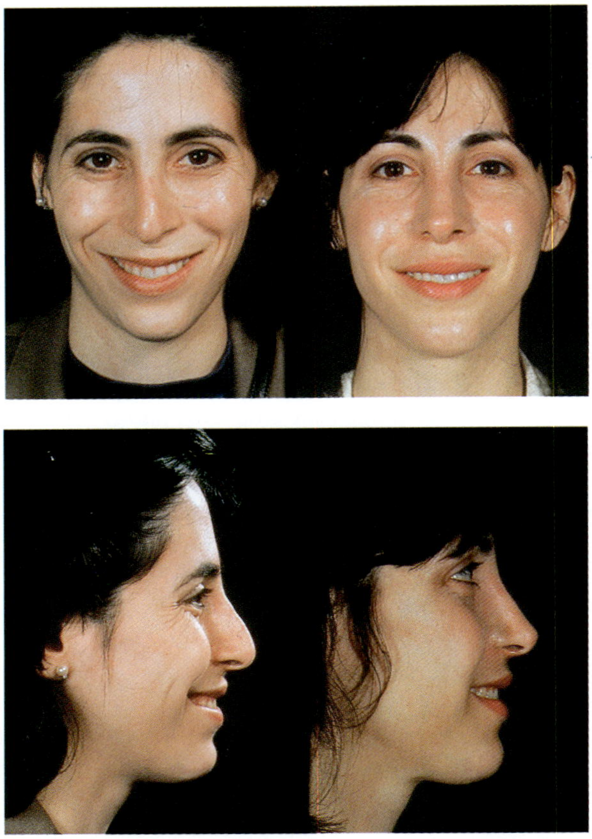

A

B

Figure 17. Patient of Jewish ancestry. Secondary rhinoplasty employing umbrella technique. **A:** Pre- and post-operative front views. Again, nasal shortening is important to achieve proper nasal aesthetics. Increased nasal length as seen pre-operatively is often observed in patients of Mediterranean backgrounds. **B:** Pre- and post-operative profile views. The foreshortened columella and lack of tip projections seen in the pre-operative photograph are characteristic of many Mediterranean patients.

External Shaving

One of the most difficult problems in rhinoplastic surgery is improving a nose that has thick, heavy, sebaceous skin. This type of skin is not elastic and will not contract around modified cartilage structures in the nasal tip pyramid. Such patients must be told that their skin type will not allow for any substantial reduction in nose size and that the primary goal of surgery will be to attempt to produce better lines. This type of nasal skin often is present in the patient of Mediterranean extraction.

The plan should begin with a routine rhinoplasty. The tip is then assessed. It is usually lacking in projection. A single or double onlay will usually improve projection. These onlays must be shorter in horizontal length (<9 mm) because of the thick skin, or they will make the tip appear too broad. If needed, a strut between the medial crura will further enhance projection.

When the skin is still so thick that the desired improvement is not obtained, in carefully selected and carefully counseled cases, the external skin may be shaved. This shaving is similar to the shaving technique used in correcting rhinophyma. The patient, of course, must be forewarned of the compromise and of the possible changes in skin color and texture. Often the skin will become whiter and the sebaceous pores more apparent.

The patient shown in the photographs was a 49-year-old woman of Italian descent. She had had three previous rhinoplasties elsewhere and represented a particularly difficult nasal reconstruction. In addition to having no tip support, she had the additional problem of a thick, heavy-skin nose, typical of many Mediterranean patients. Her reconstruction involved three procedures, including umbrella graft and shaving of the thick, heavy skin in the supratip area. The skin in the supratip area was shaved on three separate occasions, with a minimum of 9 months between procedures. The third procedure was a "touch-up" that consisted of external shave of the supratip skin as well as dermabrasion. A small cartilaginous bump was also excised. Her pre- and post-operative photographs are shown, as well as close-up views depicting satisfactory healing of the supratip skin (Fig. 18).

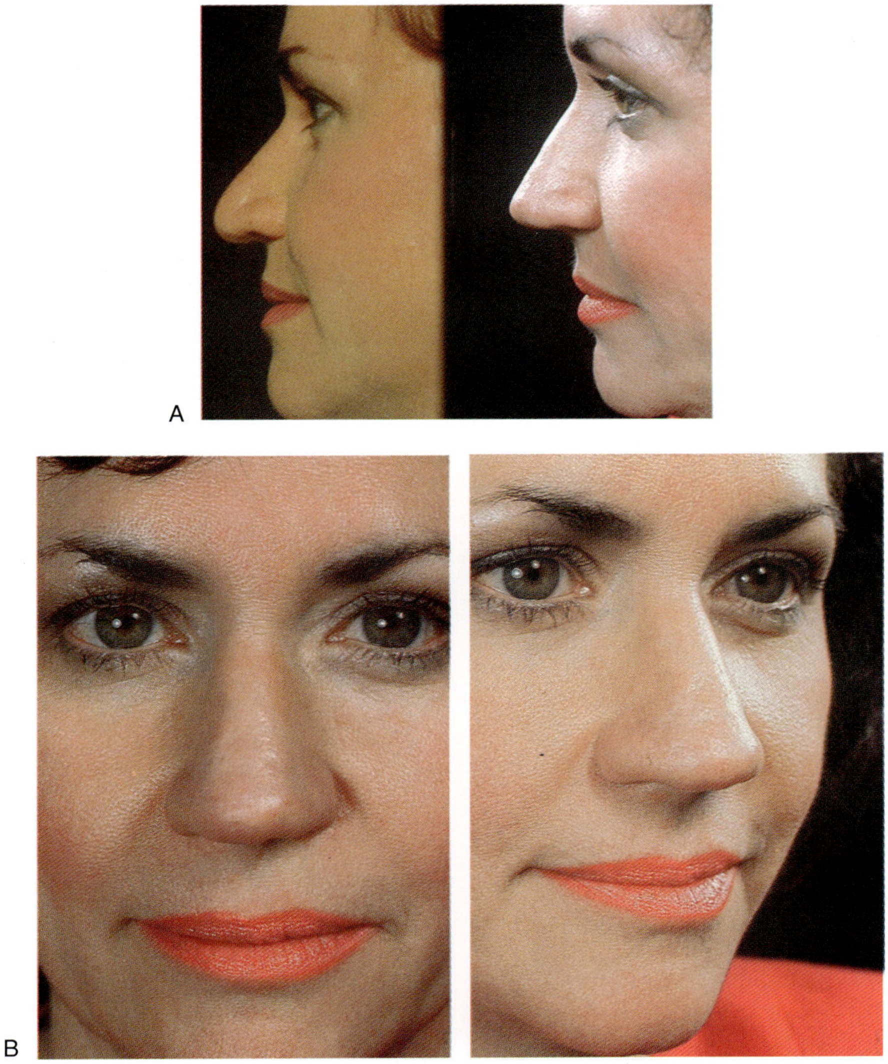

Figure 18. Patient of Italian ancestry with thick, heavily sebaceous skin characteristic of many Mediterranean patients. In addition to an umbrella graft, shaving of the thick skin in the supratip area as well as dermabrasion was performed. **A:** Pre- and post-operative profile views. **B:** Post-operative close-up views of the supratip area, depicting satisfactory healing following three external shave procedures and dermabrasion.

SUMMARY

Obtaining proper tip projection is of paramount importance in all rhinoplasties. It is rendered that much more difficult in patients of Mediterranean origin because these patients often have increased nasal length, plunging tips, foreshortened nasal pyramids, and/or thick, sebaceous skin. Our techniques for obtaining proper tip projection in these cases are outlined.

RECOMMENDED READING

Converse JM. The cartilaginous structures of the nose. *Ann Otol Rhinol Laryngol* 1955;64:220.
Peck GC. *Techniques in aesthetic rhinoplasty*. 2nd ed. Lippincott/Gower, 1990.
Rogers BO. The role of physical anthropology in plastic surgery today. *Clin Plast Surg* 1974;1.
Schmalix J. Die knorpeligen Strukturen der Nassenspitze und ihre Verbindung. *Arch Klin Exp Ohr Nase-u Kehlkopfheik* 1968;190:146

SECTION X

The Middle Eastern Patient

Ethnic Considerations in Facial Aesthetic Surgery, edited by W. Earle Matory, Jr.
Lippincott–Raven Publishers, Philadelphia © 1998.

26

The Middle Eastern Patient

Editor's Commentary

W. Earle Matory, Jr.

The exotic and alluring beauty of the Middle Eastern face is in the dark hair, prominent brows, and long neck. The most distinctive and culturally significant features, however, are the eyes (Fig. 1). The lateral canthus frequently sits 1–2 mm lower than one might find in the Caucasian. There is a dark subtleness about the eyes that draws attention; thus, one must take care to avoid excessive skin resection or overcorrection of upper lid ptosis (Fig. 2). Malar bags and festoons are quite common, with ventral herniation of the fat pads being most effectively addressed through a transconjunctival blepharoplasty, particularly in the absence of excessive lower lid skin elasticity (Fig. 3).

NOSE

The dorsal hump may be extensive, often extending to and including the glabella. Cartilaginous resection of the hump is followed by medial and midline osteotomies (Fig. 4).

Midline congenital anomalies are common, most frequently orbital diastasis and nasoencephaloceles. Cutaneous and bony reductions allow normalization of the midface (Fig. 5).

W. E. Matory, Jr.: A New You Plastic Surgery Medical Group, Irvine, California 92714

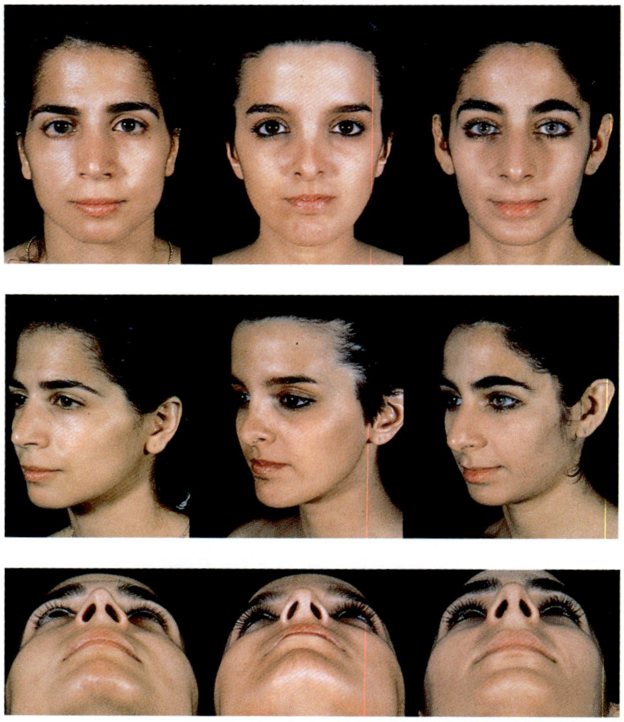

Figure 1. The facies of the Middle East tend to be highly exotic, often with a short brow to trichion, prominent cheekbones, and often a soft chin and jawline.

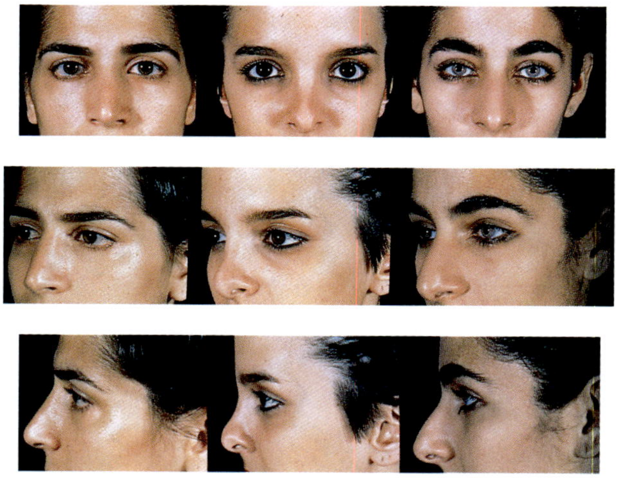

Figure 2. Attractive eyes are culturally of great significance in that in many Arab nations this is the only portion of the face that may be viewed by a suitor. The dark scalp and brow hair and the deeply pigmented orbital area bring focus on the darkly pigmented pupils and palpebral fissures. The exotic attractiveness of the peri-orbital area and the prominent malar eminence present a show of beauty that is more ethnically defined.

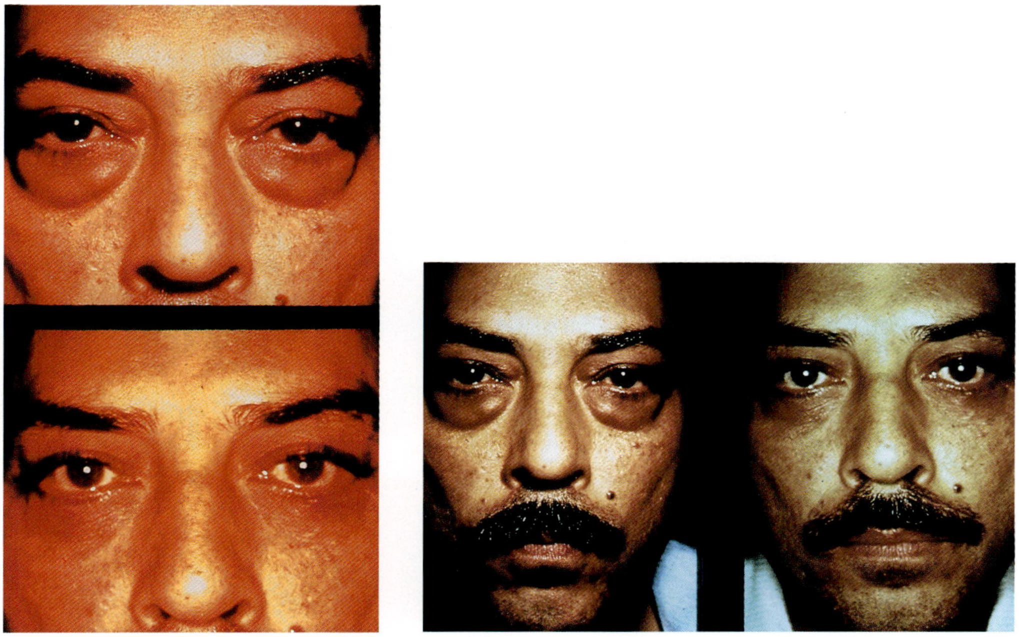

Figure 3. Upper lid skin laxity with fat eventration in the upper and lower lids is common. This presentation makes the Middle Easterner an excellent candidate for upper lid blepharoplasty with fat removal and lower lid transconjunctival blepharoplasty.

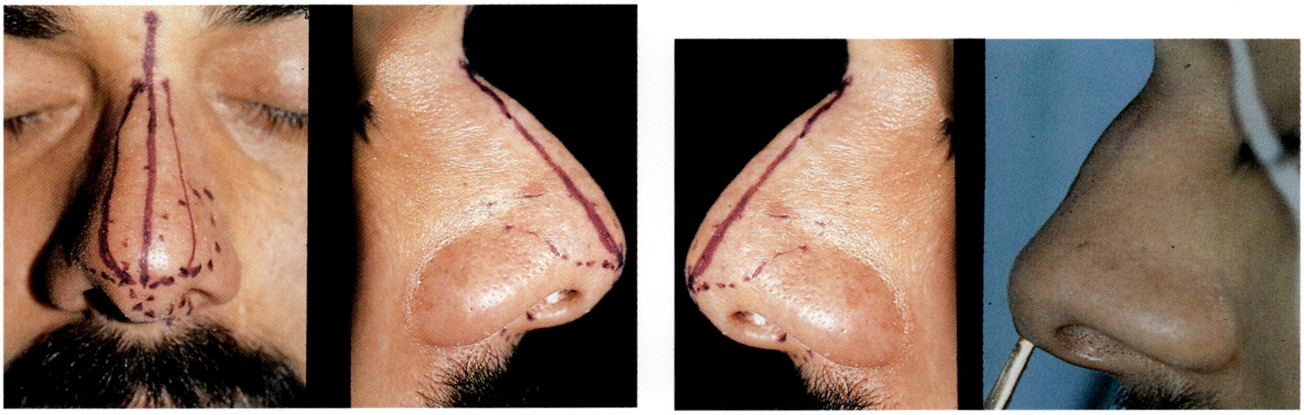

Figure 4. Bony and cartilaginous humps are very commonly noted and are often associated with thick voluminous skin cover, particularly in the tip and supratip areas. Minimal bone and cartilage resection along with dorsal and tip augmentation *(left)* is appropriate in light of the sizable skin envelope. Dorsal hump resection may need to extend to the glabella area using a combination of medial and lateral osteotomies and the Ruben osteotome *(right)*.

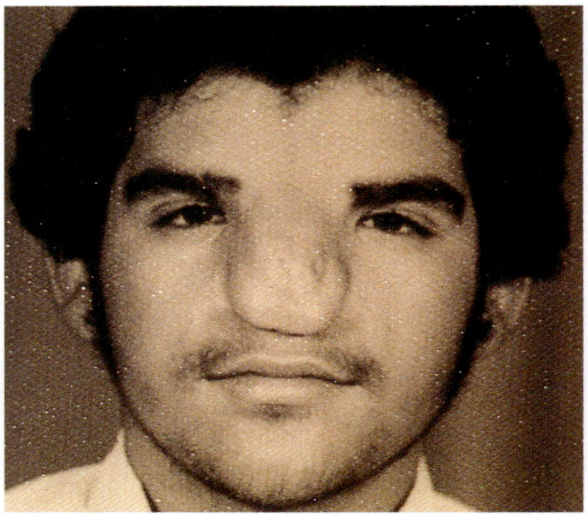

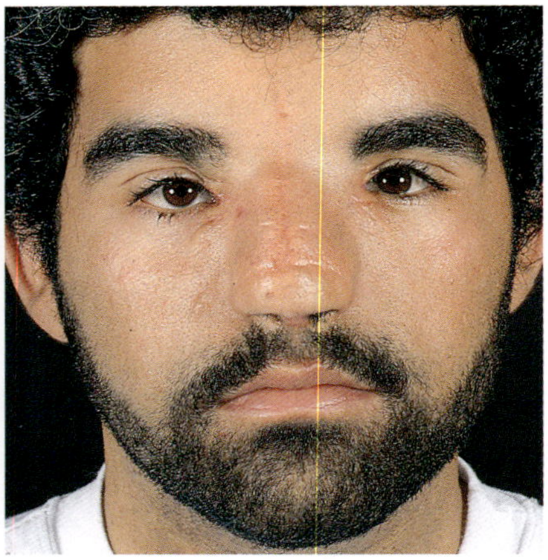

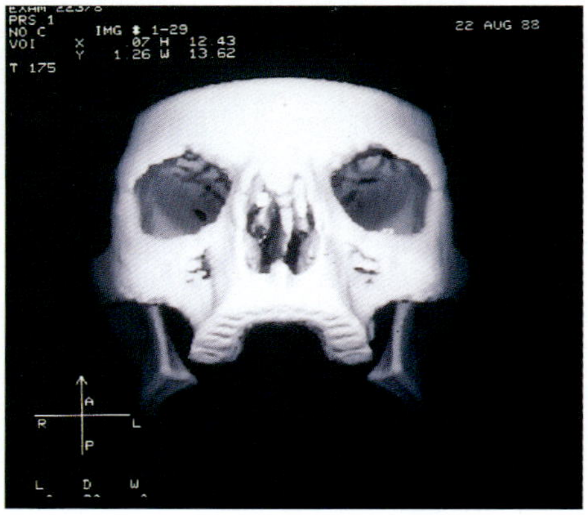

Figure 5. Midline cranial facial deformities, particularly nasoencephaloceles and telecanthus are not uncommon in the Middle East. A series of procedures led to midline soft tissue and bony reduction in this patient.

Ethnic Considerations in Facial Aesthetic Surgery, edited by W. Earle Matory, Jr.
Lippincott–Raven Publishers, Philadelphia © 1998.

27

Facial Surgery in the Middle-Eastern Patient

Bahman Teimourian and Saeed Marefat

I will suffer, but make me beautiful.
— Ancient Persian saying

By the first part of the twenty-first century, the U.S. population may include more members of ethnic groups, including groups from Southeast Asia and the Middle East, than Nordic Caucasians and other fair-skinned Europeans. It is therefore important that plastic surgeons have a good understanding of the aesthetic needs and preferences of these different populations in terms of their facial features. Each group has distinctive standards of beauty and charm that it wishes to preserve. Any individual within such a group may see him- or herself as having features that deviate from that standard and may seek surgery to bring these features closer to their view of the norm. In this practice, most of our experience with patients of different ethnic groups has been with people from the Middle East. Our approach to treating these patients is described below.

CULTURAL CONSIDERATIONS

People from the Middle East may be considered to include Israelis, Arabs, Iranians, Iraqis, Syrians, Lebanese, Jordanians, Turks, and other groups of non-Nordic Caucasians. Since members of each of these groups usually wish to retain at least some of their ethnic identity, a surgeon evaluating a Middle Eastern patient seeking facial improvement should determine the patient's ethnic origin and keep this in mind while discussing the prospective surgery. In general, it is unwise for a surgeon to transform a patient's features to the extent that the patient loses his/her racial or ethnic identity. A better approach is to emphasize the desired features and remove or reduce those features that detract from the patient's natural beauty.

B. Teimourian: Rockville, Maryland 20852
S. Marefat: Annandale, Virginia 22003-6800

There are often differences in the requests from those who reside in the West and those who live in the Middle East. In many countries of the Middle East, the eyes are the only part of a woman's face that can be seen. Expressive dark eyes for centuries have defined Islamic beauty. Thus, correction of the aging eyelids and other lid abnormalities is of particular importance to women living in the religious environment.

Age

In >30 years of practice, Dr. Teimourian has found that >90% of patients from the Middle East that seek cosmetic surgery, request aesthetic and/or functional rhinoplasty. Many are teenagers between the ages of 14 and 17 years who develop a heightened concern about their appearance. They often seek conformity with peers of the same ethnic background or, on occasion, wish their features to blend into the "melting pot." For most teenagers, softening the dorsal hump and altering the top deforming point serve as an excellent mechanism toward improved self-esteem. Among the older patients, improvement of other features, including facial rejuvenation and mentoplasty, naturally complements and enhances hidden attractive features.

Rarely are there requests for nasal surgery or protuberant otoplasty in children below the age of 12. When such requests are made, we do not vary our surgical techniques in this population.

All patients seeking cosmetic surgery require extensive preoperative counseling. Counseling must help the patients to understand the full ramifications of their desire to improve their appearance. Patients should be guided toward achieving an outcome that will be pleasing in youth as well as during maturity.

Family Approval of Surgery

As a rule, the surgeon should do the minimum amount of surgery that will meet the patient's objective. One should discourage unreasonable requests that by the surgeon's interpretation may not be in the patient's best interest. In the patient under 20–25, it is often advisable to have the family involved in the pre-operative planning or to have some indication of family approval, particularly for unusual requests. A patient's motivation for removing an ethnic feature may be perceived by the family as an effort to escape from "the group." Conversely, a reluctant patient may be pressured by the family to undergo an unwanted change. These situations rarely lead to positive outcomes. There may be other implications to the proposed changes. For example, in some countries the nose has a symbolic significance referable to the genitalia. A male patient who takes great pride in his masculinity may be distressed if the perceived strength of his pre-operative nasal form has been diminished to a smaller, "cuter" nose.

Visible Signs of Surgery

The dark skin of many Middle Eastern patients is prone to scarring and discoloration. Patients are especially interested in the surgeon leaving no evidence that any operation has been performed. It is therefore important to reassure that every effort will be made to hide the incisions and to prevent visible scarring.

GENERAL APPEARANCE

People from the Middle East usually have heavy, dark hair, light to dark brown skin, a somewhat small forehead, and sometimes a weak chin. Excess facial hair may be visible on the cheeks and around the lips. The nose often has a hump in the dorsum that some individuals feel is unsightly.

The Skin and Scarring

Many patients from the Middle East already have facial scars from their teenage years, resulting from acne or sometimes leishmaniasis, which leaves large, unsightly blemishes.

Although chemical peeling agents, dermabrasion, or CO_2 ultra-pulse laser can, in some patients, remove or improve the appearance of acne scars, we must caution against overusing this technique. The most common peeling agents used in the United States, phenol and trichloroacetic acid, are being rapidly replaced by CO_2 ultra-pulse laser. With the right dilutions and proper application, these agents can sometimes produce a smoother skin with fewer blemishes. Nevertheless, dermabrasion, chemical peel, and CO_2 ultra-pulse laser can cause depigmentation of the darker skin, leaving light or pinkish colored patches; in other patients, the treatment may result in a prolonged brownish discoloration that is a darker shade than the natural skin. This discoloration can sometimes be treated with the use of a mild steroid cream. Dermabrasion or treatment with alpha-hydroxy (lactic) acid, glycolic washes, or mild creams containing a bleaching agent such as hydroquinine (2 or 4%) or containing Retin A may also improve the appearance of the skin surface. Further information on dermabrasion is provided later in this chapter.

The Nose

The noses of people from the Middle East vary within as well as between ethnic groups. Some of the commonly seen features are as follows: (a) a high arching dorsum; (b) a low nasal tip; (c) a long contour, from root to subnasal point and from root to tip; (d) a large skin sleeve; and (e) thick skin, which is often oily, with large pores.

In general, the nose should not only be functional, but it should look good; this means that it should be proportional to the other facial features. In all ethnic groups, the nose should have an adequate dorsum, adequate tip projection, and a reasonably normal base. The hump in the dorsum in Middle Easterners stands in contrast to the depression seen in the nose of Asian patients. With a minimal amount of surgery, both conditions can be easily corrected: in the Middle Eastern patient, by removing the hump and adding cartilage to the columella and tip to improve tip projection, and in the Asian by adding tissue to the dorsum as well as to the columella and tip.

The length of the nose in the Middle Easterner can make nasal reduction difficult in the older patient because the excessive skin overlying the hump and the extended tip may not shrink to the reduced size. Usually, the skin overlying the upper part of the nose, including the dorsum, is relatively thin and easy to manipulate. Near the tip and supratip areas, however, the skin tends to be thicker, with numerous sebaceous glands. This thicker skin lacks contractile ability and may not provide the required covering for a reduced skeletal structure at the nose tip.

The Chin

In many Middle Eastern patients, both men and women, the chin is small and can benefit from augmentation mentoplasty with the use of synthetic material. For this one can use an intra-oral approach. Alternatively, one can perform advancement genioplasty. However, we have found that many patients with whom this surgery is discussed decline the operation, even though it would help to balance their facial features.

The Eyes, Forehead, and Neck

As Middle Eastern people reach their 30s, they begin to develop crow's feet around the eyes, a creased forehead, and loose skin around the neck. Compared with aging Nordic

Caucasians, these changes are not as pronounced in either the light- or dark-skinned Middle Easterners, although many of them, male and female, seek improvements at this age.

PATIENT EVALUATION AND PREPARATION

When a patient first comes to discuss the possibility of facial surgery, the surgeon should determine the primary reason for the request and, if the request is reasonable, decide on the best approach to achieve the desired results. The risks as well as the advantages of the surgical procedures should be discussed with the patient to ensure that s/he understands the immediate outcome and, most important, the expected recovery time. Information regarding the patient's general medical history should be obtained, along with any evidence of early trauma to the face. For some patients x-ray studies or a computed tomography scan may be necessary. We usually obtain a complete blood count, blood chemistry, bleeding time, urinalysis, and EKG about a week before surgery for patients who have elected to undergo facial surgery, depending on their medical history.

Viral Infection

If the patient has had a recent viral infection or if there is any indication of herpesvirus (cold sores), the patient should be put on an antiviral compound pre- and post-surgery.

Computer Imaging

Some surgeons use the results of computer imaging to show the patient what they may look like after surgery. This technique may be of some value to the patient but could also be considered a marketing tool. In our experience, a few simple Polaroid pictures taken from several angles works effectively. The surgeon marks the photographs to indicate the proposed changes, demonstrating anticipated improvements to the patient.

Anesthesia

We allow the patient to choose either local anesthesia with sedation or general anesthesia.

Evaluation of the Nose

Many patients seeking removal of the hump from the dorsum of their nose also want correction of a hooked tip, reduction of the broad base, and repair of a deviated septum. In evaluating the nose, the surgeon should determine the amount of septal deviation present or nasal obstruction if any. American immigrants from the Middle East frequently find that they have difficulty breathing in the humid climates of the eastern United States. They had no problems in the dry climates of their origin but now suffer from enlarged turbinates. Thus, the patient should be asked about allergies, allergy work-up, and any prior or current use of anti-histamines or nasal or sinus decongestants. The frequency of nasal bleeding (epistaxis) should be noted. If there is septal perforation, it is important to determine the cause. Such perforation can result from cocaine use, infection, previous surgery, or trauma to the nose. We try to find out whether the patient has been treated for nasal infection or has been treated with any antibiotics within the previous 2–3 years. We also seek information on any previous x-rays or computed tomography scans of the head.

In determining the best approach to achieving the desired result, the surgeon should bear in mind the type of surgery to be performed: whether it is to be primary, secondary, or partial. Will the incision be into the rim or inter- or intracartilaginous? Does the dorsum need reduction, an onlay graft, a change in the nasofrontal angle, or a spreader graft? Does the tip projection need to be increased or decreased, or would the tip be improved by rotation or by a change in the columella/alar relation? Is there too much flaring at the base of the alae, and, if so, how can the alae be brought together? We usually avoid entering the mucosal surface to prevent notching. Instead, we make an incision ~0.5 mm above the fold and thus minimize the visibility of the scar. For the same reason, we also avoid making incisions in the lateral aspect of the ala.

As far as the nasal bones are concerned, the surgeon should determine whether the patient needs medial, lateral, complete, or multiple osteotomy. If augmentation of the dorsum or tip is required, the graft can be obtained from the septum, ear auricle, ribs, outer table of the skull, or pelvic bone. A good source of graft material that is sometimes overlooked is the vomer bone and part of the ethmoid. Patients like the crus of the cartilage in the columella to look symmetrical, and, of course, the tip needs to be adequately projected.

Evaluation of the Eyes

For any eye surgery, the surgeon should request clearance, including a field test, from an ophthalmologist and should do a thorough examination him- or herself. The patients should be asked about any previous eye surgery, and it is imperative to check for asymmetry, ptosis, or pre-operative scleral visibility/show. The patient should be asked about symptoms of cyclic eyelid edema and dry eye syndrome, and if such symptoms are present, the surgeon may need to modify the planned surgery in a conservative direction. The surgeon should note the thickness of the eyelids, the tone of the lids, and any pigmentation differences between the orbital and palpebral parts of the lids.

Contraindications to eye surgery include significant intra- or extra-ocular pathology or malignancy. Corneal ulceration, glaucoma, or incorrectable ectropion may deter the surgeon from performing an aesthetic procedure.

Evaluation of Other Facial Features

When patients are seeking facial surgery, the surgeon should discuss all facial features with the patient and explain how each part contributes to the general appearance, often balancing or counteracting the effect of another part. Patients in their teens and early 20s usually need treatment of only one feature, the nose, but as they get older, requests for rejuvenation of the neck, forehead, and eyes become more common, with patients in their late 40s and 50s sometimes requesting a partial or complete facelift. These patients should be evaluated in the usual manner.

PRE-OPERATIVE PREPARATION

The preparation of patients from the Middle East is the same as for facial surgery in any other patient.

Just before surgery, reviewing with the patient the operating procedures to be used can help to reduce patient anxiety. Marking is done with the patient in a sitting position, and the sites of incision are verified. An antibiotic may be administered by mouth prior to surgery or intravenously during surgery. We also use a single dose of Solu-Medrol (500 mg, methylprednisolone), which appears to decrease post-operative bruising and swelling.

SURGICAL TECHNIQUES

Reduction and Contouring of the Nose (Figs. 1–4)

If local anesthesia is used, the nose is first packed with 4% liquid or powdered cocaine. If general anesthesia is used or if the patient is sedated, the entire nose is blocked with 1%

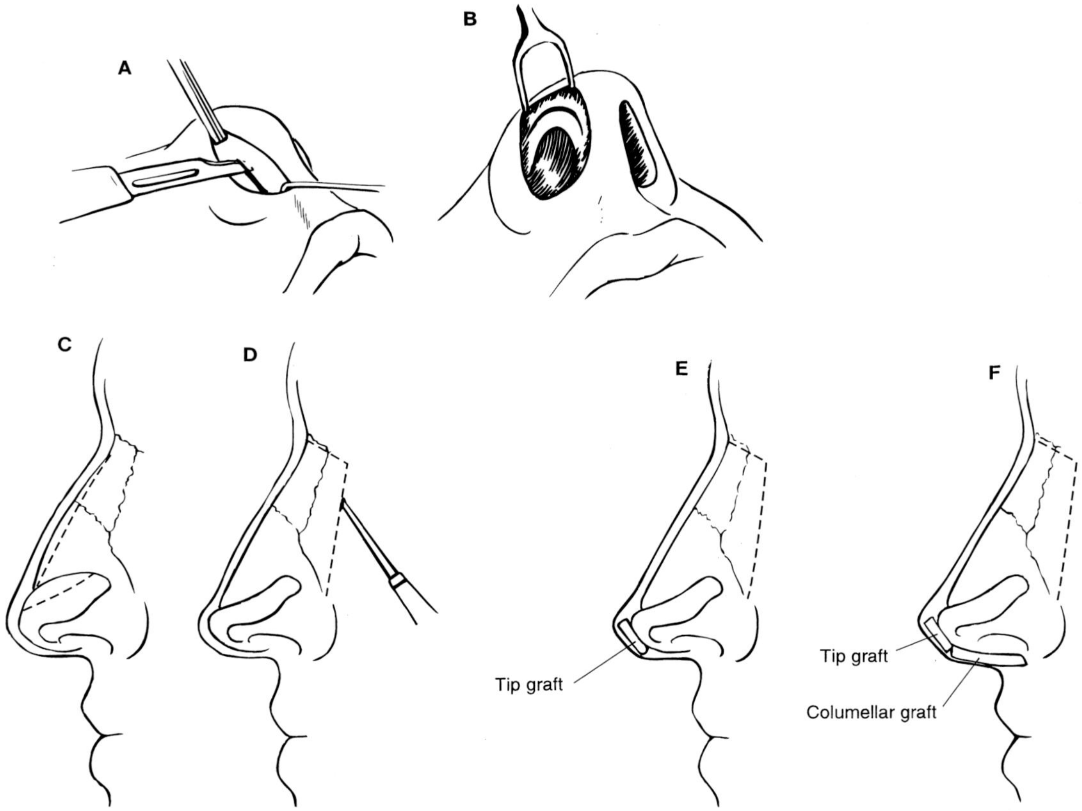

Figure 1. Diagrams showing correction of the nose. **A:** Incision in the membranous portion of the nasal septum. This incision can also be used for correcting nasal septal deviation. **B:** Intracartilaginous incision to expose the lower lateral cartilages and the upper lateral cartilages as well as the dorsum of the nose to remove the hump. **C:** Typical Middle Eastern nose with a large hump and short columella (hook nose). The dotted area of the lower lateral cartilage is the cephalo or proximal part of the lower lateral cartilage to be trimmed. The shaded area over the dorsum is where the hump is located, part of it consisting of bone and part of cartilage. **D:** Percutaneous osteotomy of the nose to separate the nasal bone from the maxilla and lacrimal bone using a 2-mm chisel. The dotted line indicates the line of osteotomy. If the nose is very wide, one has to do an osteotomy to separate the nasal bones from the septum to accomplish sufficient infracture and subsequent narrowing. **E:** Profile of the nose. The hump has been removed, the line of osteotomy is indicated, and the lower lateral cartilage has been trimmed. Tip projection has been improved by adding a cartilage graft in the columella as well as the tip. The strut is usually 2 mm wide and 2–2.5 cm long and is placed between the crus of the columella. The size of the tip graft is usually 2 × 9 mm. One or more of these grafts can be placed on top of one another through a rim incision to obtain adequate tip projection.

lidocaine containing adrenaline (epinephrine, 1:100,000). A few minutes should be allowed for the adrenaline to become effective.

Treatment of the Turbinate

The surgeon begins by straightening the septum and shrinking the turbinate, either by cryosurgery or by partial turbinectomy. A minimum amount of trimming, or no trimming, is done to the upper lateral cartilage submucosally to avoid damaging the internal nasal valve. The lower lateral cartilage can be trimmed to the desired size and shape, usually leaving at least 5-mm width, through an inter- or intracartilaginous incision or a rim incision, depending on the surgeon's ability and choice and on the agreement with the patient.

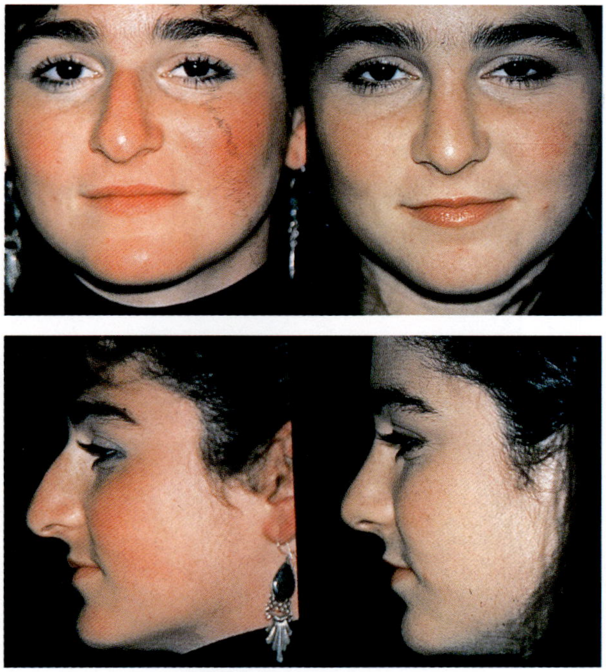

A, B

C, D

Figure 2. An 18-year-old patient who underwent septorhinoplasty with a cartilage graft to the columella and tip of the nose. **A**, **C:** Pre-operative views; **B**, **D:** post-operative views.

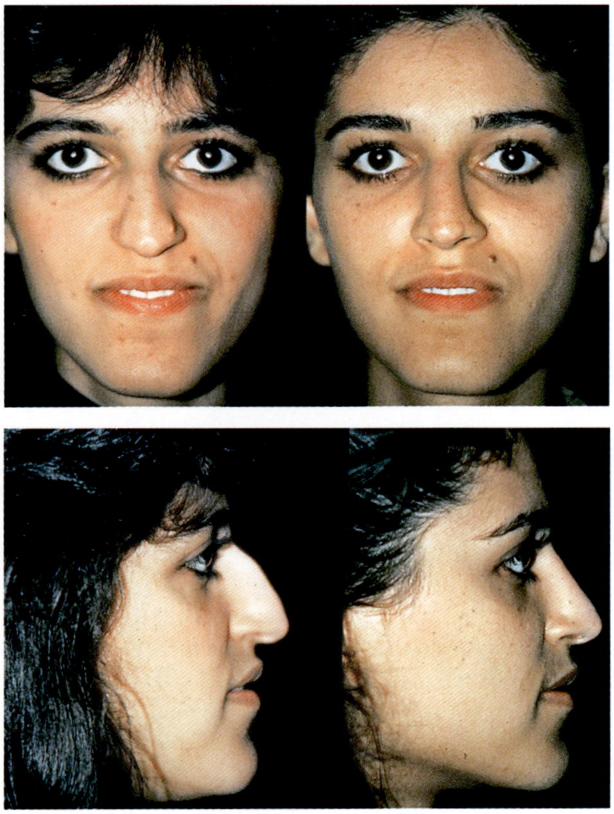

A, B

C, D

Figure 3. A 24-year-old patient who underwent septorhinoplasty with a cartilage graft to the columella and tip of the nose. **A**, **C:** Pre-operative views; **B**, **D:** post-operative views.

A, B

C, D

E, F

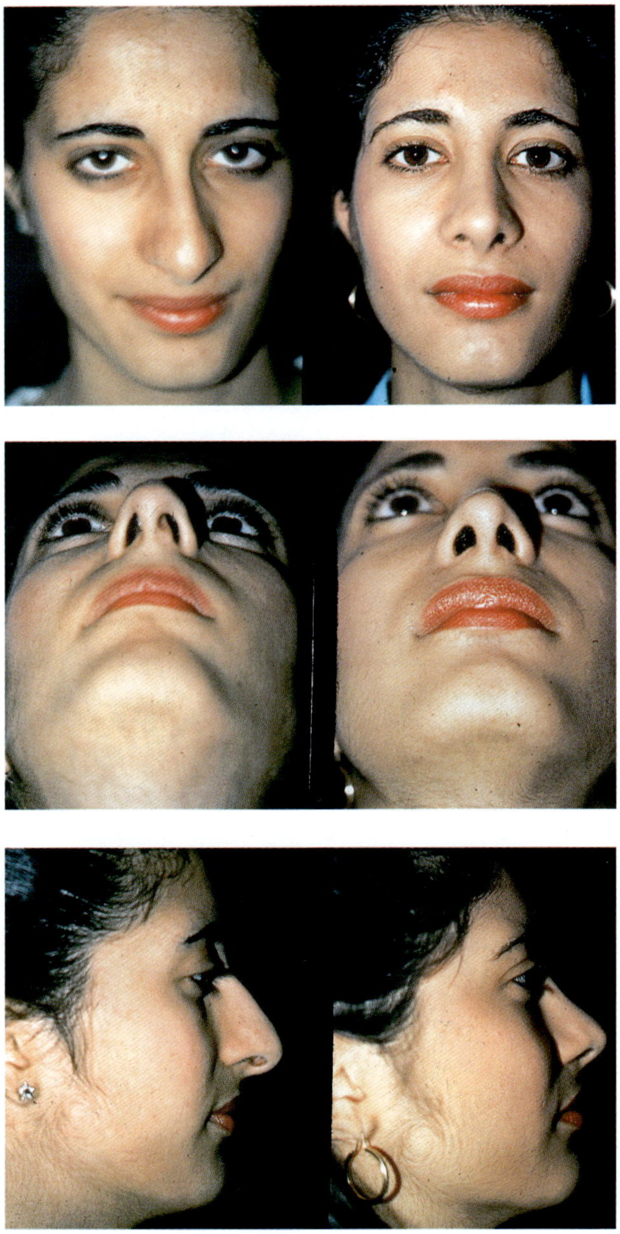

Figure 4. An 18-year-old patient who underwent septorhinoplasty with a cartilage graft to the columella and tip of the nose. **A, C, and E:** Pre-operative views; **B, D, and F:** post-operative views.

When an adequate amount of skin has been elevated over the dorsum of the nose, the hump is removed from the dorsum. Because the use of a chisel can lead to over-resection in the dorsum, the saw or rasp is the preferred instrument for this task.

Skin Reduction

The overlying skin is then made thinner from underneath by means of fine scissors or a sharp rasp, especially with a backward movement. The amount of fibroadipose tissue removed may be quite large, depending on each particular patient.

Infracture

The surgeon then performs an infracture, using an osteotome or saw at the base of the alae. Alternatively, one may perform a percutaneous osteotomy, using a 2-mm osteotome, to cause infracture of the lacrimal bone as well as the nasal bone, loosening their attachments to the maxillae. The nose is then straightened and positioned as desired. If a hump is to be removed from a nose that is very large or broad, the surgeon may have to perform an osteotomy of the nasal bone on each side to separate the bone from the septum before doing the infracture.

Nose Tip

In a woman, the angle between the lip and the columella should be between 95 and 105°; in a man we strive for an angle of 90°. In side view, the columella should fall ~2–3 mm below the alar rim.

After the infraction, the surgeon focuses on the tip of the nose, usually placing a cartilage graft between the crus to raise the base of the nose. The average size of the graft is about 2 mm wide × 2–2.5 cm, but the dimensions vary according to the patient. We usually insert an additional cartilage graft through a rim incision to improve tip projection. These grafts usually measure ~9 × 2 mm. One or several layers may be stacked one above the other.

As a rule of thumb, the sides of the triangle at the base of the nose formed between the alae and the tip should be equal. One can use the eye, a ruler, or a caliper to ensure that tip projection is adequate.

If the septum is unstable, the surgeon may apply two Reuter splints, 0.25 mm thick, on each side and suture them to each other with nylon or chromic suture. The splint is left on for a few days to achieve midline septum stability.

Post-Operative Care of the Nose

We do not support the view that post-operative packing of the nose is either necessary or desirable. Most of the severe bleeding we have encountered has occurred 7–10 days post-operatively when attempts were made to remove packing in the examining room. In the event that the turbinate has been reduced by cryosurgery or partial turbinectomy, a piece of Gel Foam or Surgicel may be placed against the turbinate. However, so long as one is careful not to damage the mucosa of the septum, there is no need for any packing to be used, and there is much less discomfort for the patient.

After completion of nose surgery, we apply a tincture of benzoin to the skin, then place a padded brown splint on the nose, keeping it in place by means of a Steri-Strip, usually 1/2 inch in width.

Post-operatively, the patient is kept in a semifowler position. If necessary, an antiemetic is administered to patients receiving a general anesthetic. Many patients do vomit blood after nose surgery because some is swallowed during the procedure. Anti-hypertensive medication may also be used if necessary.

Edema can be counteracted with steroids and by applying cold compresses to the eyes and keeping the head elevated.

The patient usually leaves the hospital 1–3 h after surgery, and the splint is removed 5–6 days later.

Patient Participation in Recovery

After the splint is removed, the patient is instructed to reapply the splint to the outside of the nose for ~30 min three times daily for 1 month and to apply pressure with an index fin-

A–C

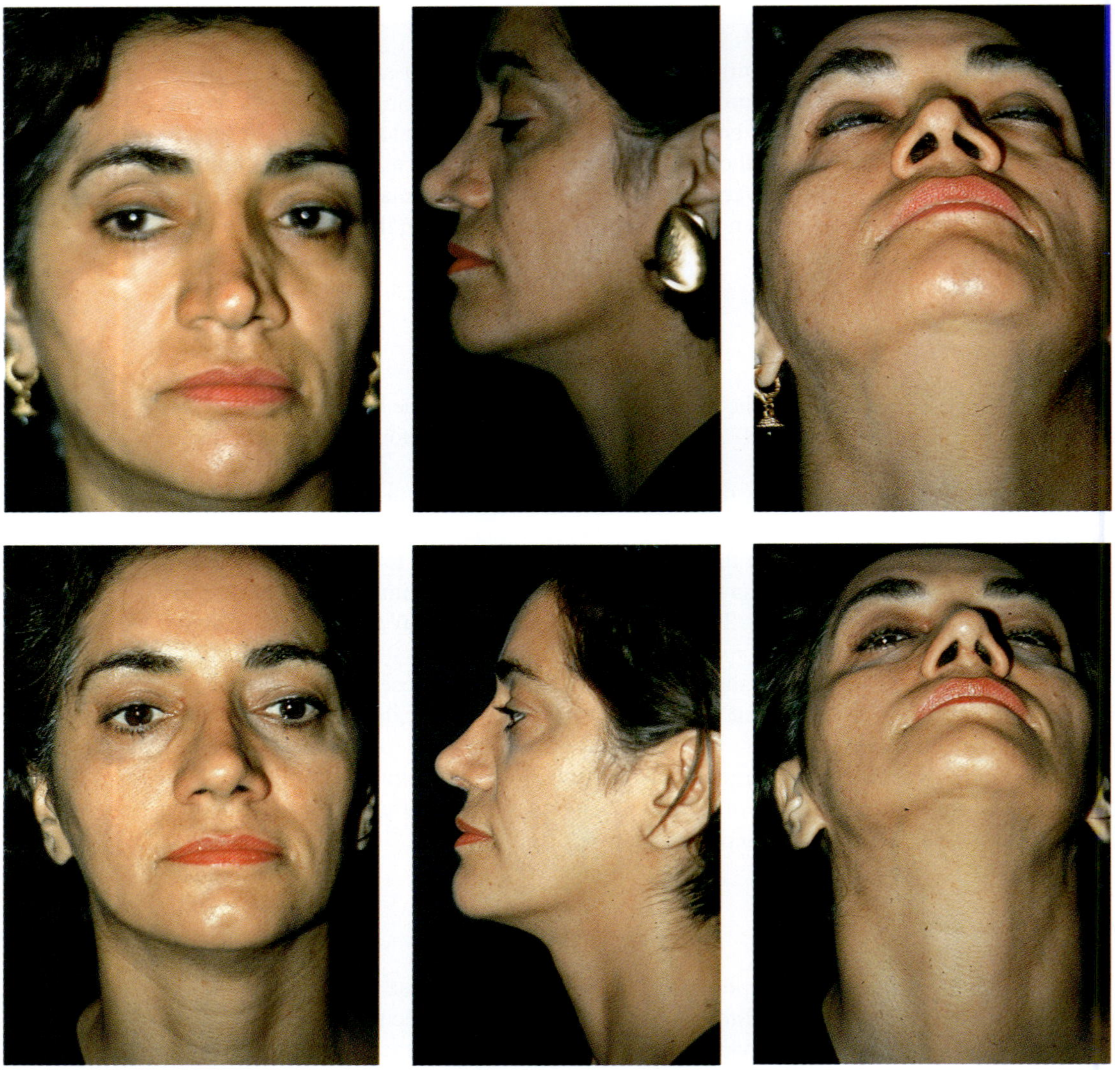

Figure 5. Secondary surgery of the nose. This 44-year-old patient had received four previous rhinoplasties with removal of too much cartilage and bone. The defects were corrected with cartilage grafts from the ears, bone grafts from the outer table of the skull, and open rhinoplasty. **A–C:** Pre-operative views; **D–F:** post-operative views.

ger to each side of the nose and to the base and the dorsum for ~10 min three or four times a day for a period of 6–8 weeks. In this way the patient participates in promoting the desired outcome and adjusts to the fact that the final shape will not be apparent for several months. Many patients become concerned when some swelling remains after 2–3 weeks and they feel that the result is not what they expected. Instructions to participate fully in the healing process for several months helps to allay their fears.

Corrective Secondary Surgery of the Nose (Fig. 5)

We usually wait at least 6–12 months before doing any secondary surgery of the nose. We find that many patients who require secondary rhinoplasty may benefit from an open or semi-open approach (alar rim incision, extending on each side of the columella, exposing the entire dorsum as well as lower lateral cartilage without cross-incision in the columella), especially if the first procedure was done by another surgeon whose techniques may differ from ours. With open rhinoplasty, one can easily see the osteocartilaginous architecture and make precise adjustments under direct vision. The risk of migration or misplacement of grafts is also minimized. However, open rhinoplasty is not without its problems and must be planned and executed meticulously to prevent loss of skin or additional bowing of the columella or other complications. If the dorsum has been over-resected by previous surgery, one can rebuild it with a bone graft. The graft is usually secured in place by means of stainless-steel pins that can be removed in a few weeks.

To repair the tip of the nose, to provide the support for adequate tip projection, one may use ear cartilage, or a "champagne glass" cartilage graft. If over-resection of the cartilaginous portion of the nose was done, a graft from the ear can be used to fill the depression. A graft from the ear can also be used as a spreader to improve breathing, depending on the patient's need.

A–C

D–F

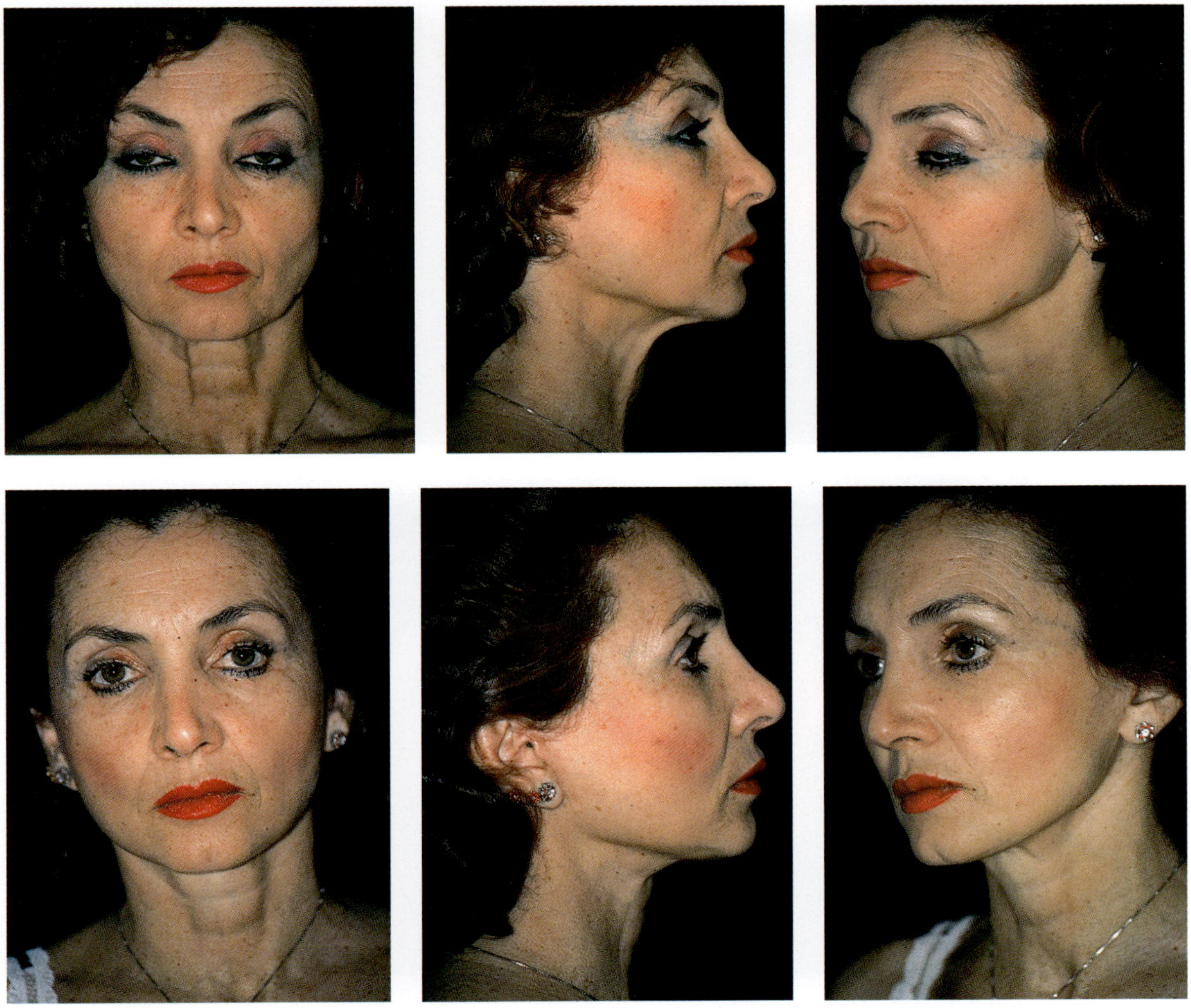

Figure 6. A 55-year-old patient who underwent a facelift, neck contouring, and upper and lower eyelid blepharoplasty. **A–C:** Pre-operative views; **D–F:** post-operative views.

Rejuvenation of the Eyes, Forehead, and Neck (Figs. 6–8)

Some Middle Eastern patients in their 20s, but many more in their late 30s or early 40s, seek improvement of their eyes and rejuvenation of their forehead and neck. In the older patients, much can often be done by improving the skin surface by the use of alpha-hydroxy acid (lactic acid) and avoidance of excess exposure to the sun. For these patients, we provide a 6-week skin rejuvenation program and instruct them to maintain treatment before, during, and after surgery.

Eyes

The goals in blepharoplasty are to remove a sufficient amount of fat and excessive eyelid skin to produce a well defined and pleasing contour of the eyelids. The surgery is done

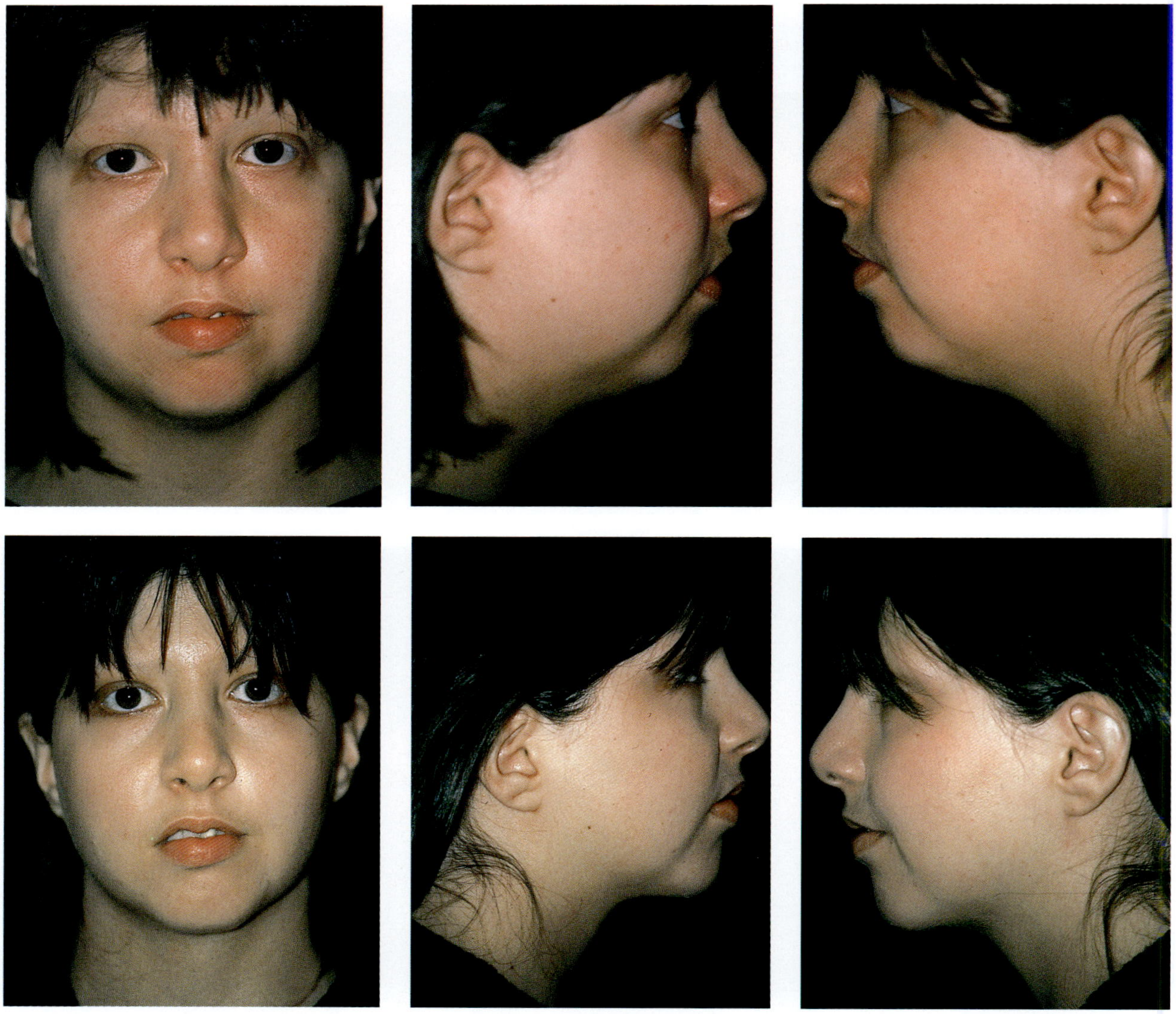

A–C

D–F

Figure 7. A 25-year-old patient who underwent neck contouring by suction lipectomy repair of the platysma muscle and augmentation mentoplasty. **A–C:** Pre-operative views; **D–F:** post-operative views.

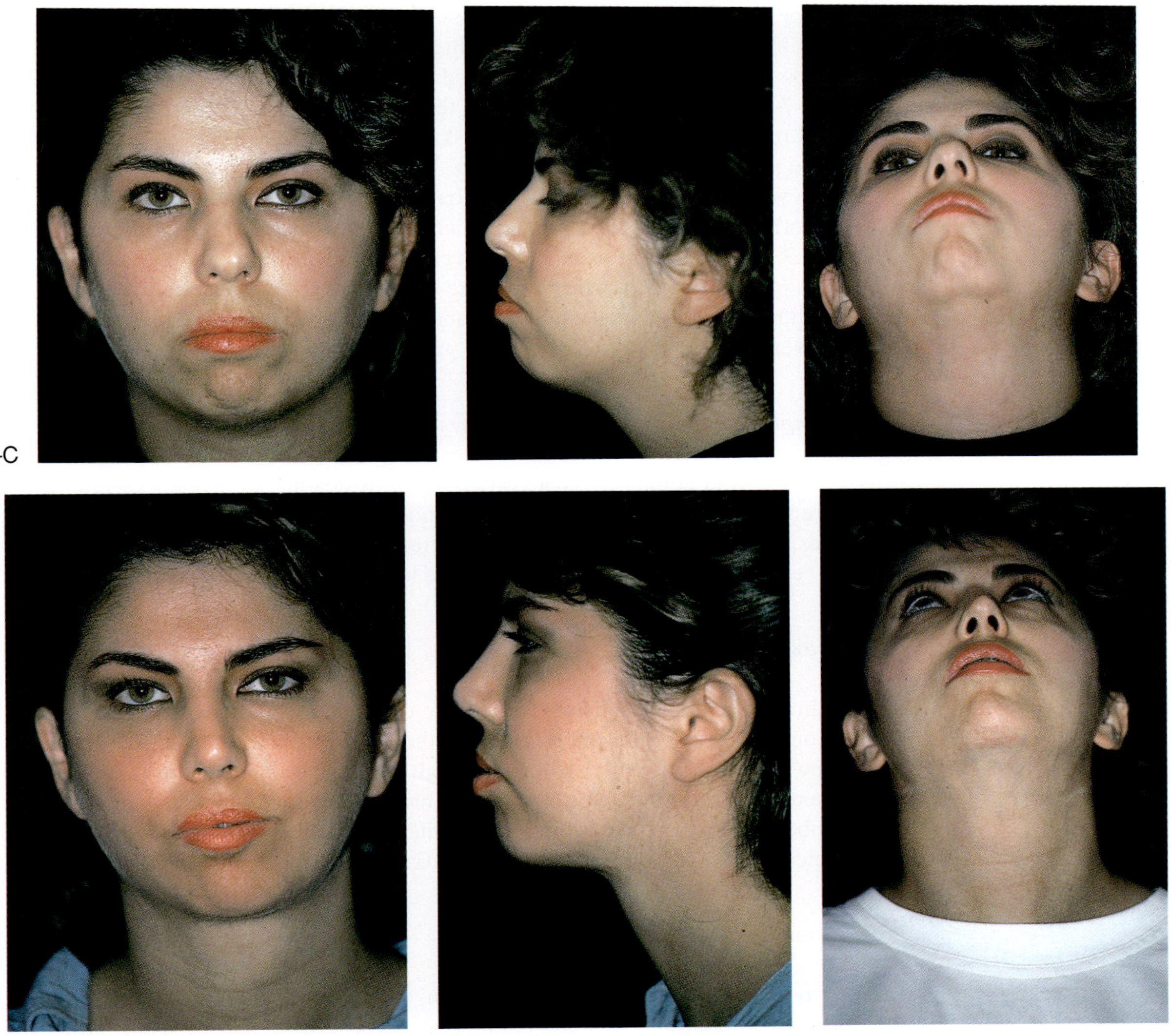

A–C

D–F

Figure 8. A 29-year-old patient who underwent neck contouring by suction lipectomy, repair of the platysma muscle, augmentation mentoplasty, and rhinoplasty. **A–C:** Pre-operative views; **D–F:** post-operative views.

in the usual manner, but with modifications to reduce scar formation and ensure scar symmetry.

The patient is marked in a sitting position. Usually, the upper incision is marked 10 mm superior to the eyelid margin and the lower lid incision, if one is absolutely necessary, ~2 mm below the ciliary margin. The eyelids are injected with 1% lidocaine containing 1:100,000 epinephrine.

For the upper eyelids, we usually perform an anchor blepharoplasty, modified so that the incision does not extend into the lateral aspect of the eyelid, unless absolutely necessary. As much skin as can be removed without pulling the eyelid upward is marked for excision. The medial extent of the excision should not invade the nasal skin. Removal of the excess skin thus removes the bags only, without causing contracture or webbing toward the nose. The amount of muscle excised varies, usually from 5 to 8 mm in width. Rather than anchoring the muscle to the tarsal plate, we achieve a modified anchorplasty by using subdermal suturing.

For the lower lids, when an external incision is necessary, we use one that is as short as possible, so that it extends no more than 2–3 mm into the crow's feet area. We take the incision laterally along one of the natural skin creases in the lateral orbital area. There should be a 7- to 8-mm skin bridge between the upper and lower eyelid incisions in the lateral orbital region. When there is minimal skin excess of the lower eyelids, we remove the bags through a transconjunctival approach.

In younger patients with minimal bags under their eyes but some loose skin, we tighten the orbital fascia to correct the herniating orbital fat pad along with minimal skin resection. Caution must be used, in that over-resection of the orbital fat pad can lead to sunken eyes (enophthalmus), which are more unsightly than bags. Attachment of the orbicularis oculi muscle to a lateral canthal ligament prior to resection of excess skin is a useful maneuver.

Complications in Treating the Eyes

We should emphasize that conservatism in treating the eyes is of utmost importance. Over-resection in treating the upper eyelids can lead to the patient being unable to close the eyes, even during sleep, and can be extremely uncomfortable, especially in patients with dry eye syndrome. Over-resection of the lower eyelid skin can lead to ectropion.

Browplasty

In many of these patients, we remove excess fat from underneath the lateral eyebrows through the same incision as used for the upper eyelids. Or, if the lateral aspects of the brows are ptotic, we place sutures through the skin, through the brow, and through the periosteum of the periorbital rim. We then bring the sutures to the outside, tying them over a rubber shod (or piece of gauze) to maintain the lateral aspect of the eyebrows in the corrected position until healed, usually 7–10 days, after which time we remove the sutures.

Forehead Rejuvenation

In some patients we do a forehead rejuvenation that is similar to the endoscopic forehead lift and is referred to as a limited incision browplasty. To avoid using a long incision that might result in an unsightly scar, we use two small incisions just behind the hairline or, if the hairline is very high, just in front of it.

The scalp and forehead are infiltrated with 0.5% lidocaine containing 1:200,000 epinephrine. A 1- to 1.5-in. incision is made on each side of the scalp near the temple. Through these incisions, one dissects the entire scalp to the vertex, subgaleally, and the forehead is elevated subperiosteally to the supra-orbital rim. The procerus and corrugator muscles are partially removed from their insertions. This can be done with a small clamp or a sharp nasal rasp. The muscles are thus weakened without causing a contour depression. As one separates the forehead from the supra-orbital rim, one actually undermines the temporal area, including the crow's feet area and upper face, as though one were doing a subperiosteal upper facelift. Periosteal elevators are used to develop the flap without resorting to any sharp dissection. In addition, the spreading action of Metzenbaum scissors is helpful. With the latter maneuver, great care must be taken in proceeding with the dissection to avoid nerve injury. It is therefore important to mark the positions of the procerus and corrugator muscles and the supra-orbital and supratrochlear nerves prior to making the incisions.

In patients with extreme curvature of the forehead, a third incision, 1/2 in. long, is made vertically in the scalp in the middle of the hairline to facilitate dissection in the area of the glabella. When dissection is completed, the entire forehead is elevated upward. The skin is grasped with an Allis clamp, and when sufficient elevation has been achieved, the skin is marked at the appropriate line of retraction and then incised at this point. To maintain flap advancement, the galea is repaired with buried 2-0 Vicryl sutures. The skin is closed with staples in the hairline area or with fine sutures if the incisions are in front of the hairline.

Microfoam tape may be applied to the forehead for 3–5 days, or until scarring has occurred, both to maintain its upward position and to minimize edema formation.

Neck Contouring

Treatment of the neck usually requires removal of adipose tissue with or without improvement of the platysma band or platysma diastasis. To achieve the desired contours, the treatment involves suctioning or direct excision of fat with scissors. Some patients require removal of fat from underneath the platysma muscle. If there is a marked or very obvious platysma band or diastasis, the band should be cut and the edges of the muscle sutured together. The skin then contracts to the new frame to give a smoother, younger appearance to the neck. This procedure can be used in young patients and in patients in their 40s and early 50s, depending on the condition of their skin.

Fat removed by suction can be used for augmentation of deficient areas in the neck or for augmentation of the cheeks or chin. Some of the fat grafted in this way survives as free fat cells and some as scar tissue. About 50% of the volume of fat injected usually remains for several years or more.

Microfoam is applied to the skin to provide pressure. It is stapled on each side just into the hairline and behind the ears. Bleeding is minimal, and when the microtape is removed the next day, there is little or no ecchymosis.

Facelifts and Neck Rejuvenation in the Older Middle Eastern Patient (Fig. 9)

In their late 30s and in their 40s, many Middle Eastern patients start to develop excess skin in the nasolabial area as well as around the eye. They often request improvement of these areas as well as a facelift and rejuvenation of the neck. We often find that we can obtain pleasing results in the neck area by using suction lipectomy alone, inserting the cannula through a small submental incision.

Facelift

A partial facelift can be achieved through an incision starting just above the ear into the post-tragus area and ending behind the earlobe. It is best not to raise the hairline. A horizontal incision, 1–2 cm long, may be made in the temporal area. We find it preferable to place the incision right over the tragus, where it will be least visible. If there is a lot of loose skin in the neck region, this incision can be carried around the back of the ear into the upper part of the mastoid and into the neck. This avoids the presence of a scar that would prevent the patient from wearing the hair tied back. However, one must also avoid a stepladder effect in the neck scar at the hairline.

In some patients one need only tighten the skin without altering the SMAS. In others, it may be necessary to undermine the skin all the way to the nasolabial area, then to remove some of the SMAS in front of the ear and raise and tighten the remaining SMAS.

Multiplane Facelift

One of the most effective techniques we use is a modification of a deep facelift in which we raise the SMAS and the overlying skin as separate flaps all the way to the nasolabial area. We refer to this technique as the multiplane facelift or fourth-generation facelift. It enables us to remove more skin than can be removed with a deep plane facelift and to achieve greater tightening without creating undue tension on the flap. There is a surprisingly good blood supply in the skin and the SMAS, which makes such tightening possible.

The success of the multiplane facelift lies in the fact that the SMAS and skin flaps are

A–C

D–F

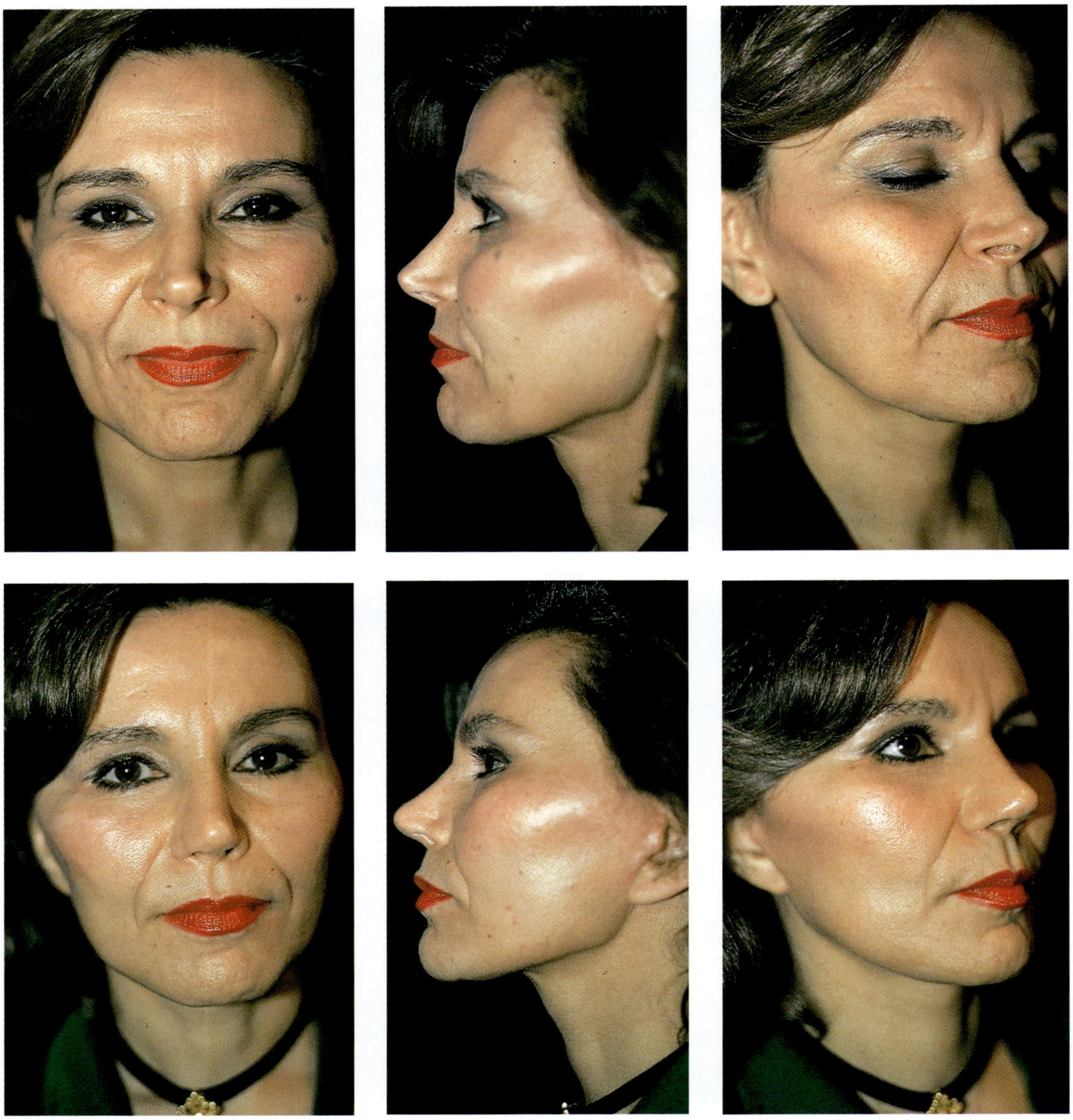

Figure 9. A 48-year-old patient who underwent a multiplane facelift, neck contouring, forehead rejuvenation, upper and lower eyelid blepharoplasty, and open rhinoplasty with cartilage and bone grafts to the nose. **A–C:** Pre-operative views; **D–F:** post-operative views.

developed separately, so that they can be treated individually, allowing for the more anterior attachment of the SMAS and more posterior anchoring of the nasolabial fold. Dissection is initiated in the peri-auricular region and after only a few centimeters descends into a sub-SMAS deep plane orientation. Dissection continues to the zygomaticus muscle and nasolabial folds, with the spreading scissor technique being used to avoid injury to the facial nerves. The flaps are then separated by starting laterally and proceeding medially across the nasolabial fold to release the zygomatic ligaments and the skin around the midface. The SMAS is advanced posteriorly and superiorly and is inset as a separate entity. The skin is then advanced and attached independently. The tragus is reconstructed by defatting the pretragal skin and recreating a normal-appearing depression.

One may close the galea with dissolvable sutures and use staples in the hair-bearing area. Sutures should be very fine: 5-0 or 6-0 in front of the ear, 4-0 chromic behind the ear, and catgut in the neck area.

Many patients receiving an extensive facelift may need further work in the central portion of the face. A fat graft may be used to fill out the junction of the vermilion of the upper and lower lips. Alternatively, a dermis graft or temporal fascia may be used to decrease the vermilion line and enhance the appearance of the lips.

Although we sometimes apply, very judiciously, trichloracetic acid to the perioral area, this can cause discoloration and should be used very rarely in Middle Eastern patients.

Earlobes

In some patients, the earlobes tend to elongate with age. The lobes can be corrected during the facelift by making an L-shaped incision through the entire width of the earlobe and repairing it in front and behind.

Postoperative Care for Facelift Patients

Tincture of benzoin is applied to the skin surface, and then Microfoam pressure dressing is placed over all surfaces that have been undermined. This eliminates the need for drains and reduces to a minimum the amount of ecchymosis that develops.

The dressing is removed the next day. Steroids, cold compresses, and elevation of the head can help to reduce swelling.

Chemical Peeling, Dermabrasion, and CO_2 Ultra-Pulse Laser (Figs. 10–12)

A surgeon discussing the possibility of treating a Middle Eastern patient with a chemical peeling agent should ensure that the patient understands and is willing to undergo the risk of permanent skin discoloration. The primary effect of peeling is depigmentation, and this may occur unevenly, depending on the patient's original skin color. Also, the darker the skin color, the more obvious will be the line of demarcation between the peeled and unpeeled skin.

The greatest beneficial effect of chemical peeling agents seems to be on light-skinned patients with sun-damaged skin. Ultraviolet radiation from the sun (or sun lamps) may unevenly increase the amount of melanin and the number of melanocytes in the skin and can lead to blotchiness. The epidermis, dermis, and basement membrane may thicken, with a disorderly arrangement of cells and dense masses of elastic fibers, and the superficial vessels may become irregular and variably dilated.

After treatment with a peeling agent, multiple spider telangiectasias may become more evident than previously and may not improve. Crusting usually disappears after 6–7 days, but there may be prolonged erythema, lasting sometimes $>$10–12 weeks. Milia may occur more frequently, beginning $\sim$6–8 weeks after treatment. The effects of dermabrasion may be similar, although not quite as severe.

For the first 24 h after dermabrasion or chemical peeling, an antibiotic ointment and moisturizers should be applied to the skin. Topical steroids (for example, Preparation H with cortisone) may be applied for a week or two. For several weeks after treatment, the skin should be kept well lubricated with moisturizers. The patient should be instructed to wash the skin vigorously, to burst the milia, and to avoid sunlight.

CO_2 ultra-pulse laser is used in a very conservative manner using millijoules per pulse with fewer passes. We prefer to use no dressing and keep the skin moist with A and E Ointment. To prevent hyperpigmentation, we instruct patients to use paste of Retin A (0.05%)

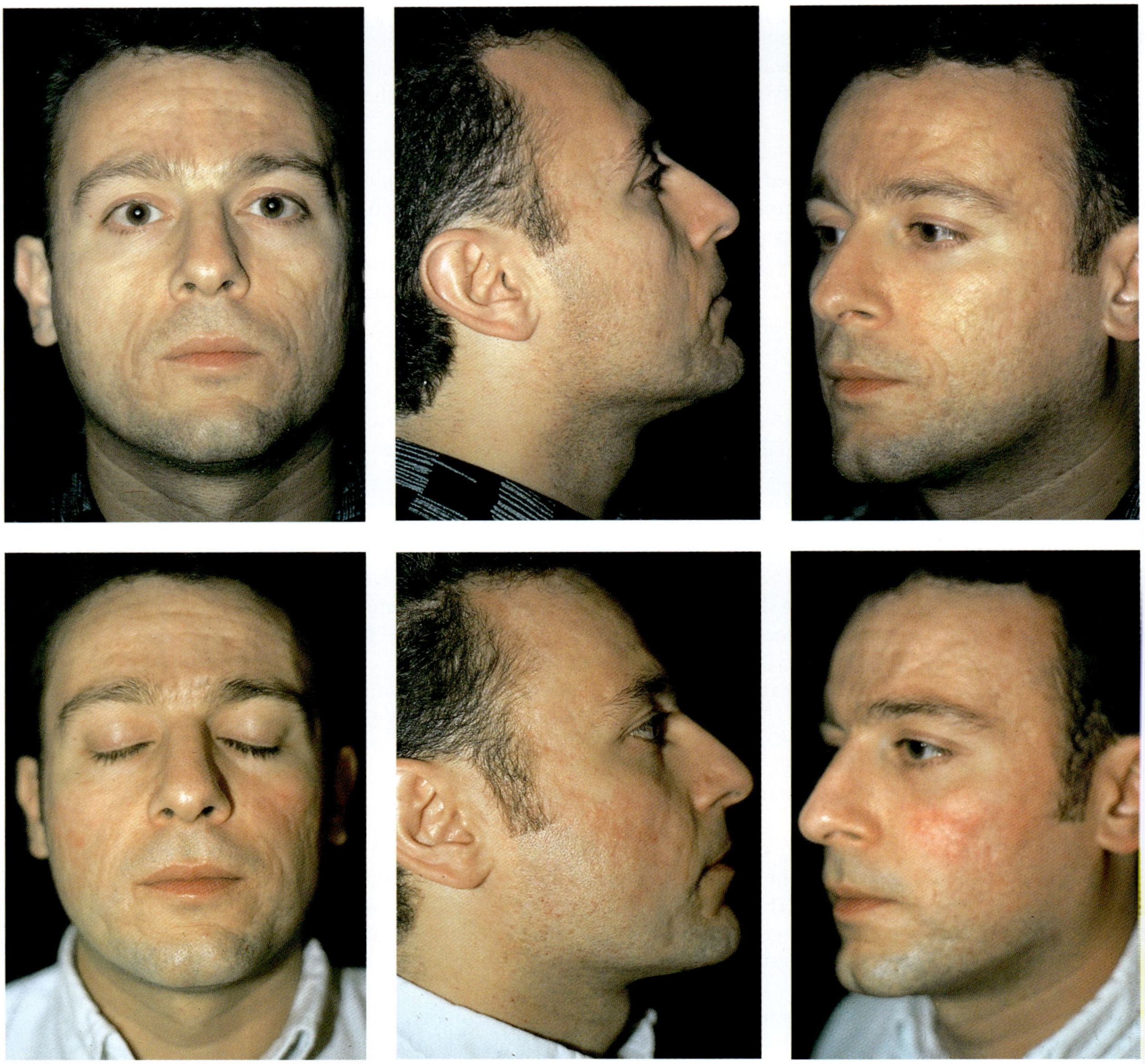

A–C

D–F

Figure 10. A 33-year-old man who underwent a single dermabrasion treatment. For further improvement, the patient may wish to undergo more treatment in the future. **A–C:** Pre-operative views; **D–F:** post-operative views.

and hydroquinine (4%) at night beginning 2 weeks after the initial treatment, for a period of 6 weeks. The patient should always use a moisturizer as well as a special make-up to cover prolonged redness (up to 4 months) during the day.

CONCLUSION

In treating patients from the Middle East, it is important to retain the natural beauty of their ethnic origins. Young patients as well as older ones need adequate counseling before

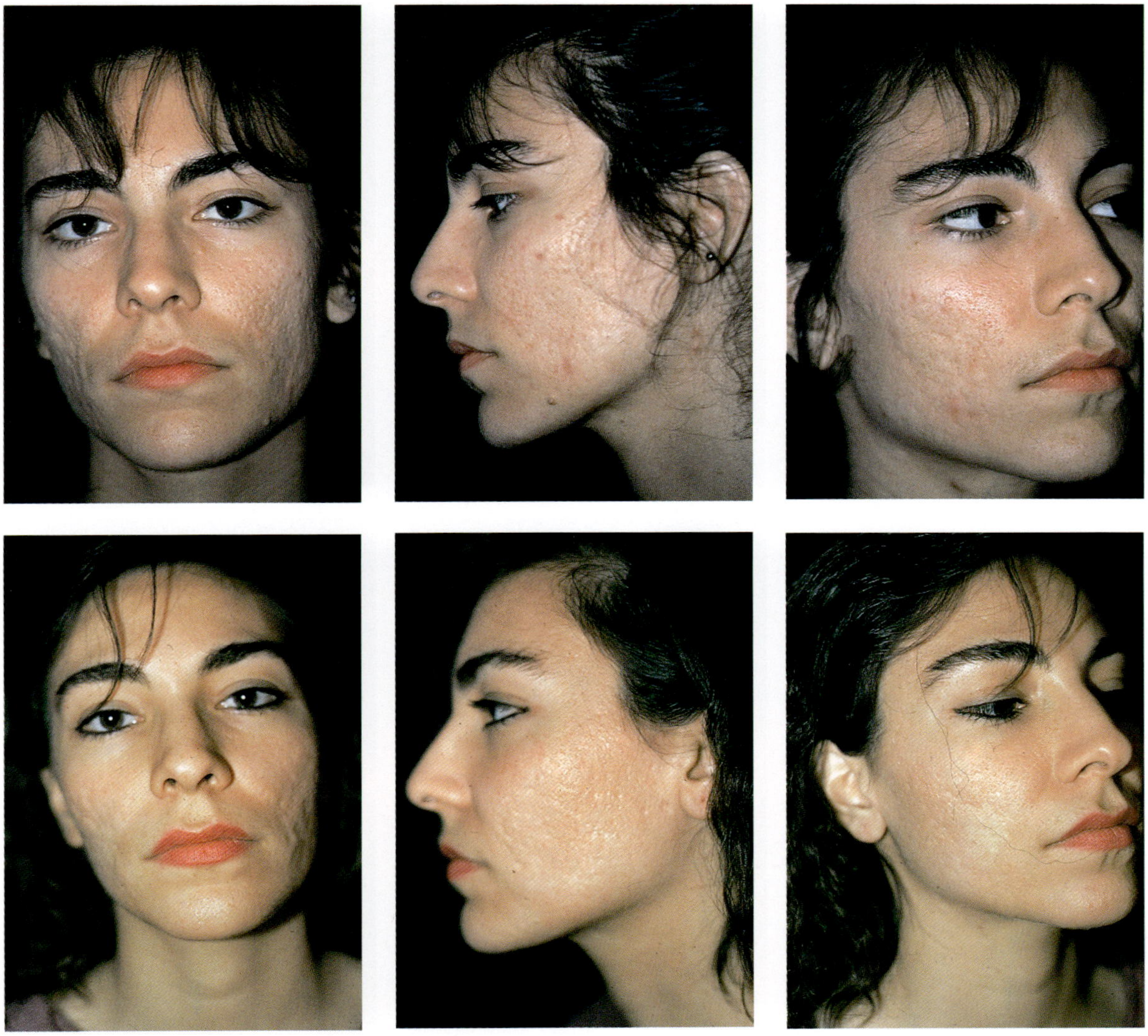

A–C

D–F

Figure 11. A 26-year-old patient who underwent dermabrasion. For further improvement, more dermabrasion will be necessary in the future. **A–C:** Pre-operative views; **D–F:** post-operative views.

surgery to determine their real wishes regarding the way they look and feel about themselves. Although it is impossible to make anyone look 30 years younger than their real age, careful minimal surgery can make the older patient appear less tired and fresher. This alone can also make them feel—and appear—12–15 years younger.

The risk of complications from facial surgery in Middle Eastern patients is no greater than in Nordic Caucasian patients and can usually be avoided by good selection of patients and by use of the best operative techniques and patient care. However, surgeons must be aware of the greater propensity for dark skin to undergo hypertrophic scarring and must make every effort to place incisions in areas where they will not be visible.

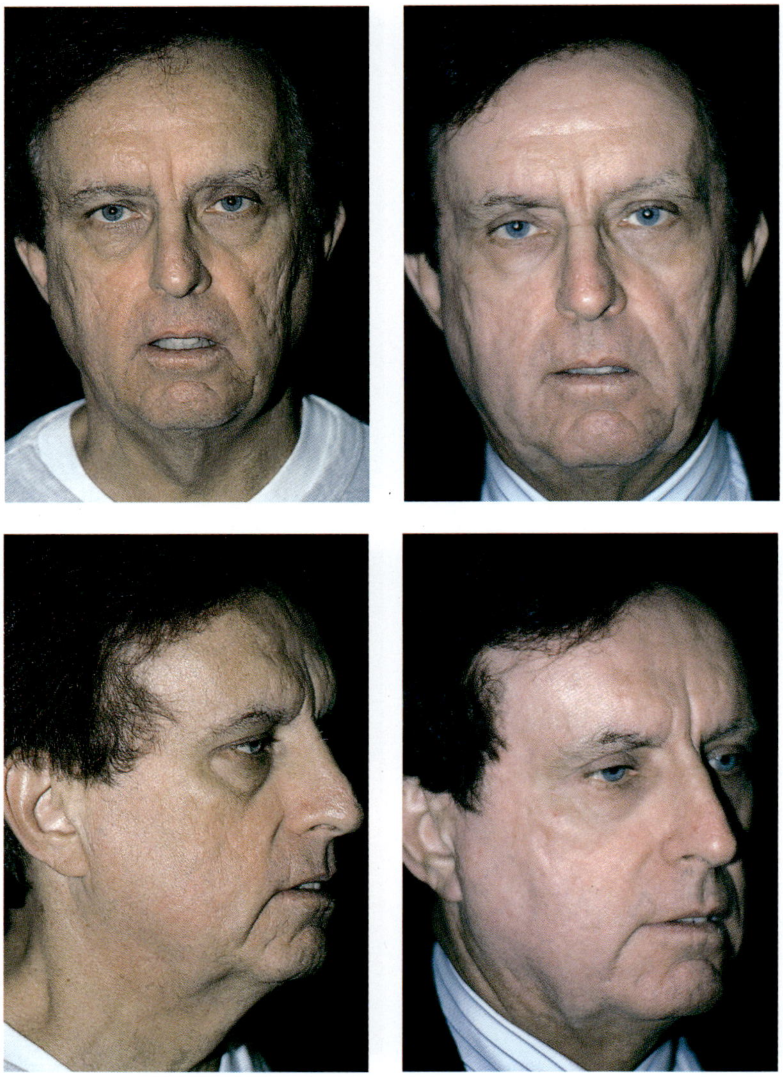

A, B

C, D

Figure 12. A 54-year-old patient who underwent CO_2 ultra-pulse laser treatment and lower eyelid blepharoplasty. **A and C:** Pre-operative views; **B and D:** post-operative views.

Suggested Reading

Baker TJ, Gordon HL. *Surgical rejuvenation of the face*. St. Louis: Mosby, 1986.

Eickelman DF. *The Middle East: an anthropological approach.* 2nd ed. Englewood Cliffs: Prentice Hall, 1989.

Goin JM, Goin MK. *Changing the body. Psychological effects of plastic surgery*. Baltimore: Williams & Wilkins, 1981:121–136.

Gonzalez-Ulloa M. The fat nose. *Aesthet Plast Surg* 1984;8:135.

Ortiz-Monasterio F, Lopez-Mas J, Araico J. Rhinoplasty in the thick-skinned nose. *Br J Plast Surg* 1974;27:19–24.

Rogers BO. The role of physical anthropology in plastic surgery today. *Clin Plast Surg* 1974;1:439–498.

Seltzer CC. Contributions to racial anthropology of the Near East. Boston: Harvard University Peabody Museum of American Archaeology and Ethnology, Papers, 1940:2.

Sheen JH, Sheen AP. *Aesthetic rhinoplasty*. 2nd ed. St. Louis: Mosby, 1987:711–719.

Stark RB. *Aesthetic plastic surgery*. 1st ed. Boston: Little, Brown.

Taheri A. *The cauldron: the Middle East behind the headlines*. London: Hutchinson, 1988:1–23.

Teimourian B, Mankani M, Stefan M. Limited-incision browplasty. Submitted.

Teimourian B. *Suction lipectomy and body contouring*. St. Louis: Mosby, 1987:34–38, 65–66, 68–69, 685–768.

Teimourian B, Wahrman A, Delia S. The multiplane facelift. *Plast Reconstr Surg* 1994;93.

Walter W. *Women in Islam*. Princeton: Weiner, 1993:183–220.

Ethnic Considerations in Facial Aesthetic Surgery, edited by W. Earle Matory, Jr.
Lippincott–Raven Publishers, Philadelphia © 1998.

28

The Middle Eastern Nose

Bahman Guyuron

There will be time to prepare a face to meet the faces you meet.
— from "The Love Song of J. Alfred Prufrock," T. S. Eliot

The last two decades have brought a more precise approach to the evaluation of soft tissue cephalometrics and the definition of ideal facial proportions (1–14). This methodology has aided in the detection and correction of imperfections of the nose without specific regard to ethnic background. By analyzing life-size photographs with the latest available techniques, one can precisely design the surgical alteration down to a fraction of 1 mm. With use of this analysis and the guidelines developed by this author, which are founded on scientific research, the surgery is performed with the highest precision (1–3). The common objective of nasal surgery is to achieve harmony and balance in the nose and face. Sharing these photographic and computer imaging results with the patient (who also needs to understand that results cannot be guaranteed) ensures a certain degree of mutual agreement of surgical goals.

On the other hand, strong emotional adherence to ethnicity may dictate alterations in the surgical plan. Some characteristics of the ethnic nose may better remain unaltered or altered less than what would be ideal for a European. These will include a lesser nasolabial angle (closer to 90°) and a straight dorsum with no supratip break for a male patient and a small supratip break for a female patient. It is not uncommon for an older Middle Eastern patient to undergo a combination of plastic surgery procedures such as facial rejuvenation and genioplasty. The ultimate surgical design is determined by a collaboration with the patient, using visual aids to minimize any misunderstandings. Awareness of the social and physical characteristics of the nose in the Middle Eastern patient is crucial to surgical planning and penultimate to a desirable outcome.

CULTURAL CONSIDERATIONS

Although an overprojected nasal tip is often observed in a patient with a Middle Eastern heritage, we find this to be more of an exception rather than a rule. Weakness of the caudal nasal frame contributes to a hanging columella.

B. Guyuron: Lyndhurst, Ohio 44124

Adolescent patients from the Mediterranean offer unique concerns. Parental influence is strong, tending to favor retention of ethnic physical stigmata. Conversely, the teens' sense of attractiveness is often altered by Western standards. One must make a concerted, often conflicting effort to satisfy the needs of the teen and parents. All decisions must be individualized. Awareness of the potential conflicts aids the surgeon in pre-operative counseling and pre-surgical planning.

Coagulopathies must be diagnosed and treated peri-operatively. If post-operative epistaxis occurs, the patient is advised to return to the medical center immediately.

Patients of Mediterranean descent may be highly critical of pre- and more importantly post-operative contour irregularities or asymmetries. In some patients, it may be appropriate to soften and reassure emotional dissatisfaction. More often than not, a judicious and sometimes expeditious correction of the deformity will lead to the quickest resolve. Surgical judgment and reassuring support are crucial to assessing and appropriately treating the patient.

In this patient population, it is crucial to define bleeding and bruising tendencies. This may disclose the need for further investigation to reveal coagulation abnormalities that may otherwise go undetected. It is the author's clinical impression that coagulation abnormalities such as Von Willebrand's disease are somewhat more prevalent in the Middle Eastern population, although this has not been scientifically documented. Further questioning may also disclose the consumption of medications that may, directly or indirectly, disturb the integrity of the coagulation system. There is a tendency to use pharmaceutical products more casually. The patient's medical history should be diligent with particular regard to those conditions that the patient may not perceive to have relevance to nose surgery, such as diabetes. The paradox between the patient's full knowledge of his/her individual nasal abnormalities and his/her abstinence from divulging information pertinent to overall health can be misleading and consequential.

FACIAL CHARACTERISTICS

Common features of the Middle Eastern face include hyperpigmented thick skin, a significantly overprojected radix (often providing an illusion of hypotelorism, with measurements of the intercanthal distance proving otherwise), absolute hypertelorism, narrow anterior dorsum, and widened nasal bones at the nasofacial junction (Table 1). The nasal bones are usually long. The upper lateral cartilages are broad, while the lower lateral cartilages are commonly thin and cephalically extended with weak domes. The tip is generally wide and amorphic with particularly thick skin. The alar bases are frequently asymmetric and cephalically displaced. The columella is disproportionately extended caudally. Nasal asymmetry and midline skeletal and cartilaginous deviation are routinely encountered.

On profile, the radix is often overprojected. This may create a straight-line transition from the forehead to the dorsum, requiring a reduction to create a 4- to 6-mm depression at the level of the upper eyelid folds. However, the radix may also be normal or underprojected. There is almost always a dorsal hump and the tip is underprojected, resulting in relative excess projection of the supratip. The lobule and the tip complex are rotated caudally. The anterior columella extends caudally and is highly visible. The nasolabial angle is acute and is usually the consequence of excess anterior nasal length or a caudally displaced columella and for hypoplasia of the anterior nasal spine. The cephalic position of the alar base is more readily appreciated in the lateral view. The slightest smile results in caudal and posterior movement of the tip and additional narrowing of the nasolabial angle. Internal nasal examination often discloses septal deviation and possibly enlargement of the inferior turbinates.

Questions concerning breathing difficulties also may result in misleading conclusions. While the patient may deny any breathing difficulties, an internal nasal examination may reveal a significant degree of obstruction. Although this is not unique to Middle Eastern patients, it is commonly observed in this patient population. This in general relates to the fact that the patients have never experienced any other way of breathing to make a comparison,

Table 1. *Preoperative evaluation of the Middle Eastern nose*

Front view	
Intercanthal distance	Increased
	Decreased
Dorsum	Asymmetric
	Narrow
	Wide
Tip	Thick skin
	Thin skin
	Narrow
	Wide
Columella	Hanging
	Retracted
Alar base	Wide
	Narrow
	Asymmetric
Intercanthal distance	Increased
	Decreased
Profile	
Radix	Underprojected
	Overprojected
Dorsum	Underprojected
	Hump
Tip	Overprojected
	Underprojected
Columella	Hanging
	Retracted
Nasal spine	Hyperplastic
	Hypoplastic
Nasolabial angle	Obtuse
	Narrow
Alar base	Cephalic displacement
	Caudal displacement

unless the problem is post-traumatic. Under the latter circumstances, the patient usually has concise statements concerning breathing difficulties, which relate to the injury.

OPERATIVE TECHNIQUE

This author prefers general anesthesia for septorhinoplasty and local anesthesia with intravenous sedation for rhinoplasty alone. Due to the complex nasal morphology, we prefer to use an open (exonasal) technique.

The nose is infiltrated with xylocaine containing 1:200,000 epinephrine. The surgical scrub will allow enough time for the vasoconstrictive effect of the epinephrine. Prior to incision, the nose is reinjected with xylocaine containing more concentrated 1:100,000 epinephrine. This optimizes vasoconstriction while minimizing systemic reabsorption of the higher epinephrine concentration.

When indicated, the septoplasty and/or turbinectomy are performed first. This will also prevent inadvertent distortion of the realigned structures during septoplasty. If the latter is conducted subsequent to rhinoplasty, nasal bleeding and swelling can be reduced by an immediate application of the packing and splint upon completion of rhinoplasty.

The nose frame is then exposed through an exonasal approach using a step columellar incision. For a nose with thick skin, the soft tissue tip flap is dissected in a deep subcutaneous plane, raising a healthy and thick flap, but leaving the excess fat and perichondrium attached to the nasal frame. The frame is then skeletonized, discarding the excess bulk of soft tissue. The cephalic margins of the lower lateral cartilages are then resected, leaving a strip of cartilage 4–5 mm wide. The lateral crura are left 6–7 mm wide for a female and even wider for a male.

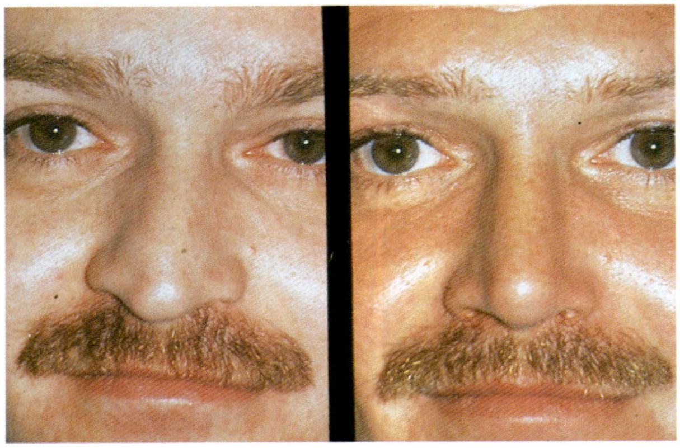

Figure 1. Patient with a typical Middle Eastern nose exhibiting asymmetric nasal bones with widened upper lateral cartilages, deviation of the nose to the right, wide alar bases, and asymmetric alar domes on frontal view *(left)*. In the year following, correction of all these abnormalities *(right)*.

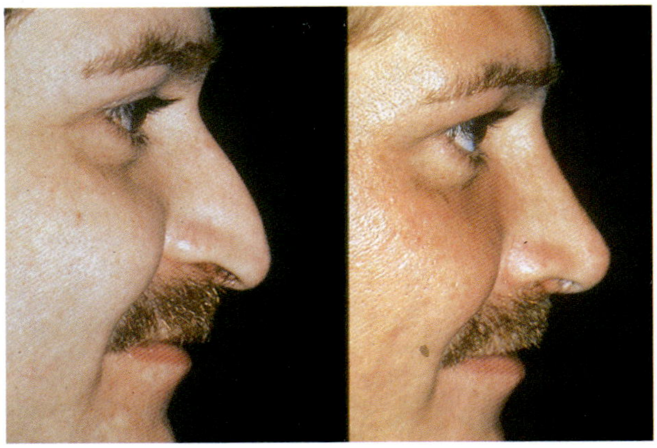

Figure 2. The profile view of the same patient pre-operatively exhibiting a low radix, a small dorsal hump, underprojected tip, narrow nasolabial angle, and weak columella with excess alar rim/columella distance pre-operatively *(left)*. The same patient following the application of a slightly crushed septal cartilage graft to the radix, removal of the dorsal hump, creation of better nasal tip projection with a columellar strut, and placement of graft in the nasal spine area *(right)*.

Removal of the lower lateral cartilage exposes the upper lateral cartilages. Careful dissection and preservation of the nasal lining reduce the necessity for the use of spreader grafts. The radix is reduced using a guarded burr as described by this author (18). The cartilaginous hump is then removed using a no. 11 blade, and the upper lateral cartilages are trimmed using a pair of serrated scissors. The dorsum is reduced to create a 34° angle with the facial plane in a female and a 36° angle in a male. A lateral low-to-low or high-to-low osteotomy using a Parkes osteotome and a vertical osteotomy using a transcutaneous 2-mm osteotome are performed (1). The osteotomy is started high to prevent moving the turbinates medially, then it is continued low to avoid step deformity. This osteotomy is taken cephalically at the level of the nasion (upper lid fold), continued caudally, and terminated at the level of medial canthus. A medial osteotomy is optional, depending on the width and thickness of the cephalic portion of the nasal bones. This, however, is often unnecessary on a Middle Eastern patient. A combination of membranous septum and septal

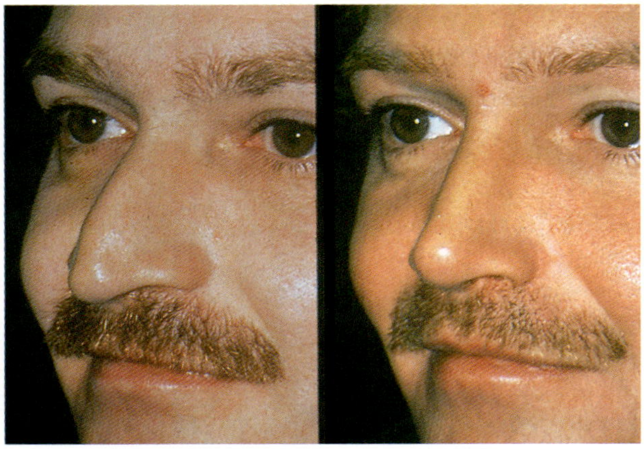

Figure 3. Pre-operative oblique view of the same patient *(left)* and following correction of the deformities *(right)*.

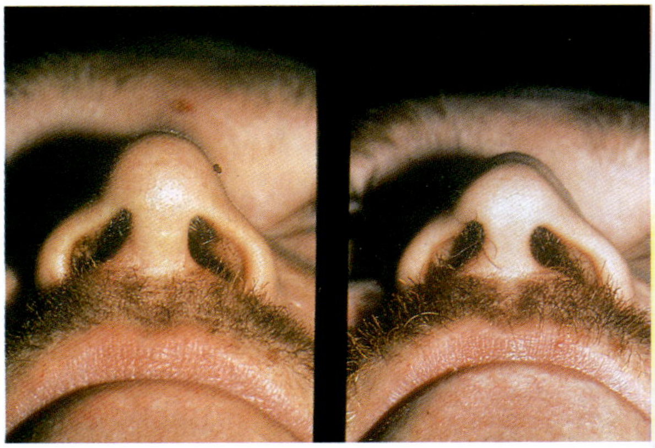

Figure 4. Pre-operative basilar view, exhibiting the short columella, underprojected lobule, and wide alar bases *(left)*. View following improvement of tip projection, lengthening of the columella, and narrowing of the alar bases *(right)*.

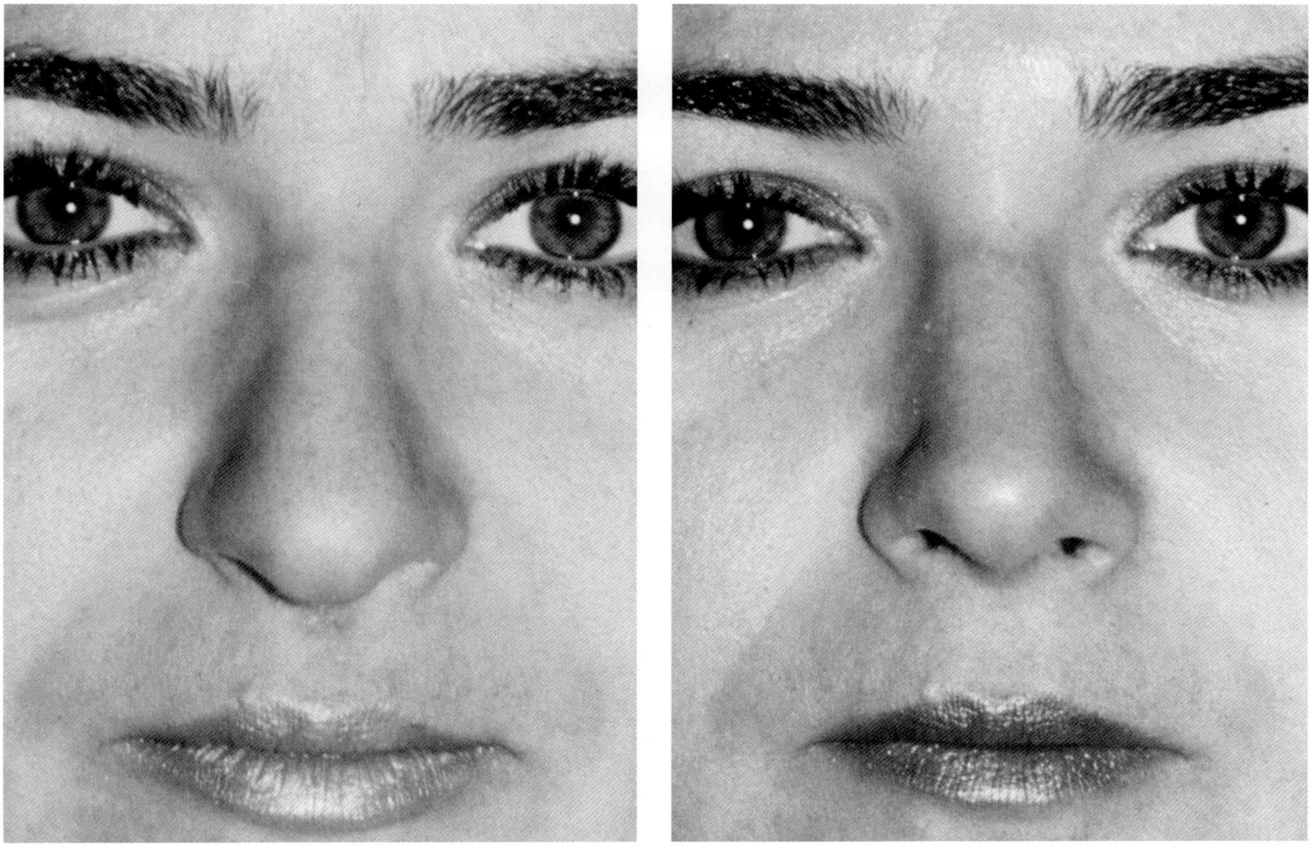

Figure 5. Pre-operative front view of patient exhibiting narrow dorsum, wide tip, and inadequate nostril show *(left)* and following rhinoplasty with removal of the hump, osteotomy, removal of the cephalic margin of the lower lateral cartilages, narrowing of the tip, and shortening of the cephalocaudal nasal dimension, illustrating a more pleasing outline of the nose *(right)*.

cartilage is resected in a wedge shape, which is based anteriorly and incorporates all of the loose tissue between the caudal septum and cephalic border of the medial crura to allow cephalic rotation of the tip, if the surgical plan demands it. Should there be an anterior deviation of the septum, which is not corrected with septoplasty, a spreader graft or an onlay graft is applied or scored to the concave side.

At this point, attention is directed to the creation of adequate tip projection and definition. This is probably one of the most crucial and difficult stages of surgery on the Middle Eastern nose. To do so, the medial crura are fully dissected. A strong, straight piece of septal cartilage is prepared as a columellar strut. If the septal cartilage is not an appropriate size or shape, conchal cartilage is utilized. The medial crura are then spread, and the columella strut is placed with the posterior end supported on the anterior nasal spine. It is important to fix the graft in position to avoid caudal rotation. It is seldom necessary to narrow the medial crura in a cephalocaudal dimension by trimming the caudal border of the cartilage in an attempt to correct the "hanging columella." More commonly, this trait is a consequence of weak medial crura buckling in. The mere introduction of a columellar strut often will correct this undesirable feature.

After the columella strut is fixed in position with 5-0 white Mersilene, the medial crura and the domes are repositioned and sewn to the columellar strut. If narrowing of the tip is intended, the sutures are placed through the domes. If the footplates are divergent, they are dissected through the transfixion incision and sewn to each other and the columellar strut with 5-0 sutures. This augments the tip projection and narrows the columellar base. How-

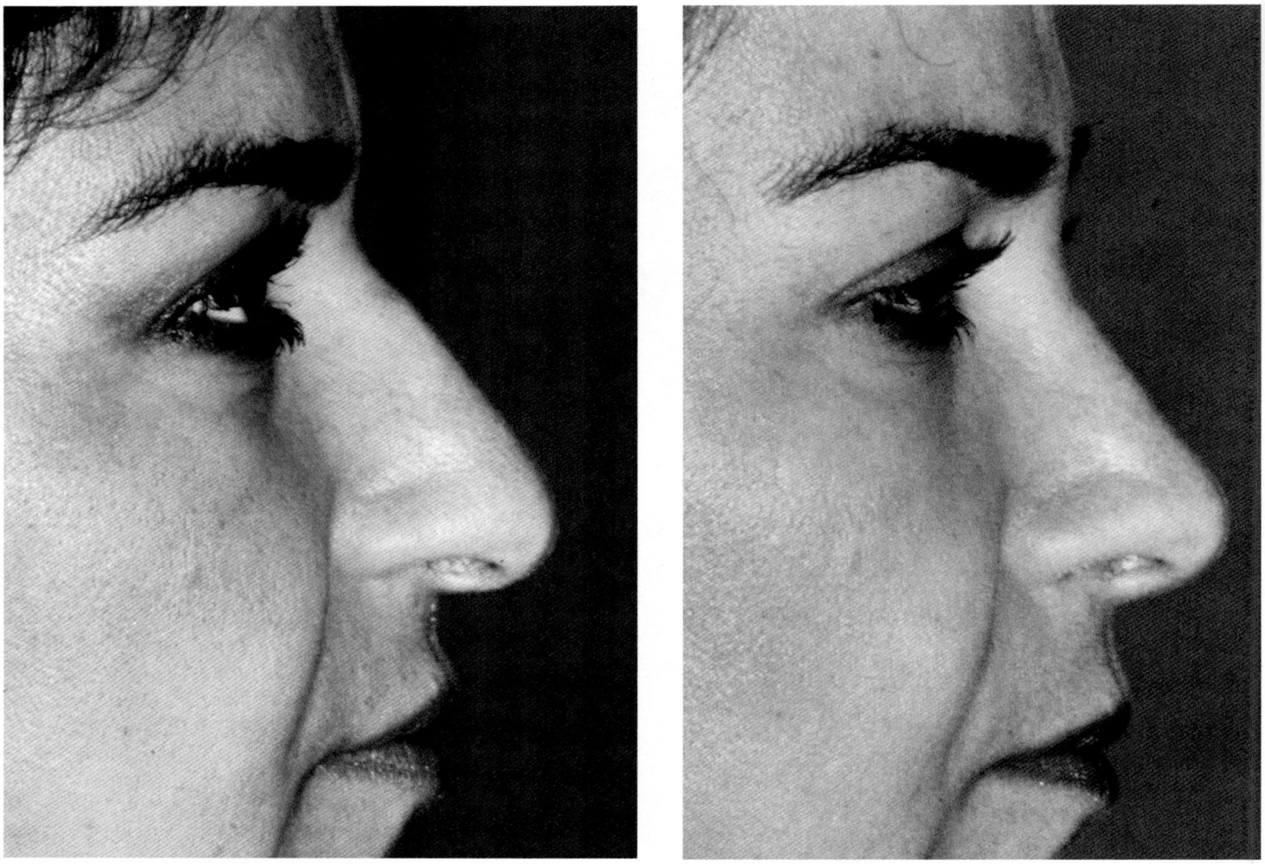

Figure 6. Pre-operative profile view of the patient demonstrating dorsal hump and a narrow nasolabial angle *(left)* and following conservative removal of the dorsal hump and cephalic rotation of the tip *(right)*.

ever, if the domes are in a desirable position, the stitch is placed through the medial genu to prevent excess narrowing of the tip. The pre-operatively wide alar bases now may or may not need narrowing, since the increased tip projection has reduced the alar base width. The alar bases can also be moved caudally, if necessary. Generally, this is necessary on a patient who also exhibits a wide alar base. Mere reduction of the base also may move the alar base caudally in some patients. Others will need an incision along the alar/facial groove and excision of the upper lip skin at the desired site for the alar base to allow caudal repositioning and repair of the alar base. The width of the alar base should be ~2 mm wider than the palpebral fissure.

Should the columella strut not provide adequate tip projection, then onlay cartilage grafts from the septum can be used (15–17). The incisions are then repaired using 6-0 plain catgut for the columellae and alar rim incision and a splint is applied (Figs. 1–8). If a septoplasty has been performed, the nose is packed. The splint is usually removed in eight days and the packing is removed in 24 h. Our studies have proved that use of packing significantly improves the airway.

DISCUSSION

The most important issue in dealing with the Middle Eastern patient is understanding the patient's objectives. Many patients of Middle Eastern background are not interested in having a nose that might satisfy a patient of European descent. Minimalism will result in greater patient satisfaction in this patient population. Often this conservatism translates into

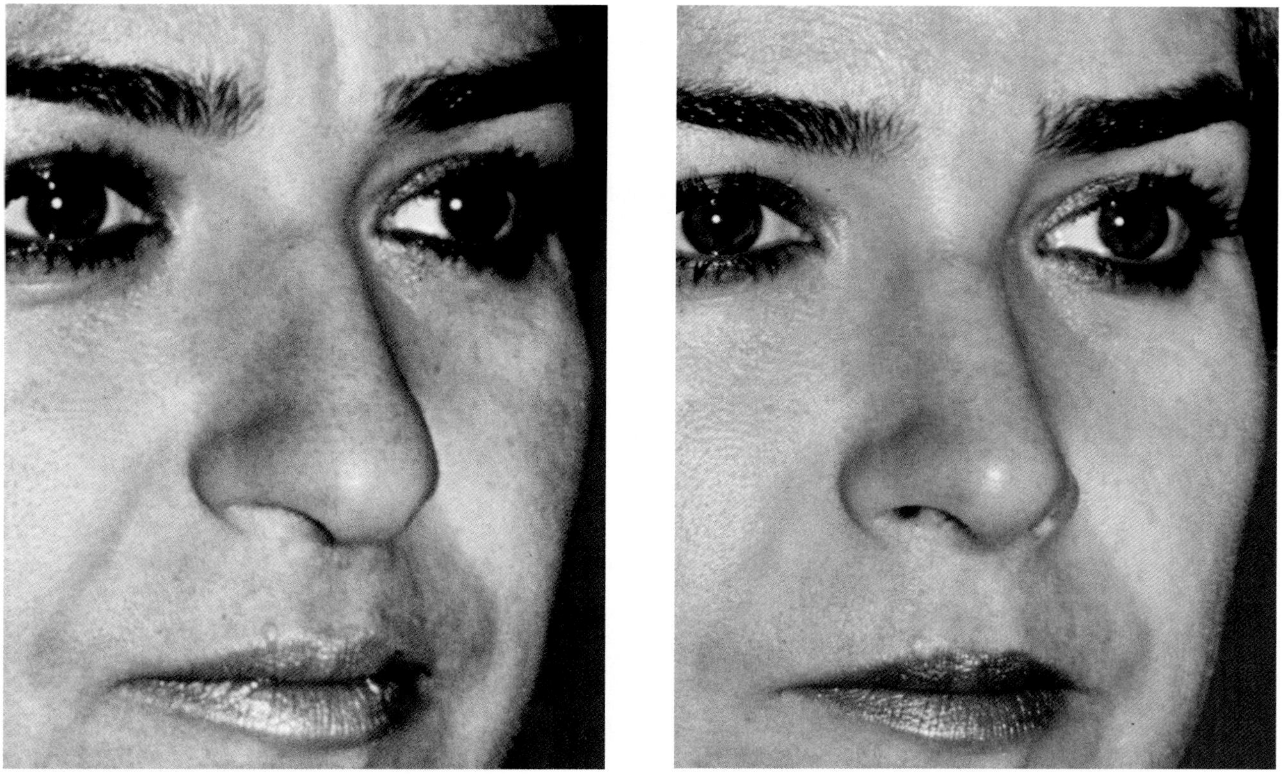

Figure 7. Oblique view of the patient pre-operatively *(left)* and following correction of the above deformities *(right)*.

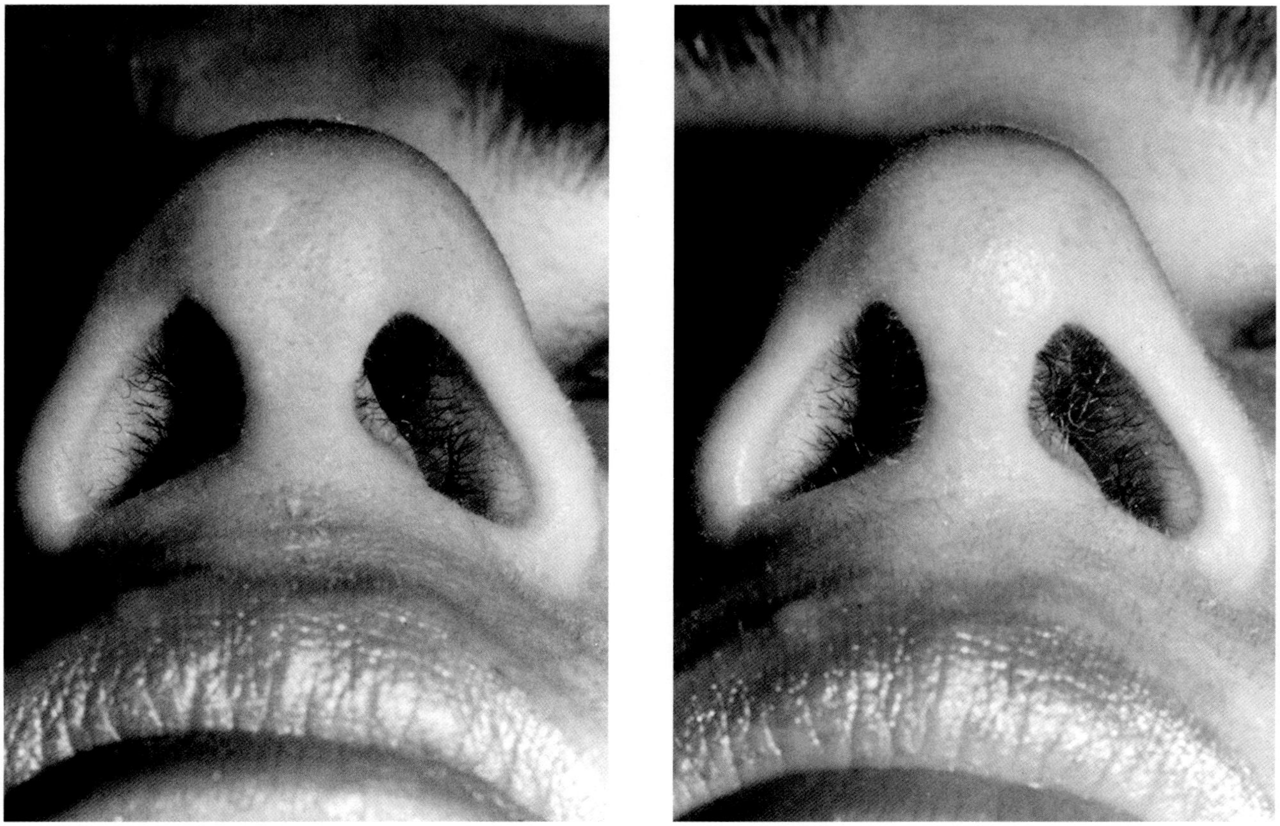

Figure 8. Basilar view exhibiting minimal abnormalities pre-operatively *(left)* and following correction of nasal disharmony *(right)*.

leaving more dorsal projection and a lesser degree of nasolabial angle than might be desired by the Caucasian. The nasolabial angle should be restored to ~90° for a male and 100° for a female. The dorsum should be as straight as possible. Familiarity with techniques that are aimed at nasal reduction is essential when encountering Middle Eastern noses.

REFERENCES

1. Guyuron B. Precision rhinoplasty I—role of life-size photographs on soft tissue cephalometric analysis. *Plast Reconstr Surg* 1988;81:489–499.
2. Guyuron B. Precision rhinoplasty II—prediction. *Plast Reconstr Surg* 1988;81:500–505.
3. Guyuron B. Dynamics of rhinoplasty. *Plast Reconstr Surg* 1991;88:970–979.
4. Guyuron B. Patient evaluation for rhinoplasty. In: Toledo LS, ed. *Annals of the recent advances in plastic surgery. III International Symposium.* Brazil: Editoria e Grafica Estadao, 1992:86–90.
5. Goetz J, Guyuron B. Cephalometrics. In: Shons AR, Jensen RM, eds. *Plastic surgery review.* Philadelphia: Saunders, 1992:264–268.
6. Guyuron B. Nasal proportions. In: Gruber RP, Peck GC, eds. Rhinoplasty: state of the art. Chicago: Mosby, 1992:13–28.
7. Guyuron B. Predictive rhinoplasty. In: Daniel RK, ed. *Aesthetic plastic surgery: rhinoplasty.* 2nd ed. Boston: Little, Brown, 1992:109–126.
8. Guyuron B, Cohen S. In: Ferraro J, ed. *Fundamentals of Maxillofacial Surgery.* New York: Springer-Verlag, 1997:224–232.
9. Colton JJ, Beekhuis GJ. Rhinoplasty analysis. *Otolaryngol Clin North Am* 1987;20:675–698.
10. Gonzales-Ulloa M. Quantitative principles in cosmetic surgery of the face (profileplasty). *Plast Reconstr Surg* 1962;29:186.
11. Larrabee WF. Facial analysis for rhinoplasty. *Otolaryngol Clin North Am* 1987;20:653–674.
12. Daniel RK, Lessard ML. Rhinoplasty: a graded aesthetic-anatomical approach. *Ann Plast Surg* 1984;13:436–451.
13. Farkas LG, Kolar JC, Munro IR. Geography of the nose: a morphometric study. *Aesthet Plast Surg* 1986;10:191–223.
14. Fontana AM. The nasofrontal angle and profile in rhinoplasty: case presentations. *Aesthet Plast Surg* 1983;7:169–170.
15. Gruber RP, Peck GC, eds. *Rhinoplasty: state of the art.* St. Louis: Mosby Year Book, 1993.
16. Peck GC. *Techniques in aesthetic rhinoplasty.* New York: Thieme-Stratton, 1984.
17. Peck GC. *Techniques in aesthetic rhinoplasty.* 2nd ed. Philadelphia: Lippincott, 1990.

SECTION XI

The Northern European Patient

Ethnic Considerations in Facial Aesthetic Surgery, edited by W. Earle Matory, Jr.
Lippincott–Raven Publishers, Philadelphia © 1998.

29

The Northern European Patient

Editor's Commentary

W. Earle Matory, Jr.

The concept of broad, narrow, and moderate facial features can be depicted in the Caucasian model (Fig. 1). Similar features are noted in the teen (Fig. 2).

NOSE

The thick amorphous tip with diastasis or boxiness can be addressed using some of the same techniques noted within this text. In Fig. 3, slight dorsal rasping, nasal infracture, along with cephalic resection of the lower lateral cartilage was followed by use of an M-strut to lengthen and define the nasal tip. Interalar reduction was performed for alar base narrowing.

A similar technique was used in Fig. 4 incorporating cephalic rotation of the nasal tip and suture fixation of the lower lateral cartilage to the septum. Dorsal hump deformity and septal deviation were corrected by submucous resection and spreader graft fixation to the septum (Fig. 5). Thinness of the dorsal skin may show dorsal deformities following rasping or osteotomy. Use of a crushed septal cartilage graft can cover grafted areas.

W. E. Matory, Jr.: A New You Plastic Surgery Medical Group, Irvine, California 92714

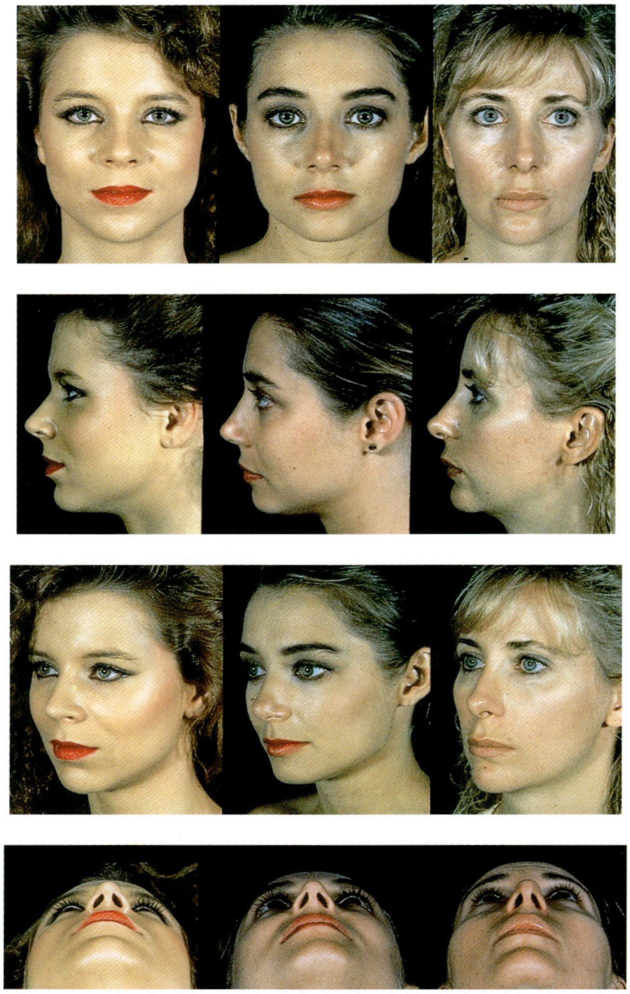

Figure 1. The facies of Northern European descent have many features common to attractiveness in any ethnic group, including an oval face, prominent cheekbones, a smooth, natural jawline, and a nose in proportion to the eyes, lips, and face.

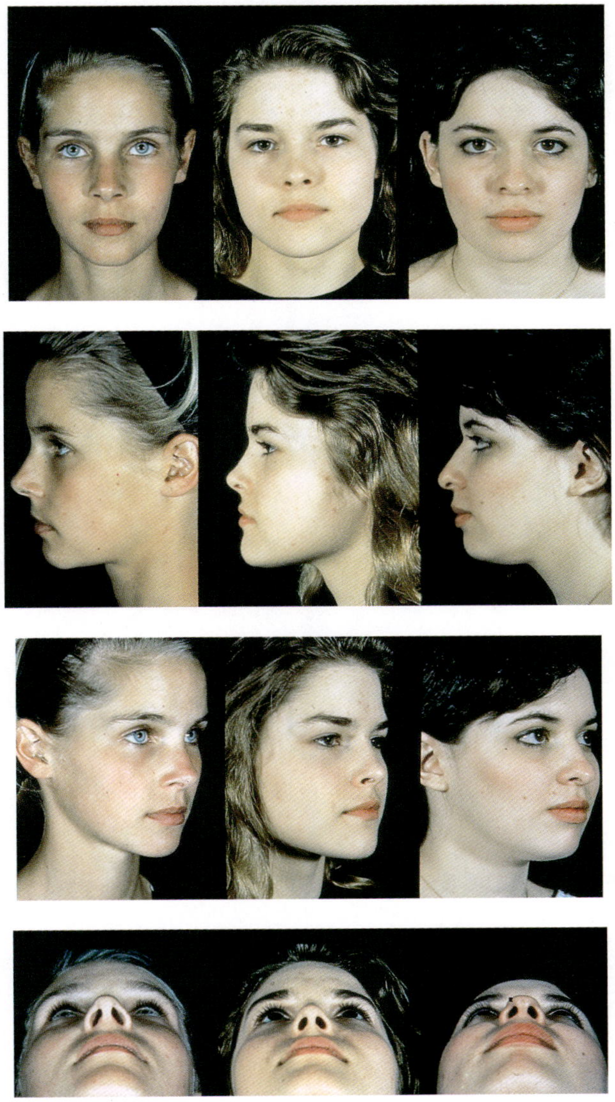

Figure 2. These same features are prevalent in the attractive teen. However, the lower third of the face tends to be somewhat delayed in its development of fullness to achieve an oval contour.

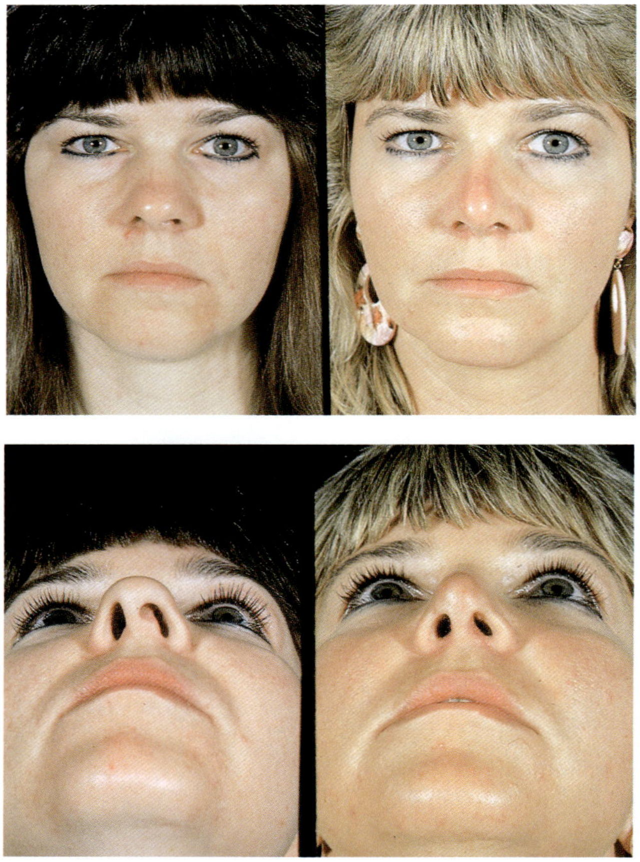

Figure 3. The case with an amorphous, poorly defined, and bifid tip with septal deviation and asymmetry of the columella is preferably addressed using an open approach to allow tip contouring with suture fixation of a domal spanning graft. Septal cartilage is used to augment the dorsum using a 28 × 4 × 3–mm crushed septal cartilage graft. Mattress sutures were used to bring the medial footplates to the midline. An M-strut was used to optimize tip projection and length. Results are noted at 18 months.

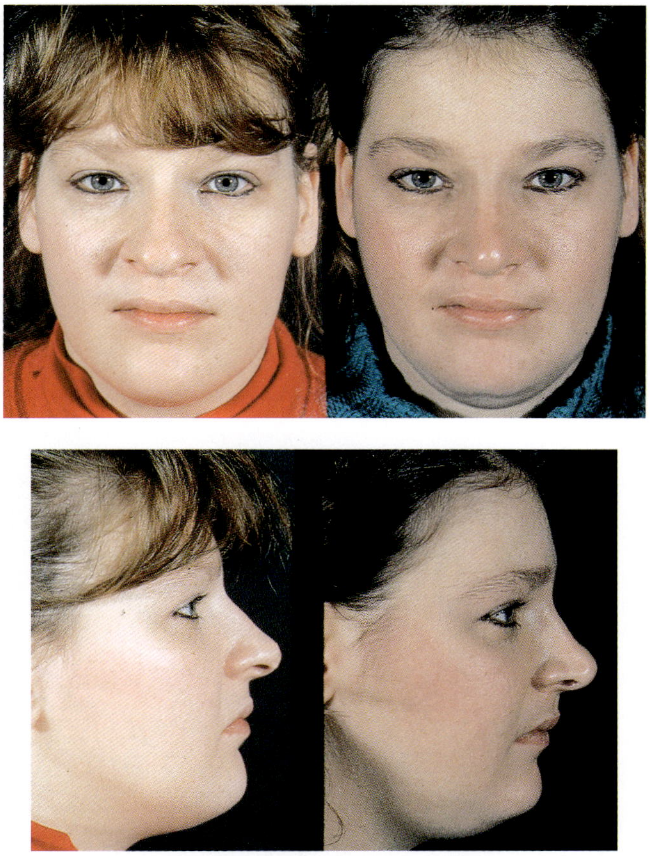

Figure 4. This bifid tip with alar notching was addressed with cephalic resection of the lower lateral cartilage and 2-mm trimming of the distal septal cartilage to achieve cephalic rotation of the tip. Light dorsal rasping was also accomplished. Results are shown at 16 months *(bottom)*.

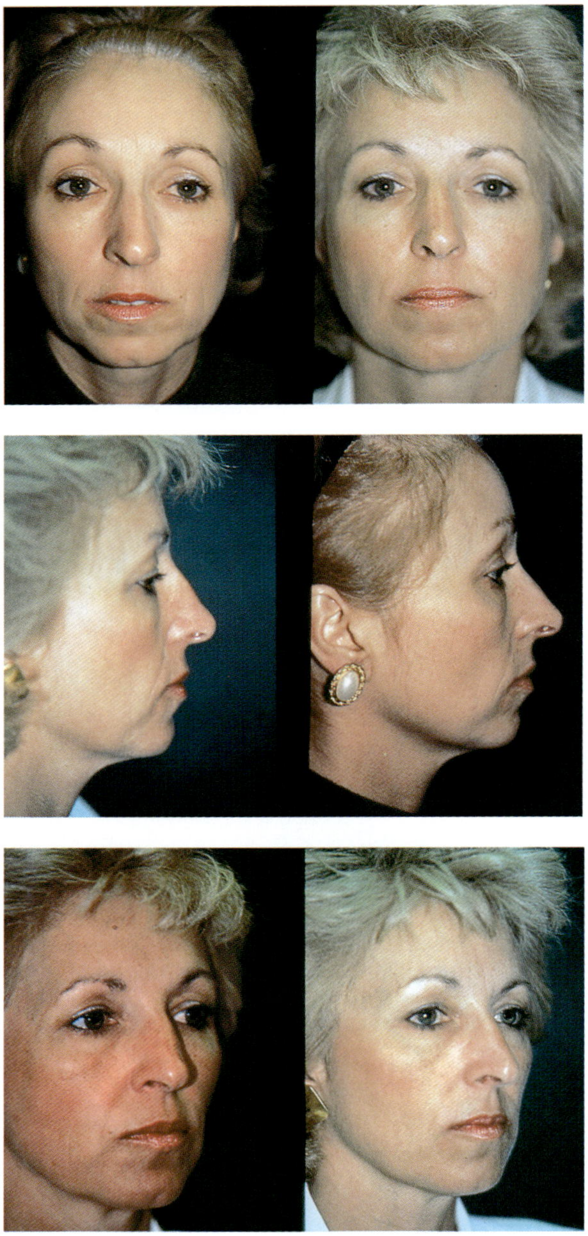

Figure 5. Physiologic obstruction of the nasal valve caused by a deviated nasal septum was addressed using cartilage scoring of the septum and fixation with mattress sutures. Dorsal rasping with a small cartilaginous hump resection achieved this result noted at 18 months.

Ethnic Considerations in Facial Aesthetic Surgery, edited by W. Earle Matory, Jr.
Lippincott–Raven Publishers, Philadelphia © 1998.

30

Rhinoplasty in the Northern European Patient

Brian P. Maloney
and E. Gaylon McCollough

We are what we repeatedly do. Excellence, then, is not an act, but a habit.
— Aristotle

The region known as Northern Europe generally refers to the countries of Germany, Poland, Belgium, Norway, Finland, Denmark, the Netherlands, and possibly portions of Russia. The physical characteristics of the people of this region are as heterogeneous as the geography of this scenic region of the globe. Although rhinoplasty is a patient-specific operation, some generalities can be made regarding the procedure when performed in certain ethnic populations within this region. This chapter will focus on individuals of European descent that have platyrrhine features.

THE LEPTORRHINE NOSE

Many patients of Northern European ancestry have tall, slender, or leptorrhine noses. The term "leptorrhine" (Greek *leptos*—slender, Greek *rhis*—nose) was originally used by anthropologists to differentiate this classic Caucasian nose from flatter, broader noses and wider nostrils, i.e., platyrrhine and mesorrhine noses. The leptorrhine nose has a high nasal dorsum, with long medial and lateral crural legs that provide support to the nasal tip. The nasal skin is thin, frequently allowing the experienced eye to discern the outline of the lower lateral cartilages, or thick, obscuring the underlying structures.

The general conditions to be corrected involve reducing structures that contribute to the excessive length of the nose, projection of the tip, and height of the dorsum. This fact gen-

B. P. Maloney: Atlanta, Georgia 30338
E. G. McCollough: Birmingham, Alabama 35205-4916

erally places the surgeon in better control of the operation in that the vagaries of healing associated with grafts and augmentation materials may be lessened (2–6).

PLATYRRHINE AND LEPTORRHINE NOSES—SURGICAL ANATOMY

One key to successful rhinoplasty lies in a working knowledge of the dynamic anatomy of the nose. This includes an understanding of which structures are producing the undesirable characteristics of the nose in question and which surgical maneuvers have the resulting effect of creating the desired postoperative architecture.

Bony Cartilaginous Vault

Analysis of the bony cartilaginous vault can be performed by gently palpating the structures. The paired nasal bones generally make up less than one-third of the osseocartilaginous hump. The cartilaginous vault, composed of the paired upper lateral cartilages and the nasal septum, generally makes up the majority of the osseocartilaginous hump. The upper lateral cartilages extend cephalically several millimeters underneath the nasal bones. The cartilages fuse to the septum in the midline and extend laterally to the frontal process of the maxilla. The caudal end of the upper lateral cartilage attaches to the cephalic edge of the lower lateral cartilage in a scroll or S-shaped fashion (Fig. 1).

The cartilaginous septum connects the ethmoid bone posteriorly to the nasal spine, providing midline support to the nasal bones and upper and lower lateral cartilages. The attachment of the quadrangular cartilage to the undersurface of the nasal bones becomes an important area of support after submucous resection. A continuous strip of cartilage must be maintained from the ethmoid bone to the insertion at the nasal spine; otherwise collapse of the nasal dorsum may need augmenting. Since the dorsal nasal height is generally not excessive, the surgeon should plan a conservative submucous resection anticipating the amount of dorsal cantilever to be preserved for support (Fig. 2).

The soft tissues of the nose are thickest at the nasion and supratip area and thinnest at the

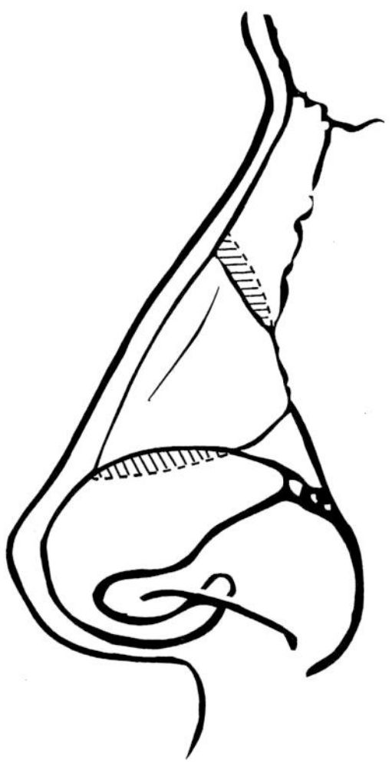

Figure 1. The upper lateral cartilages attach to the undersurface of the nasal bones superiorly (striped area) and the undersurface of the lower lateral cartilages inferiorly (striped area). After hump removal and tip modifications, the only remaining support for the upper lateral cartilage is superiorly under the nasal bones and laterally at the pyriform aperture.

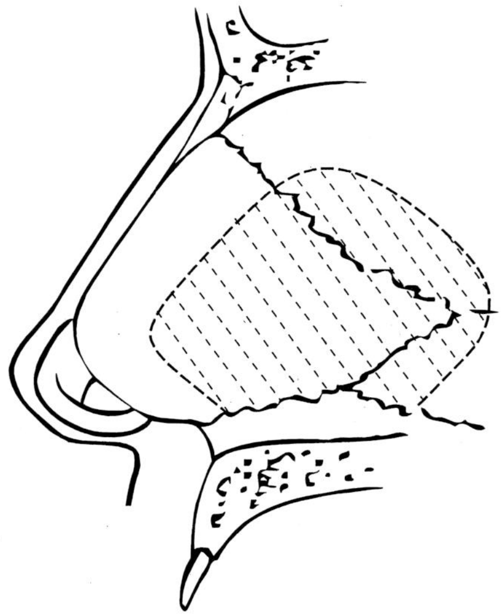

Figure 2. Striped area shows area removed with submucous resection. When lowering the dorsum in the Northern European patient, it is important to remember to preserve a continuous strip of cartilage extending from the nasal bones to the nasal spine. This will help prevent collapse of the central nose post-operatively.

rhinion. Skin thickness can vary from thin to thick among Northern European noses. The thinner the skin, the more irregularities are potentially visible. The procerus muscle can contribute to the soft tissue thickness at the nasion and Pitanguy's ligament can contribute to supratip fullness. The size of the lobule is not necessarily indicative of skin thickness. Large alar cartilages and thin skin may be as contributory as thick skin and thin frail cartilages.

Dorsal augmentation may be achieved by a number of methods. Autologous materials (septal or auricular cartilage) are preferable; however, in some cases, alloplastic materials and homologous materials may be used.

Nasal Tip

Due to the extreme variation in nasal tip anatomy in the Northern European population, the surgeon needs a working knowledge of tip relationships. The dynamics of tip modification are based upon the tripod concept of projection and rotation. The combined anatomical conformation of the two alar cartilages and the thickness of the overlying skin determine the extent of nasal tip definition that can be attained. Changing the shape of the tip is achieved by modifying the length and strength of the legs as well as the base, which supports this limb of the tripod. Experience has shown that noses with thick skin generally require more aggressive tip cartilage-narrowing techniques to obtain the desired post-operative refinements. Generally, the thicker the skin, the longer the post-operative tip edema will persist, commonly up to 12–18 months in cases of thick skin.

The shape and intrinsic strength of the medial crura can play a more crucial role in the tip support than is often appreciated, especially when their length extends to the columellar base. This factor is usually lacking in the platyrrhine nose. If the medial crura extend only a short distance along the length of the columella, disruption of their attachment to the caudal septum destroys much of this critical support mechanism. After surgery and during healing, the feet of the medial crura may settle until they rest at a level that will become the new columellar base, resulting in loss of tip projection. To prevent extreme settling when it is necessary to detach the medial crura from the caudal septum by a complete and/or lateral transfixion incision, additional support can be provided by inserting plumping grafts or supporting cartilaginous struts or by placing permanent suspension sutures extending from the medial crura to the caudal end of the septum.

The right and left lateral crura comprise two legs of the tripod, and the two conjoined medical crura function as the third leg. Anatomically, the medial crura are shorter than the lateral crura. This condition is more prevalent in platyrrhine-type noses. The medial crural leg is supported by its attachment to the inferior (caudal) margin of the nasal septum and suspended superiorly by Pitanguy's ligament.

The effect of a bilateral transfixation incision, interruption of Pitanguy's ligament, and freeing soft tissues at the dorsal septal angle is a loss of tip projection. Top ptosis and the emergence of a more acute nasolabial angle are also predictable sequelae. These phenomena occur because the medial leg of the tripod's support is disrupted, allowing it to tilt in the direction of the shorter leg. These potential sequelae are more apt to occur in patients who may already have small nasal spines, a retrusive premaxilla, and large perioral features; therefore, it behooves the surgeon to preserve or reconstruct these important tip supports—and augment when indicated.

If the lateral crura are shortened and a bilateral transfixation incision is extended inferiorly past the medial crural footplates, the end result can be a reduction of tip projection. Tip ptosis is minimized because a taller tripod has been converted on all three sides to one with shorter legs. The net effect is often tip retrodisplacement. Additional nostril flaring is usually noted because the skin and soft tissue covering are deprived of their support, and alar sill resections may be required.

A limited or no transfixion incision along with shortening of the lateral legs (lateral crura) helps to maintain much of the pre-operative tip support. This allows for upward rotation of the tip and produces a more obtuse nasolabial angle. When the medical crura are supported by a cartilaginous columellar suture, plumping grafts, or permanent buried septocolumellar suture, the medial leg of the tripod becomes the dominant leg, allowing for tip projection and sometimes causing cephalad rotation of the tip. This is especially important in platyrrhine noses that need projection but generally do not need shortening. A geometric tenet is that nasal height and width influence each other. If one increases projection, the lower one-third of the nose will be narrowed. Conversely, when tip projection is reduced, the lower one-third of the nose becomes wider. In like manner, when the nasal dorsum is augmented, the nose generally appears more narrow. However, when the nasal dorsum lacks dorsal height, the middle and upper third of the nose appears wide.

Because most patients view their own noses several times each day from the front, they are more often critical of the post-operative shape and symmetry of the lobule, nostrils, and width of the bony pyramid of the nose.

It must be remembered that the skin is a drape that covers the nasal. The soft tissues of the nose are thickest at the nasion and supratip area and thinnest at the rhinion. Skin thickness can vary from thin to moderate in most Northern European noses. The thinner the skin, the more irregularities are potentially visible. Conversely, thick skin will camouflage sharp curves and projection. The procerus muscle can contribute to the soft tissue thickness at the nasion and Pitanguy's ligament can contribute to undesirable supratip fullness.

CONSULTATION

Pre-operatively, the patient's aesthetic goals and motivations need to be understood as specifically as possible. The experienced surgeon frequently uses mirrors, photographs, and computer imaging to help better define the patient's desires. This allows both parties to have similar aesthetic goals. It is important to ascertain whether the patient desires simply modification or refinement in the existing features or significant change consistent with more leptorrhine characteristics. The surgeon must be realistic in determining whether it is possible to achieve the goals that are set and discuss the limitations openly. The patient's nose should also be evaluated for asymmetries as they relate to the other facial features.

The bony and cartilaginous components of the nose can be assessed by gentle palpation and visual inspection. It is helpful to demonstrate anatomical structures to the patient and point to any areas that may exhibit special challenges—to explain what might and might not be achievable at surgery. Pointing these limitations out at this time will be construed by the patient as informed consent; later bringing attention to these things may be looked upon as an excuse.

OPERATIVE TECHNIQUE

Rhinoplasty can be performed under general or intravenous conscious sedation depending on the patient and surgeon desires. In either case, cocaine 4% solution is generally applied to the nasal membranes. No other medication provides both vasoconstriction and anesthesia as does topical cocaine. That fact makes its use desirable and appropriate.

Limited quantities of 2% lidocaine with 1:75,000 epinephrine are injected in the anticipated planes of dissection to enhance local anesthesia.

The Nasal Dorsum

The degree of dorsal modification, if appropriate, is generally assessed prior to performing the septoplasty so that dorsal support will not be compromised after anterior reduction with hump removal and posterior reduction with submucous resection of the septum. A conservative submucous resection of the obstructing septum is then performed through the appropriate transfixion incision. When satisfactory cartilage and bony septal correction has been achieved, the mucoperichondrial flaps are reapproximated with a running dissolvable horizontal mattress suture.

Access to the dorsal cartilaginous and bony portions is obtained when the soft tissues overlying the upper lateral cartilages are elevated sharply using a no. 15 Bard Parker knife blade and a Converse retractor. Over the dorsal septum and upper lateral cartilages, the plane of dissection is immediately supraperichondrial regardless of whether the rhinoplasty is being performed endonasally through an intercartilaginous or transcolumellar incision. Adhering to this plane of dissection generally limits intra-operative bleeding and decreases post-operative swelling and scarring. The tissues are elevated 1–2 mm cephalad to the caudal edge of the nasal bones. At this point, a round knife is used to incise the periosteum on each nasal bone. A limited subperiosteal pocket just overlying the dorsal hump is created, and the periosteum is raised in continuity with the overlying soft tissues of the nasal dorsum. Extensive elevation could compromise support for the lateral nasal bone complex, and this should be avoided. Following hump removal and osteotomy, a significant support mechanism for the nasal bones will be the remaining attached periosteum externally and the endonasal portions.

During the elevation of the soft tissues, one must be careful not to detach the upper lateral cartilages from the undersurface of the nasal bones. If this occurs and goes undetected, the only support for the upper lateral cartilage after hump removal will be laterally at their attachment to the nasal bony complex and the remaining soft tissue connections. Should they become detached at surgery, the upper lateral cartilage may fall inward, creating an inverted V appearance to the external nose at the caudal end of the nasal bones (Fig. 3).

The estimate of how much, if any, of the nasal dorsum to remove involves many elements, such as the patient's aesthetic desires, the nasal and facial anatomy, and the surgeon's experience. In females, the dorsum should be relatively straight or slightly concave, creating a slight supratip break relative to the tip. In males, the ideal nasal dorsum gener-

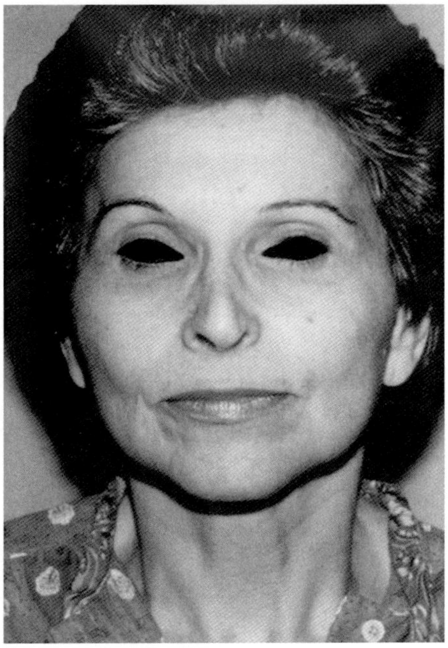

Figure 3. A post-operative patient who underwent rhinoplasty by another surgeon presents for revision surgery. In addition to a pinched asymmetric tip, this patient demonstrated collapse of the upper lateral cartilages evidenced by the inverted V deformity in the central portion of the nose.

ally parallels a straight or slightly convex line beginning at the nasion and ending at the nasal tip.

If dorsal reduction is required, the sharp tip of a no. 11 Bard Parker knife blade is passed through the upper lateral cartilages and septum at the caudal end of the nasal bones. The knife is advanced caudally with a sawing motion to remove the desired amount of cartilage. Although not generally present in platyrrhine-type noses, when a large cartilaginous hump is incised, it generally remains attached to the nasal bones. In these cases, the Rubin osteotome can be inserted between the incised portions of the cartilage and seated at the caudal end of the nasal bones. The surgeon guides the osteotome on a parallel course to the ideal dorsal line, while an assistant gently taps the osteotome with a mallet. It is prudent to underestimate the degree of profile reduction with the osteotome and fine-tune the dorsum with a rasp.

When minimal degrees of dorsal reduction are required (as is generally the case in patients with platyrrhine characteristics), a sharp rasp is usually the instrument of choice. For more efficient use, the bone can be roughened with a Joseph saw. The saw abrades the surface of the nasal bones, allowing the rasp to be more effective. Fine-tuning the dorsum is accomplished using fine, sharp rasps on the bony pyramid and sharp dissection on the cartilaginous pyramid.

Once reduction of the osseocartilaginous hump has been accomplished, lateral osteotomies are performed to reduce the open roof deformity and narrow the nasal side walls. Medial osteotomies are seldom necessary.

It is important to check the dorsal line following the lateral osteotomies because the medial edges of the upper lateral cartilages may spring up, creating dorsal irregularities. The caudal scroll of the upper lateral cartilage can contribute to supratip fullness or pollybeak post-operatively. Therefore, they should be examined and modified accordingly. To evaluate the height of the cartilaginous septum in the supratip area, digital pressure is placed on

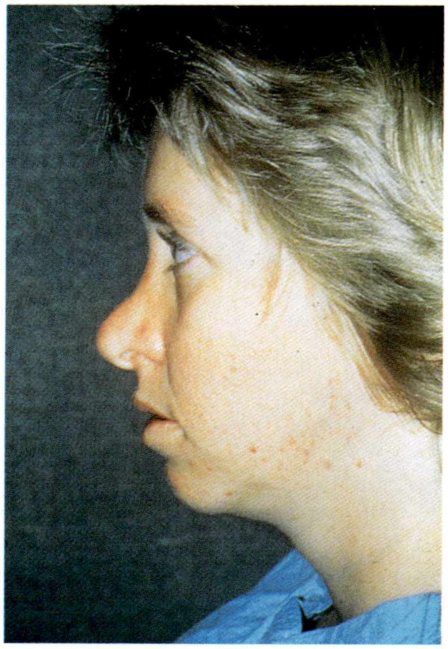

Figure 4. Patient demonstrating post-operative pollybeak deformity secondary to inadequate lowering of cartilaginous septum. Other possible causes of post-operative pollybeak include scar formation, inadequate trimming of lower lateral cartilages, and prominent caudal scroll of upper lateral cartilage.

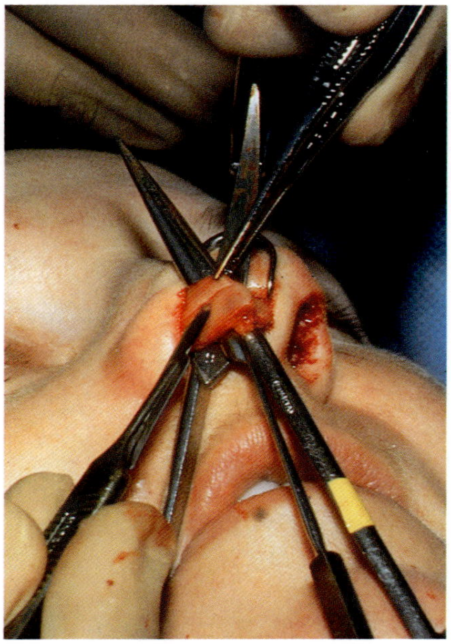

Figure 5. Intra-operative photograph showing delivery of lower lateral cartilages through marginal and intercartilagenous incisions and excising a complete strip. The scissors provide a stable surface upon which the cartilage can be trimmed. Note an adequate continuous strip of cartilage remains to prevent post-operative alar notching.

the tip cartilages, displacing them inferiorly. If the superior septal angle appears as a distinct, angulated structure during forceful tip depression, it should be lowered to help reduce the chances of having a cartilage pollybeak post-operatively (Fig. 4).

The Nasal Tip

In the author's operative sequence, tip refinements are performed after hump removal and osteotomies so as not to disturb any grafts or delicate tip sutures while modifying the dorsum. Due to the considerable variation of noses in individuals from Northern European regions, a working knowledge of the progressive or cascading approach to tip-plasty is very useful. The cascade begins with the simplest means of narrowing the tip, that is, a complete strip technique. If additional refinements are necessary, the surgeon can progressively advance to the next level, single-dome unit, then double-dome unit, and finally dome division, if necessary. This cascade allows the rhinoplasty surgeon to proceed in a controlled stepwise fashion until the desired degree of tip narrowing is achieved. To illustrate the cascade and highlight some of the challenges found within the Northern European population, each level will be examined in sequence.

Complete Strip

By definition, a complete strip procedure requires that the caudal margin of the lower lateral cartilage be preserved and intact from the foot of the medial crus to the most lateral extension of the lateral crus. The excessive portion of the lateral crus is excised following a line parallel to its caudal (or inferior) border (Fig. 5). A reduction on the superoinferior dimension of the lateral crus reduces supratip fullness. Unless the cartilages are thin and frail

A

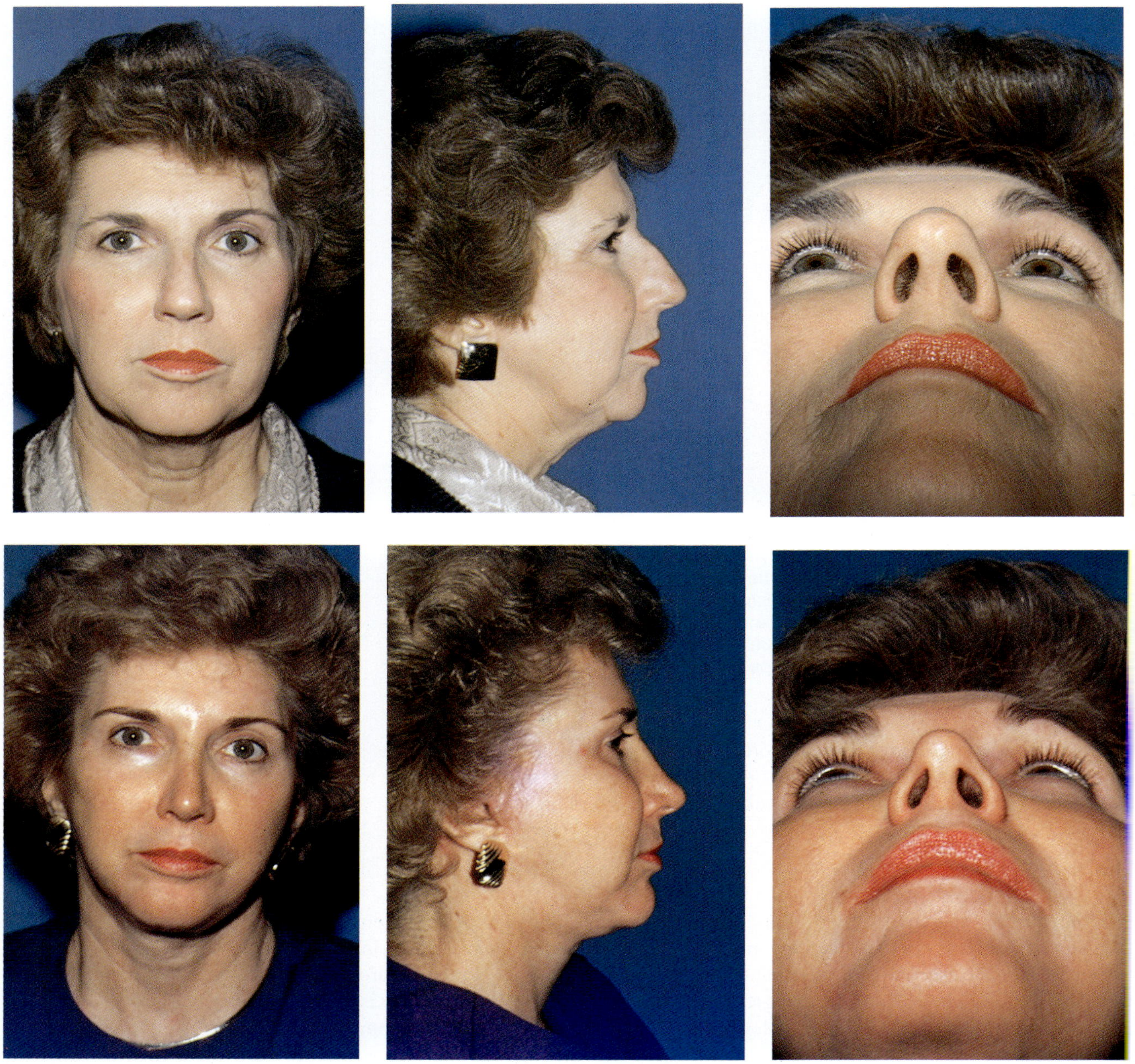

B, C

D

E, F

Figure 6. A–C: Pre-operative views of a 52-year-old patient with a wide nose with dorsal convexity. **D–F:** Patient after rhinoplasty, facelift, and chin implant. After reduction of the dorsum with a Rubin osteotome, a cephalic strip was removed from each lower lateral cartilage to achieve the desired tip refinement.

and the overlying skin is thick and non-compliant, the result is supra-alar definition. Generally, no superior rotation occurs when that lateral crus is not incised (or excised). The complete strip technique tends to prevent alar notching and unwanted upward rotation in noses that are already short. Flaring of the nostrils may also result when upward rotation is caused by increasing the length and strength of the medial crura. In most tip-plasties, the complete strip maneuver is all that is necessary to produce an aesthetically pleasing nasal tip (Fig. 6); however, in platyrrhine-type noses, more aggressive techniques are often required. Even noses that are narrowed sufficiently with a complete strip may need additional central support. This can often be accomplished by placement of a long, strong, cartilage strut between the medial crura.

Single-Dome Intact Unit

In the progressive tip-plasty approach and when more lobular refinement is desired, a single-dome procedure may be created. The single-dome unit is created by suture fixation of the medial crus to the lateral crus at the dome. The more acute some angle created by a double horizontal mattress suture provides additional tip refinement. The integrity of the remaining complete strip of alar cartilage remains intact. An absorbable polyglycolic suture (5-0 Vicryl) is used to hold the cartilages in position until a capsule of fibrous tissue forms.

The most crucial step in dome reconstruction is accurate identification of the junction of the medial with the lateral crus of the lower lateral cartilage. The dome is identified after the lower lateral cartilage is delivered (or visualized) and the cephalic border trimmed (complete strip). The anatomical dome is determined to be that portion of the cartilage between the external soft triangle (facet) inferiorly and the internal soft triangle superiorly. Identification of this juncture can usually be achieved by both observation and by placing a blunt instrument on the vestibular skin surface of the chondrocutaneous flap and lifting upward. The highest point of projection can be grasped with forceps and secured for suture placement. If minor asymmetry is present, a new dome angle can be created by this suture fixation technique (Fig. 7).

In double-dome creation, the underlying vestibular skin is preserved and a horizontal mattress suture of 5-0 Vicryl or Dexon is used to create more acute dome angles. Each dome is examined and sutured independently. This technique narrows the tip and, to a lesser degree, increases the height of the lobule. In addition, a slight increase in tip projection can generally be observed.

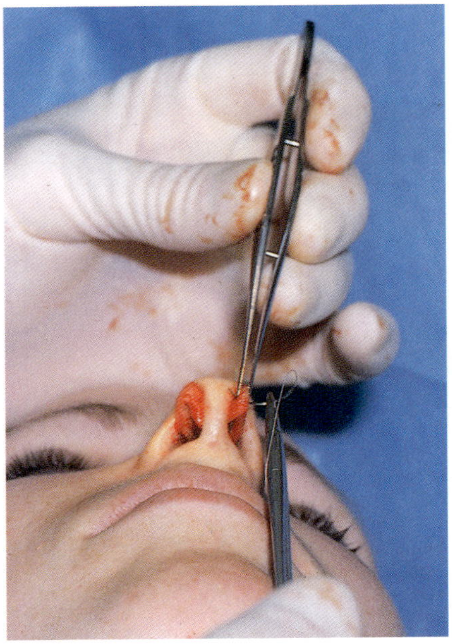

Figure 7. Intra-operative photograph showing newly constructed single-dome units. Minor asymmetries can be corrected sometimes with suture fixation. Major asymmetries would probably be better served with an alternative tip technique.

If significant asymmetry is present pre-operatively, cartilage memory can return (to varying degrees) during the post-operative period, resulting in post-operative asymmetry. In some cases, a strong central support is afforded by a cartilaginous strut or I-beam graft and may prevent twisting of the medial crura. In all cases employing single/double-dome techniques, the final result almost totally depends on the capsule of fibrous tissue that holds the cartilages in their new positions. Therefore, the single-dome unit is usually contraindicated in asymmetric tips because it does not provide for correction of significant unilateral cartilage asymmetries. Other tip techniques are recommended.

Double-Dome Intact Unit

If, after creation of single-dome units, a double-dome unit may be indicated, additional lobule narrowing is desirable. A 5-0 Dexon (or Vicryl) mattress suture that passes through both newly produced single-dome units will create the double-dome unit when tied together (Figs. 8 and 9).

A cartilaginous strut also can be placed in the columella between the medial crura of the mattressed complex to further enhance tip projection and help maintain support in the post-operative period. It may be desirable to extend the cartilaginous graft into the lobule and between the two newly created single-dome units to which it too can be sutured.

In both the single- and double-dome units, suture fixation secures the desired location of the tip cartilages until scar formation stabilizes them. Early attempts at morselizing the domes prior to suturing were found to be unpredictable. The morselized areas sometimes stiffen during the healing period, commonly resulting in asymmetry. This fact led to the abandonment of morselization of the dome for the most part.

The authors generally resort to a more predictable dome division procedure in the cases of significant asymmetry (Fig. 10). It has, however, been found helpful in cases of twisted medial crural components to gently morselize the portions of these cartilages that extend into the columella and splint them with a strut or I-beam cartilage graft.

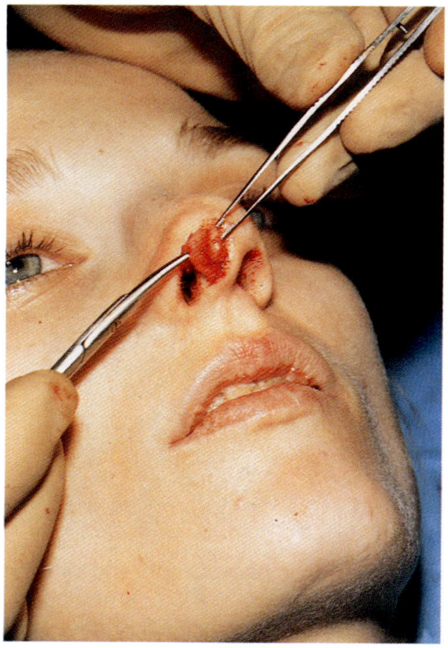

Figure 8. Intra-operative photograph of double-dome unit.

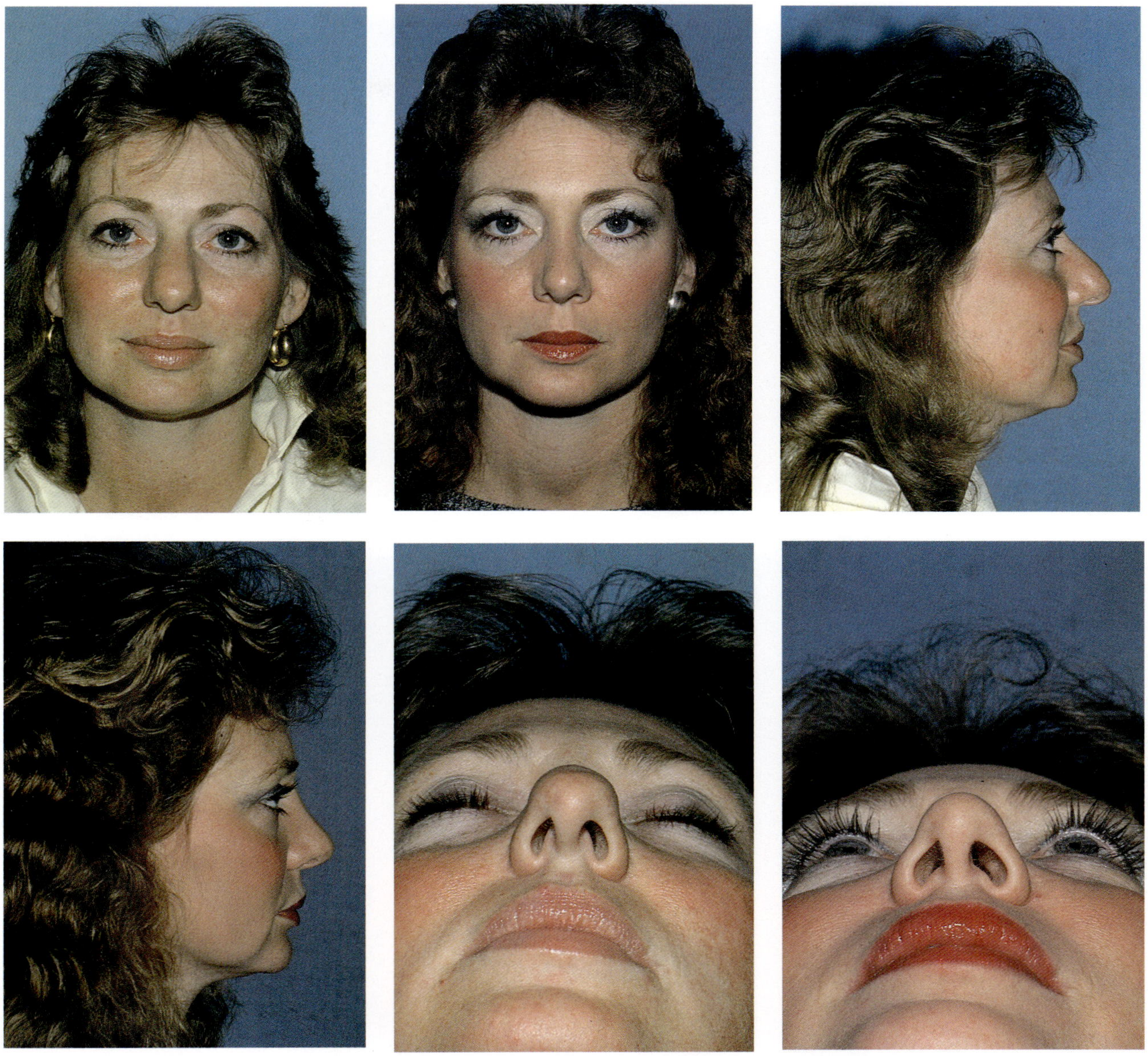

A B, C D E, F

Figure 9. A, C, and E: Thick rhinophymatomus skin in this 34-year-old White woman contributed to the amorphous appearance of her nasal tip and middle one-third of her nose. Tip ptosis and supratip fullness and the flaring of the medial crura feet can also be noted. **B, E, and F:** After bilateral osteotomies and double-dome tip-plasty, narrowing and definition were achieved. Minimal hump removal is required when tip projection/rotation can be attained, and the columellar deformity was corrected by suturing the feet of the medial crura to each other.

Dome Division

Unlike the previous techniques, this one completely interrupts the remaining caudal strip of the lower lateral cartilages in the region of the domes (Fig. 11). This technique is utilized when increased projection or rotation is required or narrowing of the nasal tip is necessary. When gross asymmetry between the lower lateral cartilages exists, this technique can be used to neutralize the differences.

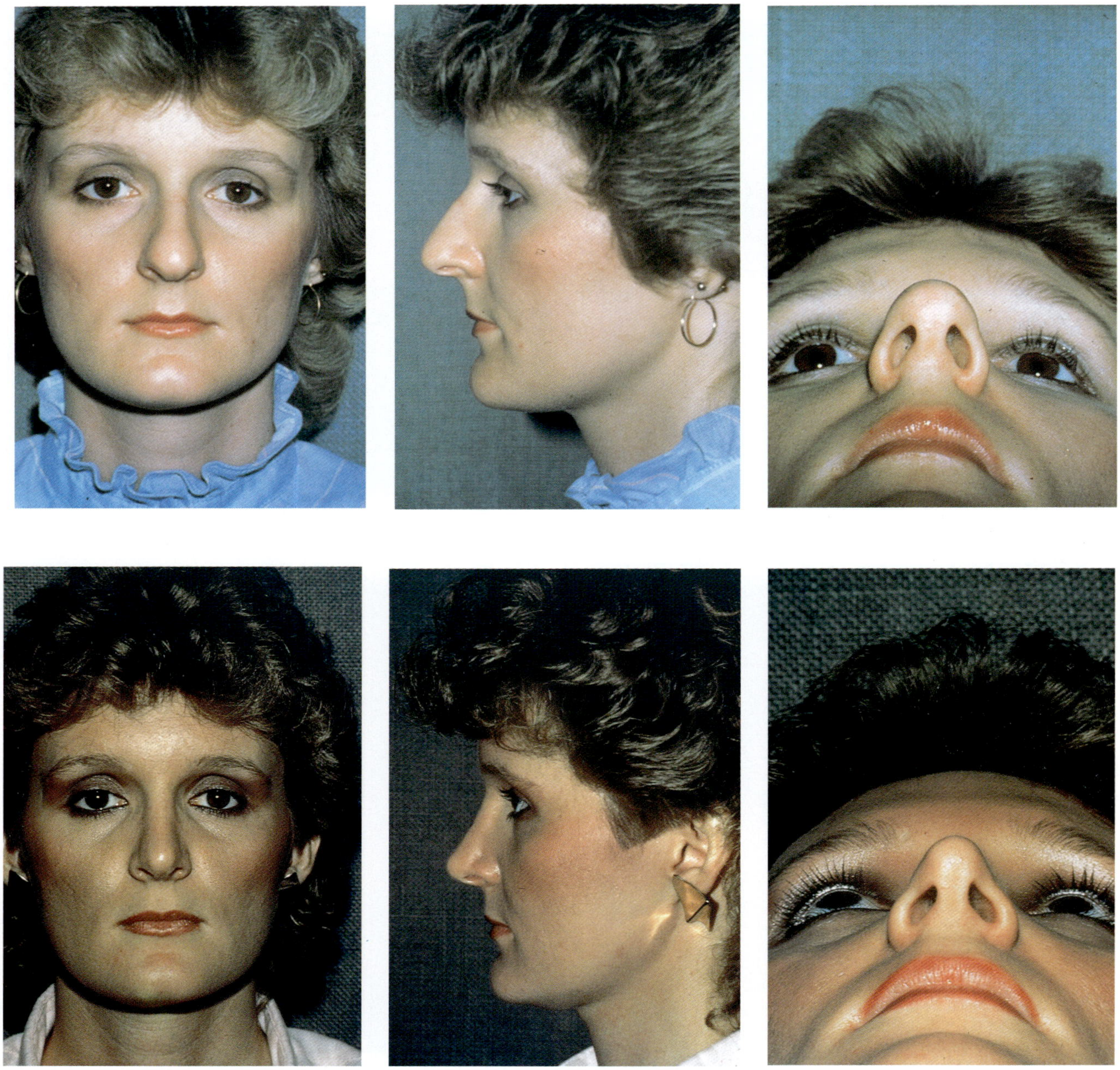

A

B, C

D

E, F

Figure 10. Pre-operative photographs of frontal **(A)**, lateral **(B)**, and base **(C)** views of a patient with ptotic wide nasal tip. Post-operative photographs of frontal **(D)**, lateral **(E)**, and base **(F)** views showing increase in rotation and narrowing with dome division and strut cartilaginous techniques. The patient's caudal septum was shortened as well to aid in upward tip rotation.

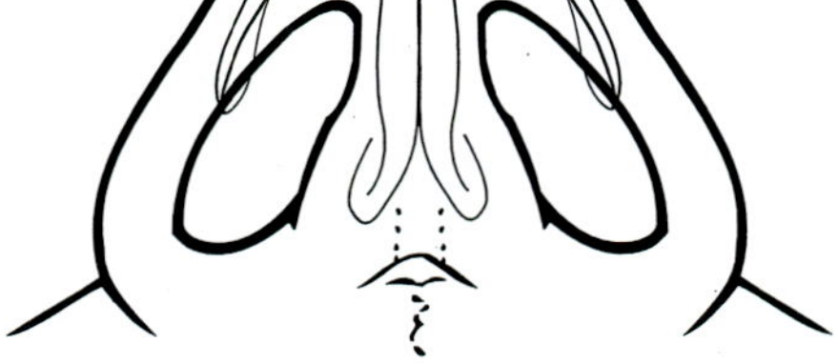

Figure 11. Illustration showing interruption of inferior crural margins with dome division or Goldman technique. Central support is created by suturing medial crura if additional support is needed.

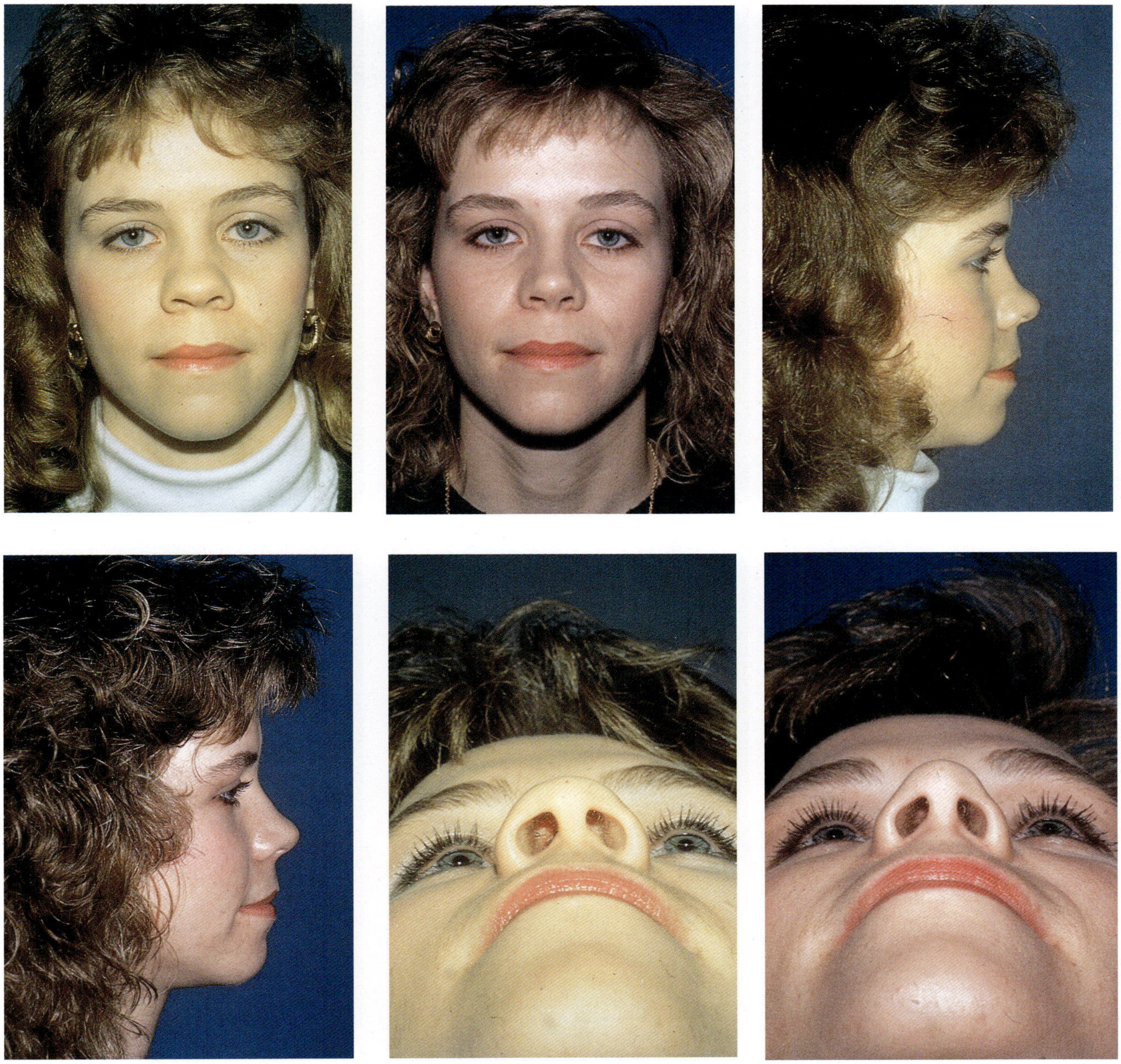

A B, C D E, F

Figure 12. A, C, and E: Pre-operative views of 20-year-old White woman who presented with a number of platyrrhine features of her nose and middle one-third of her face, including a low nasal dorsum, bulbous tip, wide nasolabial angle, and wide lobule and alae. **B, D, and F:** Rhinoplasty alone was performed and osseous narrowing and dorsal nasal grafting coupled with tip-plasty gave her a more leptorrhine-like appearance. Dome division tip-plasty utilizing an I-beam columellar graft with premaxillary plumping grafts and alar base resections was also performed.

After a conservative horizontal portion of the lateral crus is removed, the remaining caudal segment is divided at the domes if no increase in projection is required. If, however, increased projection is needed, the cartilages are divided lateral to the dome; but, no more than 2–3 mm of lateral crus should be borrowed. If additional support is needed to enhance the support of the newly created central complex, a cartilaginous strut may be placed in a pocket between the medial crura (Figs. 12 and 13). The Northern European patient with a platyrrhine-type nose will, in most cases, not require shortening of the caudal septum. Most, in fact, are deficient in the caudal, septal, and nasal spine regions. To access whether the

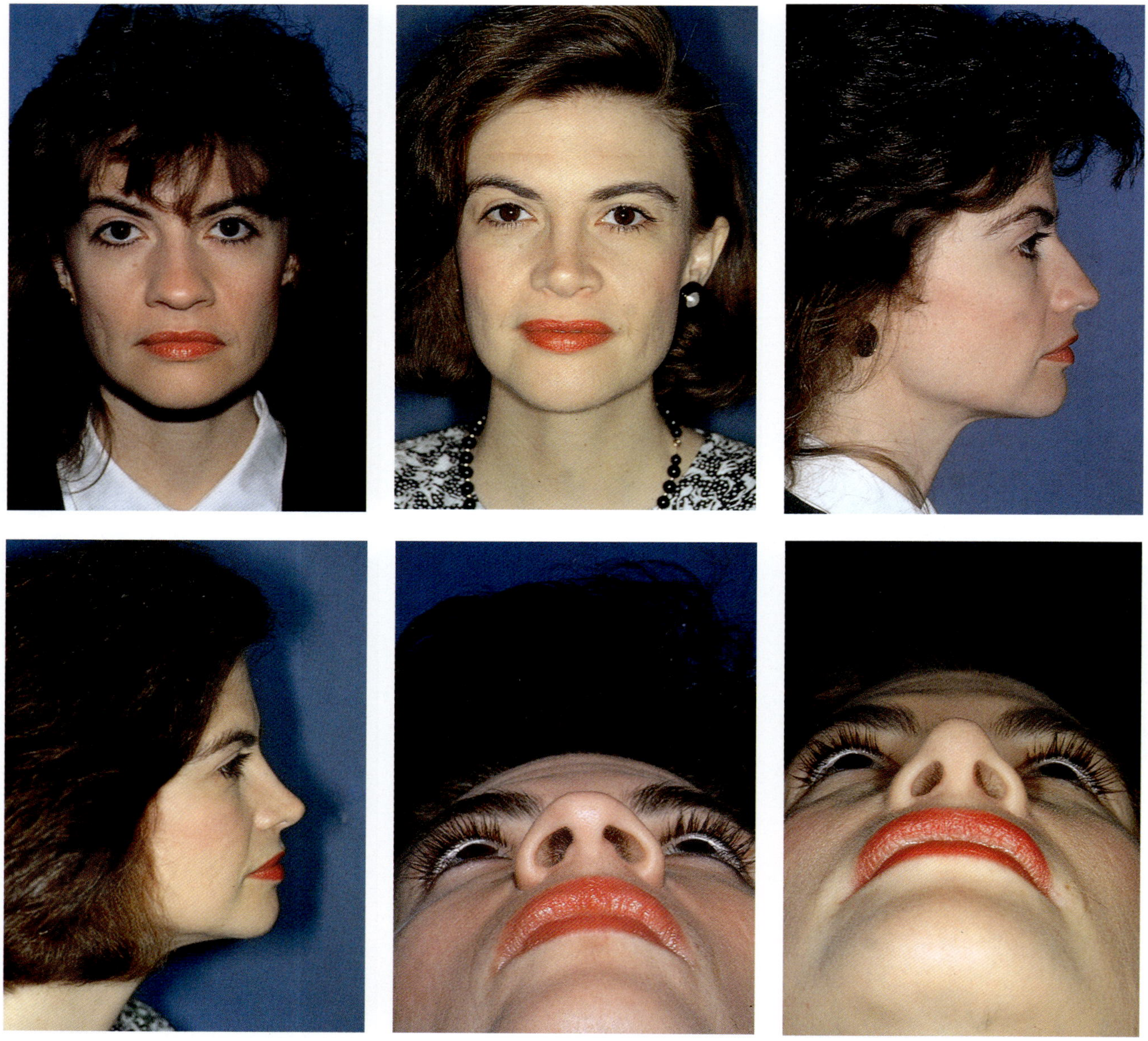

A B, C D E, F

Figure 13. A, C, and E: Pre-operative view of a 33-year-old White woman with a wide nose, a slight dorsal hump, a wide lobule, and wide, flaring alae. **B, D, and F:** Alar base resections provided correction of nostril flaring and narrowing and projection of the lobule were achieved by a dome division technique, supported by a central I-beam graft. Alar base resections provided more symmetry and narrowing of the nasal width.

membranous or cartilaginous septum requires shortening, one should press upward on the base of the tip. If one encounters firm resistance, the caudal cartilage may require shortening, especially if a strut or I-beam graft is to be used (Figs. 14–18).

EXTERNAL RHINOPLASTY

External rhinoplasty is not required for most nasal plastic operations; however, it is extremely helpful in difficult revisional cases and complicated primary procedures that require maximum visibility for diagnosis and correction. Exposure is most easily accomplished by first carrying out the classic delivery technique and then connecting the marginal incisions with an inverted V transcolumellar incision within the thinnest portion of the columellar skin. The post-operative scar is usually inconspicuous but may be more prominent when the incision is placed in the thicker skin toward the base of the columella.

The authors generally perform intercartilaginous and transfixion incision so that most of the operation can be carried out in the more conventional manner. However, reflecting the tip and dorsal nasal skin following a transcolumellar incision provides panoramic exposure and generally facilitates diagnosis and correction of the more complex deformity (Fig. 19). Any of the previously described tip procedures can be performed precisely and accurately under direct vision through an external approach. Its use in training programs and by inexperienced surgeons is recommended until the surgical dynamics and anatomical relations of the nasal components are more thoroughly understood.

The only disadvantage of external rhinoplasty is the resulting transcolumellar scar. In most cases, adherence to classic plastic surgical principles should allow the tissues to heal precisely and with minimal deformity. The resulting scar is usually thin and narrow and follows the natural contour lines of the base of the nose; therefore, surgeons with all degrees of experience should not hesitate to add the transcolumellar incision to an evolving armamentarium.

In patients with platyrrhine-like nasal features, the lower lateral cartilages may be thin and frail. Because the skin is often thicker, irregularities or post-operative asymmetry may not be readily visible. Dome division with or without central grafting provides maximum projection and narrowing. Thicker skin blankets sharp edges. External rhinoplasty conversion may be the most predictable way to ensure accurate approximation of structures along with fixation of grafting materials.

Thin skin requires more accurate sculpting. The transcolumellar scar generally heals well and is often less noticeable in the thin skinned tip.

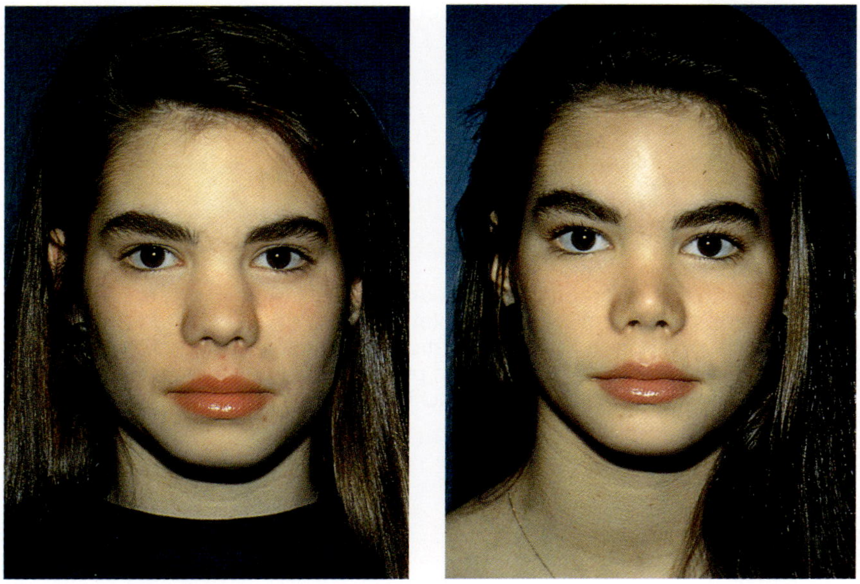

Figure 14. A: Pre-operative photograph of a 15-year-old White girl with platyrrhine-like features. **B:** Narrowing of the upper one-half of the nose was achieved with lateral osteotomies alone. Tip definition was obtained with dome division and suturing the transected ends of the medial crura together.

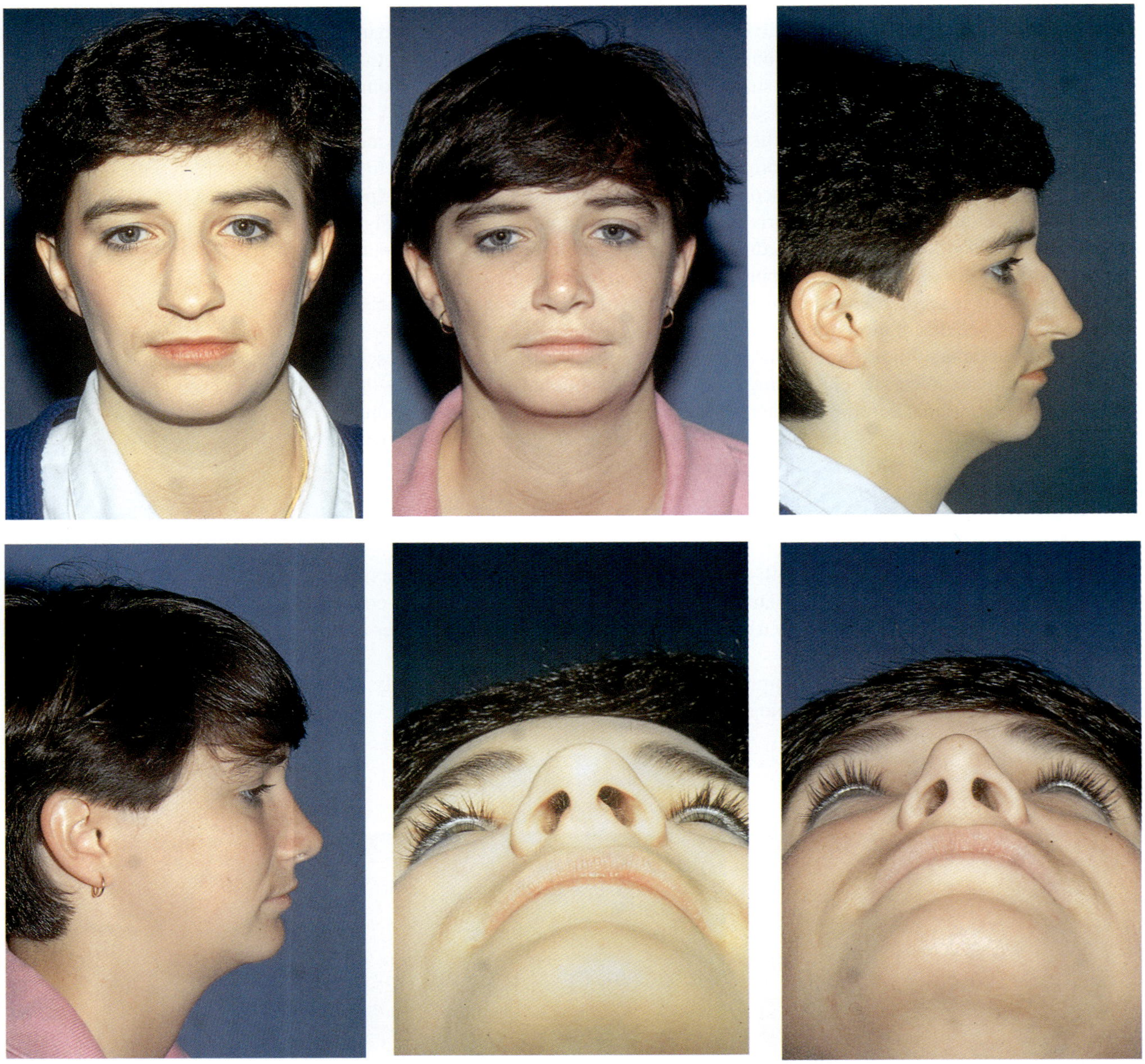

A B, C D E, F

Figure 15. A, C, and E: Pre-operative photograph of a 21-year-old White woman with a wide nose and asymmetrical face, a small dorsal hump and ptotic tip, and an asymmetric broad lobule, coupled with flaring alae. **B, D, and F:** Post-operatively, the nose is more narrow and has better tip definition. Hump removal and tip rotation provide better balance and harmony. Correction of the broad lobule and flaring alae was achieved with dome divisions and alar base resections.

ALAR SILL RESECTIONS

If, after obtaining desired projection of the tip, additional narrowing is desired, an alarplasty can be considered.

If possible, incisions and excisions should be restricted to the sill region (Fig. 20). The incision should be planned to preserve a portion of the natural curvature of the alae.

An effective and efficient method of resecting the unwanted portion of tissue can be carried out with an Adson Brown or Griffis Brown forceps and a no. 11 blade.

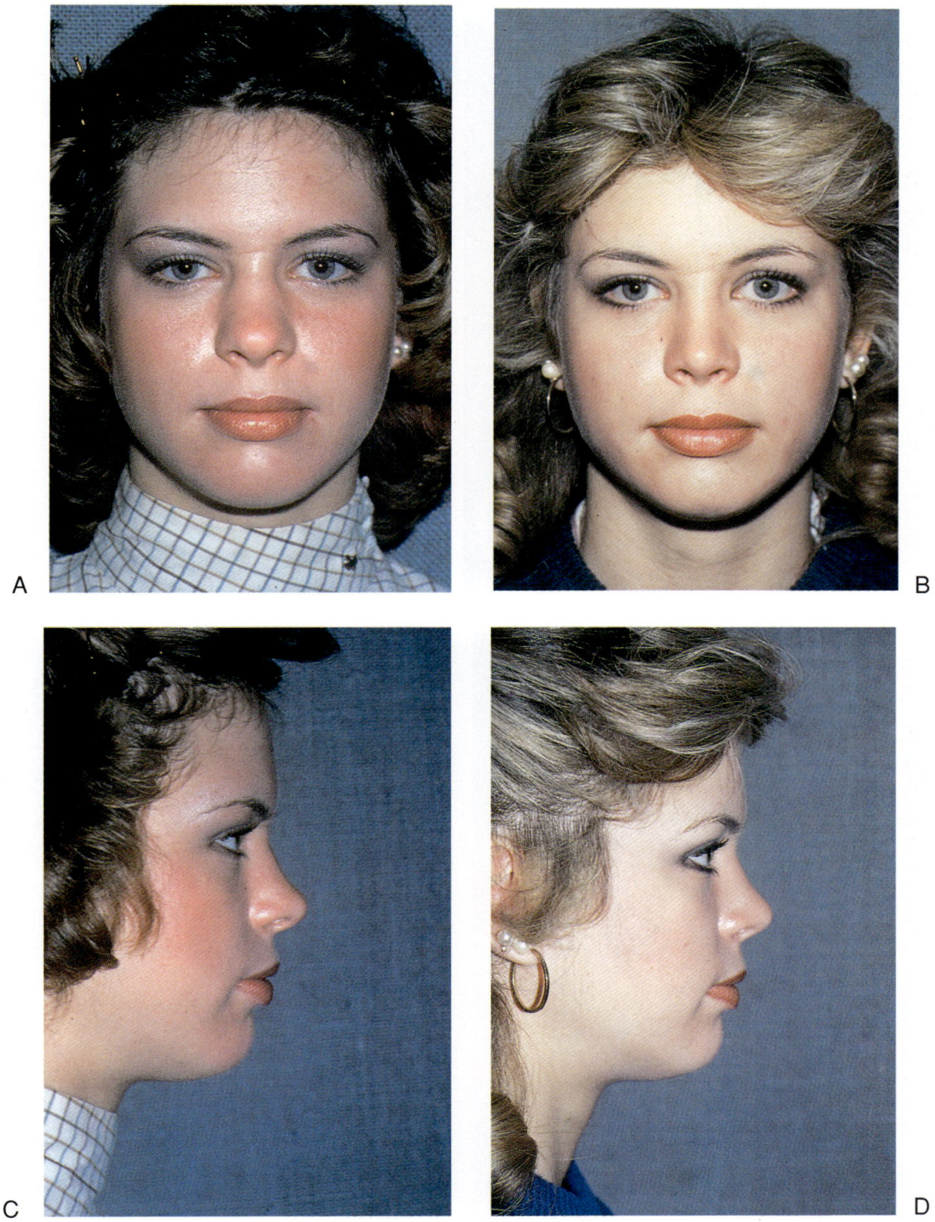

Figure 16. A and C: Pre-operative views of 18-year-old White woman who presented with a wide, short nose, no dorsal hump, and an obtuse nasolabial angle. **B and D:** Post-operatively the nose fits well within the intercanthal one-fifth of the face. Osteotomies alone provided narrowing of the bony and midcartilage portions and dome division tip-plasty provided definition of the lobule. No alar base resection was carried out, nor were hump removal, augmentation, or additional tip rotation.

Soft tissue resection should be carried into the floor of the vestibule. Only when a relatively large amount of tissue has been removed is an incision carried into the nasofacial crease. This extended maneuver can create an advancement/rotation flap and may help to prevent post-operative widening. Excision of a crescent-shaped portion of ala as described by Weir is seldom indicated. Complications can result when this type of excision is carried to the extreme.

Closure of the wound is a prerequisite to obtaining pleasing scars. Deep or buried sutures usually are not necessary. Accurate wound edge approximation and eversion can be ac-

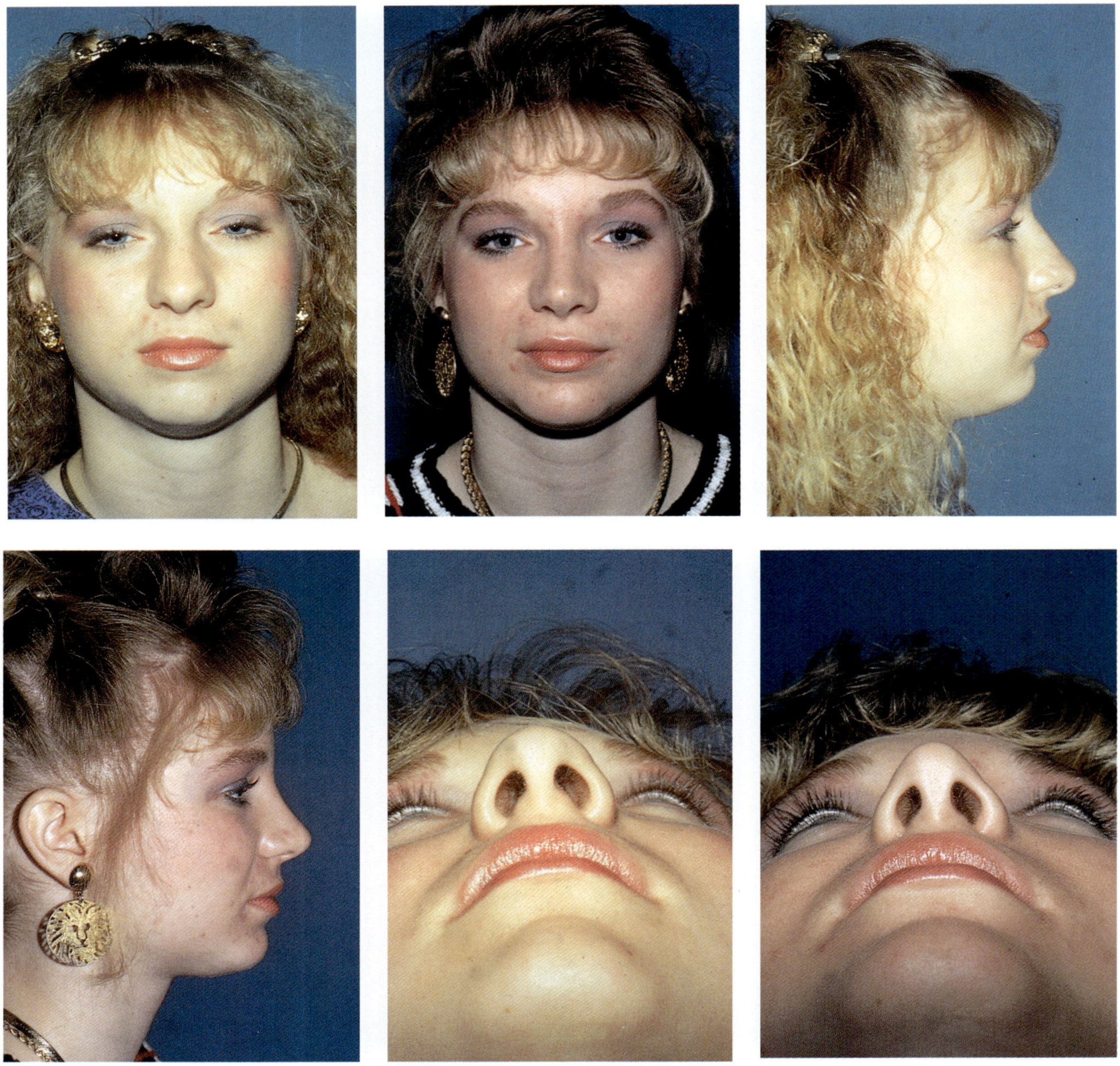

A B, C D E, F

Figure 17. A, C, and E: Pre-operative appearance of a 14-year-old White girl with a broad nose, a slight dorsal hump exaggerated by the presence of microgenia, and a wide alar base. **B, D, and F:** Post-operatively the side walls have been narrowed and there is greater tip definition. Hump removal and chin augmentation with a Mersilene mesh implant provided improved facial harmony. The alar base was narrowed with dome division tip-plasty alone.

complished with 5-0 plain catgut sutures. If the sutures are saturated with hydrogen peroxide six to eight times daily and kept moist with a mild antibiotic ointment during the post-operative period, most of the suture material disintegrates during the first 5–6 days.

At the end of the operation, customized external dressing is molded to the nose to help keep the components in alignment during the early post-operative course. When properly applied, the conforming dressing often helps to reduce the chance of soft tissue pollybeak post-operatively.

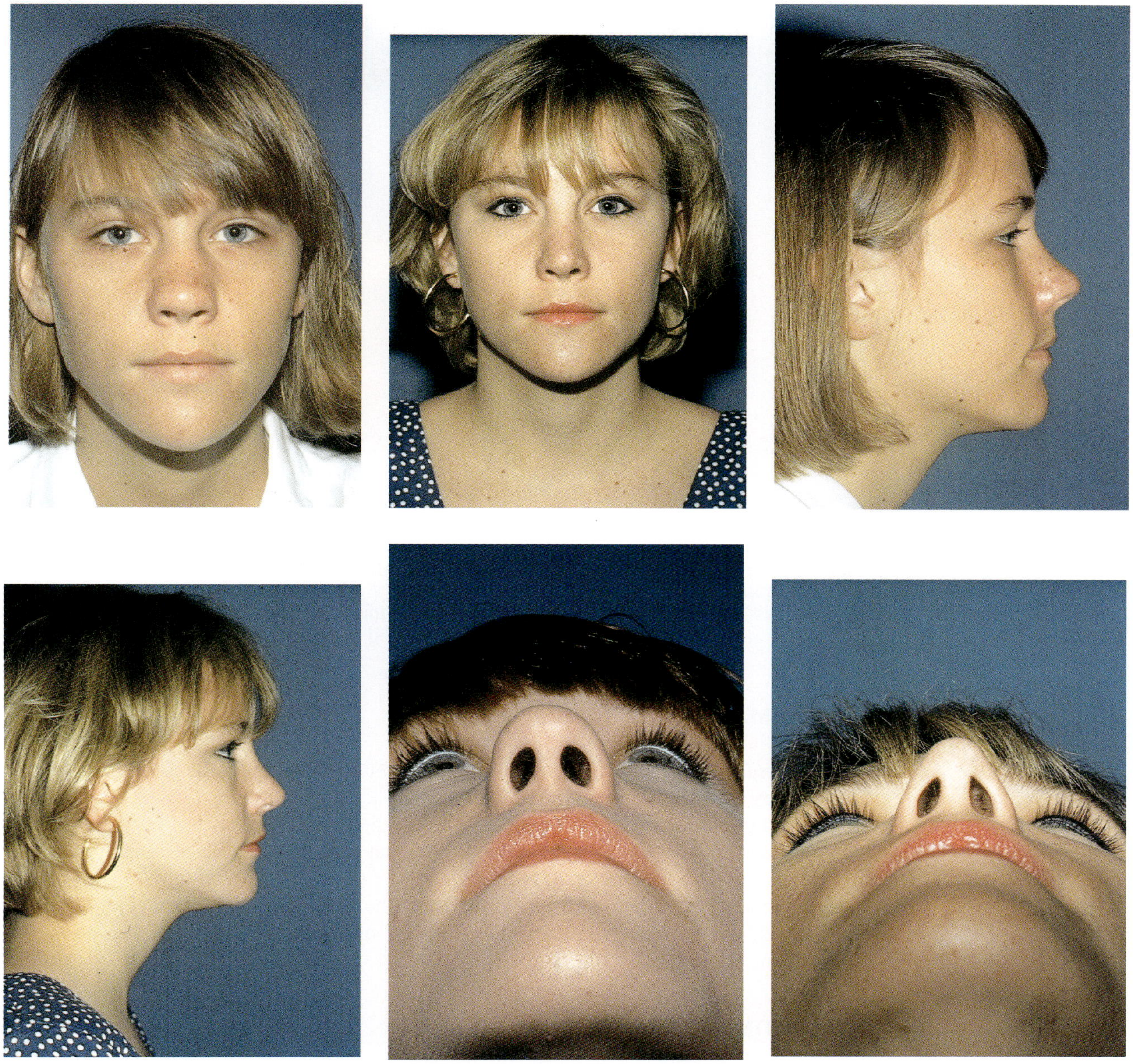

A B, C D E, F

Figure 18. A, C, and E: Pre-operative photographs of a 22-year-old White woman who presented with a wide nose and amorphous tip and supratip fullness due to thick skin and abundance of subcutaneous tissue. **B, D, and F:** Five years post-operatively, the narrowing and improved tip definition are shown. Tip projection was achieved by dome division tip-plasty and crushed cartilage overlay grafting over the two sutured ends of the medial crura. Intralesional triamcinolone was also required to soften supratip fullness.

When tip projection is either maintained or increased, alar base resections are required less frequently. Conversely, as tip retrodisplacement occurs, the alae flare. Keloids and/or hypertrophic scars seldom occur in the nasolabial fold. This dreaded complication, although it may be presented to the patient, is highly unlikely, provided observation of appropriate principles of wound closure are followed.

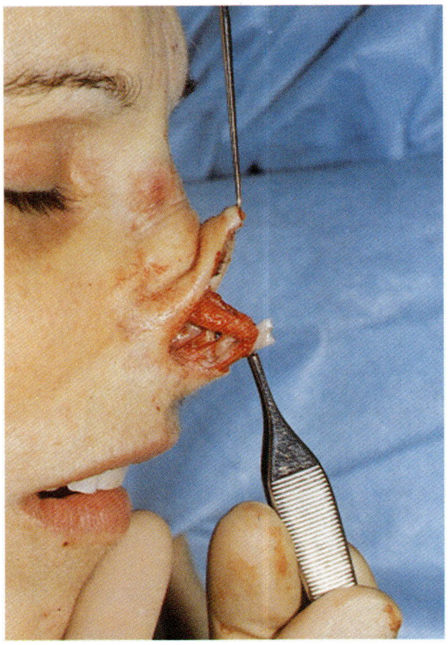

Figure 19. Intra-operative view showing the excellent exposure that can be obtained with an open rhinoplasty technique. Placement and suturing of tip grafts can easily be performed.

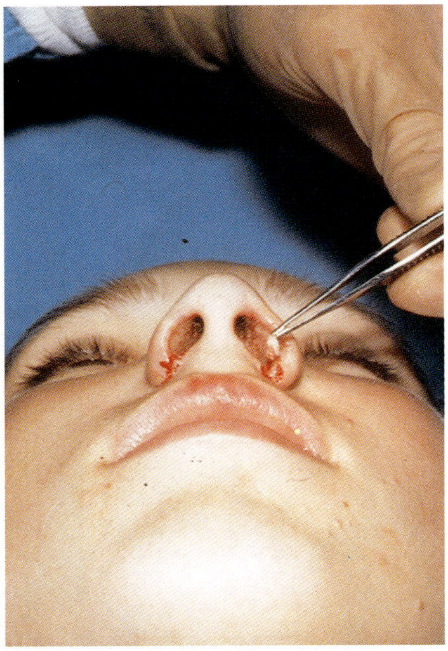

Figure 20. Intra-operative photograph showing a completed alar sill resection *(right)* and excision of a portion of the sill *(left)*. Note that in this patient the incision did not extend to the alar but was limited to the sill.

SUMMARY

A prudent surgeon chooses the simplest technique that will get the job done. Experience teaches that less is better. The cascading approach to the nasal tip affords the surgeon the opportunity to recognize the point in the operation when one has reached the peak of the plastic surgery risk/benefit curve and knows that s/he has achieved the greatest amount of good with the least amount of harm.

The most important aspect in approaching the patient with white skin and platyrrhine-like features is to ascertain what s/he wishes the operation to do, for success is measured as a happy patient.

RECOMMENDED READING

1. Peter LJ. Peter's Quotations. New York: Bantam, 1987.
2. Berman WE. *Rhinoplastic surgery*. St. Louis: Mosby, 1989.
3. Colton JJ and Beekhuis GJ. Rhinoplasty. *Otolaryngol Clin North Am* 1987;20:4.
4. Rees TD, Baker DC, Tabbal N. *Rhinoplasty problems and controversies*. St. Louis: Mosby, 1988.
5. Meyer R. *Secondary and functional rhinoplasty: the difficult nose*. Orlando: Grune and Stratton, 1988.
6. Facial plastic surgery of North America. *Adv Rhinoplasty* 1994;2:4.

Subject Index

Note: *f* following page number denotes figure; *t* following page number denotes table.

A

Abscesses, 106–109, 110*f*, 111
Accutane, 110*f*, 111, 112–113, 114, 122, 127–128, 140, 141
Acne, 99, 103–106, 121, 122, 123, 124*t*, 125–129, 139–140
  Filipinos and Polynesians, 287
  medications and, 106, 111
  Middle Easterners, 345
  and pigment abnormalities, 101
  pomade, 122, 123, 139
  pre- and postoperative care, 131, 136
  and scarring, 122, 131, 174*f*, 183*f*, 185
  treatment, 103, 111, 129
    alpha-hydroxy acids for, 112
    benzoyl peroxide for, 115
Acne cosmetica, 126
Acne keloiditis, 122, 131, 183*f*, 185
Acne mechanica, 106, 126
Acne medicamentosa, 106
Adenoma sebaceum, 111
Adolescents
  African American, 207, 208*f*, 210
  Middle Eastern, 344, 347, 364
  Northern European, 375*f*
Advancement genioplasty, 57, 345
Adverse outcomes. *See* Complications
Aesthetician, 26, 29, 103, 132
Aesthetics, 12, 13
  African American. *See* African Americans, aesthetics
  Asian, 247–249, 254, 255, 257, 264–265
    double eyelid creation, 267–268
    rhinoplasty, 282
  Caucasian, 39–58
    appraisal, 42–45, 46*f*
    cephalometrics/Frankfort horizontal, 46–49
    cheek, 57–58
    chin, 56–57
    eyes, 50–52
    forehead, 50, 51*f*
    golden proportion, 41–42, 43*f*
    historic evolution, 39–40
    mouth, 54–55, 56*f*
    nose, 52–53, 54*f*
    objective standards/criteria, 40–41
    preferred, 49–50
    proportions, 45–46
  cultural factors, 3. *See also* Cultural considerations
  ethnic diversity, 61–83
    cephalometrics/Frankfort horizontal, 64*t*, 65
    eyes, 74–79
    facial (phi) relationships, 79
    golden proportions, 64*t*, 66–73, 67*f*, 67*t*, 70*t*, 71*t*, 72*t*
    media representations, 61, 62*f*, 62*t*
    medical risk factors, 79, 81
    neoclassical canons of proportions, 64*t*, 65–66
    nose, 73
    objective standards and criteria, 64*t*, 65–73
    outcomes and goals of surgery, 81, 82*f*, 83*f*
    study population, 61, 63, 63*t*, 64*t*
  harmony as surgical goal, 21
  Hispanics, 310, 311*f*
  Mediterranean nose, 328
  Middle Eastern, 339, 340*f*, 344–346
  Northern European, 85–96
    lip and chin relationships, 95
    nasal proportions, 89–95
    nostrils, 85, 86*f*
African Americans
  aesthetics, 61, 62*f*, 63*t*, 64*t*, 80*f*, 82*f*, 85
    defining elements, 13
    eye, 76*f*, 77, 78–79
    facial proportions, 88
    Frankfort horizontal, 65*f*
    golden proportions, 64*t*, 66–73, 67*f*, 67*t*, 70*t*, 71*t*, 72*t*
    individualization of approach, 197–199
    nose, 85, 86*f*, 86*t*, 88, 89, 91*f*, 92–95
  aging, 100, 151, 152*f*, 153*f*, 153*t*, 154*t*, 155, 156, 169*t*, 170*t*
    facelifts, 165*f*
    lips, 168–169
    lower face and neck, 162
  anatomy, 200–201, 213–214
  anthropological and physiological comparisons, 31–34
  cheiloplasty, 208*f*, 210, 241–242*f*
  chin augmentation, 233–235, 236, 238*f*
  lash liner, permanent, 159
  medical risk factors, 79
  patient selection, 25
  rhinoplasty
    adolescent and pediatric patients, 207, 208*f*, 210
    alar base techniques, 203
    alar flaring, 221–227, 228*f*
    anatomic considerations, 213–214
    cultural considerations, 195
    dorsal augmentation, 228–236
    dorsum, 204–207
    historical considerations, 214, 215*f*, 216*f*, 217*f*
    individualization of approach, 197–199
    open approach, 236–237
    psychosocial considerations, 199–200
    rhinophyma, 209*f*, 210
    skin thickness, 237–242
    suboptimal results, 242–244
    surgical description, 201–202

African Americans, rhinoplasty *(contd.)*
surgical maneuvers, 210–211, 210*t*, 211*t*
techniques, 215, 218–220*f*, 220–221
tip defatting, 215, 218*f*
tip projection techniques, 202–203
tip surgery, 203–204
skin disorders, 131
acne. See Acne
acne treatment, 129
keratosis pilaris, 133–134
pseudofolliculitis barbae, 141–143
skin sensitivity, 127
African phenotype, Hispanics, 310, 313*f*, 315, 316*f*
Africans, 32
Age
and facial hair, 123
Middle Eastern patients, 344
Aging, 3, 99–101
African Americans, 207, 214
changes, 151–154, 152*t*, 153*t*, 154*t*
eye and eyelid changes, 77, 78, 79
Hispanics, 303, 305*f*, 311
lateral face and neck, 162, 164*f*, 165*f*, 166–168*f*
lips, 55, 168–169
malar fat pad, 160–162, 163*f*
Middle Easterners, 345–346
nasolabial, 162*f*, 163*f*, 164
periorbital area, 155–160
scalp, 155
and skin conditions, 119
variations among ethnic groups, 34
Alar base
aesthetics, 68
Asians, 258, 263
Filipinos and Polynesians, 288
Middle Easterners, 364, 365*t*, 367, 368
Alar base surgery, 222
African Americans, 203
and airway, 228*f*
anatomy, 201
versus Caucasians, 211*t*
long-term effects, 200
Filipinos and Polynesians, 292–293*f*
Hispanics, 312
Northern Europeans, 373, 376*f*, 391*f*, 392*f*
Alar cartilage grafts, 318*f*, 319, 331
Alar cartilage surgery. *See also* Alar wedge excision/resection
African Americans, 210, 227, 243*f*
Asians, 259–260*f*
Mediterraneans, 327, 328*f*, 329
Alar dome onlay grafts, 330–331
Alar flare
aesthetics, 89, 90*f*, 91*f*
African Americans, 68, 69
Caucasians, 53
African Americans, 199, 199*t*, 200, 200*t*, 221–227, 228*f*, 233–235*f*
aesthetics, 68, 69
incisions and fixation techniques, 202
Asians, 258
Northern Europeans, 392*f*, 394*f*
Alar notching, 377*f*
Alar rim, 92
Alar rim incision, 368
Alar rim surgery, African Americans, 238*f*, 239–240*f*, 242
skin thickness and, 237–242
suboptimal results, 244
tip enhancement with, 225, 225*f*, 226*f*
Alar sill advancement, 223
Alar sill resection
African Americans, 225
Northern Europeans, 381, 394–397, 398*f*
Alar structure. *See also* Alar flare; Alar width
Filipinos and Polynesians, 287, 288
Hispanics, 315, 316*f*
Alar wedge excision/resection
Asian rhinoplasty, 261
Filipinos and Polynesian rhinoplasty, 294–295*f*
Hispanics, 312, 314*f*, 315, 316*f*, 319*f*, 320
Alar width. *See also* Alar flare
aesthetics, 69*f*, 89, 90*f*, 91*f*
African Americans, 213–214
Asians, 247, 258
Hispanics, 305*f*
Northern Europeans, 89, 90*f*, 91*f*, 373, 376*f*
Allantoin, 132, 133
Allergy/hypersensitivity, skin, 121, 122, 123, 127, 141
to benzoyl peroxide, 129
to hydroquinone, 103
and infraorbital shadowing, 131
keratosis pilaris management, 134
preoperative assessment, 346
preoperative testing, 132
Alloplastic implants. *See* Synthetic materials
Aloe vera, 128, 130, 132, 133
Alopecia, 122, 155
Alpha-hydroxy acids, 102, 133, 213, 354
acne keloiditis, 131
and hyperpigmentation, 145
keratosis pilaris management, 134
pre- and postoperative skin care, 131, 132, 136
for skin conditions, 99, 111–112, 113, 122
acne, 127, 128–129
pigmentation abnormalities, 123
Anatomy. *See specific ethnic groups*
Anchor blepharoplasty, 254, 355
Androgens, 132
Anesthesia, 8, 288, 346
blepharoplasty, 355
Asians, 269, 271
Middle Easterners, 355
rhinoplasty, 279, 347–348, 365
Anterior maxillary spine, 201
Anthropological differences, 31–34, 44*f*
Anthropometrics, 85
Antibiotics
after chemical peels, 359
for hidradenitis suppurativa, 143
and pigment abnormalities, 101, 125
postoperative, 133
prophylactic, before rhinoplasty, 279
Filipinos and Polynesians, 288
graft and implant material pretreatment, 207
Middle Easterners, 347
for skin conditions, 105, 115, 122, 127
acne, 127, 128, 140–141
acne keloiditis, 131
pseudofolliculitis barbae, 107*f*
Anti-fungal creams, 135
Antihistamines, 131, 346
Anti-inflammatory agents
botanical, 132, 133
steroidal. *See* Corticosteroids
Antimicrobials, 115. *See also* Benzoyl peroxide
acne treatment, 126–127
aloe vera properties, 132
Antioxidants, 115
Antiviral agents, 115
Apocrine glands. *See* Hidradenitis suppurativa
Arnica montana, 133
Ascorbic acid, 123, 133
Ashy skin, 122
Asian phenotypes, Filipinos, 286–287
Asians
aesthetics, 64*t*, 70*t*, 72*f*, 81*f*, 82*f*, 83*f*, 247–249, 264–265
defining elements, 13
eye, 74, 75*f*, 76*f*, 77–78
facial proportions, 88
nose, 73, 86*f*, 86*t*, 91*f*, 92, 95
aging, 100, 151, 152*f*, 154*f*, 155
lips, 168
lower face and neck, 162
anatomy, 254, 263
anthropological and physiological comparisons, 31–34
cultural considerations, 253, 264, 265–267
eyelid surgery, 251–252, 254–257
anatomy, 263
epicanthoplasty, 274–277
lower lid blepharoplasty, 277
upper lid blepharoplasty, 267–274
facial characteristics, 247–249, 254
malar prominence, 247, 248*f*, 249–251
septal cartilage thickness in, 290
maxillary implants, 283–284
medical risk factors, 79
patient selection, 25
rhinoplasty, 249, 250*f*, 251, 257–261, 278–283
skin, 105*f*, 263–264
acne treatment, 129
keratosis pilaris, 133–134
scarring and keloid formation, 184
sensitivity/hypersensitivity of, 127
Asymmetry. *See also* Complications; Symmetry
African Americans
alar base resection complications, 227, 228*f*
preoperative studies, 222
Asians
after blepharoplasty, 273–274
epicanthoplasty and, 276–277
Middle Easterners
eyelid, 347

rhinoplasty, 364, 366*f*
Augmentation mentoplasty, 82*f*, 345, 354*f*, 355*f*
Augmentation of dorsum. *See* Dorsal augmentation
Autogenous tissue grafts. *See also specific tissues*
African American chin augmentation, 236
African American rhinoplasty, 202–203, 211
dorsal augmentation, 229–236
open approach, 236, 238*f*
Asian rhinoplasty, 278
Filipinos and Polynesians, 290–291, 299
Hispanics, 309
Middle Easterners, 347, 358*f*
Autoimmunity, vitiligo, 146

B

Baldness. *See* Hair loss
Balms, 132
Beauty. *See also* Aesthetics; Cultural considerations
Asian values, 264–265
Benzoin, tincture of, 351, 359
Benzophenone, 124
Benzoyl peroxide, 105, 111, 115, 121, 122, 128, 130
acne treatment, 127, 127*t*, 128, 129, 140
complications, 145
keratosis pilaris management, 134
pseudofolliculitis barbae, 107*f*
Bichat's fat pad excision, 315
Bimaxillary protrusion, 88, 309, 310, 313, 319–320
Bimaxillary surgery, Hispanics, 319–320
Bioflavonoids, 133
Birth control pills, 101, 105, 125, 126, 140
Birth defects. *See* Congenital deformities
Bizygomatic distance, Hispanics, 310, 311*f*, 318*f*, 319
Blackheads, 122, 139
Bleeding disorders, 364
Blepharoplasty, 81*f*, 118*f*, 157, 158*f*, 159, 161*f*, 167*f*
Asians, 251, 252*f*, 254–257
lower lid, 277
upper lid, 267–274
Asian patient, 251, 252*f*, 254–257
Hispanics, 310, 313
Middle Easterners, 339, 341*f*, 347, 353*f*, 354–356, 353, 358*f*, 362*f*
Blood disorders, 364
Body image, 4
Bone grafts, rhinoplasty
Asians, 260
Filipinos and Polynesians, 290
Middle Easterners, 347, 358*f*
secondary, 352–353
Botanicals, 132, 133
Brachycephaly, 44*f*
Broadbent and Matthews canons of beauty, 68, 69*f*
Brow. *See* Forehead/brow
Browplasty, 356–357
Byrd, facial analysis of, 88

C

Calcium antagonists, 188, 189*f*
Calcium thioglycolate, 142
Caldwell-Luc-like incision, 202
Canthal ligament, lateral, 356
Carbon dioxide ultrapulse laser, 359–360, 362*f*
Cartilage grafts
African American rhinoplasty, 202–203
dorsal augmentation, 229–236
open approach, 236
septal cartilage material, 217
suboptimal results, 242, 243*f*, 244*f*
Asian rhinoplasty, 260, 278
East Indians, 80*f*
Filipinos and Polynesians, 292–293*f*, 294–295*f*, 296*f*
dorsal augmentation, 291
tip enhancement, 289
Hispanics, 309, 312, 314*f*, 315, 316*f*
Middle Easterners, 347, 349*f*, 353, 358*f*, 367, 368
Northern Europeans, 373, 376*f*, 388
Cartilage splitting, 198
Castilians, 70*t*, 78*f*, 79*f*, 92, 95, 303, 304*f*
Caucasians. *See also* Northern Europeans
aesthetics, 39–58, 64*t*
appraisal, 42–45, 46*f*
cephalometrics/Frankfort horizontal, 46–49, 65*f*
cheek, 57–58
chin, 56–57
comparison with African Americans, 63*t*, 66, 67*t*, 69*f*, 70*t*, 71*f*, 71*t*
eyes, 50–52, 74, 75*f*, 78
facial relationships, 79
forehead, 50, 51*f*
golden proportion, 41–42, 43*f*, 66, 67*t*
historic evolution, 39–40
middle crura, 72*f*
mouth, 54–55, 56*f*
nose, 52–53, 54*f*, 73, 86*f*, 86*t*, 95
objective standards/criteria, 40–41
preferred, 49–50
proportions, 45–46
aging, 346
anthropological and physiological comparisons, 31–34
eyelid anatomy, 254*f*
keloids in, 184
lash liner, permanent, 159
rhinoplasty, 200, 199*t*, 200*t*
Caudate septum, 95
Cautery. *See* Electrocautery
Cellulitis
African American patient, 213
scalp, 109
Cephalic resection
African Americans, 204, 217, 219*f*
Asians, 260
Mediterraneans, 323, 324*f*, 325*f*
Cephalic rotation of tip
African American patient, 214, 215*f*, 217*f*, 240*f*
Filipinos and Polynesians, 287
Mediterraneans, 323, 324*f*
Middle Eastern nose, 368
Northern Europeans, 373, 377*f*, 389*f*, 390*f*
Cephalometry
Caucasians, 46–49
ethnic groups, 64*t*, 65
Hispanics, 309, 311–312
Cervicoplasty. *See* Neck
Cheek
aesthetics, 49, 50, 57–58
augmentation, 58
Hispanics, 315
Middle Easterners, 357
Cheekbones
aesthetics, 41, 78–79
Hispanics, 310, 311*f*, 318*f*, 319
Cheiloplasty, African Americans, 208*f*, 210, 241–242*f*
Chemical depilatories, 142
Chemical irritation, 123, 124
earring keloids, 185–186
skin reactions, 101, 106, 126, 132
Chemical peels, 121, 123, 130, 131, 145
acne treatment, 141
dressings, 132–133
Hispanics, 315
Middle Easterners, 345, 359–360
for pigment problems, 112, 113*f*, 114*f*
pre- and postoperative skin care, 131, 132, 136
skin care after, 116
Children
aging changes, 169*t*, 170*t*
circles under eyes, 131
epicanthal webbing, 77
keratosis pilaris, 133–134
Middle Eastern patients, 344
Chin
aesthetics, 41, 96
Caucasian, 49–50, 56–57
ethnic groups, 68
Northern Europeans, 95
aging, 153*t*, 154*t*, 169*t*, 170*t*
Asians, 247
Chin augmentation, 57, 82*f*, 167f. *See also* Mentoplasty
African Americans, 233–235f, 236, 238*f*
Filipinos and Polynesians, 292*f*, 299–300
Frankfort horizontal as guideline, 65
Hispanics, 309, 310, 315, 316*f*
Mediterraneans, 325*f*
Middle Easterners, 345, 357
Northern Europeans, 386*f*, 395*f*
rejuvenation techniques, 166
Chinese national characteristics, 266–267
Cholasma, 101, 122
Circles under eyes, 130–131, 153*t*, 157, 166
Citric acid, 111
Cleansing, 101
acne treatment, 127*t*
cleansers and moisturizers, 103, 121
hidradenitis suppurativa management, 143
pre- and postoperative care, 131–132, 136
Cleft lip and palate, 5, 32, 208*f*, 210, 241–242*f*
Clindamycin, 115, 128
Clotrimazole, 135
Coagulation abnormalities, 364

Cocaine, 106, 126, 346, 347, 382
Collagenase, 145, 188
Collagen implants, acne scars, 141
Color of nasal implants, 281
Columella
  aesthetics, 92
    Caucasian, 53
    ethnic groups, 73
    Northern European, 85
  African Americans, 73, 201, 233*f*, 239–240*f*
    anatomy, 200–201
    versus Caucasian patient perceptions, 199, 199*t*, 200, 200*t*
    skin thickness and, 242
  Asians, 258, 261, 263
  Filipinos and Polynesians, 287
  Hispanic patient ethnic variations, 310, 312
  Mediterraneans, 327, 333, 334*f*
  Middle Easterners, 345, 347, 348*f*, 349*f*, 363, 364, 365*t*, 366*f*, 367, 368
  Northern Europeans, 388, 389*f*
Columellar angle, 93*f*, 95
  African Americans, 69, 72*t*, 73
  ethnic groups, 63*f*
  facial relationships, 79
  Filipinos and Polynesians, 288
Columellar grafts
  Hispanics, 312, 315, 316*f*, 319–320
  Northern Europeans, 391*f*
Columellar incision, 201
Columellar splitting, 202
Columellar struts
  African Americans, 203, 206*f*, 211*t*, 214
  Asians, 279, 280, 281
  Middle Easterners, 367, 368
Comedonal acne, 139, 140
Comedones, 106, 139, 140, 145
  extraction of, 122, 131, 141
  glycolic acid and, 133
Common disorders, 122
Complete strip procedure, 385–386
Compliance/noncompliance of patient
  acne management, 140
  patient selection considerations, 23, 24–25
  pre- and postoperative skin care, 131
Complications. *See also* Pigmentation abnormalities; Scarring
  with African American rhinoplasty patients, 199, 207
    alar base resection caveats, 227
    cephalad rotation of tip, 214, 215*f*, 217*f*
    dorsal augmentation with L-shaped struts, 228
    long-term effects of tip enhancement grafts, 226*f*, 227
    skin thickness and, 242
    tip defatting, 215
  with Asian patients
    aesthetic values, 265
    blepharoplasty, 257, 273–274
    epicanthoplasty, 276
    rhinoplasty, 258, 281–283
  with Filipinos and Polynesian patients, 295–300
  with Hispanic patients, 315
  inflammatory skin conditions and, 110*f*
  of L-shaped implants, 295–298
  with Middle Easterner patients, 361
    dermabrasion, chemical peels, and laser treatment, 359–360
    orbital fat removal, 356
  with Northern European patients
    alar sill resection, 395
    nasal grafts, 373
    rhinoplasty, 381, 384–385
  orbital fat removal, 273, 356
  preoperative discussions concerning, 8
Compression dressings, keloid prevention, 176, 177*f*
Computer imaging. *See* Imaging
Conchal cartilage grafts
  African Americans, 229, 230*f*
  Filipinos and Polynesians, 289, 292–293*f*, 294–295*f*, 296*f*
  Mediterraneans, 331, 332
Congenital deformities
  cleft lip and palate, 5, 32, 208*f*, 210, 241–242*f*
  of Middle Easterners, 339, 342*f*
  patient motivations, 5
  preauricular cysts and sinuses, 31
  retinoid side effects, 128, 141
  variations among ethnic groups, 33–34
Connective tissue. *See also* Fatty/fibrofatty tissue; Scarring; Skin thickness
  Asian, 263–264
  cellulitis, 109, 213
  scalp, 109
  wound healing, 179–182
Corneal ulceration, 347
Coronal incision, malar ostectomy, 248*f*
Corrective surgery. *See* Secondary rhinoplasty
Corset platysmaplasty, 306*f*
Corticosteroids, 124*t*, 130, 131, 133, 345, 347, 351
  and acne, 126
  for acne, 140
  after dermabrasion, chemical peel, or facelift, 359
  for hidradenitis suppurativa, 143
  keloid management, 145, 187, 188, 189*f*
  keloid prevention, 176, 190
  for pseudofolliculitis barbae, 143
  and tinea versicolor, 135
  for vitiligo, 137, 146
Cosmetics and personal care products, 166, 121, 122–123, 124, 124*t*, 145, 146
  allergy and hypersensitivity. *See also* Hidradenitis suppurativa
    and acne, 104, 122, 123, 126, 139
    pigmentation changes caused by, 101, 130–131
  after chemical peels and dermabrasion, 132
  postoperative, 133, 136
  psoralens, 117
Costs/fees, 8, 306
  financially stressed patient, 28–29
  secondary surgery, 26, 29
Craniofacial anomalies
  anthropological differences, 31, 32
  Middle Easterners, 339, 342*f*
Cranium
  aesthetics, 43–44
  anthropological variations, 33
Crouzon's disease, 33
Crura
  aesthetics, 53, 72*f*
  African Americans
    anatomy, 200
    crural diastasis, 219*f*
    fixation of, 214, 215*f*
    infracartilagenous incisions and, 215, 217, 219*f*
    tip surgery, 203–204
  Asians, 258, 259–260*f*
  Filipinos and Polynesians
    excision of, 292–293*f*
    lowering by transection, 300
  Hispanic patient ethnic variations, 310
  Mediterraneans, umbrella graft, 332
  Middle Easterners, 365, 367, 368
  Northern Europeans, 379, 381, 382
    dome division procedure, 389, 390*f*
    dome reconstruction, 387, 388, 389, 390*f*
    tip plasty, 385, 386–387
Crural advancement, 259–260*f*
Crural dissection, 367
Crushed cartilage overlay grafts, 397*f*
Cryosurgery
  acne treatment, 141
  keloids, 145
  skin conditions, 119, 136
  turbinate, 348, 351
Cryptotia, 32
Cultural considerations. *See also* Aesthetics; Family
  African Americans, 195
  Asians, 255, 257, 264, 265–268
  Filipinos and Polynesians, 286–287
  Hispanics, 307
  Mediterraneans, 327–328
  Middle Easterners, 343–344, 363–364
Curvilinear consideration, 44
Cystic acne, 110*f*, 127
Cysts, inflammatory, 111

D

Decongestants, 346
Decortication, 201, 202
Dehydroepiandrosterone, 132
Demerol, 288
Dental arch, 310, 313, 319–320
Deodorant bumps. *See* Hidradenitis suppurativa
Depilatories, chemical, 142
Depressed scars, 177, 178*f*
Deproteinized hemodialysate, 132, 133
Dermablend, 146
Dermabrasion, 335
  acne treatment, 141
  Middle Easterners, 345, 359–360, 361*f*
  pre- and postoperative care, 131, 132, 136
Dermal deepithelialization, medial advancement and septal fixation, 225
Dermal tattoos, 117, 118, 119
Dermatochalasis, 77

Dermatosis papulosa nigra, 118*f*, 119, 122, 135–136
Dermis. *See also* Scarring
  aging, 154
  scarring, 174*f*
Desquamators, 121. *See also* Alpha-hydroxy acids; Retin A
Deviated septum or dorsum (crooked nose)
  African American versus Caucasian patient perceptions, 199, 200*t*
  Mediterraneans, 324*f*
Deviation, septal
  Filipinos and Polynesians, 287
  Middle Easterners, 364, 366*f*
  Northern Europeans, 378*f*
Dexamethasone, 187
Diabetes, 364
Diastasis, 373, 376*f*
Diathermy, 143
Diathesis, platysma, 357
Diazepam, contraindicated for blepharoplasty, 271
Diet/foods
  antibiotic absorption, 141
  postoperative, 133
  skin reactions, 105, 106, 121, 126
Discoid lupus erythematosus, 117
Dissatisfied patient. *See also* Complications; Patient expectations; Patient satisfaction
  dealing with, 19
  hostile rage, 26
  litigation potential, 28, 29
  prediction of, 18–19
DNA, 132
Dolichocephaly, 44*f*
Dome division, 389, 390*f*, 391–392, 393, 393*f*
Dome onlay grafts, 330–331
Dome reconstruction, Northern Europeans, 387–393, 393*f*
Domes, 93*f*
  Mediterraneans, 330
  Middle Eastern nose, 364, 367, 368
Dome spanning graft, 376*f*
Dorsal augmentation, 82*f*, 167*f*
  aesthetics, 80*f*
  African Americans, 220*f*, 228–236
    versus Caucasians, 211*t*
    limiting and interacting factors, 199
    open approach, 236
    tip projection and, 200
  Asians, 258, 259–260*f*, 260
  Filipinos and Polynesians, 80*f*, 290, 291, 292–293*f*, 294–295*f*, 298–299
  Hispanics, 312, 319–320
  Middle Easterners, 347
  Northern Europeans, 376*f*, 381
Dorsal hump
  aesthetics, 69, 73
  African Americans, 199, 199*t*, 200, 200*t*, 205*f*, 211*t*
  Asian rhinoplasty, 280
  Hispanics, 309, 314*f*, 318*f*, 319
  implant positioning, 298
  Mediterraneans, 323, 324*f*, 325*f*, 327
  Middle Easterners, 339, 341*f*, 344, 348*f*, 349, 364, 366*f*, 367*f*
  Northern Europeans, 373, 376*f*, 377*f*, 378*f*, 380, 394*f*, 395*f*
Dorsal rasping, Northern Europeans, 373, 376*f*, 377*f*, 378*f*
Dorsal width
  aesthetics, 91*f*
  African Americans, 214
  Northern Europeans, 391*f*, 392*f*
Dorsum
  aesthetics, 21, 69, 73, 80*f*, 88, 92, 93*f*
  African Americans, 204–207
    augmentation of. *See* Dorsal augmentation
    versus Caucasian patient perceptions, 199, 199*t*, 200, 200*t*, 211*t*
    narrowing of, 216*f*
    resection of, 242
    width of, 214
  Asians, 249, 250*f*, 251, 258
  complications of L-shaped implants, 297
  Hispanics, 309, 310, 311, 312, 314*f*, 315, 316*f*, 318*f*, 319
  Mediterraneans, 323, 324*f*, 325*f*, 327
  Middle Easterners, 345, 363, 364, 365*t*, 367*f*, 370
  Northern Europeans, 379, 382–385, 386*f*
Double dome creation, 387
Dressings
  keloid prevention, 176, 189–190
  scar prevention, 132, 133
Drug reactions, 101, 106, 111, 123, 125, 126
Dry eye syndrome, 347, 356
Dyoderm, 146
Dyschromias. *See* Pigmentation abnormalities

E

Ear area
  aging, 154, 162
  facelift scars, 165
  keloid repair, 176–177
  preauricular anomalies, 31, 32
Ear cartilage grafts
  African American rhinoplasty, 229, 231*f*
  Filipinos and Polynesians
    dorsal augmentation, 291
    tip augmentation, 290
  Hispanics, 312
  Mediterraneans, 333
Earring keloids, 185–186
Ears, 5
  ethnic differences, 31, 32
  keloids, 177*f*, 188
  lobe shortening, 333
  otoplasty, 82*f*
  variations among ethnic groups, 34
Eastern Europeans, 64*t*
East Indians
  aesthetics, 64*t*, 80*f*
  aging, 100
Eccrine syringomas, 277
Economic status, 13, 14, 22
Ectropion, 257, 347, 356
Eczema, 123
Edema
  eyelid, 347
  keloid prevention, 190
  postoperative
    after blepharoplasty, 273, 274, 347
    after facelift, Middle Eastern patients, 359
    methylprednisolone and, 347, 351
    patient concerns, 352
    after rhinoplasty, 351, 352
  silicone-induced, 299
  wound healing, 181, 182
Elasticity, skin. *See* Skin elasticity/laxity
Elastin, vitamin A derivatives and, 112–113
Elastosis, 154, 306*f*
Electrocautery
  dermatosis papulosa nigra, 136
  preseptal fat removal in Asians, 57
  skin conditions, 118, 119, 136
  supratarsal fold creation, 254
Electrolysis, 123, 143
Enophthalmus, 356
Enzyme peels, 121, 130
Epicanthal folds, 77–78
  aesthetic conventions, 255
  Asian, 251, 263, 269, 271
Epicanthoplasty, 273, 274–277
Epicanthus supraciliaris, 78
Epidermal growth factor, 132, 133
Epilation, 143
Epinephrine, 288, 355, 382
Epiphora, 157, 158*f*
Erythromycin, 115, 128, 140–141, 143
Ethmoid bone, 347
Ethnicity, mixed. *See* Mixed ethnicity
Euriprosopus, 310
European nose, 327–328
Exfoliants, 101, 124*t*, 130
  acne treatment, 126–127
  keratosis pilaris management, 134
  pre- and postoperative skin care, 131, 132
External rhinoplasty
  African Americans, 198, 201–202, 210*t*, 215
  Northern Europeans, 392–393, 398*f*
  secondary procedures, 295
Eye area/orbit
  aesthetics, 50–52, 57, 74–79
  aging, 153*t*, 155–160
  infraorbital hollowing, 161*f*
  infraorbital shadowing, 130–131, 153*f*, 157, 166
  malar fat pad resuspension, 162
  orbital diastasis, 339, 342*f*
  orbital rim implant, 313
  pigment changes, 130–131
  skin care, 125
Eyebrows
  aesthetics, 51–52
  aging, 151, 157, 169*t*, 170*t*
Eyelid ptosis
  Asians, 255, 273
  in Middle Easterners, 339, 340*f*
  upper, 255
Eyelids
  aesthetics
    Caucasian, 52
    ethnic groups, 74–78
  aging, 34, 100, 151, 153*t*, 154*t*, 156*f*, 157, 158*f*, 159, 169*t*, 170*t*

Eyelids *(contd.)*
Asians, 251–252, 254–257
anatomy, 263
epicanthoplasty, 274–277
lower lid blepharoplasty, 277
supratarsal fold, 251–252
upper lid blepharoplasty, 267–274
Hispanics, 310, 311
Middle Easterners, 339, 340*f*, 341*f*, 347, 353*f*, 354–356
skin conditions, 116*f*
Eyeliner, permanent, 12, 303, 306*f*
Eyes
aesthetics, 41
Caucasian, 50–52
defining elements of beauty, 13
ethnic groups, 68, 74–79
aging, 157, 158*f*
Middle Easterners, 339, 340*f*, 341*f*, 344, 345–346, 347, 353*f*, 354–359
UV protection, 131

F

Fabric softeners, 104, 121, 126
Facelifts, 165*f*, 166–167, 168*f*
Hispanics, 303, 306*f*, 313
Middle Easterners, 347, 353, 357–359
Northern Europeans, 386*f*
Facial characteristics. *See also* Aesthetics; *specific ethnic groups*
aesthetics, 41, 44, 45*f*
African Americans, 69, 72*t*
ethnic groups, 67–73, 79
Filipinos and Polynesian feature calibration, 299–300
Hispanics, 308, 310, 311*f*, 312, 313
Middle Easterners, 363, 364–365, 365*t*
Northern Europeans, 86–88
Facial cleansers. *See* Cleansing
Facial hair, 123, 344. *See also* Pseudofolliculitis barbae
Facial rejuvenation. *See* Chemical peels; Dermabrasion; Facelifts
Family, 27
communication with, 8
patient selection, 7, 18, 22–23
and personality, 12
Fascia grafts, 229, 231*f*, 232*f*, 299
Fat, dietary, 106
Fat grafts
African Americans
chin, 236, 238*f*
tip modification, 203, 204
malar prominence, 160, 161*f*, 162*f*
Middle Easterners, 357, 359
scar repair, 178
Fats and oils
acne cosmetica, 126
skin-care products, 114*t*
skin sensitivity to, 123
Fatty acids, 126, 140
Fatty/fibrofatty tissue, 94f. *See also* Suction lipectomy
African Americans, defatting rhinoplasty, 202, 203, 204, 215, 218*f*
aging, 169*t*, 179*t*
Asians, 263
lower eyelid, 277
nose, 257
orbit and eye region, 74, 75*f*, 76*f*, 255, 256*f*, 267, 272*f*, 273
Filipinos and Polynesians, 287, 289, 291
Hispanics, 311
defatting with rhinoplasty, 317*f*, 318–319
ethnic variations, 310
eyelid, 313
suction lipectomy, 303, 305*f*, 315
malar fat pads, 78, 79
Mediterranean nose, 329, 330
Middle Easterners
blepharoplasty, 354
eyelid, 339, 341*f*
neck rejuvenation, 354*f*, 355*f*, 357
orbital, 356
rhinoplasty, 365
orbital area, 156*f*, 157, 157
variations among ethnic groups, 34
Fatty tissue augmentation. *See* Fat grafts
Fees/costs, 8, 308
Fentamyl, 288
Filipinos and Polynesians, 285–300
aesthetics, 64*t*, 80*f*
anatomy, 286
chin augmentation, 292*f*
cultural considerations, 286–287
national characteristics, 267
preoperative evaluation, 287–288
rhinoplasty, 287–299
perioperative details, 288
pitfalls and complications, 298–299
preoperative evaluation, 287–288, 299–300
secondary, 395–298
rhinoplasty techniques
dorsal augmentation, 290, 291, 292–293*f*, 294–295*f*
grafting, 290–291, 292*f*
tip enhancement, 289, 290–291, 292–293*f*
Finances, 8, 26, 28–29, 308
Fixation of graft
African American rhinoplasty, 202, 236, 239–240*f*, 242
Asian rhinoplasty, 250*f*
Fixation sutures
Asian blepharoplasty, 272*f*, 273
epicanthoplasty, Asians, 275
Hispanics, 313*f*
Northern Europeans, 378*f*
Flesh moles (dermatosis papulosa nigra), 135–136
Floating method, tip augmentation, 290–291
Flurouracil, 137
Folliculitis. *See* Pseudofolliculitis barbae
Follow-up, 8, 26, 29
Foods. *See* Diet/foods
Footplates, medial, 373, 376*f*
Forehead/brow
aesthetics, 50, 51–52
aging, 151, 153*t*, 154*t*, 156, 157, 169*t*, 170*t*
Asian patient, 247
Hispanics, 311
Middle Easterners, 345–346, 347, 353*f*, 354*f*, 356–357
Foreign body reaction. *See* Scarring
Fractures, nasal, 207, 210
Frankfort horizontal
African Americans, 72*t*
Caucasians, 44, 46*f*, 47, 48, 49, 57–58
ethnic groups, 63*f*, 64*t*, 65, 64*t*
Freezing. *See* Cryosurgery
Frontal angle elevation, 299
Fronto-orbital modeling, 310

G

Gender, patient selection, 25
Genetics
and facial hair, 123
and personality, 11, 12
and skin disorders
hidradenitis suppurativa, 109
keloid formation, 184
keratosis pilaris, 133–134
tinea versicolor, 135
Genioplasty
advancement, 57
Hispanics, 309, 310, 313, 317*f*, 318–319
Middle Easterners, 345
sliding, 313, 317*f*, 318–31
Genu
African American tip definition, 217*f*
Asians, 258, 260, 261
German nose, 327–328
Glabella, Middle Easterners, 341*f*
Glabellar angle, 45*f*, 63*f*, 69, 72*t*
Glabrene, 102
Glabridin, 102
Glaucoma, 347
Glucocorticoids. *See* Corticosteroids
Glucose-6-phosphate dehydrogenase, 81
Glycolic acid, 103, 105, 110*f*, 112, 122, 124*t*, 125, 130, 133
acne treatment, 127*t*
hypersensitivity testing, 132
keratosis pilaris management, 134
pseudofolliculitis barbae, 107*f*
Glycolic acid peels, 102, 110*f*, 129, 131
hyperpigmentation treatment, 123
pre- and post-operative care, 136
Golden proportions
Caucasians, 41–42, 43*f*
ethnic groups, 64*t*, 66–73, 67*f*, 67*t*, 70*t*, 71*t*, 72*t*
Goldman technique, 389, 390*f*, 391–392, 393*f*
Gortex grafts, 203, 279
Grafts
African American chin augmentation, 233–235*f*, 236, 238*f*
African American rhinoplasty
versus Caucasians, 211*t*
dorsal augmentation, 214, 228–236
hump augmentation, 204, 206*f*, 207
open approach, 236
suboptimal outcomes, 242–244
tip enhancement, 201, 202, 202–203
tip enhancement complications, 225
tip enhancement long-term effects, 226*f*, 227
Asians, 250*f*, 251, 258, 260, 278
Filipinos and Polynesians, 290–291, 292*f*, 292–293*f*, 294–295*f*, 296*f*
dorsal augmentation, 291

tip enhancement, 289
Hispanics, 309, 312, 314*f*, 315, 316*f*
Mediterraneans, 329*t*, 330–333, 332*t*, 334*f*
Middle Easterners, 347, 352–353, 358*f*, 366
Northern European rhinoplasty, 373, 376*f*
secondary rhinoplasty, 352–353
skin, 100, 141, 144, 147
Growth factors
keloid formation, 186
keloid treatment, experimental, 145, 187, 188, 189*f*
wound healing, 132, 133, 180–181, 182
Guinta implants, 284

H

Hair, 14
acne keloiditis, 131
aesthetics, 41, 43
baldness and hair loss, 14
defining elements of beauty, 13
keratosis pilaris, 133–134
Middle Easterners, 344
pseudofolliculitis barbae, 106–109, 110*f*, 141–143
Hair, facial, 123, 344. *See also* Pseudofolliculitis barbae
Hair-care products, 105, 123, 126
acne cosmetica, 126
pomade acne, 122, 123, 139
Hair loss
aging, 153*t*, 154*t*, 155, 169*t*, 170*t*
Hispanics, 311
Hamilton Assessment of Life Balance test, 17
Hamilton Assessment of Self Esteem test, 17
Hamilton Standards of Beauty Questionnaire, 17–18
Han Chinese, 247
Hanging columella, 367
Harmony. *See* Aesthetics
Head form, 33, 43–44
Healing by secondary intent, 109, 110*f*
Hematein, 102
Hematological abnormalities, 33
Hemodialysate, deproteinized, 132, 133
Hemoglobinopathies, 81
Hemolytic anemia, 81
Herpesvirus infections, 115, 346
Hidradenitis suppurativa, 99, 109, 111, 122, 123, 124*t*, 143–144
alpha-hydroxy acids for, 112
benzoyl peroxide for, 115
Hispanics
aesthetics, 64*t*, 69, 70*f*, 70*t*, 78*f*, 93*f*
defining elements, 13
facial proportions, 88
Frankfort horizontal, 65*f*
middle crura, 72*f*
nose, 73, 88, 89, 92, 95
study group, 61, 63
aging, 151, 152*f*, 154*f*, 155, 311
facelifts, 165*f*
lips, 168
lower face and neck, 162
blepharoplasty, 313
case studies, 315–320
cheek augmentation, 315
chemical peeling, 315
complications, 315
contraindications for procedures, 308
cultural considerations, 307
diagnostic and therapeutic approaches, 312–313
ethnic specifics, 310–311
face and neck contouring, 303, 305*f*, 306
facelift, 313
facial characteristics, 308
features, 303, 304*f*, 305*f*
indications for procedures, 308
lash liner, permanent, 159–160
orthognatic procedure, 313
patient satisfaction, 310
patient selection, 25
pre-operative evaluation, 308–309
rhinoplasty, 312, 313*f*, 314*f*
skin disorders, 105*f*, 131
acne treatment, 129
keratosis pilaris, 133–134
skin sensitivity, 127
suction lipectomy, 315
History. *See* Medical history
Holoprogin, 135
Hormonal factors
and acne, 105, 126
and facial hair, 123
and hidradenitis suppurativa, 143
and keloid formation, 186
and pigment abnormalities, 101
and vitiligo, 146
Hostile patient, 26
Hump deformity. *See* Dorsal hump
Hyaluronic acid, 115
Hydrocortisone, 130, 131, 133, 187
Hydroquinone, 101, 102, 105, 114, 123, 125, 130, 213, 345, 360
acne treatment, 127*t*
allergy to, 103, 132
keratosis pilaris management, 134
pseudofolliculitis barbae, 107*f*
Hydroxyapatite graft material, 203
Hygiene. *See* Cleansing
Hyperkeratosis, 127, 140
Hyperpigmentation/discoloration, 101–103, 123. *See also* Pigmentation abnormalities
retinoid side effects, 128
sun sensitivity and, 127
Hypersensitivity, skin. *See* Allergy/hypersensitivity, skin
Hypertrophic scars, 122, 184–186
Hypopigmentation
tinea versicolor, 122, 134–135
vitiligo, 116–119, 122, 137, 146–147, 178*f*

I

I-beam cartilage grafts, 388, 391*f*, 392, 392*f*
Identity
body image, 4
ethnic, patient attitudes, 4, 5, 6
psychological considerations, 11–19
Imaging
aesthetics, 81*f*, 83*f*
African Americans, 222, 244*f*
Asians, blepharoplasty planning, 269, 270*f*, 271*f*, 274
clarification of patient goals and expectations, 21, 22
Filipinos and Polynesians, 287, 299–300
Hispanics, 309
informed consent, 29
Middle Easterners, 346, 363
Northern European rhinoplasty, 382
Imidazole anti-fungals, 135
Immune system, 135, 146, 179–182
Immunosuppression, 135
Implantech, 291
Implants. *See also* Grafts; Synthetic materials
African American rhinoplasty
versus Caucasians, 211*t*
hump augmentation, 204, 206*f*, 207
Asian rhinoplasty, 278, 279–283
chin augmentation, 82*f*
complications, 295, 296*f*
Incisal angle, 63*f*, 69, 72*t*
Incisions. *See also specific procedures*
dressings, 132–133
facelift, 165*f*
Indian. *See* East Indians; Native Americans
Infection
Asian rhinoplasty, 281
fungal, 122, 134–135
and pigment abnormalities, 101
post-inflammatory hyperpigmentation, 122
preoperative assessment, 346
pseudofolliculitis barbae, 106–109, 110*f*
rhinoplasty complications in Filipinos and Polynesians, 293, 298
Inflammation. *See also* Scarring
electrolysis and, 123
keloid prevention, 190
post-inflammatory hyperpigmentation, 101, 102, 122, 123, 139–140, 145, 146
skin lesions, 105. *See also* Skin problems
pre- and post-operative care, 136
pseudofolliculitis barbae, 106–109, 110*f*
wound healing, 179–182
Inflammatory acne, 139, 140
Informed consent, 29
Infracture
Hispanics, 312
lateral
African Americans, 214, 236
Filipinos and Polynesians, 80*f*
Middle Eastern rhinoplasty, 351
septal, Asians, 250*f*, 251
Infraorbital hollowing, 161*f*
Infraorbital shadowing, 130–131, 153*t*, 157, 166
Interalar cinch procedure, 225
Interalar dimensions
aesthetics, 68, 69, 70*f*
Filipinos and Polynesians, 287
Northern Europeans, 89, 90*f*, 373, 376*f*

Intercanthal dimensions
aesthetics, 89
Caucasian, 51
ethnic groups, 62*f*
Asians, 247
Middle Easterners, 365*t*
Intercrural fixation, 219*f*
Intercrural grafts, 291
Interferons, 145
Interleukin-1, 145
Internal approach
African American rhinoplasty, 215, 217, 219*f*
Hispanics, 312, 313*f*
Intra-oral approach. *See* Internal approach
Inverted V transcolumellar incision, 393
Iodide, 105
Isotretinoin (Accutane), 110*f*, 111, 112–113, 114, 122, 127–128, 140, 141
Italian phenotypes, 333, 335
Italians. *See* Mediterraneans

J

Japanese national characteristics, 265–266
Jaw/jawline. *See also* Hypogonia
aesthetics, 41, 44*f*, 82*f*, 95
African Americans, 69–70
Caucasian, 49–50
cephalometrics, 48, 49
aging, 81*f*, 82*f*, 168*f*
Asians, 247
fat grafts, 162, 164*f*
Hispanics, 303, 305*f*
Middle Easterners, 340*f*
Jewish phenotypes, 333, 334*f*
Jobst pressure garment, 132
Jowls, 82*f*, 162, 164*f*, 168*f*

K

Keloid, 122, 144–145
African Americans. *See* Scarring
Asians, 264
Northern Europeans, 397
pre- and postoperative prophylaxis, 132–133
Keloiditis, acne, 131
Kenalog, 312
Keratolytics, 130
Keratoses
Asians, 277
seborrheic, 135
Keratosis pilaris, 122, 133–134
Ketoconazole, 135
Koebnerization of skin grafts, 147
Kojic acid, 101, 102, 114, 123, 125, 130, 132, 133
Kolite cream, 102
Korean national characteristics, 266

L

Lactic acid, 103, 111, 134, 354
Lapps, 31
Laser treatment
keloids, 145
Middle Easterners, 359–360, 362*f*
pigment abnormalities, 103
skin lesions, 102
Lash liner, permanent, 159–160, 303, 306
Lateral canthus suspension, 159, 356
Lateral cartilage, 93*f*
African Americans, 214, 219*f*, 239–240*f*
anatomy, 200
cartilage-splitting techniques, 199
tip anatomy and, 203
Asians, 260, 278, 279, 283
Mediterraneans, 323, 324*f*, 325*f*, 325*f*, 328–330, 329*t*
Middle Easterners, 348*f*, 364, 366*f*
Northern Europeans, 373, 376*f*, 380*f*, 384, 385, 389, 393
Lateral face, age changes, 162, 164*f*, 165*f*, 166–168*f*
Lateral genu, infracartilagenous incisions and, 217
Lateral infracture
African Americans, 214, 236
Filipinos and Polynesians, 80*f*
Lateral osteotomy, 211*t*
Leforte I setback osteotomy, 88
Leishmaniasis, 345
Lentiges, 277
Leptorrhine nose, 32, 379–380
Levator anguli plication, 82*f*
Levator aponeurosis, 75*f*, 76*f*, 77, 254*f*, 255, 256*f*, 268, 272*f*
Liability issues, 6–7
Lichen planus, 145
Licorice derivatives, 102
Lidocaine, 355, 382
Lightening creams, 13, 14
Limited incision browplasty, 356–357
Lipectomy/liposuction. *See* Suction lipectomy
Lipids. *See* Fats and oils; Fatty/fibrofatty tissue
Lips
aesthetics, 41
Caucasian, 54–55
ethnic groups, 62*f*, 68
Northern Europeans, 95
aging, 101, 153*t*, 154*t*, 168–169, 169*t*, 170*t*
augmentation/repair
African Americans, 208*f*, 210, 241–242*f*
Filipinos, 287
cleft lip and palate, 5, 32, 208*f*, 210, 241–242*f*
defining elements of beauty, 13
Hispanic patient ethnic variations, 311
reduction of, 82*f*
skin care, 125
Litigation, 5, 19, 27–29
Lobular columella angle, Filipinos and Polynesians, 288
Lobular projection, Asian rhinoplasty, 280–281
Long-term effects
African American rhinoplasty, 200
alar base modification, 203
dermal thinning, 203, 204
graft resorption, 203
hump augmentation and tip ptosis, 207
tip blunting and drooping, 242
tip enhancement, 221
Hispanic patient facelifts, 313
tip grafts, floating, 290–291
L-shaped implants
African Americans, 228
Filipinos and Polynesians, complications, 295, 296*f*
Lupus erythematosus, 117

M

Make-up. *See* Cosmetics and personal care products
Malar area
aging, 151, 155, 157, 160–162, 163*f*, 169*t*, 170*t*
of Asians, 247, 248*f*, 249–251
fat pad, 162
aging and, 151, 157, 160–162, 163*f*
resuspension of, 81*f*, 306*f*
of Filipinos with Asian features, 286–287
hypoplasia
aesthetics, 69–70, 72*f*, 78–79
African Americans, 233–235*f*, 236, 238*f*
aging, 155
of Middle Easterners, 339, 340*f*
Malar augmentation/implants, 160, 161*f*, 167*f*
aging changes and, 161*f*
fat grafts, 162
Filipinos and Polynesians, 299–300
Frankfort horizontal as guideline, 65
Mediterraneans, 324*f*
rejuvenation techniques, 166
Malar bags, 339
Malar eminence, 340*f*
Malar sag, 306*f*
Malays. *See* Filipinos and Polynesians
Males
aesthetics, 64*t*, 70*f*, 80*f*
African Americans, 66, 67*t*, 69*f*
Caucasians, 49, 50, 54–55
defining elements, 13
ethnic groups, 62*f*
golden proportions, 66–67, 68
nose, 92
African American
alar base resection caveats, 227
cephalic rim resection in, 219*f*
aging, 153, 154*t*, 170*t*
Asian
double eyelid creation, 267
lower lid blepharoplasty, 277
Hispanic, 307, 311
Middle Eastern, 366*f*
Northern European rhinoplasty, 383–384
patient expectations, 5
patient selection, 25
preauricular cysts and sinuses, 31
skin conditions, 105, 111. *See also* *specific skin conditions*
Malic acid, 111
Mandible. *See also* Hypogonia
aesthetics, 49–50, 88
rocker jaw, 285
Mandibular angles, 95
Mandibular augmentation, Filipinos, 287
Mandibular osteotomy, 319–320
Mandibular setback, 311

Maori, 285
Marcaine, 288
Marquart overlay, 42, 43*f*
Mauro technique, 254
Maxilla
  aesthetics, 49
  Asian, 263
Maxillary augmentation
  Asians, 283–284
  Filipinos and Polynesians, 299–300
Maxillary osteotomy, 88, 319–320
Maxillary spine, 201
Meatoplasty, 211*t*
Mechanical stress
  and acne, 106, 126
  graft material, 203
  and scarring, 181, 182, 184*f*
    keloid formation, 189
    keloid prevention, 189–190
  skin reactions, 123
Medial advancement, 225
Mediation, 26
Medical conditions
  ethnic groups, 79, 81
  physiological comparisons of ethnic groups, 31–34
Medical history, 22
  hyperpigmentation problems, 123
  Middle Eastern patients, 364
Medications, skin reactions, 101, 106, 111, 123, 125, 126
Mediterraneans, 33, 323, 324–325*f*
  acne, 129
  cultural considerations, 327–328
  medical risk factors, 79
  rhinoplasty, 323, 324*f*, 325*f*, 327–336
    external shaving, 334–335
    lower lateral cartilage sculpturing, 328–330
    onlay graft, 330–331
    tip projection, 328–335, 328*t*
    umbrella graft, 332–333, 332*t*, 334*f*
  skin sensitivity, 127
Melanesians, 31. *See also* Filipinos and Polynesians
Melanocyte transplants, 147
Melasma, 101, 113*f*, 114*f*, 122, 123
Menstrual cycles, 126, 143
Mental and submental fullness, aging and, 162, 164*f*, 165*f*
Mental illness, 16
Menton, aesthetics, 79
Mentoplasty, 82*f*, 344, 354*f*, 355f. *See also* Chin augmentation
Mersilene mesh, 367
  African American rhinoplasty, 204, 207
  Asians
    maxillary implants, 284
    rhinoplasty, 279
  secondary procedures, 295, 296*f*
Mesorrhine nose, 32, 379
Mestizo features, 307, 309, 310, 313
Methyl anthranilate, 124
Methylprednisolone, 347
Miconazole, 135
Microfoam dressing, 357, 359
Microgenia
  African Americans, 69–70, 72*f*, 233–235*f*
  Hispanics, 313, 315, 316*f*, 317*f*, 318–320
  Mediterraneans, 325*f*
  Northern European, 395*f*
Microorganisms
  and hidradenitis suppurativa, 143
  skin flora, 140
Micropigmentation procedure, 117, 137, 147
Midazolam, 271
Midcolumellar incisions, 259*f*
Midcolumellar strut, 214
Middle Easterners
  aesthetics and features of, 64*t*, 80*f*, 339, 340*f*, 344–346
    eyelids, 339, 340*f*, 341*f*
    eyes, 344
    general appearance, 344–346
    nose, 73, 92, 95, 339, 341*f*, 342*f*
  age, 344
  chemical peel, dermabrasion, and laser treatment, 359–360, 361*f*, 362*f*
  cultural considerations, 343–344
  patient evaluation and preparation, 346–347
  preoperative preparation, 347
  rejuvenation of eyes, forehead, and neck, 353*f*, 354–359
  rhinoplasty, 363–370
    cultural considerations, 363–364
    facial characteristics, 364–365, 365*t*
    operative techniques, 347–353, 354*f*, 355*f*, 365–368, 369
    patient expectations and objectives, 368, 370
    preoperative evaluation, 365*t*
Mikamo technique, 254
Milia, 111, 133, 213, 359
Miltex Shamberg extractor, 122
Minerals, 133
Mini-facelift, 165*f*, 166–167, 168*f*, 303, 306*f*
Minocycline, 125, 131, 140
Mixed ethnicity, 33
  aesthetic study populations, 63*f*, 64*t*
  Hispanics, 309, 310–311, 315, 316*f*, 317*f*, 318–319
Moisturizers, 99, 116, 124*t*, 125
  after chemical peels and dermabrasion, 132
  postoperative, 133
Mongolian spots, 122
Morphometrics, 85
Motivation, patient. *See* Patient expectations; Patient selection
Mouth. *See also* Lips
  aesthetics, 44*f*, 54–55, 56*f*
  Asians, 247
  dental arch, 310, 313, 319–320
M-struts, 167*f*
  African American rhinoplasty, 219*f*, 220–221, 221*f*, 243*f*, 244*f*
    dorsal augmentation, 229, 232–235*f*
    tip augmentation, 236–237
    tip revision, 239–240*f*
  Asian rhinoplasty, 250*f*, 251
  Northern Europeans, 373, 376*f*
Multiplane facelift, 357–359

N

Nasal decortication, 201
Nasal length
  aesthetics, 69, 88, 93*f*, 96
    Caucasians, 53
    ethnic groups, 62*f*
  African Americans, 214, 215*f*
    complications of medial crural fixation in African Americans, 214, 215*f*
    skin thickness and, 242
  Mediterraneans, 323, 324*f*, 325*f*, 333, 334*f*
  Middle Easterners, 345, 364
  Northern Europeans, 379
Nasal obstruction, African American versus Caucasian patient perceptions, 199, 199*t*, 200, 200*t*
Nasal templates, 73
Nasal tip. *See* Tip augmentation/ enhancement; Tip structure
Nasal valve collapse
  Hispanics, 312, 315, 317*f*, 318–319
  Mediterraneans, 324*f*
Nasal valve obstruction, Northern Europeans, 378*f*
Nasal valve support, Hispanics, 317*f*, 319
Nasal width
  aesthetics, 62*f*
  variations among ethnic groups, 33
Nasion, aesthetics, 69, 70*t*, 71, 73
Nasoencephalocoeles, 339, 342*f*
Nasofrontal angle
  aesthetics, 92
  Filipinos and Polynesians, 288
  Middle Easterners, 347
Nasoglabellar angle, 312
Nasolabial angle, 95
  aesthetics, 53, 93*f*, 94*f*
  African Americans, 200
  Asians, 258
  Filipinos and Polynesians, 287, 288
  Hispanics, 309, 310, 312, 313*f*, 314*f*, 315, 316*f*
  Mediterraneans, 327
  Middle Easterners, 363, 364, 365*t*, 370
  Northern Europeans, 382, 391*f*
Nasolabial fold
  aging, 153*t*, 157. 160, 162*f*, 163*f*, 164, 166, 167*f*, 169*t*, 170*t*
  Hispanics, 306*f*, 311
Nasolabial implants, 211*t*
Nasolabial problems, African American versus Caucasian patient perceptions, 199, 199*t*, 200, 200*t*
National characteristics, Asian, 265–267
Native American phenotype, Hispanics, 314*f*, 315, 316*f*, 317*f*, 318–319
Native Americans, 32
  aesthetics, 64*t*, 73
  aging, 100
  skin disorders, 105*f*
Nd-Yag laser, 102, 103
Neck
  aging, 153*t*, 154*t*, 162, 164*f*, 165*f*, 166–168*f*, 169*f*, 169*t*, 170*t*
  rejuvenation, 81*f*, 82*f*
    Hispanics, 310
    Middle Easterners, 345–346, 347, 353, 354, 357, 358*f*

Neck *(contd.)*
skin conditions, 117*f*
acne keloiditis, 131
pseudofolliculitis barbae, 106–109, 110*f*
Necrosis of tip, 312
Negroid phenotype, 310, 313*f*, 315, 316*f*
Neoclassical canon of proportions, 64*t*, 65–66, 78
Niacinamide, 102
Nifedipine, 188
Nodulocystic acne, 139, 140
Normocephaly, 44*f*
Northern Europeans. *See also* Caucasians
aging, 346
aesthetics, 13, 85–96
facial features, 373, 374*f*, 375*f*
nose characteristics, 327–328
rhinoplasty, 379–398
alar sill resections, 394–397, 398*f*
anatomy, 380–382
dorsum, 382–385, 386*f*
external, 392–393, 398*f*
features of nose, 373, 376*f*, 377*f*, 378*f*
leptorrhine nose, 379–380
preoperative consultation, 382
tip, 385–392, 393*f*, 394*f*, 395*f*, 396*f*, 397*f*, 398*f*
Nose. *See also* Alar cartilage surgery; Alar wedge excision/resection; Dorsum; Rhinoplasty
aesthetics, 41
Caucasian, 52–53, 54*f*
defining elements of beauty, 13
ethnic groups, 68–69, 70*t*, 71, 73
facial relationships, 79
Northern Europeans, 85–95
African Americans, 201
aging, 100, 153*t*, 154*t*, 169*t*, 170*t*
anthropological comparisons, 32
Asian, 247, 263, 274, 277, 278
dimensions of. *See* Nasal length; Nasal width; Nostrils; Tip structure
Hispanics, 303, 305*f*, 310–311, 312, 315, 316*f*, 319–320
Middle Easterners, 339, 341*f*, 342*f*, 346–353, 354*f*, 355*f*, 364, 365*t*
Northern Europeans, 379–398
skin conditions, 110*f*
Nostrils. *See also* Alar cartilage surgery; Alar wedge excision/resection
aesthetics, 53, 85, 86*f*, 86*t*, 92
African Americans, 199, 199*t*, 200, 200*t*
alar flaring. *See* Alar flare
Asians, 258
comparison of ethnic groups, 32–33
Filipinos and Polynesians, 287
Hispanics, 309, 310, 311, 312
Northern Europeans, 379, 381, 392*f*
Nostril wedge excision. *See* Alar wedge excision/resection
Nutrition, 133. *See also* Diet/foods

O

Occlusion (dental)
cephalometrics, 48–49, 50
Hispanics, 309, 312, 313
Oceania. *See* Filipinos and Polynesians
Ochronosis, 123
Octyl methoxycinnamate, 124
Octyl salicylate, 124
Ohashi technique, 254
Oils. *See* Fats and oils
Oily skin, 110*f*, 121
Onlay grafts, 80*f*, 82*f*
African Americans, 221
Mediterraneans, 329*t*, 330–331
Middle Easterners, 347, 368
Open bite deformities, 72*f*
Open rhinoplasty
African Americans, 215, 236–237
Filipinos and Polynesians, tip enhancement, 289
Middle Easterners, 358*f*
Northern Europeans, 376*f*
secondary procedures, 295, 296*f*, 352–353
Operating room etiquette, 8
Oral contraceptives, 101, 105, 125, 126, 140
Orbicularis oculi, 75*f*, 76*f*
attachment to lateral canthal ligament, 356
palpebral fold creation in Asians, 268
suturing of in Asians, 272*f*, 273
Orbit. *See* Eye area/orbit
Orbital diastasis, 339, 342*f*
Orbital rim implant, 313
Orthodontics
cephalometry, 48–49, 50
Hispanics, 309, 312, 313
Orthognathic occlusion, 48
Orthognatic surgery, Hispanics, 309, 310, 312, 313
Ostectomy, 248*f*
Osteotomy
African American versus Caucasians, 211*t*
Asians, malar reduction, 249, 249*f*, 250*f*
Hispanics, 313, 318–319, 319*f*, 320
Leforte I setback, 88
Middle Easterners, 339, 341*f*, 347, 348*f*, 366, 367*f*
Northern Europeans, 373, 376*f*, 383, 384, 393*f*
Otoplasty, 5, 82*f*
keloid formation, 174*f*
Middle Eastern patients, 344
Oxybenzone, 124

P

Packing, after septoplasty, 368
Padimate O, 124
Palpebral fissure, 70*t*
Palpebral fold, 267, 268, 274
Paraben, 132
Paraminobenzoic acid, 124
Patient care coordinator, 26, 29
Patient evaluation. *See* Patient selection; Preoperative evaluation
Patient expectations, 3, 4, 5, 6. *See also* Dissatisfied patient; Patient satisfaction
Asian rhinoplasty, 279
clarification of goals, 21
Hispanics, 308–309
imaging and, 83*f*
Middle Easterners, 363, 368, 370
Northern Europeans, 382
outcomes and goals of surgery, 81, 82*f*, 83*f*
physician-patient communication, 19
unrealistic, 23
Patient satisfaction, 21–26, 398. *See also* Complications; Dissatisfied patient; Patient selection
African American rhinoplasty, 242–244
Asians, 254
aesthetic values, 265
blepharoplasty planning, 269, 270*f*, 271*f*, 274
cultural values, 266–267
preparation for changes after blepharoplasty, 252*f*
Hispanics, 310
litigation, 27–29
Northern European rhinoplasty, 382
pre- and postoperative skin care, 131
Patient selection, 3–8
assessing suitability, 16–18
contraindications, 4
dealing with dissatisfied patient, 19
demand/market for surgery, 3
emotional (in)adequacy, 5
gender, 25
ideal candidate, 3–4
liability potential, 6–7
personality growth and development, 11–12
physician-patient relationship, 19, 22
preoperative visits, 23
prevention of problems, 8
problem personality characteristics, 23–25
psychological considerations, 11–19
screening and elimination criteria, 18–19
self-criticism, dynamics of, 12–14
social support system, 22–23
stability, defining, 14–15
Pedestal graft, 203
Pediatric patients. *See* Adolescents; Children
Peer support. *See* Family
Penicillin, 143
Perifolliculitis capitis abscendens et suffidiens, 109
Pernicious anemia, 33
Personality disorders, 16
Personality, patient. *See* Patient selection
Phenol peels, 112, 145, 345
Phenylalanine, 137
Phi (Phidias), 58
Asians, 247, 248*f*
defined, 41, 42*f*
ethnic groups, 64*t*, 66–73, 67*f*, 67*t*, 70*t*, 71*t*, 72*t*, 79
Asians, 247, 248*f*
Phospholipid-containing skin care products, 116
Photoaging. *See* Sun damage
Photography. *See* Imaging
Photosensitivity, 122, 125
antibiotics and, 127
medications causing, 115*t*
retinoids and, 128, 141
Phototherapy, 137, 145, 147

Physician-patient relationship, 140
  Asians, 264, 265, 266–267
  clarification of goals, 21
  communicating with patient, 19
  informed consent, 29
  litigation, 27–29
  patient selection, 7, 19
    key questions, 22
    red flags, 23–25
Physiological differences, 31–34
Pigmentation, 13, 14. *See also* Skin color
Pigmentation abnormalities, 121, 122, 141
  acne and, 103
  in African Americans
    dermal thinning and, 203–204
    normal variation in, 145, 146*f*
    rib cartilage donor site, 242, 244*f*
  in Asians, 254, 263, 264
  causes of, 100, 105
  chemical peel or laser treatment complications, 345, 359–360
  in Hispanics, 312, 315
  hyperpigmentation/discoloration, 101–103, 123
  infraorbital shadowing, 130–131, 153*f*, 157, 166
  keratosis pilaris and, 134
  micropigmentation procedure, 117, 137, 147
  in Middle Eastern patients, 344, 345, 359–360
  retinoid side effects, 114, 128
  sun sensitivity and, 127
  supratip skin shaving and, 335
  vitiligo, 116–119, 146–147
Pigmented lesions, in Asians, 277
Pigment neutralizers. *See* Skin lighteners
Piriformis, 310, 311
Pitanguy's ligament, 381, 382
Pityriasis rosea, 145
Pityrosporon orbiculare, 134
Platyrrhine nose, 32, 379, 381, 374, 382, 386, 391, 393*f*
Platysma, suction lipectomy, 354*f*
Platysma banding, 162, 166, 168*f*, 357
Platysmaplasty, corset, 306*f*
Platysma repair
  Hispanics, 306*f*
  Middle Easterners, 354*f*, 355*f*
Platysma resection, 167
Pollybeak deformity, 384–385, 395
Polyamide grafts, 203, 204, 207. *See also* Synthetic materials
Polynesians. *See* Filipinos and Polynesians
Polytetrafluoroethylene materials, 228, 229*f*
Pomade acne, 122, 123, 139
Portugese. *See* Mediterraneans
Portugese phenotype, Hispanics, 317*f*, 318–319
Post-inflammatory hyperpigmentation, 122
Postoperative care, 131–133, 136
  Middle Easterners, 359
    of nose, 351
    skin regimen, 354
  patient follow-up, 8, 26, 29
Preauricular area
  aging, 154, 162
  cysts, sinuses, appendages, 31
Pregnancy, 125, 126
  and pigment abnormalities, 101
  retinoid side effects, 128, 141
  and tinea versicolor, 135
Preoperative care, 131–133, 136
Preoperative consultations, 23
Preoperative evaluation
  Asians
    blepharoplasty, 269, 270*f*, 271*f*, 274
    communication with and counseling of, 254
    epicanthoplasty, 277
    rhinoplasty, 279, 282
  Filipinos and Polynesians, 287–288, 299–300
  Hispanics, 308–309, 315
  Middle Easterners, 346–347, 360–361, 363, 365*t*
  Northern Europeans for rhinoplasty, 382
  psychological, 16–18
Preoperative imaging. *See* Imaging
Pressure dressings and garments, 132, 176
Procerus muscle, 381, 382
Profile, aesthetics, 41, 44, 45*f*, 46*f*, 47, 49–50
Prognathic occlusion, 48, 310
Progonion, facial convexity angle, 45*f*
Propionibacterium acnes, 140
Proplast grafts, 203, 242, 243*f*, 324*f*
Proptosis
  aging, 155, 156, 158*f*
  lower lid, 79
Pseudofolliculitis barbae, 99, 103, 106–109, 110*f*, 122, 130, 140–143
  alpha-hydroxy acids for, 112
  benzoyl peroxide for, 115
Pseudofolliculitis nuchae, 108*f*
Psilosebaceous occlusive diseases, 106–111, 115, 135–144
Psoralens, 115*t*, 117, 137, 145, 147
Psychiatric consultation, patient approval, 4
Psychiatric illness, 22, 24
Psychology. *See* Patient selection
Psychosocial considerations, African Americans, 199–200
PTFL-xomed, 228, 229*f*
Punch grafting, acne treatment, 141
Pustular acne, 128
PUVA (psoralens), 137, 145, 147

R

Radiation therapies, 143, 188–189
Razor bumps. *See* Pseudofolliculitis barbae
Remedial surgery. *See* Secondary rhinoplasty
Resorcinol, 121, 130, 134
Resorption of cartilage grafts, 203
Retention hyperkeratosis, 127
Retin A/retinoids, 102, 103, 111, 121, 122, 124*t*, 128, 345
  acne treatment, 140
  African American patient pretreatment, 213
  complications, 145
  keratosis pilaris management, 134
  after laser treatment, 359–360
  photosensitivity with, 125
  pre- and postoperative skin care, 131
  pseudofolliculitis barbae, 143
  for tinea versicolor, 135
Retrognathic occlusion, 48
Revisions. *See* Secondary rhinoplasty
Rhinophyma, 111, 209*f*, 210, 334
Rhinoplasty
  aesthetics, 80*f*, 81, 82*f*, 83*f*
  African Americans
    adolescent and pediatrics, 207, 208*f*, 210
    alar base techniques, 203
    alar flaring, 221–227, 228*f*
    anatomic considerations, 213–214
    cultural considerations, 195
    dorsal augmentation, 228–236
    dorsum, 204–207
    historical considerations, 214, 215*f*, 216*f*, 217*f*
    individualization of approach, 197–199
    open approach, 236–237
    psychosocial considerations, 199–200
    rhinophyma, 209*f*, 210
    skin thickness, 237–242
    suboptimal results, 242–244
    surgical description, 201–202
    surgical maneuvers, 210–211, 210*t*, 211*t*
    techniques, 215, 218–221
    tip defatting, 215, 218*f*
    tip projection techniques, 202–203
    tip surgery, 203–204
    topographical anatomy, 200–201
  Asians, 249, 250*f*, 251, 257–261, 278–283
  Filipinos and Polynesians, 287–299
    dorsal augmentation, 290, 291, 292–293*f*, 294–295*f*
    grafting, 290–291, 292*f*
    perioperative details, 288
    pitfalls and complications, 298–299
    preoperative evaluation, 287–288, 299–300
    secondary, 295–298
    tip enhancement, 289, 290–291, 292–293*f*
  Hispanics, 303, 308, 309, 310, 312, 313*f*, 314*f*, 315, 316*f*, 317*f*, 318–319
  Mediterraneans, 323, 324*f*, 325*f*, 327–336
    cultural considerations, 327–328
    operative techniques, 328–335, 328*t*
  Middle Easterners, 339, 341*f*, 342*f*, 345, 347–353, 354*f*, 355*f*, 363–370
    age and, 344
    cultural considerations, 363–364
    evaluation of, 346–347
    facial characteristics, 364–365, 365*t*
    operative techniques, 365–368, 369
    patient expectations and objectives, 368, 370
    preoperative evaluation, 365*t*
  Northern Europeans, 85–96
    alar sill resections, 394–397, 398*f*
    anatomy, 380–382
    dorsum, 382–385, 386*f*
    external, 392–393, 398*f*

Rhinoplasty, Northern Europeans *(contd.)*
features of nose, 373
leptorrhine nose, 379–380
nasal proportions, 89–95
nostrils, 85, 86*f*
preoperative consultation, 382
tip, 385–392, 393*f*, 394*f*, 395*f*, 396*f*, 397*f*, 398*f*
patient motivations, 5
templates for different ethnic groups, 73
Rhytidectomy, 165*f*, 166–167, 168*f*
Asians, 254, 264
Hispanics, 303, 306*f*, 315
scarring, 165*f*, 166
Rhytides, 99, 100, 151, 154, 277
Rib cartilage grafts
African American rhinoplasty, 239–240*f*
dorsal augmentation, 229, 232–235*f*
open approach, 236
skin stretching, 238*f*
suboptimal results, 242, 243*f*, 244*f*
Asian rhinoplasty, 251, 260
Filipinos and Polynesians, 290
Hispanics, 309
Middle Easterners, 347
Ricketts caliper, 66
Ricketts method, 58
Rocker jaw, 285
Rosacea, 101, 111, 112, 115

S
Saddle deformity
African American rhinoplasty, 199, 199*t*, 200, 200*t*, 220*f*
Hispanics, 315
Sagging
Hispanics, 313
Salicylic acid, 127, 129, 140, 141
Samoans, 64*t*
Scalp
acne keloiditis, 122, 131
aging, 153*t*, 154*t*, 155, 169*t*, 170*t*
cellulitis of, 109
pseudofolliculitis barbae, 106–109, 110*f*
skin problems, 122
Scarring, 14, 122, 173–178, 179–190
acne, 103, 131, 141
acne keloiditis, 131
African American rhinoplasty, 201, 202
alar base incisions and, 203, 223*f*
open approach and, 237
Asians, 263–264, 276
causes, contributing factors, pathogenesis, 173, 174*f*, 175*f*, 182–184, 183*t*
chemical peels and, 145
clinical manifestations, 184–186
depressed scars, 177, 178*f*
facelift considerations, 165*f*, 166, 313
Hispanics, 303, 310, 312, 313, 315
Mediterraneans, 330
Middle Easterners, 344, 345, 355, 361
normal wound healing, 179–182
Northern Europeans, 397
preoperative discussion and postoperative regimen, 132
prevention, 189–190
pseudofolliculitis barbae and, 109
rhinoplasty
external, 393
secondary, 298
sites where keloids do not occur, 173, 176
skin color and, 184
skin disorders, 105*f*
treatment, 174*f*, 176–177, 186–189
Screening, patient. *See* Patient selection
Scrubs, 130
Seborrhea, 122
Seborrheic keratoses, 135, 277
Secondary procedures
Hispanics, 308
preoperative discussion of potential need for, 26, 29
Secondary rhinoplasty
Filipinos and Polynesians, 293, 295–298
Hispanics, 308, 309, 317*f*, 318–320
Mediterraneans, 331
Middle Easterner, 352–353
Northern Europeans, 383, 384, 392–393
Second opinion, 26, 29
Sedation, 8, 288
Selenium sulfide, 135
Self-criticism, dynamics of, 12–14
Self-image. *See* Identity
Septal cartilage grafts
African Americans, 202–203, 217, 229, 231
Asians, 250*f*, 251, 260
Filipinos and Polynesians, 289, 290
Hispanics, 315, 316*f*
Mediterraneans, 324*f*
Middle Easterners, 347, 367
Northern Europeans, 373, 376*f*
Septal deformities, 207
Septal deviation, 32
Middle Easterners, 364
Northern Europeans, 376*f*, 378*f*
Septal infracture, Asians, 250*f*, 251
Septal perforation, 346
Septoplasty
African Americans, 210, 211*t*, 220
Middle Easterners, 349*f*, 365, 367, 368
Northern Europeans, 382
Septum
African Americans, 214
Northern Europeans, 380–381, 389*f*, 390*f*
Shaving of supratip area, 328, 329*t*, 334–335
Shield grafts, 289
Sickle cell disease, 81
Silicone/Silastic materials
aging changes and, 160
Asians
maxillary augmentation, 282–283
rhinoplasty, 258, 278, 279–283
complications, 298
dressings, 132, 133, 176, 190
Filipinos and Polynesians, 291, 292–293*f*, 294–295*f*, 299
Mediterraneans, 325*f*
Silicone injections, 299
SIL-K, 133
Sill incisions, 202
SIMON (acronym), 5
Single-coat Jessner's, 129
Single-dome intact unit, tip-plasty, 387–388
Sinus infections, 346
Skeletonization of tissue
African Americans, 203–204
Filipinos and Polynesians, 289
Middle Easterner, 365
Skin
aesthetics, 41
African Americans
adolescents, 210
rhinophyma, 209*f*, 210
subdermal fibrofatty tissue removal, 203–204
supratip corrugation, 214
aging, 151, 153*t*, 154*t*
Asians, 263–264, 277
anatomic features, 263
eye lid, 267
nose, 257
defining elements of beauty, 13
Filipinos and Polynesians, 287, 291
Hispanics, 310
Mediterraneans, 327
Middle Easterners, 339, 342*f*, 345–346, 345
dermabrasion, chemical peels, and laser treatment, 359–360, 361*f*, 362*f*
rejuvenation program, 354
variations among ethnic groups, 33, 34
Skin cancer, 101
Skin care, 101–102, 124–125, 124*t*
Skin-care products, 121, 124–125, 124*t*
acne cosmetica, 126
acne treatment, 127*t*
ingredients to avoid, 114*t*, 123
Skin color, 13, 14, 122. *See also* Pigmentation abnormalities
micropigmentation tattoos, 117, 137, 147
and scarring, 184
Skin elasticity/laxity, 100, 121
aging and, 169*t*, 170*t*
eyelid skin of Middle Easterners, 339, 342*f*
variations among ethnic groups, 34
Skin grafts, 100, 141, 144, 147, 144, 147
Skin lighteners, 13, 14, 101, 102, 103, 114 123, 124*t*, 125, 130, 131, 145
Skin problems, 99–119
acne, 125–129, 139–140
acne and oily skin, 103–106
acne keloiditis, 131
aging, 99–101
ashy skin, 122
caveats, 121, 122
chemical peels, 145
common disorders, 122
dermatosis papulosa nigra, 118*f*, 119, 135–136
electrolysis, 123
hidradenitis suppurativa, 109, 111, 143–144
keloids, 144–145
keratosis pilaris, 133–134
make-up, 122–123
perioperative care, 131–133, 136, 288
pigmentation
hyperpigmentation/discoloration, 101–103, 123

infraorbital shadowing, 130–131, 153*f*, 157, 166
micropigmentation procedure, 117, 137, 147
normal variation in, 145, 146*f*
vitiligo, 116–119, 146–147
pseudofolliculitis barbae, 106–109, 110*f*, 130, 140–143
psilosebaceous occlusive diseases, 106–111, 135–144
scarring. *See* Scarring
sensitivity/allergic reactions, 121
skin care, 124–125
skin tags, 118*f*, 119, 135–136
sun damage, 125
tinea versicolor, 122, 134–135
treatments, 111–116. *See also specific compounds and approaches*
alpha-hydroxy acids, 111–112, 113
antibiotics, 115
benzoyl peroxide, 115
hyaluronic acid, 115
isotretinoin (Retin A), 112, 114
micropigmentation, 117, 137, 147
moisturizers, 116
pre- and postoperative, 131–133, 136, 288
skin lighteners, 114
Skin sensitivity. *See* Allergy/hypersensitivity, skin
Skin tags, 118*f*, 119, 135–136
Skin thickness, 121
aesthetics, 73, 80*f*
African Americans, 213–214, 237–242
and onlay grafts, 221
tip defatting, 218*f*
Asian nose, 278, 279, 281
Filipinos and Polynesians, 298, 299
Hispanics, 308, 309, 310, 312, 314*f*, 315, 316*f*
ethnic variations, 310, 311
facelift considerations, 313
and inflammatory skin conditions, 110*f*
Mediterraneans, 328
and onlay graft thickness, 331
supratip shaving, 334–335
Middle Easterners, 345, 364
Northern Europeans, 373, 376*f*, 379, 381, 382, 389*f*, 393, 397*f*
Skin tone, 121, 122, 132
Skin transplantation, 137
Slavic nose, 327–328
Sleep disturbances, 104, 105
Sliding genioplasty, 309, 310, 313, 317*f*, 318–319
SMAS, 151, 167, 357–359
Smoking, 22, 100, 157, 312
Snap test, 157
Social status, 13, 14, 40–41
Social support system. *See* Family
Sodium hyposulfite, 135
Soft tissue. *See also* Fatty/fibrofatty tissue
African Americans, 201
Hispanics, 313
Middle Easterners, 339, 342*f*
Northern Europeans, 380–381, 382, 395
variations among ethnic groups, 34
Solar acne, 126
Solar elastosis, 154
Solu-Medrol, 347
Spaniards. *See* Mediterraneans
Spider telangiectasias, 359
Spironolactone, 140
Spouse. *See* Family
Spreader grafts
Hispanics, 312, 315, 316*f*, 317*f*, 319, 319–320
Mediterraneans, 324*f*
Middle Easterners, 347, 366
Northern Europeans, 373, 376*f*
Staff
operating room etiquette, 8
patient interactions with, 22, 24
Staphylococcus aureus, 143
Step-off deformity, dorsal implant, 298
Steroids. *See* Corticosteroids
Stress
and acne, 103, 125
financial, 28–29
patient selection considerations, 22
Stretch relaxation, Hispanics, 313
Strip procedure, lateral crus, 385–386
Struts
African American rhinoplasty, 219*f*, 220, 244*f*
columellar, 203, 214
dorsal augmentation, 228, 229, 232–235*f*
tip augmentation, 220–221, 221*f*, 236
Asian rhinoplasty, 279, 280, 281
Mediterraneans, 332
Middle Easterners, 348*f*, 367
Northern European rhinoplasty, 388, 392
Submental area
aging, 153*t*, 154*t*
Hispanics, 311
Submental plication, 166
Submucous resection, Northern European nose, 373, 380
Subnasion, facial convexity angle, 45*f*
Suboptimal results. *See* Complications; Patient satisfaction
Subperiosteal facelift, 313
Substance abuse, 22, 126
Suction lipectomy, 82*f*
Hispanics, 303, 305*f*, 315
Middle Easterners, 354*f*, 355*f*, 357
nasolabial fold, 163*f*, 238*f*
neck and jawline improvement, 165*f*
submental area, 166, 167*f*
Sulfur, skin preparations, 111, 124*t*, 127*t*, 129, 134
Sun avoidance, 354
Sunblock, 101, 102, 122, 123, 124, 130, 133
acne treatment, 127*t*
pre- and postoperative skin care, 131, 132, 136
Sun damage, 99–100, 101, 121, 125
chemical peels, 359
solar acne, 126
solar elastosis, 154
Sun exposure, 123
after chemical peels, 359
and skin conditions, 106
Sunscreen. *See* Sunblock
Sun sensitivity. *See* Photosensitivity
Supratarsal fold, 70*t*
aesthetic, 74, 75*f*, 76*f*, 79
Asians, 251, 252*f*, 255
Hispanics, 311
Supratip structure and modification
African Americans, 237–242
Hispanics, 315
Mediterraneans, 328, 329*t*, 334–335
Middle Easterners, 364
Northern Europeans, 381, 384, 389*f*, 397*f*
Surgery
keloid prevention, 189–190
keloid repair, 176–177, 187
operating room etiquette, 8
skin abnormalities after, 123
treatment of skin conditions
acne, 141
dermatosis papulosa nigra, 136
hidradenitis suppurativa, 143–144
Surgiholic patient, 8
Sutures. *See also specific procedures*
facelift, 167
scarring, 173, 174*f*
Swelling, *See* Edema
Symmetry
aesthetics, 41, 41, 43, 50
African Americans
alar base resection complications, 227, 228*f*
individualization of proportions, 198
Asian aesthetic values, 265
Asian blepharoplasty, upper lid, 273
Hispanics, 310, 315, 319–320
Northern European rhinoplasty, 382, 387, 388, 389, 391
Synthetic materials, 203. *See also specific grafts and materials*
African American rhinoplasty
dorsal augmentation, 204, 207, 228, 229*f*
rib cartilage donor site, 242, 244*f*
Asians
maxillary augmentation, 282–283
rhinoplasty, 258, 278, 279–283
chin augmentation, 345
Mediterraneans, 325*f*
Syringomas, 111, 277
Systemic lupus erythematosus, 117

T

Tarsal wedge resection, 158*f*
Tarsus
aesthetics, 74, 75*f*, 76*f*, 77
palpebral fold creation in Asians, 255, 256*f*, 268, 272*f*
Tartaric acid, 111
Tattoos, micropigmentation procedures, 117, 137, 147
Teeth
aesthetics, 41, 48–49, 50, 54
orthodontics, 309, 312, 313
Telangiectasia, 101, 154*f*
Telecanthus, 342*f*
Templates, nasal, 73
Temporal area fat grafts, 162, 164*f*
Temporal fascia grafts
African American rhinoplasty, 229, 231*f*, 232*f*
Filipinos and Polynesians, 299

Teratogenicity, retinoids, 128, 141
Testosterone, 105
Tetracycline, 102, 125, 140, 143
Thai national characteristics, 267
Thalassemia, 33
Tinea versicolor, 122, 134–135
Tip augmentation/enhancement
  African Americans, 203–204, 219*f*, 220–221, 221*f*
    with alar base resection, 225, 225*f*, 226*f*
    alar flare reduction with, 223, 224*f*, 225
    complications, 226*f*, 227
  Asians, 258
  Filipinos and Polynesians, 289, 290–291, 292–293*f*, 294–295*f*, 292–293*f*
  Hispanics, 315, 316*f*, 317*f*, 319
  Middle Easterners, 347
  Northern Europeans, 373, 376*f*
Tip definition. *See* Tip structure
Tip deformity
  African American versus Caucasian patient perceptions, 199, 199*t*, 200, 200*t*
  alar flare reduction and, 222
  as complication of L-shaped implants, 297
Tip dimensions. *See* Tip structure
Tip drooping. *See* Tip lengthening/drooping/ptosis
Tip enhancement. *See* Tip augmentation/enhancement
Tip grafts, 80*f*
  African Americans
    versus Caucasians, 211*t*
    dorsal augmentation, 229, 232–233*f*
  Hispanics, 312, 317*f*, 319, 319–320
  Middle Easterners, 239*f*, 350*f*, 351
Tip lengthening/drooping/ptosis
  African Americans
    long-term effects, 242
    suboptimal results, 244
    tip grafts and, 221
  Hispanics, 314*f*
  Northern Europeans, 381, 389*f*, 390*f*, 394*f*
Tip modification. *See also* Tip augmentation/enhancement
  African Americans, 236–237*f*
  Asians, 278–279
  cascading approach to, 398
  East Indians, 80*f*
  Hispanics, 312, 318*f*, 319
  Middle Easterner, 349*f*, 350*f*
Tip projection
  aesthetics, 85, 88, 92, 93*f*, 94*f*, 95, 93*f*
  African Americans, 214
    anatomy, 200, 201
    long-term effects, 200
    techniques, 202–203
  Asians, 278, 281
  dome reconstruction and, 387
  and dorsal augmentation, 200
  Filipinos and Polynesians, 287, 292–293*f*
  Hispanics, 310
  limitations and interactions with other parameters, 199
  Mediterraneans, 327, 328–335, 329*t*, 328
  Middle Easterners, 345, 348*f*, 352–353, 366, 367
  Northern Europeans, 379
Tip rotation, 21, 95
  Filipinos and Polynesians, 288
  Mediterraneans, 323, 324*f*, 325*f*
  Middle Easterners, 368
  Northern Europeans, 373, 377*f*, 389*f*, 390*f*
Tip skin. *See also* Skin thickness
  aging, 153*t*, 154*t*, 169*t*, 170*t*
  defatting
    African Americans, 202, 203, 204, 215, 218*f*
    Asians, 259–260*f*
Tip softening, 216*f*
Tip stasis, 236–237*f*
Tip structure
  aesthetics, 32, 69, 73, 91*f*, 92, 96
    ethnic groups, 68, 69*f*
    facial relationships, 79
  African Americans, 214, 217*f*, 233–234*f*, 236–237*f*, 237–242
    preoperative imaging and planning, 244*f*
    skin thickness and, 242
  Asians, 249, 250*f*, 258
  Filipinos and Polynesians, 287
  Hispanics, 305*f*, 309, 311, 314*f*, 319–320, 315, 316*f*
  Mediterraneans, 327, 334–335
  Middle Easterners, 363, 364, 365*t*
  Northern Europeans, 373, 376*f*, 377*f*, 379, 381–382, 385–392, 393*f*, 394*f*, 395*f*, 396*f*, 397*f*, 398*f*
  variations among ethnic groups, 34
Titanium dioxide, 124, 125, 132, 136
Tolnaftate, 135
Transcolumellar incision, 202, 289, 393
Transconjunctival blepharoplasty, 277, 339, 341*f*
Transfixing incision, 219*f*, 312, 381, 382
Transplantation, epidermis, 137
Trauma
  nose, 207, 210, 346
  skin response, hyperpigmentation, 101
Tretinoin, 111. *See also* Retin A/retinoids
Triamcinolone, 109, 133, 397*f*
  keloid management, 145, 187, 188
  keloid prevention, 176, 190
Trichloracetic acid, 112, 113*f*, 114*f*, 130, 145, 345
Tumescent suction lipectomy. *See* Suction lipectomy
Tumor necrosis factor, 145
Turbinates, 33
Turbinate surgery
  African Americans versus Caucasians, 211*t*
  Middle Easterners, 348, 351, 365
  partial turbinectomy, 348, 351

U

Ultraviolet radiation, 101. *See also* Sun damage
  eye protection, 131
  skin protection. *See* Sunblock
Umbrella graft, 290, 328, 329*t*, 332–333, 332*t*, 334*f*, 335*f*
Unhappy patient. *See* Complications; Dissatisfied patient; Patient satisfaction

V

Valium, 288
Verapamil, 188
Versed, 288
Video imaging. *See* Imaging
Viral infections, 101, 123, 346
Vistaril, 288
Vitadye, 146
Vitamin A derivatives, 112, 114, 127–128, 133. *See also* Isotretinoin; Retin A
Vitamin C, 115, 133
Vitamin E, 115, 123, 132, 133, 189*f*, 190
Vitamin K, 132, 133
Vitiligo, 116–119, 122, 137, 146–147
Vomer bone, 347
Von Willebrand's disease, 364

W

Warts, 136
Wedge resection
  alar. *See* Alar wedge excision/resection
  tarsal, 158*f*
Weir resection, 222, 227, 395
Whiteheads, 139
Wood's light, 145
Wound closure, keloid prevention, 189–190
Wound healing, 179–182. *See also* Scarring
  Asian, 263–264
  skin conditions and, 111
W-plasty, 275–276, 277*f*
Wrinkling, 99, 100, 151, 154, 277. *See also* Rhytidectomy

X

X-ray epilation, 143
Xylocaine, 365

Z

Zinc picolinolate, 133
Zinc pyrithione, 135
Zovirax, 115
Z-plasty, epicanthal folds, 275